ATLAS OF
INTERNAL
MEDICINE
SECOND EDITION

EDITOR-IN-CHIEF

Eugene Braunwald, MD, MD (Hon), ScD (Hon)
Distinguished Hersey Professor of Medicine
Harvard Medical School
Faculty Dean for Academics
Brigham and Women's Hospital
Massachusetts General Hospital
Vice President for Academic Programs
Partners Healthcare System
Boston, Massachusetts

With 13 contributors
Developed by Current Medicine, Inc.
Philadelphia

McGraw-Hill
Medical Publishing Division

New York Chicago San Francisco Lisbon
London Madrid Mexico City Milan New Delhi
San Juan Seoul Singapore Sydney Toronto

McGraw-Hill

A Division of The McGraw·Hill Companies

Current Medicine, Inc.

400 Market Street
Suite 700
Philadelphia, PA 19106

Developmental Editor: Teresa M. Giuliana
Commissioning Supervisor, Books: Annmarie D'Ortona
Illustrators: Wieslawa Langenfeld and Maureen Looney
Design: Jennifer Knight
Assistant Production Manager: Penny Weisman
Indexing: Linda Herr Hallinger

Library of Congress Cataloging-in-Publication Data
Atlas of internal medicine / editor-in-chief, Eugene Braunwald; with 13 contributors. — 2nd ed.
               p.;   cm.
        Includes bibliographical references and index.
        ISBN 0-07-140240-3 (HB : alk. paper)
         1. Internal medicine—Atlases.   I. Title: Internal medicine. II. Braunwald,
  Eugene, 1929–   .
         [DNLM: 1. Internal Medicine—methods—Atlases. 2. Disease—Atlases.
    WB 17 A8822 2001]
    RC46 .A.86   2001
    616—dc21

                         2001047168

NOTICE

Printed in Thailand by Imago Productions (FE) Pte Ltd.
10 9 8 7 6 5
Developed by Current Medicine, Inc., Philadelphia

PREFACE

There are three principal approaches to learning medicine and keeping abreast of new developments: the printed word, in the form of textbooks and journals; the spoken word, in the form of lectures and audiotapes; and the picture, in the form of atlases, slides, and video and computer images. Each approach has its place in the educational armamentarium, and each lends itself to imparting certain facts, ideas, and concepts best. Many aspects of internal medicine require the visual approach. How better to describe a rash, a management algorithm, an echocardiogram, or the appearance of a duodenal ulcer?

In the present healthcare milieu, a solid foundation in internal medicine has assumed greater significance as the role of the primary care physician has expanded. This second edition of the *Atlas of Internal Medicine* is well-suited as a resource in this expanded role of health maintenance advisor and provider of many services that in the past were often carried out in hospital or in the care of a specialist.

This volume encompasses all the major fields of internal medicine, including cardiology, pulmonary and critical care medicine, gastroenterology, hematology, oncology, dermatology, hepatology, rheumatology, nephrology, neurology, allergy and immunology, endocrinology, and infectious diseases. It is a unique compilation of over 1500 images, selected as the "best of the best" from the work of the highly respected colleagues who have joined me in the preparation of this volume.

The content of each chapter has been carefully selected to be useful to the primary care physician in identifying both common and more rare disease entities. The color photographs provide visual confirmation of disease, while the algorithms, charts, schematics, and tables guide the physician in the decision-making process concerning diagnostic tests, treatment, and follow-up.

I trust that this second edition of the *Atlas of Internal Medicine* will be useful to the broad array of physicians who wish to remain current in internal medicine and have at their fingertips the most up-to-date reference available.

Eugene Braunwald, MD

CONTRIBUTORS

WILLIAM M. BENNETT, MD

Professor
Department of Medicine
Oregon Health Sciences University
Medical Director, Solid Organ and Cellular
  Transplantation
Northwest Renal Clinic
Legacy Good Samaritan Hospital
Portland, Oregon

EUGENE BRAUNWALD, MD, MD (HON), ScD (HON)

Distinguished Hersey Professor of Medicine
Harvard Medical School
Faculty Dean for Academics
Brigham and Women's Hospital
Massachusetts General Hospital
Vice President for Academic Programs
Partners Healthcare System
Boston, Massachusetts

JEFFREY P. CALLEN, MD, FACP

Professor
Department of Medicine/Dermatology
University of Louisville School of Medicine
Chief, Division of Dermatology
University of Louisville Health Sciences Center
Louisville, Kentucky

THOMAS P. DUFFY, MD

Professor
Department of Medicine
Yale University School of Medicine
New Haven, Connecticut

DAVID S. ETTINGER, MD

Professor
Department of Medicine/Oncology
Johns Hopkins University School of Medicine
Associate Director for Clinical Research
The Johns Hopkins Oncology Center
Baltimore, Maryland

MARK FELDMAN, MD

Chairman
Department of Internal Medicine
Presbyterian Hospital of Dallas
Clinical Professor of Internal Medicine
University of Texas Southwestern Medical School at
  Dallas
Dallas, Texas

GENE G. HUNDER, MD

Professor Emeritus
Department of Medicine
Mayo Medical School
Consultant, Division of Rheumatology
Mayo Clinic
Rochester, Minnesota

STANLEY G. KORENMAN, MD

Professor
Department of Endocrinology
Associate Dean for Ethics and Medical Scientist Training
UCLA School of Medicine
Los Angeles, California

PHILLIP L. LIEBERMAN, MD

Clinical Professor
Department of Medicine/Pediatrics
University of Tennessee
Memphis, Tennessee

WILLIS C. MADDREY, MD

Professor
Department of Internal Medicine
University of Texas Southwestern Medical School
Executive Vice President for Clinical Affairs
Aston Ambulatory Care Center
Dallas, Texas

GERALD L. MANDELL, MD

Professor of Medicine
Owen R. Cheatham Professor of the Sciences
Chief, Division of Infectious Diseases
University of Virginia Health Sciences Center
Charlottesville, Virginia

D. KEITH PAYNE, MD

Professor
Department of Medicine
Acting Chief
Division of Pulmonary and Critical Care Medicine
Louisiana State University Health Sciences Center
Shreveport, Louisiana

ROGER N. ROSENBERG, MD

Professor of Neurology and Physiology
Zale Distinguished Chair in Neurology
The University of Texas Southwestern Medical Center
Senior Neurologist
Zale-Lipshy University Hospital and Parkland Memorial
  Hospital
Dallas, Texas

CONTENTS

9 Oncology

David S. Ettinger

10 Hematology

Thomas P. Duffy

11 Gastroenterology

Mark Feldman

Cardiology

EUGENE BRAUNWALD

Disorders of the cardiovascular system are the most common causes of death and serious morbidity in the industrialized world. A total of three quarters of a million deaths in the United States, more than 40% of all deaths, are attributed to cardiac and vascular diseases. These conditions account for almost 5 million years of potential life lost.

Despite these sobering statistics, progress in cardiovascular medicine has been immense and is, in fact, accelerating. Our understanding of the pathobiology of most forms of heart disease has advanced steadily, and there have been enormous advances in the diagnosis, treatment, and prevention of cardiovascular disorders. For example, during just one decade, from 1990 to 2000, the overall death rates from cardiovascular disease declined by 26%, and death rates from acute myocardial infarction declined by 32%. Similar progress has been made in other major cardiovascular disorders, including hypertension, valvular and congenital heart disease, congestive heart failure, and the arrhythmias.

Physicians responsible for the care of patients with cardiovascular disease—both primary care physicians and specialists—now have available numerous publications for obtaining up-to-date information, including excellent journals and textbooks of every conceivable size, scope, and depth. In developing new strategies for transmitting information about these conditions, it is important to consider that cardiovascular medicine is one of the most visual of medical specialties. Cardiovascular diagnosis is based on the recognition and understanding of a variety of graphic waveforms, images, decision trees, and microscopic sections. Treatment increasingly involves the intelligent use of algorithms, which are most effectively portrayed visually. Likewise, mechanical correction of cardiovascular disorders, whether catheter-based or surgical, can best be described pictorially. This chapter has been designed to provide visual exposition of those aspects of cardiovascular medicine of greatest interest to the general internist.

■ ATHEROSCLEROSIS: RISK FACTORS AND TREATMENT

FORMATION OF THE ATHEROSCLEROTIC PLAQUE

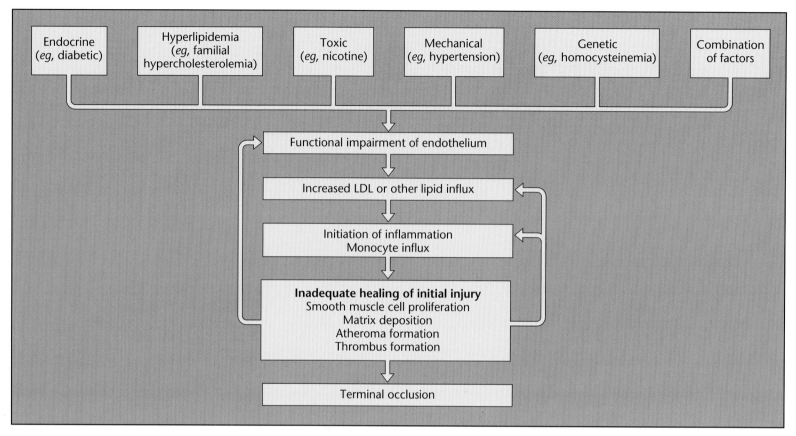

FIGURE 1-1.

Mechanisms in arteriosclerotic lesion formation. Multiple risk factors and pathologic states have been correlated with early lesion formation and lesion progression. It is hypothesized that these factors all induce functional impairment of the arterial endothelium resulting in either increased lipid influx or initiation of an inflammatory vessel wall response. This process is propagated by additional accumulation of inflammatory cells such as monocytes within the vessel wall. Consequently, under persistence of the noxious agent(s), chronic inflammation persists, leading to inadequate healing of initial injury. Ultimately terminal occlusion of the vessel by a thrombus occurs. LDL—low-density lipoprotein. (*Courtesy of* Marschall S. Runge and Andreas R. Huber.)

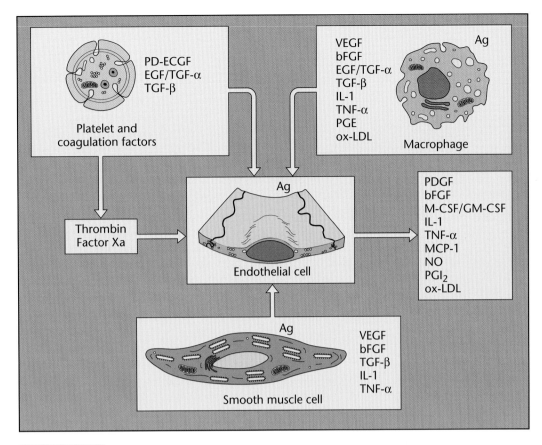

FIGURE 1-2.

Platelet, macrophage, and smooth muscle products in the endothelial response to vascular injury. During atherogenesis, the endothelium interacts with macrophages, platelets, smooth muscle cells, and T lymphocytes. These interactions result in the expression and secretion of several potential mediators of vascular lesion formation. Macrophages produce endothelial mitogens including vascular endothelial growth factor (VEGF), fibroblast growth factor (FGF), interleukin-1 (IL-1), and transforming growth factor-α and -β (TGF-α, TGF-β). IL-1 and both TGF-α and TGF-β can inhibit endothelial proliferation and induce secondary gene expression by the endothelium of such growth factors as platelet-derived growth factor (PDGF) and other potential regulators of vascular lesion formation. TGF-β also induces synthesis and secretion of connective tissue by the endothelium.

The endothelium and macrophages can produce oxidized low-density lipoprotein (ox-LDL), causing further injury to endothelial cells. Platelets produce TGF-α, TGF-β, and platelet-derived endothelial cell growth factor (PD-ECGF), a potent mitogen. A procoagulant state of the endothelium can be stimulated by thrombin and factor Xa, present in plasma. Several of the same molecules formed by macrophages and platelets are also generated in the artery wall or in atherosclerotic lesions underlying the endothelium by smooth muscle cells. Endothelial cells in injured vessels express several growth-regulatory molecules, including those that cause connective tissue to proliferate (PDGF, bFGF, TGF-β) and those that induce secondary gene expression for PDGF in smooth muscle and endothelial cells. Further, endothelial cells produce macrophage colony-stimulating factor (M-CSF), granulocyte-macrophage-colony stimulating factor (GM-CSF), and ox-LDL, which are mitogenic and activating factors for underlying macrophages. Endothelial cells also provide potent chemotactic factors that affect leukocyte chemotaxis, including ox-LDL and monocyte chemotactic protein-1 (MCP-1), and modulate vasomotor tone through the formation of nitric oxide (NO) and prostacyclin (PGI$_2$).

Thus, multiple interactions among platelets, macrophages, and smooth muscle cells have been documented and are likely to provide the inflammatory and growth-promoting milieu necessary for repair of vascular injury. In abnormal arteries, it is likely these same mechanisms stimulate formation of pathologic vascular lesions. Ag—antigen; EGF—epidermal growth factor; PGE—prostaglandin E; TNF—tumor necrosis factor. (*Adapted from* Ross *et al.* [1].)

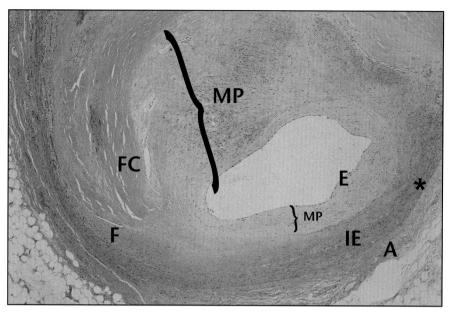

FIGURE 1-3.

Plaque development and localization. Lesion progression in a fibrofatty plaque in the left anterior descending coronary artery of a 51-year-old man who died from a cardiac ischemic episode. The eccentric fibrofatty calcified plaque occupies approximately two thirds of the arterial circumference. Luminal to the plaque, there is a concentric, relatively cellular proliferation of fibromuscular tissue that stains lighter than the underlying plaque. Similar fibromuscular tissue is also recognized extending between the fibrous cap of the original plaque (FC) and the media (*asterisk*)

through an obvious fissure (F) of the FC at the shoulder region. Besides being the site of growth (recruitment of monocytes), the plaque "shoulders" also show significant neovascularization (angiogenesis). Mechanical transmural shearing forces, secondary to the cardiac cycle, are likely to be maximal at these sites, probably due to differences in compliance of the diseased versus nondiseased segment of the arterial wall. Plaques in which the lipid core is situated eccentrically are also associated with fissuring [2]. Arterial wall reaction to fissuring of a plaque may contribute to the growth of the lesion by either a neointimal proliferation or organization of a thrombus formed at the site of plaque fissuring. In the section shown, fingerprints of a preceded thrombotic episode (hemosiderin deposition, neovascularity) are lacking. The "thrombogenic" or "encrustation" hypothesis proposes that fibrin deposition and thrombus organization on an atheromatous plaque may play a role in plaque development. Evidence that thrombus incorporation contributes to the plaque progression has been demonstrated with monoclonal antibodies, which have identified fibrin, fibrinogen, and their split products [3].

This case clearly demonstrates that the atheromatous plaque is not a static structure, but is subject to either growth or dynamic modification and remodeling (original magnification, X 80). A—adventitia; E—endothelium; IE—interna elastica; MP—myofibroblastic proliferation. (*Courtesy of* Michael B. Gravanis.)

LOW-DENSITY LIPOPROTEINS

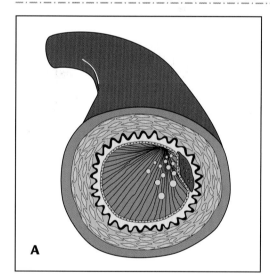

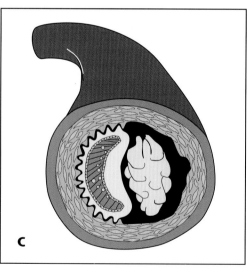

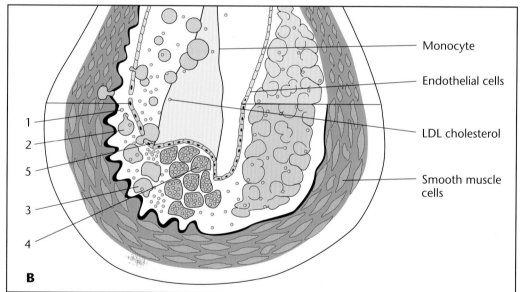

FIGURE 1-4.

The atherosclerotic process. **A,** Artery depicting early fatty streak development. **B,** *1,* low-density lipoprotein (LDL) becomes oxidized within the arterial subendothelial space. *2,* Circulating monocytes are recruited to the subendothelial space by chemoattractants including oxidized LDL. *3,* These monocytes undergo differentiation, becoming macrophages, which are scavenger cells that recognize and accumulate oxidized LDL. *4,* The lipid-laden macrophages then become foam cells, which cluster under the endothelial lining to form a bulge into the artery. *5,* This bulge is called a fatty streak and is the first overt sign of atherosclerotic change. **C,** Cross-section of an artery with an atherosclerotic lesion with a narrowed lumen. (*Courtesy of* Merrell Dow Pharmaceuticals Inc, Cincinnati, OH.)

HIGH-DENSITY LIPOPROTEINS

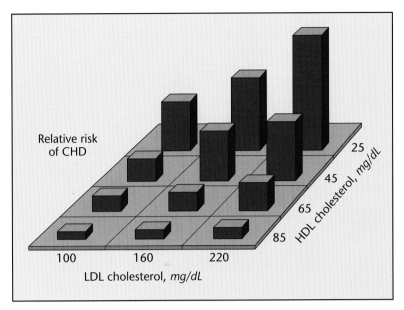

Relative risk of CHD

HDL cholesterol, mg/dL — 25, 45, 65, 85

LDL cholesterol, mg/dL — 100, 160, 220

FIGURE 1-5.

The Framingham Heart Study: risk of coronary heart disease (CHD) by high-density lipoprotein (HDL) and low-density lipoprotein (LDL) cholesterol. Epidemiologic studies have definitely established that total and LDL cholesterol concentrations are directly correlated with clinical coronary atherosclerosis [4]. The inverse association of HDL cholesterol concentrations with CHD endpoints has also been established in both cross-sectional and prospective epidemiologic studies [5]. In the Framingham Heart Study, the interrelationship between LDL and HDL cholesterol concentrations and the relative risk of developing CHD is particularly striking [6]. For individuals with HDL cholesterol concentrations of 45 mg/dL or less, the risk of CHD increases as the LDL cholesterol concentrations increase. However, patients with elevated HDL cholesterol concentrations appear protected. This protection is striking at 65 mg/dL, and at 85 mg/dL even high concentrations of LDL may increase CHD risk only modestly. Therefore, high concentrations of HDL cholesterol in the blood are associated with a remarkably lower risk for developing vascular disease. (*Courtesy of* H. Bryan Brewer, Jr. and Jeffrey M. Hoeg.)

TRIGLYCERIDE-RICH LIPOPROTEINS

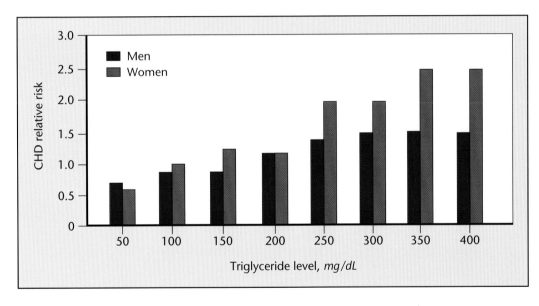

■ Men
■ Women

CHD relative risk

Triglyceride level, mg/dL — 50, 100, 150, 200, 250, 300, 350, 400

FIGURE 1-6.

The incidence of coronary heart disease (CHD)–induced events, such as myocardial infarction and cardiac death, was found to be higher in both men and women with triglyceride levels above the mean for the population. The increase is most obvious as the baseline levels rise from approximately 150 to 350 mg/dL. This relationship of plasma triglycerides to risk of CHD is often stronger in women than in men, as was found in the Framingham Heart Study [6]. (*Courtesy of* Ngoc-Anh Le and W. Virgil Brown.)

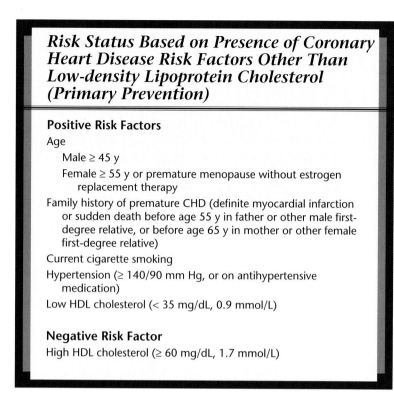

Risk Status Based on Presence of Coronary Heart Disease Risk Factors Other Than Low-density Lipoprotein Cholesterol (Primary Prevention)

Positive Risk Factors

Age

    Male ≥ 45 y

    Female ≥ 55 y or premature menopause without estrogen replacement therapy

Family history of premature CHD (definite myocardial infarction or sudden death before age 55 y in father or other male first-degree relative, or before age 65 y in mother or other female first-degree relative)

Current cigarette smoking

Hypertension (≥ 140/90 mm Hg, or on antihypertensive medication)

Low HDL cholesterol (< 35 mg/dL, 0.9 mmol/L)

Negative Risk Factor

High HDL cholesterol (≥ 60 mg/dL, 1.7 mmol/L)

FIGURE 1-7.

Guidelines for drug treatment of atherosclerosis. *High risk*, defined as a net of two or more coronary heart disease (CHD) risk factors, leads to more vigorous intervention. Age (defined differently for men and women) is treated as a risk factor because rates of CHD are higher in the elderly than the young, and in men than women of the same age. Use of antihypertensive medication has not produced the expected reduction in CHD risk and, thus, treated hypertension continues as a risk factor. High-density lipoprotein (HDL) cholesterol levels decrease CHD risk and, thus, one risk factor is subtracted. Although obesity is not listed as a risk factor because it operates through other risk factors that are included (hypertension, hyperlipidemia, decreased HDL cholesterol, and diabetes mellitus), it should be considered a target for intervention. Physical inactivity is similarly not listed as a risk factor, but it too should be considered a target for intervention. (*Courtesy of* Donald B. Hunninghake.)

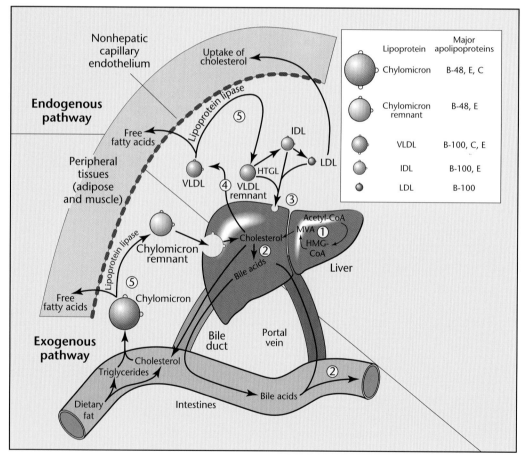

FIGURE 1-8.

Overview of lipoprotein metabolism [7]. The five major sites for drug action that are associated with low-density lipoprotein (LDL) or triglyceride lowering are shown. The major mechanism for lowering LDL involves an increase in LDL receptor numbers (3). Increases in the number of LDL receptors occur when there is a decrease in the cholesterol content of hepatic and other cells. This can occur either by decreasing the rate-limiting enzyme in cholesterol synthesis (hydroxymethyl glutaryl-coenzyme A [HMG-CoA] reductase) (1) or increasing the fecal excretion of bile acids with the resulting decrease in the bile acid pool (2). Enhanced receptor activity (3) increases the removal of LDL plus the precursors of LDL, very low-density lipoprotein (VLDL) remnants, and intermediate-density lipoprotein (IDL). Thus, the formation of LDL can also be decreased. VLDL remnants and IDL also contain triglycerides and thus a modest decrease in triglycerides may be observed. Inhibition of lipoprotein synthesis (4) decreases the synthesis or secretion of VLDL, the major triglyceride-carrying lipoprotein. Secondarily, the formation of VLDL remnants, IDL, and LDL are decreased and both LDL cholesterol and triglyceride levels are reduced. Increased lipoprotein lipase activity (5) facilitates the removal of triglycerides from both chylomicrons and VLDL. These smaller particles may then be removed from the circulation by the remnant receptor. Moreover, the VLDL remnants can proceed to the formation of IDL and LDL, which can be removed by the LDL receptor. Acetyl-CoA—acetyl coenzyme A; HTGL—hepatic triglyceride lipase; MVA—mevalonate. (*Courtesy of* Donald B. Hunninghake.)

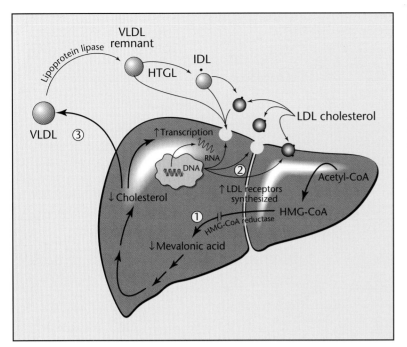

FIGURE 1-9.

Mechanism of action of statins [8,9]. The statins inhibit the rate-limiting enzyme, hydroxymethyl glutaryl-coenzyme A (HMG-CoA) reductase, in cholesterol biosynthesis (1). The major organs for cholesterol biosynthesis are the small intestine and liver. The associated decrease in hepatic and cellular cholesterol concentration stimulates the production of low-density lipoprotein (LDL) receptors, which increase the rate of removal of LDL from the plasma (2). There is also increased removal of very low-density lipoprotein (VLDL) remnants and intermediate-density lipoprotein (IDL), which are precursors to LDL formation. In some patients, there may also be a decrease in lipoprotein synthesis (3). The enhanced removal of VLDL remnants and IDL and the inhibition of lipoprotein synthesis may contribute to the modest triglyceride-lowering effect of the statins. Acetyl-CoA—acetyl coenzyme A; HTGL—hepatic triglyceride lipase. (*Courtesy of* Donald B. Hunninghake.)

Recommended Combination Therapy of Elevated Low-density Lipoprotein Cholesterol and Triglycerides

Statin + nicotinic acid
  Effect of two drugs is additive
  Low HDL cholesterol is common, and nicotinic acid increases HDL cholesterol
  Risk of myopathy small
Statin + fibric acid derivative
  If nicotinic acid is not tolerated
  Fibric acid has little effect on LDL cholesterol levels, but decreases triglycerides and increases HDL cholesterol
  Risk of myopathy greater
  Useful in non–insulin-dependent diabetes mellitus
Fibric acid + nicotinic acid
  Dose of nicotinic acid that is tolerated is usually insufficient to control LDL cholesterol levels

FIGURE 1-10.

Combination therapy. Recommended drug combinations for patients with elevations of both low-density lipoprotein (LDL) cholesterol and triglycerides (200 to 400 mg/dL) [10]. (*Courtesy of* Donald B. Hunninghake.)

ACUTE MYOCARDIAL INFARCTION AND OTHER ACUTE ISCHEMIC SYNDROMES

TRIGGERING OF ACUTE MYOCARDIAL INFARCTION

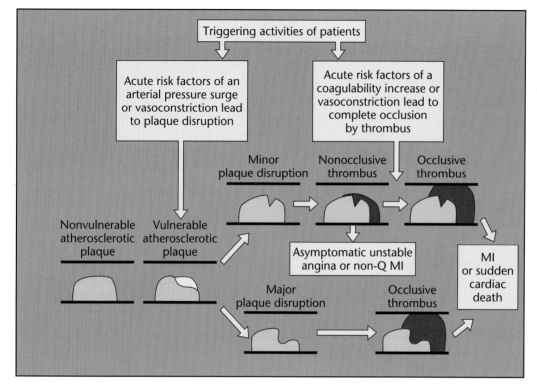

FIGURE 1-11.
Hypothetical steps in the triggering of coronary thrombosis [11]. Plaque disruption with thrombus formation occurs at a critical moment when a threshold combination of hemodynamic, prothrombotic, and vaso-constrictive forces (acute risk factors) is rapidly generated by external stressors (triggers) during a period of plaque vulnerability. Development of such vulnerability—perhaps the most critical step leading to coronary thrombosis—is a poorly understood process. If the trigger does not exert its effect during vulnerability, the plaque may change and become nonvulnerable. Disruption of the plaque may be severe enough to produce a thrombogenic stimulus sufficiently intense to cause occlusive coronary thrombosis, leading to myocardial infarction (MI) or sudden cardiac death. A minor rupture may lead only to a mural thrombus, which may fail to produce symptoms or lead to unstable angina or a non–Q-wave MI. (*Courtesy of* Sergio Waxman and James E. Muller.)

PATHOLOGY OF ACUTE ISCHEMIC SYNDROMES

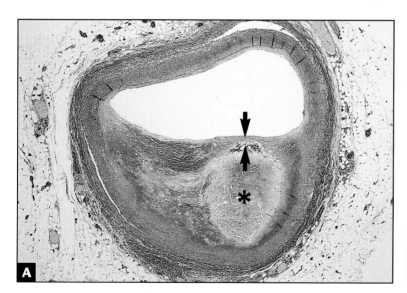

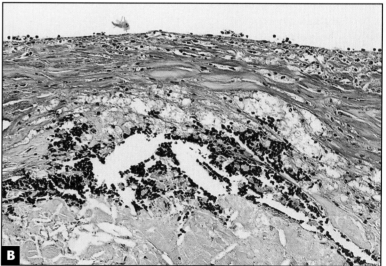

FIGURE 1-12.
The consistency of coronary plaques and their vulnerability to rupture differ. Whereas the collagen-rich sclerotic plaque component is hard and stable, the lipid-rich atheromatous component is soft and unstable. **A** and **B**, A thin cap of fibrous tissue (*between arrows*) separates the soft, lipid-rich pool (*asterisk*) from the lumen. Such a thin fibrous cap, infiltrated with macrophage foam cells (clearly seen in *B*), overlying an extracellular lipid pool is mechanically weak and vulnerable to rupture. The presence of erythrocytes just beneath the cap indicates that the cap is ruptured nearby. (*From* Falk and Andersen [12]; with permission.)

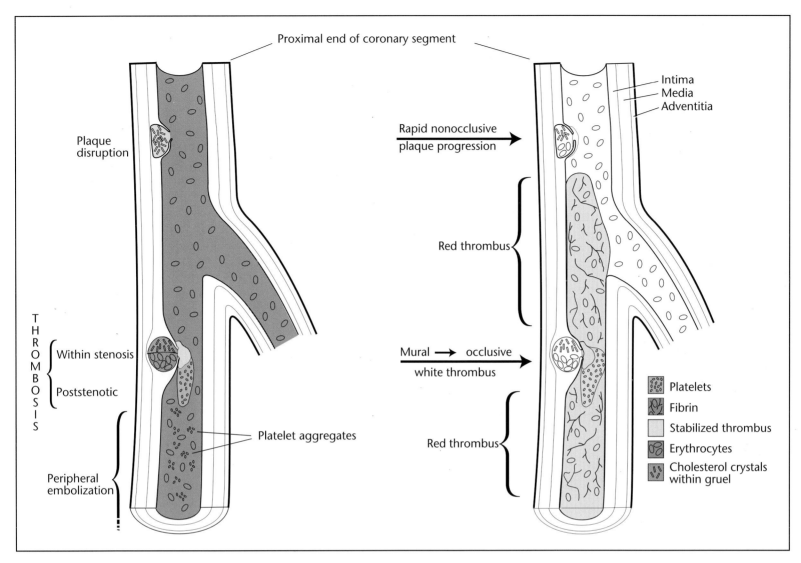

FIGURE 1-13.

Pathogenesis of a coronary thrombus. Most coronary thrombi (about three-fourths) are initiated by plaque rupture, exposing thrombogenic material to the flowing blood; the atheromatous gruel appears to be highly thrombogenic. The thrombus is platelet-rich and usually gray-white at the rupture site; severe stenosis, if present, promotes thrombosis via shear-induced platelet activation. Fibrin soon enmeshes the platelets, stabilizing the thrombus. Thrombus formation is dynamic: recurrent thrombosis,

thrombolysis, and peripheral embolization occur simultaneously, with or without concomitant vasospasm, causing intermittent flow obstruction. Nonoccluding thrombi may extend poststenotically, and if the platelet-rich thrombus occludes the vessel, the blood proximal and distal to the occlusion may stagnate and coagulate, giving rise to upstream and/or downstream propagation of a red, fibrin-dependent, venous-like thrombus. Upstream thrombus propagation does not occlude major side branches. (*Adapted from* Falk [13].)

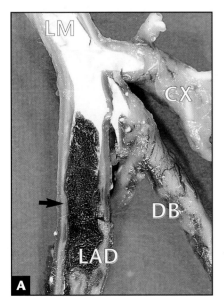

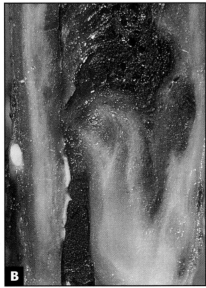

FIGURE 1-14.

Coronary occlusion: propagation of thrombosis. Secondary to flow reduction, a red stagnation thrombus may propagate upstream. **A** and **B**, The proximal left anterior descending coronary artery (LAD) has been cut open longitudinally. A ruptured plaque with a gray-white occluding thrombus (platelet-rich) can be seen at the *arrow* in *A* (magnified in *B*), and a red thrombus (erythrocyte-rich) is seen propagating upstream up to the first diagonal branch (DB). (Panel A *from* Falk [13]; with permission; panel B *courtesy of* Erling Falk and Prediman K. Shah.)

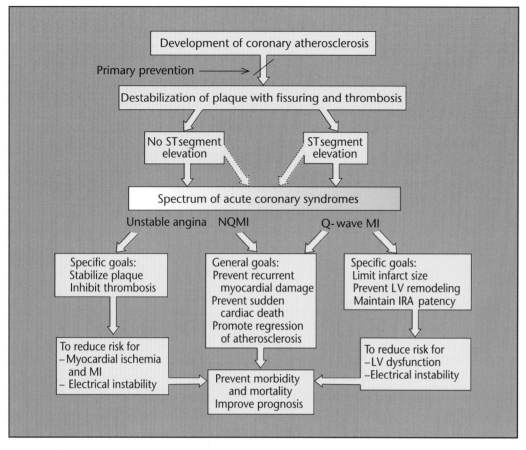

FIGURE 1-15.

Major goals of medical therapy for acute coronary syndromes. Efforts at primary prevention of coronary atherosclerosis are fundamental to reversing the epidemic of coronary heart disease in the industrialized nations of the world. Once coronary atherosclerosis has developed, however, patients may present with chronic exertional angina pectoris or one of the features of the acute coronary syndromes: unstable angina pectoris/non–Q-wave myocardial infarction (NQMI) or Q-wave myocardial infarction (MI). A common pathophysiologic mechanism precipitating the acute coronary syndromes is destabilization of an atherosclerotic plaque due to fissuring of its surface, with exposure of its contents to the local microvascular environment and varying degrees of coronary thrombosis (subtotal occlusion in the case of unstable angina/NQMI and complete thrombotic occlusion in the case of Q-wave MI).

Patients usually present with a worsening pattern or prolonged episode of ischemic pain at rest and can be divided into two categories based on the electrocardiogram (ECG): those without persistent ST-segment elevation, who have myocardial ischemia with or without some degree of myocardial necrosis, and those with persistent ST-segment elevation (a marker of acute coronary occlu-

sion), the majority of whom evolve a Q-wave MI (*solid arrows*). The former group can be further subdivided into those with unstable angina or NQMI on the basis of measurements of serum markers (*eg,* cardiac enzymes, proteins); however, these two subgroups are often considered together because of their similar clinical presentation and treatment strategy and because it is difficult to discriminate the two syndromes prospectively. Furthermore, some patients with no ST-segment elevation on the initial ECG ultimately evolve a Q-wave MI (*dashed arrows*).

Preventing recurrent myocardial damage and sudden cardiac death and promoting regression of atherosclerosis are goals common to the treatment of both unstable angina/NQMI and Q-wave MI, but additional considerations come into play when one is treating patients at the two ends of the spectrum. Patients with unstable angina/NQMI are at markedly increased risk for recurrent myocardial ischemia and infarction because of an unstable plaque with recurrent reductions in coronary blood flow due to subtotal coronary thrombosis. Efforts directed toward stabilizing the plaque (antiplatelet therapy) and inhibiting coronary thrombosis are critical to reduce morbidity and mortality (due in part to electrical instability) in this group of patients. For patients with Q-wave MI, an effort should be made to limit infarct size, prevent left ventricular (LV) remodeling and subsequent congestive heart failure (with angiotensin-converting enzyme [ACE] inhibitors), and maintain patency of the infarct-related artery (IRA) (with aspirin, antithrombins). By reducing the degree of LV dysfunction and minimizing the size of a myocardial scar that could otherwise lead to electrical instability, clinicians can markedly improve the long-term prognosis of patients with Q-wave MI. (*Courtesy of* Elliott M. Antman.)

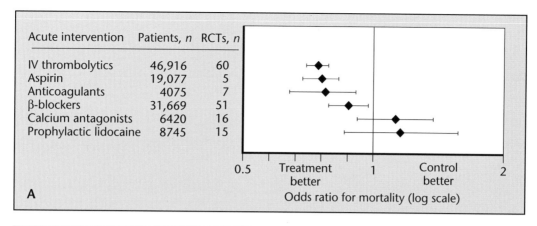

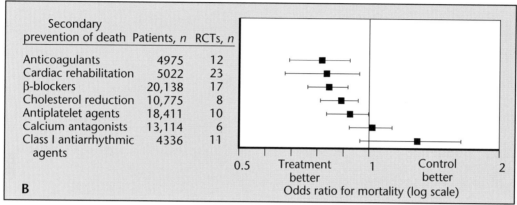

FIGURE 1-16.

Pooled results of randomized controlled trials in *acute* myocardial infarction (MI) [14].
A, Meta-analysis of several trials of acute therapy for MI. This graph presents the pooled estimate of the odds of reducing (or increasing) mortality with the test intervention versus control. The 95% confidence intervals (CI) around these point estimates are indicated by the width of the horizontal lines. Therapies that reduce mortality are plotted to the left of the vertical line (*Treatment better*), and those that increase mortality are plotted to the right (*Control better*). For example, intravenous (IV) thrombolytic agents were evaluated in 60 trials that collectively enrolled 46,916 patients; the pooled odds ratio for mortality was 0.75 (CI, 0.71 to 0.79), indicating a reduction in the odds of dying by about 25% in those patients who received thrombolytic therapy versus placebo. The pooled data from trials of calcium antagonists and prophylactic lidocaine show a trend toward increased mortality in patients who received active therapy. B, Meta-analysis of trials of *secondary prevention* of mortality following MI conducted between 1960 and 1990 [14]. Whereas long-term therapy with calcium antagonists shows no significant evidence of benefit, class I antiarrhythmic agents are associated with increased mortality. The other therapies studied were all associated with improvements in survival, although precise dose-ranging information has not been established definitively for important drugs such as warfarin and aspirin. This has set the stage for new clinical trials (*eg*, the ongoing CARS [Coumadin-Aspirin Reinfarction Study] and CHAMP [Combination Hemotherapy and Mortality Prevention] studies) to refine further the optimal dose and combination of agents that can be used widely in the treatment of patients with infarction. (*Adapted from* Lau *et al.* [14].)

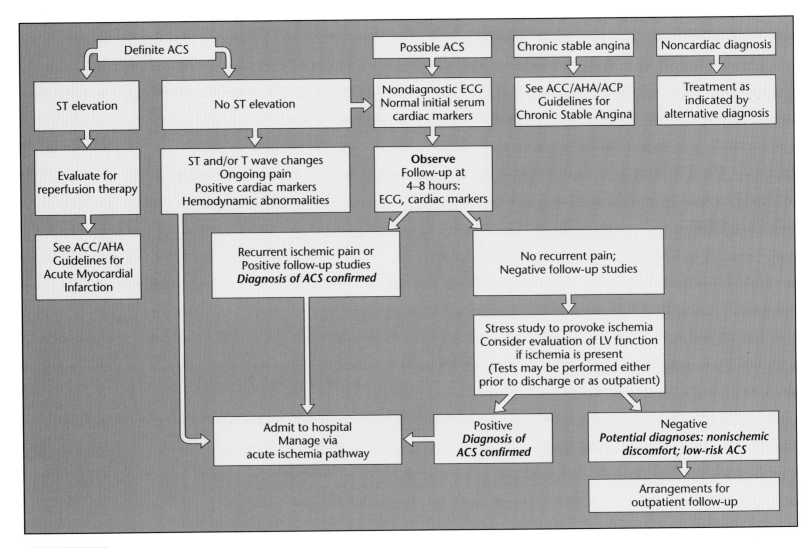

FIGURE 1-17.

Algorithm for the evaluation and management of patients suspected of having acute coronary syndrome (ACS). Guidelines for the management of patients with unstable angina and non-ST segment elevation myocardial infarction have recently been developed by the American College of Cardiology and the American Heart Association [15]. In patients presenting to the hospital with symptoms suggestive of ACS, the information from the history, physical examination, 12-lead electrocardiogram (ECG), and initial biochemical cardiac marker tests allow clinicians to assign patients to one of four categories: noncardiac diagnosis, chronic stable angina, possible ACS, and definite ACS. Patients with possible ACS are those with an episode of chest discomfort at rest not entirely typical of ischemia but who are pain free when initially evaluated, and have a normal or unchanged ECG and no elevations of cardiac markers. Patients with a recent episode of chest discomfort typical of ischemia that is either severe or of new onset and accelerates should initially be considered to have definite ACS. Such patients may be at low risk if the ECG obtained at presentation has no diagnostic abnormalities and the initial cardiac-specific troponin is negative [16–18]. Patients with definite ACS are triaged based on the pattern of the 12-lead ECG. Patients with ST-segment elevation are managed with either admission to the hospital or additional observation at home. During such observation, patients who experience recurrent ischemic discomfort, evolve abnormalities on a follow-up 12-lead ECG or cardiac troponin, or develop worsening congestive heart failure should be admitted to the hospital. The patient at low risk may be considered for an early stress test to provoke ischemia if he does not experience any further ischemic discomfort and the follow-up ECG and cardiac troponin after 6 to 8 hours of observation remain normal. (*Adapted from* Braunwald *et al.* [15].)

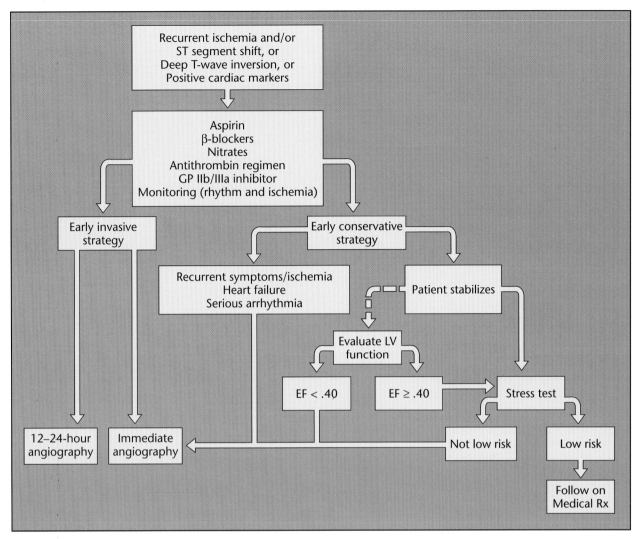

FIGURE 1-18.

American College of Cardiology/American Heart Association guidelines [15] for the hospital care of patients with unstable angina and non-ST segment elevation myocardial infarction. Patients should initially be placed at bed rest, and those with cyanosis, respiratory distress, or other high-risk features should receive supplemental oxygen. Patients should undergo continuous electrocardiographic (ECG) monitoring during their early hospital phase. Patients whose symptoms are not relieved by three 0.4-mg sublingual nitroglycerin (NTG) tablets taken 5 minutes apart should be started on intravenous (IV) NTG unless they are hypotensive.

Morphine sulfate (1–5 mg IV) is recommended for patients whose symptoms are not relieved after three serial sublingual NTG tablets or whose symptoms recur despite adequate anti-ischemic therapy. β-blockers should be started early in the absence of contraindications (bradycardia, heart failure, or bronchospasm). In patients with ongoing rest pain, these agents should be administered intravenously followed by oral administration; in intermediate- and low-risk patients, oral administration alone is sufficient.

Calcium antagonists may be used in patients receiving adequate doses of nitrates and β-blockers with continuing or recurrent ischemia and in patients who are unable to tolerate adequate doses of one or both of these agents [16]. (*Adapted from* Braunwald *et al.* [15]).

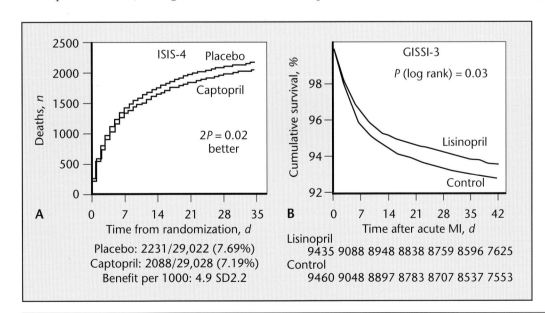

FIGURE 1-19.

Angiotensin-converting enzyme (ACE) inhibition. Results of treatment with ACE inhibitors after acute myocardial infarction (MI). Two trials of acute therapy in unselected patients (*ie*, both with and without evidence of left ventricular dysfunction) have shown that ACE inhibitors reduce mortality at 4 to 6 weeks [19,20]. This effect was seen in two different patient populations and with two different ACE inhibitors, captopril (**A**) and lisinopril (**B**), attesting to the consistency and generalizability of the observations. (Panel A *adapted from* ISIS-4 Collaborative Group [19]; panel B *adapted from* Gruppo Italiano per lo Studio della Sopravvivenza nell'Infarto Miocardico [20].)

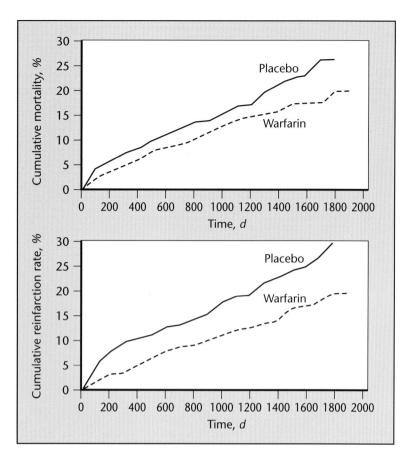

FIGURE 1-20.
Warfarin therapy. The Warfarin Reinfarction Study (WARIS) demonstrated reductions in mortality and the rate of reinfarction in patients given active therapy with warfarin compared with placebo (*Adapted from* Smith *et al.* [21].)

CONSEQUENCES OF CORONARY OCCLUSION AND REPERFUSION

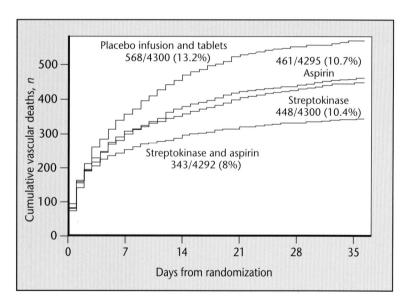

FIGURE 1-21.
Effect of thrombolytic therapy on mortality. The ISIS-2 (Second International Study of Infarct Survival [22]) trial confirmed the results of GISSI-1 (Gruppo Italiano per lo Studio della Streptochinasi nell'Infarto Miocardico [23]) by finding a decrease in 5-week mortality from 12.0% with placebo to 9.2% with streptokinase, which indicates a 25% relative reduction. Moreover, aspirin alone resulted in a 23% relative reduction in mortality, and the combination of streptokinase and aspirin resulted in an even more impressive additive effect, with a 42% relative reduction in mortality from 13.2% to 8.0%. (*Adapted from* ISIS-2 Collaborative Group [22].)

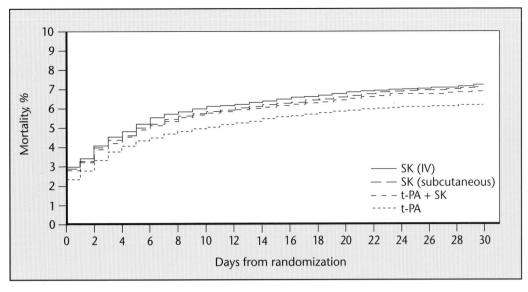

FIGURE 1-22.

Accelerated tissue plasminogen activator (t-PA) was associated with the lowest 30-day mortality in the GUSTO trial at 6.30%, compared with 7.25% with streptokinase (SK) with sub-cutaneous heparin, 7.35% with streptokinase with intravenous (IV) heparin, and 7.0% for the combination of streptokinase and t-PA [24]. The protocol called for combining the streptokinase groups if there was no significant difference between the two in order to get a more reliable estimate of the overall effect of streptokinase. Compared with streptokinase, there was a relative reduction in 30-day mortality of 14% with accelerated t-PA (*P*< 0.001). This corresponds to 10 additional lives saved with accelerated t-PA (compared with streptokinase) per 1000 patients treated, or one of every seven deaths prevented that would have occurred with streptokinase. The survival advantage seems to be explained by the difference in 90-minute patency between the strategies. (*Courtesy of* Christopher B. Granger.)

PLATELETS AND THE MECHANISMS OF ARTERIAL THROMBOSIS

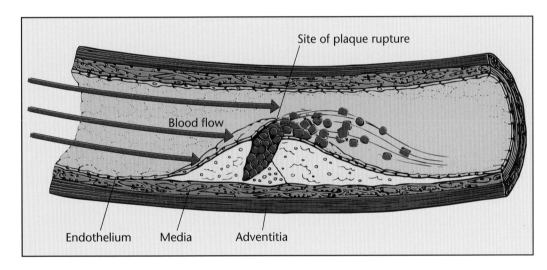

FIGURE 1-23.

Diagram of arterial thrombus responsible for acute myocardial infarction (MI). Platelet adhesion and aggregation occur at the site of plaque rupture ("white thrombus"). Activated platelets exert procoagulant effects and the soluble coagulation cascade is activated. Fibrin strands and erythrocytes predominate within the lumen of the vessel and downstream in the "body" and "tail" of the thrombus [25]. (*Courtesy of* Neal S. Kleiman.)

◼ CHRONIC ISCHEMIC HEART DISEASE

PATHOPHYSIOLOGY OF ANGINA

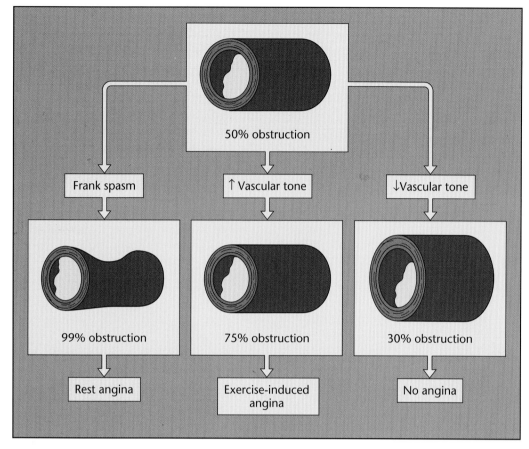

FIGURE 1-24.

Coronary stenosis as a cause of angina. It is now recognized that coronary artery obstructions are capable of changing caliber, and constriction or narrowing of a preexisting lesion can be a factor in precipitating angina and myocardial ischemia.

If the coronary segment has sufficient smooth muscle (media) that is not involved in the atherosclerotic process, the vessel can dilate or constrict at the site of the stenosis. In general, vasoconstriction is most likely to occur with eccentric or asymmetric lesions, which consist of coronary atherosclerotic plaque in a segment of the vessel wall, with some relatively normal media intact. Concentric stenoses are less likely to constrict further or dilate. In concentric atherosclerosis, the atherosclerotic plaque circumferentially involves the entire area of the vessel. It is believed that at least 25% of an arc or rim of media in the coronary artery must be preserved to allow for stenosis vasomotion.

This figure shows how the caliber of eccentric coronary artery stenoses may change, with considerable variation in the degree of stenosis resistance and the propensity to produce angina. Both increased vascular tone (first two examples) and decreased vascular tone (third example) are depicted. This phenomenon has been called dynamic coronary obstruction by some, emphasizing the variability and transitory nature of the actual "obstruction." (*Adapted from* Epstein and Talbot [26].)

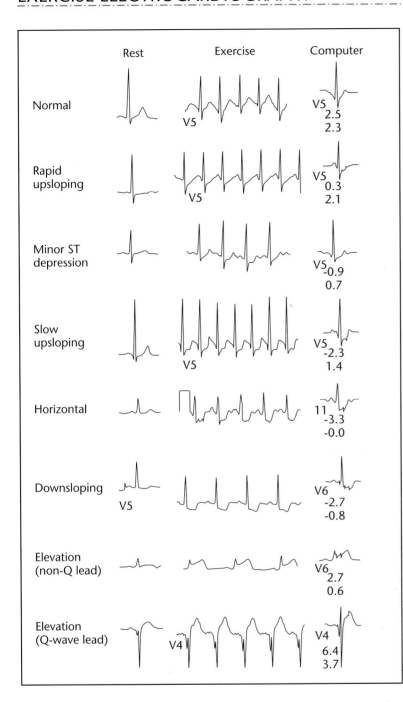

FIGURE 1-25.

Typical exercise electrocardiographic (ECG) patterns at rest and at peak exertion. The computer-processed incrementally averaged beat corresponds with the raw data taken at the same time during exercise. The patterns represent a gradient of worsening ECG response to myocardial ischemia. In the column of computer-averaged beats, ST-80 displacement (*top number*) indicates the magnitude of ST-segment displacement 80 ms after the J-point relative to the PQ junction or E point. ST-segment slope measurement (*bottom number*) indicates the ST-segment slope at a fixed time after the J-point to the ST-80 measurement. At least three noncomputer averaged complexes with a stable baseline should meet criteria for abnormality before the exercise ECG can be considered abnormal.

The first two tracings illustrate normal and rapid upsloping ST segments; both are normal responses to exercise. Minor ST depression can occur occasionally at submaximal workloads in patients with coronary disease; in the illustration, the ST segment is depressed 0.9 mm (0.09 mV) 80 ms after the J-point. A slow upsloping ST-segment pattern often demonstrates an ischemic response in patients with known coronary disease or those with a high clinical risk before testing. Criteria for slow upsloping ST-segment depression include J-point and ST-80 depression of 1.5 mV/s or greater and an ST segment slope of 0.7 to 1.0 mV/s or greater.

Classic criteria for myocardial ischemia include horizontal ST-segment depression observed when J-point and ST-80 depression are 0.1 mV or greater and the ST-segment slope is within the range of ± 0.7 to 1.0 mV/s. Downsloping ST-segment depression occurs when J-point and ST-80 depression are 0.1 mV or greater and ST-segment slope is -0.7 to -1.0 mV/s or greater. ST-segment elevation in a non–Q-wave non-infarct territory lead occurs when J-point and ST-60 are 1.0 mV or greater and represents a severe ischemic response. ST-segment elevation in an infarct territory (Q-wave lead) indicates a severe wall motion abnormality and is usually not an ischemic response. (*Courtesy of* Bernard R. Chaitman.)

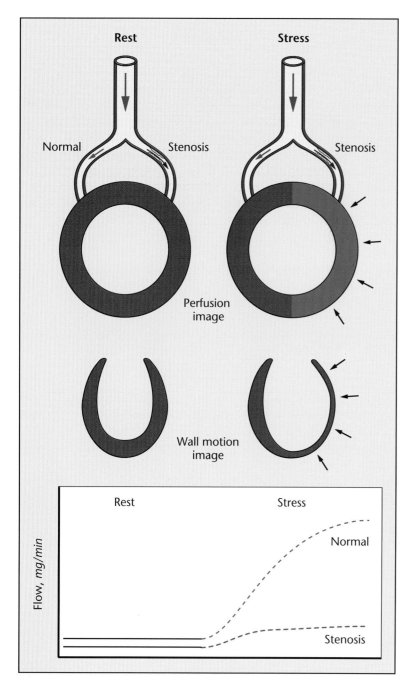

FIGURE 1-26.

Principle of stress radionuclide imaging for the detection of coronary artery disease. Shown are 1) a normal coronary artery and an artery with significant stenosis (top), 2) the myocardial territory (perfusion image), and 3) the ventricular wall (wall motion image) supplied by each artery. The graph (bottom) depicts coronary blood flow both at rest and during stress. At rest, coronary blood flow is similar in the normal artery and in the artery with stenosis. Resting coronary blood flow in the diseased artery is maintained at a normal level and is sufficient to meet resting metabolic myocardial demands because of recruitment of coronary reserve (dilatation of the resistance vasculature) in the distal coronary bed. If the patient does not have angina pectoris, coronary myocardial perfusion is homogeneous and global and regional left ventricular function is normal.

During exercise, myocardial metabolic demands increase and more myocardial nutrient blood flow is required. Coronary reserve is increased as a result of dilatation of the coronary resistance vessels in the peripheral coronary bed. In the territory of the normal coronary artery, the resistance vessels dilate and coronary blood flow is increased by 2 to 2.5 times. In the abnormal coronary bed, which is distal to the significant coronary stenosis, resistance vessels are already dilated and little if any further dilatation is possible. Increased metabolic demands thus cannot be met, and the relatively hypoperfused myocardium becomes ischemic.

The distribution of regional myocardial blood flow in the myocardium is heterogeneous, *ie*, there is less blood flowing in the ischemic myocardial bed (blue area) than in the normal myocardial bed. This heterogeneity of myocardial perfusion can be visualized noninvasively using radionuclide imaging with Tl-201 or a Tc-99m perfusion agent like sestamibi. When exercise-induced ischemia is severe enough, regional and global left ventricular dysfunction occurs. This can be assessed noninvasively using radionuclide ventriculography by either first-pass radionuclide angiocardiography or equilibrium radionuclide angiocardiography. (*Courtesy of* Frans J. Th. Wackers.)

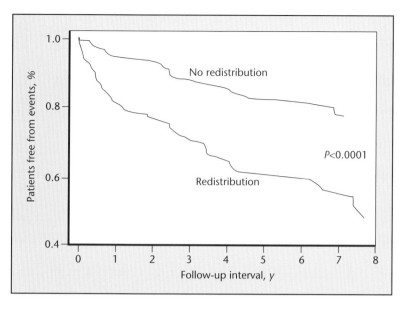

FIGURE 1-27.

Event-free survival of patients with and without Tl-201 redistribution. Numerous investigators have shown that, in addition to detection of coronary artery disease, important prognostic and functional information can be obtained from exercise and rest myocardial perfusion images. This illustration demonstrates the significant difference in event-free survival in patients who had angiographic coronary artery disease with and without evidence of Tl-201 redistribution. "Event-free" indicates freedom from death, nonfatal myocardial infarction, coronary bypass surgery, or angioplasty for 3 months or longer after completion of the study. Five-year event-free survival was 82% for patients with no redistribution and 60% for patients with redistribution [27]. (*Courtesy of* Frans J. Th. Wackers.)

ASSESSMENT OF LEFT VENTRICULAR FUNCTION

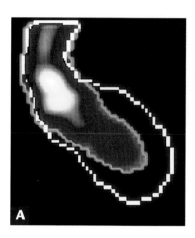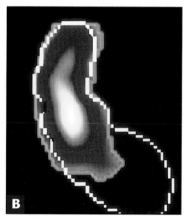

FIGURE 1-28.

Normal first-pass radionuclide angiography at rest and during exercise. In this illustration the left ventricular end-diastolic (ED) outline (white) in the anterior position is superimposed on the end-systolic (ES) image. This display allows assessment of regional wall motion from a static image; such images are best interpreted by dynamic display as an endless loop cine on a computer screen. Here, maximum count activity is yellow and the lowest activity is green. Resting left ventricular ejection fraction (LVEF) in this patient is 60% (**A**), and peak exercise LVEF is 80% (**B**). Regional wall motion shows uniformly increased contraction. In order to meet the increased demand during exercise, cardiac output must increase; this is achieved by increasing heart rate and LVEF (LVEF = ED volume - ES volume/ED volume). A normal LVEF response is defined as an increase in LVEF of 5% or greater compared with baseline LVEF and a uniform increase of regional wall motion. (*Courtesy of* Frans J. Th. Wackers.)

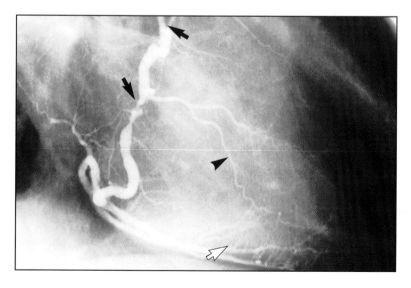

FIGURE 1-29.

Coronary arteriography for right coronary artery disease. Complex stenosis in the right coronary artery of a patient with a long-standing history of chronic stable angina, which progressed to rest pain and resulted in hospitalization, is depicted. After initial angiography demonstrated a tight complex stenosis (*lower arrow*), successful balloon angioplasty was performed. Shown here is a right anterior oblique angiogram. *Upper arrow* indicates coronary catheter; *arrowhead* indicates right ventricular branch; and *open arrow* indicates posterior descending artery. (*Courtesy of* Eric R. Powers.)

Anti-ischemic Mechanisms of Medical Therapy in Stable Angina

Action	Nitroglycerin or Nitrates	β-Blockers	Calcium Antagonists
	Drug Class		
Decreased myocardial demand	++	+++	+ to ++
Increased coronary blood supply	+++	0 to +	++ to +++
Prevent coronary spasm or vasoconstriction	++	0 to -	++ to +++
Coronary stenosis enlargement	++	0 to +	+ to ++
Left ventricular function	Improves	- to 0	- to 0
Other	Reverses disordered endothelial function; antiplatelet action	Electrical stabilization; antiarrhythmic; antihypertensive	Antihypertensive

0—no effects; -—negative effects or may worsen; +—minor effects; ++—moderate effects; +++—major effects.

FIGURE 1-30.

Anti-ischemic mechanisms of medical therapy in stable angina. It is traditionally believed that all classes of drugs act predominantly through lowering myocardial oxygen consumption, thereby lessening cardiac energy demands. The β-blockers are the most potent in this regard. The nitrates and calcium antagonists increase coronary blood flow and thus are used in the presence of coronary artery vasoconstriction. Coronary atherosclerotic stenosis constriction is believed to be an important cause of angina in some patients. Data regarding drugs other than the nitrates in preventing or reversing stenosis constriction are limited. The nitrates are the favored drugs for patients with angina and left ventricular dysfunction or congestive heart failure. The β-blockers and calcium antagonists are ideal for angina occurring in the presence of hypertension. (*Courtesy of* Jonathan Abrams.)

DETECTION OF SILENT ISCHEMIA

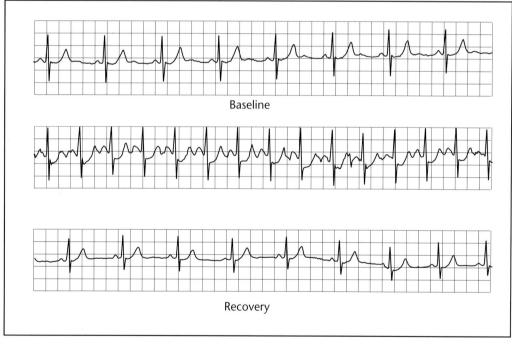

Baseline

Recovery

FIGURE 1-31.

Detection of silent myocardial ischemia (SMI): exercise testing. Exercise stress testing is the most useful single test currently available for the evaluation of SMI. It is well standardized, relatively inexpensive, and readily available. SMI should be considered when, in the absence of symptoms, 1 mm or greater horizontal ST-segment depression occurs at least 80 ms after the J point in a lead that was initially isoelectric, as shown in this example. ST-segment depression serves as a marker of transient ischemia in the absence of other less specific causes. Exercise stress testing done in patients with a known or high likelihood of coronary artery disease (CAD) can provide information helpful to access risk outcome. The following findings suggest high risk for CAD events (*eg*, worsening angina, myocardial infarction) or sudden death: a failure to complete 6.5 METs or to achieve a heart rate of 120 bpm or higher; a flat or declining systolic blood pressure response to exercise; a 1-mm or greater ST-segment depression or elevation; exercise-induced arrhythmia; and ischemic changes at low heart rates (< 120 bpm), for prolonged periods (> 6 min), or in multiple leads. (*Courtesy of* Barry D. Bertolet and Carl J. Pepine.)

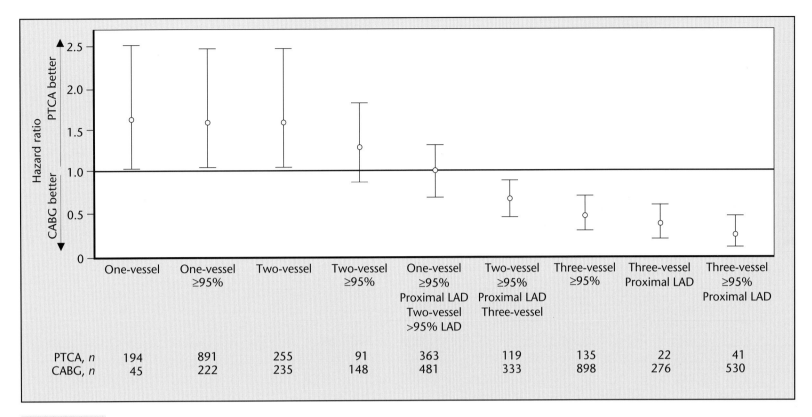

	One-vessel	One-vessel ≥95%	Two-vessel	Two-vessel ≥95%	One-vessel ≥95% Proximal LAD Two-vessel >95% LAD	Two-vessel ≥95% Proximal LAD Three-vessel	Three-vessel ≥95%	Three-vessel Proximal LAD	Three-vessel ≥95% Proximal LAD
PTCA, *n*	194	891	255	91	363	119	135	22	41
CABG, *n*	45	222	235	148	481	333	898	276	530

FIGURE 1-32.

Results from the Duke trial comparing percutaneous transluminal coronary angioplasty (PTCA) and coronary artery bypass grafting (CABG). The preferred method of therapy depends on the extent and severity of coronary disease. Whereas PTCA seems to be suprior in patients with less extensive disease, CABG is more advantageous for patients with more extensive coronary disease [28,29].

NORMAL CONTRACTION

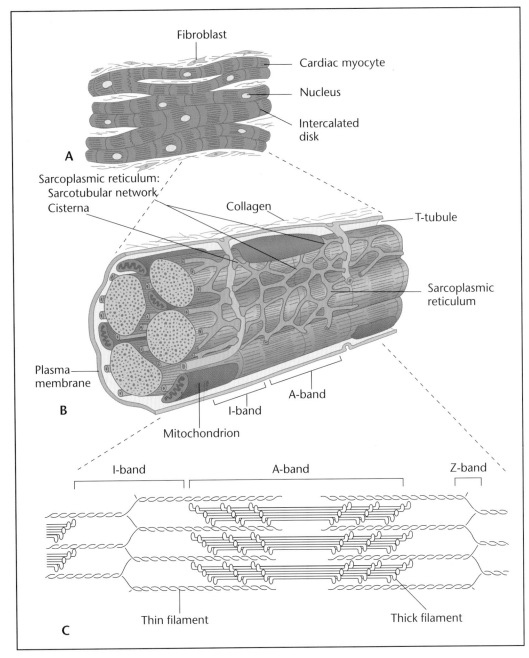

FIGURE 1-33.

Structure of the heart. The heart is composed of both myocytes and nonmyoctes. **A,** Nonmyocytes include connective tissue cells (mainly fibroblasts), vascular smooth muscle cells, and endothelial cells. Whereas large cardiac myocytes make up most of the heart's mass, the majority of the cells of the heart (approximately 70%) are smaller nonmyocytes. The large, branched cardiac myocytes, which are enmeshed in a collagen network, are separated longitudinally by intercalated discs, which represent specialized cell-cell junctions. The intercalated discs provide strong mechanical connections between adjacent cells and contain gap junctions that provide low-resistance pathways for electrical conduction.

B, Cardiac myocytes that are specialized for contraction contain myofilaments whose organization in a regular array of thick and thin filaments gives rise to the characteristic striated appearance. Also prominent within these cells are two membrane structures: energy-producing mitochondria and the sarcoplasmic reticulum, which regulates cytosolic Ca^{2+} concentration. The latter is an intracellular membrane system that contains the calcium channels that initiate systole by delivering activator calcium to the myofilaments, and calcium pumps that, by removing calcium from the cytosol, dissociate this activator cation from its binding sites on the thin filament.

Myofilaments contain about 70% of the protein of the cardiac myocytes, and most of the membrane surface is found in the mitochondria. Other important membranes include the plasma membrane, which is continuous with the transverse tubular membranes (t-tubules) that extend toward the center of the cell and carry depolarizing currents into the myocardial cell. C, Each sarcomere, which is delimited by two Z-bands, contains one A-band and two half I-bands. The A-bands are made up of thick, myosin-containing filaments into which thin filaments interdigitate from the adjacent two half I-bands. The latter are made up of actin and the regulatory proteins, tropomyosin and the troponin complex. Bisecting each Z-band is a lattice of axial and cross-connecting filaments that includes the overlapping ends of thin filaments from adjacent sarcomeres. (*Adapted from* Katz [30].)

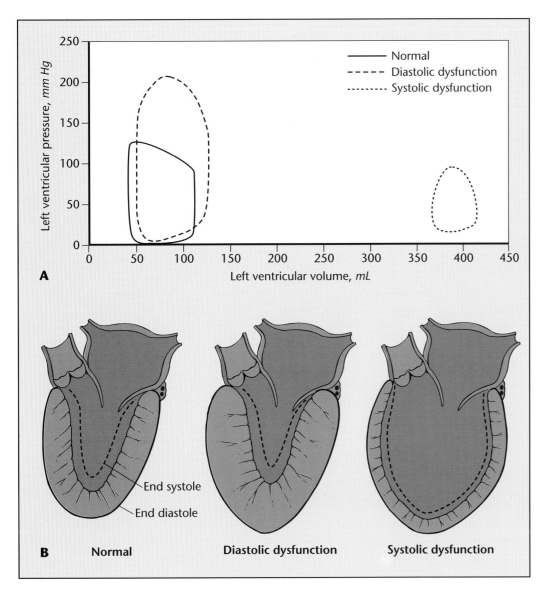

A

B Normal Diastolic dysfunction Systolic dysfunction

FIGURE 1-34.
Heart failure resulting from systolic and diastolic dysfunction.

A, The hemodynamic profiles, illustrated as the relationship between ventricular pressure and volume throughout a representative cardiac cycle, for the three hearts shown in shown in **B.** Digitalis has value in the treatment of systolic dysfunction, but it has no value and may be detrimental in predominantly diastolic dysfunction.

VENTRICULAR REMODELING

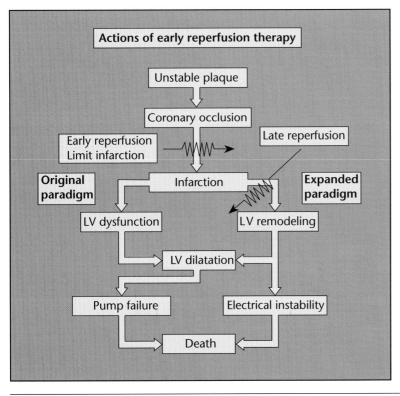

Actions of early reperfusion therapy

Unstable plaque

Coronary occlusion

Early reperfusion
Limit infarction   Late reperfusion

Original paradigm   Infarction   **Expanded paradigm**

LV dysfunction   LV remodeling

LV dilatation

Pump failure   Electrical instability

Death

FIGURE 1-35.
Expansion of the paradigm of the beneficial actions of early reperfusion therapy. The original paradigm appears on the left and the expanded paradigm is on the right. Restoration of coronary flow during the early (salvage) phase of acute myocardial infarction (MI) is administered to reduce MI size and transmurality. This preservation of myocardium was anticipated to reduce the wall motion abnormality, improve the ejection fraction, and ultimately lead to a reduction in mortality. Although these observations are accurate, the reduction in death appears to be out of proportion to the improvement in ejection fraction observed in the large placebo-controlled trials [31]. However, recent observations of the influence of infarct vessel patency on left ventricular (LV) remodeling and electrical stability led to an expansion of the original paradigm. The favorable effects of reperfusion therapy in reducing LV dilatation have a prominent role in the more current hypothesis explaining the beneficial actions of reperfusion therapy. (*Adapted from* Kim and Braunwald [32].)

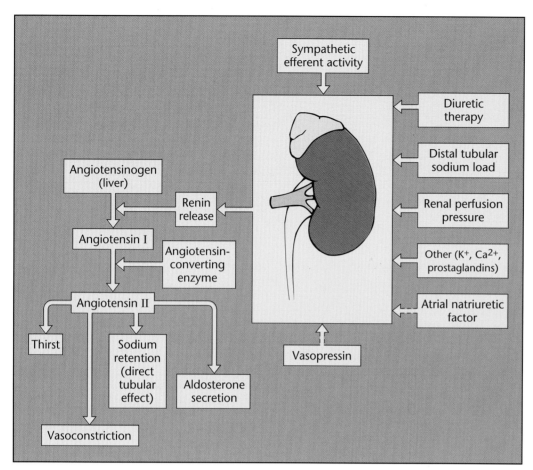

FIGURE 1-36.

The renin-angiotensin-aldosterone system
The renin-angiotensin system is activated in
patients with congestive heart failure. The
major site of release of circulating renin is the
juxtaglomerular apparatus of the kidney,
where multiple stimuli may contribute to
renal release of renin into the systemic circulation, including increased renal sympathetic
efferent activity, decreased distal tubular
sodium delivery, reduced renal perfusion pressure, and diuretic therapy. Atrial natriuretic
factor and vasopressin (*dashed arrows*) may
inhibit the release of renin. Renin enzymati-
cally cleaves angiotensinogen, a tetrapeptide
produced in the liver, to form the inactive
decapeptide angiotensin I. Angiotensin I is
converted to the octapeptide angiotensin II
by the angiotensin-converting enzyme.
Angiotensin II is a potent vasoconstrictor; it
promotes sodium reabsorption by increasing
aldosterone secretion and by a direct effect on
the tubules, and it stimulates water intake by
acting on the thirst center. Angiotensin II
causes vasoconstriction directly and may
also facilitate the release of norepinephrine
by acting on sympathetic nerve endings.
(*Adapted from* Paganelli *et al.* [33].)

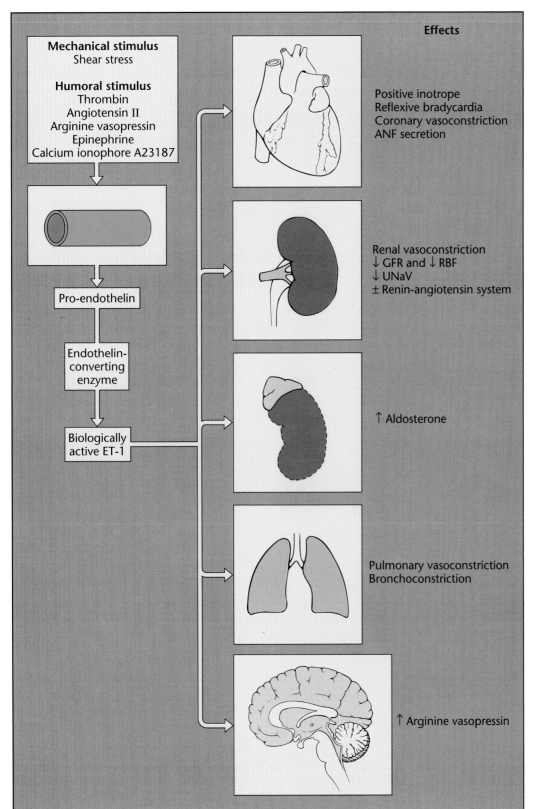

Effects

Positive inotrope
Reflexive bradycardia
Coronary vasoconstriction
ANF secretion

Renal vasoconstriction
↓ GFR and ↓ RBF
↓ UNaV
± Renin-angiotensin system

↑ Aldosterone

Pulmonary vasoconstriction
Bronchoconstriction

↑ Arginine vasopressin

Mechanical stimulus
Shear stress

Humoral stimulus
Thrombin
Angiotensin II
Arginine vasopressin
Epinephrine
Calcium ionophore A23187

Pro-endothelin

Endothelin-
converting
enzyme

Biologically
active ET-1

FIGURE 1-37.

Summary of the stimuli for endothelin secretion and effects of endothelin in several organs. Mechanical (shear stress) and humoral (thrombin, angiotensin II, vasopressin, epinephrine, calcium ionophore A23187) stimuli may cause the release of endothelin-1 (ET-1). Endothelin increases circulating levels of atrial natriuretic factor (ANF), vasopressin, and aldosterone. It also modulates renin release. Endothelin has a positive inotropic effect and produces coronary and systemic vasoconstriction. These responses produce an increase in blood pressure that is associated with a reflex decrease in heart rate. ET-1 constricts human pulmonary resistance vessels and has a potent bronchoconstrictor effect. Furthermore, ET-1 causes renal vasoconstriction, leading to a reduction in renal blood flow (RBF) and glomerular filtration rate (GFR) and a decrease in urinary sodium excretion (UNaV). (*Adapted from* Underwood *et al.* [34].)

CLINICAL FEATURES

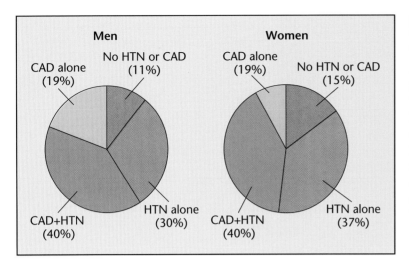

Men

CAD alone (19%)

No HTN or CAD (11%)

CAD+HTN (40%)

HTN alone (30%)

Women

CAD alone (19%)

No HTN or CAD (15%)

CAD+HTN (40%)

HTN alone (37%)

FIGURE 1-38.

The epidemiology of congestive heart failure in the United States. The Framingham Heart Study, which followed a cohort of 9405 Americans over a 40-year period, has provided valuable information regarding the etiologic basis of congestive heart failure in the United States [35]. Of 331 men and 321 women who developed heart failure, the majority had coronary artery disease (CAD) with or without hypertension (HTN), and approximately one third had HTN alone. At present, idiopathic dilated cardiomyopathy has replaced HTN as the second most important etiologic factor in the development of heart failure. CAD continues to be the most common risk factor for the development of heart failure in the United States. (*Adapted from* Ho *et al.* [35].)

MANAGEMENT OF HEART FAILURE

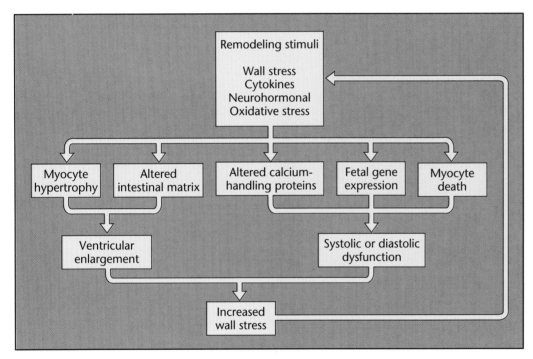

Remodeling stimuli

Wall stress
Cytokines
Neurohormonal
Oxidative stress

Myocyte hypertrophy

Altered intestinal matrix

Altered calcium-handling proteins

Fetal gene expression

Myocyte death

Ventricular enlargement

Systolic or diastolic dysfunction

Increased wall stress

FIGURE 1-39.

Pathophysiology of myocardial remodeling. Chronic hemodynamic stimuli such as pressure and volume overload lead to ventricular remodeling through increased mechanical wall stress and neuroendocrine activation. The myocardium responds with adaptive as well as maladaptive changes. Myocyte hypertrophy and changes in the quantity and nature of the interstitial matrix might at first normalize the wall stress, but these occur at the expense of ventricular compliance. Re-expression of fetal programs and calcium handling proteins may contribute to impaired contraction and relaxation. Myocytes unable to adapt might be triggered to undergo programmed cell death. These events lead to changes in the structure and function of the ventricle, which may result in further pump dysfunction and increased wall stresses, thereby promoting further pathologic remodeling [36,37]. (*Adapted from* Sawyer and Colucci [38].)

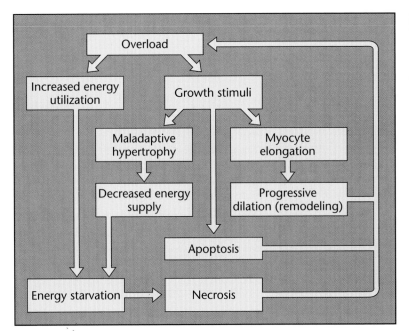

FIGURE 1-40.

Vicious cycles in the overloaded heart. Overload both increases energy utilization and stimulates growth [39]. Increased energy utilization contributes directly to energy starvation, which is worsened by several consequences of maladaptive hypertrophy that decrease energy supply. Growth stimuli include myocyte elongation, which causes remodeling, a progressive dilatation that raises wall tension and increases the overload. Growth stimuli also promote programmed cell death (apoptosis), which by decreasing the number of viable cardiac myocytes increases the load on those that survive. Hypertrophy also causes architectural changes that reduce the energy supply to working cardiac myocytes [39].

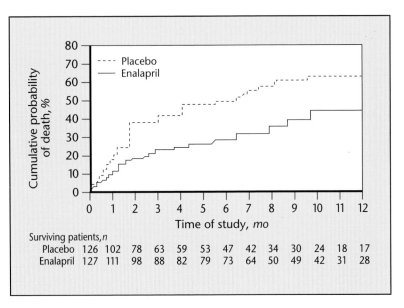

Surviving patients, *n*

Placebo	126	102	78	63	59	53	47	42	34	30	24	18	17
Enalapril	127	111	98	88	82	79	73	64	50	49	42	31	28

FIGURE 1-41.

Angiotensin-converting enzyme (ACE) inhibitors. The CONSENSUS (Cooperative North Scandinavian Enalapril Survival Study) trial, the first mortality study of an ACE inhibitor in patients with congestive heart failure, demonstrated that an ACE inhibitor improved mortality compared with placebo. A lesser-known aspect of the study was that the mean age of the patients at randomization was 70 years. In addition, the majority of patients were elderly and belonged to New York Heart Association functional class IV despite digoxin and diuretic therapy. Approximately 25% of the patients in this trial were also receiving other vasodilators, such as nitrates, before randomization. Early diagnosis of the placebo and enalapril treatment groups prompted early termination of the study. The mean dose of enalapril was just under 20 mg/d. Careful dose titration obviated the excess hypotension observed in early stages of the study. (*Adapted from* CONSENSUS Trial Study Group [40].)

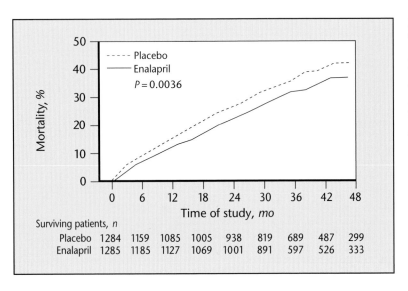

Surviving patients, *n*

Placebo	1284	1159	1085	1005	938	819	689	487	299
Enalapril	1285	1185	1127	1069	1001	891	597	526	333

FIGURE 1-42.

The SOLVD (Studies of Left Ventricular Dysfunction) treatment subgroup demonstrated mortality benefit in moderate heart failure. The treatment subgroup included patients who already had symptomatic congestive heart failure and were randomized to either placebo or enalapril therapy. Criteria for randomization were a baseline ejection fraction of 35% or less and symptomatic heart failure. The majority of patients in this study had functional class II congestive heart failure. Enalapril was associated with a significant reduction in mortality compared with placebo in these patients. This mortality benefit was primarily the result of reducing mortality due to congestive heart failure. Mortality due to presumed arrhythmic death was not significantly different from placebo. (*Adapted from* the SOLVD Investigators [41].)

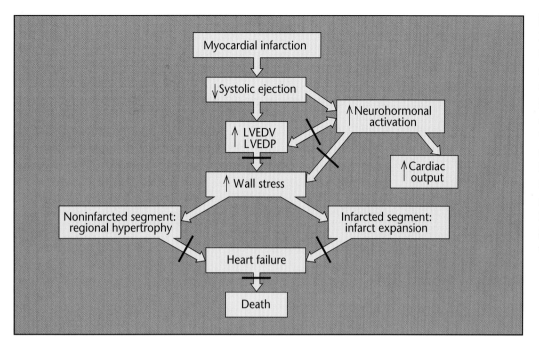

FIGURE 1-43.

Potential role of angiotension-converting enzyme (ACE) inhibitors in left ventricular remodeling. Although the pathophysiology of infarct healing is complex, there are several potential mechanisms by which an ACE inhibitor may favorably improve left ventricular remodeling. Shown with *intersecting bars* are sites at which an ACE inhibitor may interrupt an adverse consequence of myocardial infarction that would contribute to heart failure or death. LVEDP—left ventricular end-diastolic pressure; LVEDV—left ventricular end-diastolic volume. (*Adapted from* McKay *et al.* [42].)

Drugs with Vasodilator Properties and Their Use in Chronic Congestive Heart Failure

ACE inhibitors
  The only vasodilator class approved for CHF
  Efficacy has been demonstrated in exercise and mortality trials
Direct-acting vasodilators
  The combination of hydralazine and isosorbide dinitrate has also demonstrated clinical and mortality benefit
  Flosequinan was initially approved, then withdrawn due to increased mortality and increased heart rate during surgery
α-Adrenergic blockers
  Associated with hemodynamic tachyphylaxis
  No mortality benefit
Calcium antagonists
  Benefit thus far limited to subgroups, such as diastolic heart failure in hypertension or ongoing coronary ischemia
  Mortality studies currently in progress will assess the benefit of this class when added to standard therapy
Inodilators (*eg*, milrinone)
  Increased exercise capacity
  Increased mortality during chronic oral therapy in severe heart failure
Potential newer approaches
  Augmentation of circulating natriuretic properties
  Inhibition of endothelin by use of specific antagonists

FIGURE 1-44.

The current status of oral vasodilators for the treatment of congestive heart failure (CHF). Angiotensin-converting enzyme (ACE) inhibitors are the only class of vasodilators that has been approved by the Food and Drug Administration for treatment of CHF. In addition, ACE inhibitors have proven effective in large clinical trials of CHF, with both a mortality benefit and an improvement of functional capacity. The direct-acting vasodilators have not had a uniformly successful course in the treatment of CHF. The combination of hydralazine–isosorbide dinitrate has been effective in large clinical trials of CHF, demonstrating either improved clinical benefit or an improved mortality outcome versus placebo. Historically, minoxidil has not been successful in treatment of CHF despite its proven vasodilating properties.

More recently, flosequinan was initially approved for the treatment of CHF, and then later withdrawn, because of evidence of increased mortality in a placebo-controlled study that compared flosequinan with placebo against background therapy with digoxin, diuretics, and an ACE inhibitor. In addition, flosequinan was associated with an inexplicable heart rate increase during chronic therapy.

α-Adrenergic blocking agents are associated with tachyphylaxis during chronic use. In addition, prazosin did not demonstrate a mortality benefit compared with placebo in the original VHeFT (Veterans Administration Cooperative Vasodilator Heart Failure Trial) study. The reason for this is not clear but may involve the activation of neurohormonal pathways. For the calcium antagonists, evidence of clinical benefit thus far is limited to subgroups such as diastolic heart failure in patients with hypertension or ongoing coronary artery ischemia. Mortality studies are currently in progress that will assess the benefit of the calcium antagonists as adjunctive therapy in patients receiving digoxin, diuretic, and ACE inhibitor therapy. Another group of vasodilator substances are the "inodilators." This class is best represented by milrinone, a bipyridine. These compounds, by inhibiting peak III phosphodiesterase, produce a positive inotropic effect as well as a vasodilating effect. However, milrinone was associated with increased mortality during chronic oral therapy in severe heart failure, possibly due to an excessive increase in myocardial cAMP.

It is now recognized that pure vasodilators may not be of long-term benefit in CHF. However, compounds that produce vasodilatation as part of a profile related to modulation of neurohormonal factors may be of benefit. Examples of potential new approaches in this area are now evident. For example, augmentation of circulating natriuretic peptides produces vasodilatation. Inhibition of adverse neurohormonal vasoconstrictors, such as endothelin, by specific antagonists is also a therapeutic approach under development. (*Courtesy of* Robert J. Cody.)

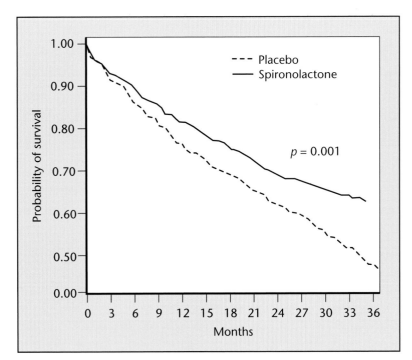

FIGURE 1-45.
Results of the Randomized Aldactone Evaluation Study (RALES) trial. In this double-blinded randomized trial spironolactone improved survival in patients with heart failure [43,44]. (*Adapted from* Pitt *et al.* [44].)

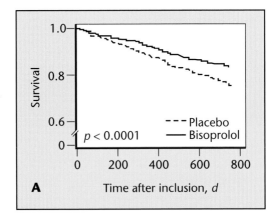

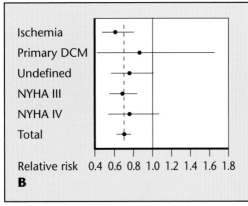

FIGURE 1-46.
Results of the Cardiac Insufficiency Bisoprolol Study II (CIBIS-II) trial.
A, Survival curves in the double-blinded randomized CIBIS-II trial. **B**, Relative risk of treatment effect on mortality by etiology and functional class at baseline in the CIBIS-II trial. Horizontal bars represent 95% confidence intervals. The beta blocker bisoprolol improved survival in patients with heart failure [43,45]. (*Adapted from* [45].)

Pharmacologic Properties and Therapeutic Considerations in Using Inotropic-Vasopressor Agents

Pharmacologic Features	Dobutamine	Dopamine Low Dose	Dopamine High Dose	Norepinephrine
Receptor agonism				
α	+	+	+++	++++
β₁	++++	+	++	+
β₂	++	0	0	0
Dopaminergic	0	+++	++	0
Systemic vascular resistance	↓↓	↓	↑↑	↑↑↑↑
Stroke volume and cardiac output	↓↓↓↓	↑	↑↑	↑
Ability to increase systemic blood pressure	→ to ↑	→	↑↑↑	↑↑↑↑
Ventricular filling pressure	↓↓	↓ to →	→ to ↑↑	→ to ↑↑
Chronotropic	→ to ↑↑	→	→ to ↑↑↑	→ to ↑
Myocardial oxygen demand/supply	→ to ↑	→	→ to ↑↑	→ to ↑↑

FIGURE 1-47.
Principal pharmacologic properties and therapeutic considerations in the use of the major inotropic/vasopressor agents in acute or severe heart failure. (*Courtesy of* Carl V. Leier.)

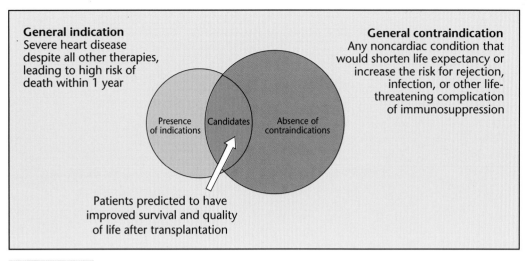

General indication
Severe heart disease despite all other therapies, leading to high risk of death within 1 year

General contraindication
Any noncardiac condition that would shorten life expectancy or increase the risk for rejection, infection, or other life-threatening complication of immunosuppression

Presence of indications | Candidates | Absence of contraindications

Patients predicted to have improved survival and quality of life after transplantation

FIGURE 1-48.

The rationale and arithmetic of the selection process for cardiac transplantation. During the first decade of cardiac transplantation, selection of candidates was focused on the definition of contraindications, the indications being considered obvious in the absence of other options. With increasing sophistication of alternative medical therapy with vasodilators and diuretics tailored to hemodynamic and neurohormonal goals for advanced heart failure, many patients previously relegated to transplantation can now enjoy functional status and prognosis similar to those achieved by transplantation. The challenge is to select those patients with sufficient cardiovascular limitation but also adequate noncardiac organ function and psychosocial support to derive major benefit from transplantation in terms of both quality of life and survival [46,47]. (*Courtesy of* Lynne Warner Stevenson.)

Contraindications to Cardiac Transplantation

Older age (usual limit 60–65 y)
Active infection
Severe diabetes mellitus with other end-organ disease
Pulmonary function > 60%* predicted, or chronic bronchitis
Serum creatinine > 2 mg/dL or clearance > 40 mL/min*
Bilirubin > 2.5 mg/dL, transaminases 2 X normal*
PAS > 60 mm Hg, TPG > 15 mm Hg*
High risk of life-threatening noncompliance

FIGURE 1-49.

Specific contraindications to cardiac transplantation [47]. These vary slightly among programs, particularly with regard to age. Older patients have been shown in large studies to have a slightly higher mortality during extended follow-up [48–50]. Relative or borderline contraindications are usually weighed more heavily in the older potential candidate. Chronically elevated filling pressures lead to pulmonary hypertension and compromised pulmonary and hepatic function. Renal function is usually impaired to some degree in cardiac transplant candidates. Several days of intravenous therapy to optimize hemodynamics are frequently required to determine whether pulmonary hypertension and organ dysfunction (*asterisks*) are intrinsic or are secondary to hemodynamic compromise (and therefore presumably reversible). The patient and family are considered together as a unit that requires extensive psychological and social work evaluation regarding the potential for good outcome. Non-compliance remains a major cause of late mortality. PAS—pulmonary artery systolic pressure. TPG—transpulmonary gradient: mean pulmonary artery pressure minus capillary wedge pressure. (*Courtesy of* Lynne Warner Stevenson.)

CARDIOMYOPATHY, MYOCARDITIS, AND PERICARDIAL DISEASE

HYPERTROPHIC CARDIOMYOPATHY

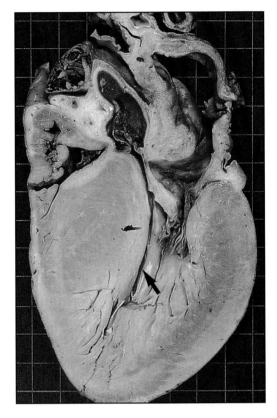

FIGURE 1-50.

Asymmetric septal hypertrophy. Longitudinal section of the heart of a 31-year-old woman with subaortic obstructive HCM who died suddenly while on propranolol therapy. Hemodynamic investigation confirmed subaortic obstruction as well as mitral regurgitation. The regurgitation was partially due to an abnormal mitral valve (insertion of an anomalous papillary muscle (*arrow*) onto the ventricular surface of the anterior mitral leaflet). Note the asymmetric hypertrophy with a grossly thickened ventricular septum. A narrowed outflow tract between the upper septum and the anterior mitral leaflet, which is very thickened and fibrosed from repeated contact with the septum, can also be seen. There was microscopic evidence of extensive myocardial fiber disarray involving the septum and free wall of the left ventricle. (*From* Wigle *et al.* [51]; *courtesy of* L. Horlick.)

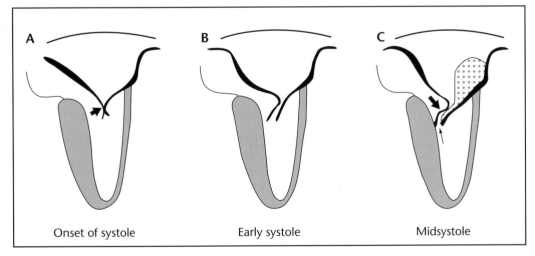

A	**B**	**C**
Onset of systole	Early systole	Midsystole

FIGURE 1-51.

Functional anatomy of mitral leaflet systolic anterior motion and mitral regurgitation in subaortic obstructive HCM. Drawing of a transesophageal echocardiogram (frontal long-axis plane) demonstrating the anterior and superior motion of the anterior mitral leaflet to produce mitral leaflet–septal contact and failure of leaflet coaptation in midsystole. **A,** At the onset of systole, the coaptation point (*arrow*) is in the body of the anterior and posterior leaflets rather than at the tip of the leaflets, as in normal subjects [52,53]. The portion of the leaflets beyond the coaptation point is referred to as the residual length of the leaflet [52,53]. During early systole (**B**) and midsystole (**C**) there is anterior and superior movement of the residual length of the anterior mitral leaflet (*thick arrow* in *C*), with septal contact and failure of leaflet coaptation (*thin arrow* in *C*) with consequent mitral regurgitation directed posteriorly into the left atrium (*dotted area*). (*Adapted from* Grigg *et al.* [53].)

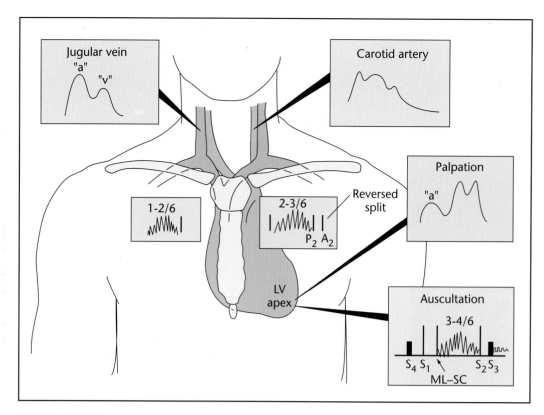

FIGURE 1-52.

Physical examination in subaortic obstructive HCM. There are seven physical signs in subaortic obstructive HCM that are not found in nonobstructive HCM. On palpation, a spike-and-dome arterial pulse can often be felt in the carotid artery or in a peripheral pulse. On palpation of the left ventricular (LV) apex, there may be a triple apex beat caused by a palpable left atrial gallop and a double systolic impulse—one impulse comes before the onset of obstruction and the other after. On auscultation, at or just medial to the LV apex, there is a late onset, diamond-shaped systolic murmur of grade 3 to 4/6 in intensity. This murmur is caused by both the subaortic obstruction and the concomitant mitral regurgitation, causing the murmur to radiate to both the left sternal border and to the axilla. Because of the mitral regurgitation, there is often a short diastolic inflow murmur after the third heart sound. Rarely, a mitral leaflet–septal contact (ML–SC) sound may be heard preceding the systolic murmur at the apex. Finally, if there is severe subaortic obstruction, reversed splitting of the second heart sound may occur. In nonobstructive HCM, there is often a third or fourth heart sound at the apex, depending on the type of diastolic dysfunction. If the fourth heart sound is palpable, there will be a double apex beat, which is quite different in timing and significance from the double *systolic* apex beat that occurs in subaortic obstructive HCM. In nonobstructive HCM, there is either no apical systolic murmur or at most a grade 1 to 2/6 murmur of mitral regurgitation. In any type of HCM, a grade 1 to 3/6 systolic ejection murmur at or below the pulmonary area may be heard. This murmur may reflect obstruction to right ventricular (RV) outflow. Examining the jugular venous pulse frequently reveals a prominent a-wave that rises on inspiration, reflecting RV diastolic dysfunction. Rarely, this is accompanied by an RV fourth heart sound. (*Courtesy of E. Douglas Wigle, Allan D. Kitching, and Harry Rakowski.*)

IDIOPATHIC DILATED CARDIOMYOPATHY

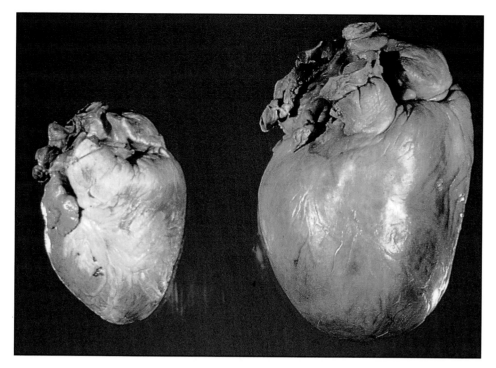

FIGURE 1-53

Gross pathology. In contrast to the normal heart (*left*), the heart in idiopathic dilated cardiomyopathy (*right*) is characterized by biventricular hypertrophy and four-chamber enlargement. The weight is often 25% to 50% above normal. Enlargement of the heart can be seen easily on chest radiography or cardiac echocardiography. (*Courtesy of* Edward K. Kasper, Ralph H. Hruban, and Kenneth L. Baughman.)

SPECIFIC HEART MUSCLE DISEASE

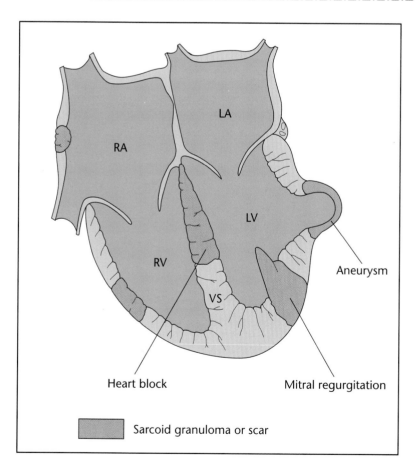

FIGURE 1-54.

Cardiac sarcoidosis. Distribution and consequences of sarcoid granulomas in sarcoid heart disease. In an autopsy series of 26 patients reported by Roberts *et al.* [54], cardiac granulomas were observed grossly in 25 hearts. Sarcoid granulomas were present in the left ventricular (LV) free wall of all 25 patients, in the right ventricular (RV) septum in 19, in the RV wall in 12, in the right atrial (RA) wall in three patients, and in the left atrial (LA) wall in two. Involvement of the cephalad portion of the muscular ventricular septum was associated with complete heart block. Important consequences of the involvement of the LV wall were aneurysm formation and mitral regurgitation. VS—ventricular septum. (*Adapted from* Roberts *et al.* [54].)

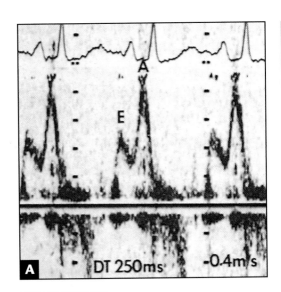 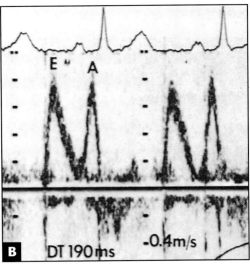 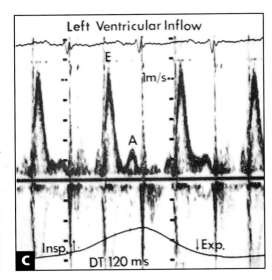

FIGURE 1-55.

Cardiac amyloidosis. The spectrum of abnormal Doppler echocardiographic patterns in cardiac amyloidosis. Echocardiography is of considerable value in the diagnosis of infiltrative amyloid heart disease [55]. Typical features on two-dimensional echocardiography include a granular appearance of the myocardium and increased thickness of the myocardial walls. A number of studies have clearly shown that diastolic dysfunction in cardiac amyloidosis exhibits a spectrum of abnormalities that can be followed up serially by Doppler echocardiography. In earlier stages of amyloid heart disease, abnormal relaxation is the Doppler pattern seen (**A**). The E wave is of lower magnitude than the a-wave and the deceleration time is prolonged. As the disease progresses, a pseudonormalization Doppler pattern may emerge (**B**, the same patient as in *panel A*, taken 6 months later). Eventually, a restrictive pattern (**C**) emerges. As shown in this example (pulsed-wave Doppler recording of a left ventricular inflow profile), there is increased E/A ratio (3.7) and short deceleration time (120 ms). (*From* Klein *et al.* [55]; with permission.)

RESTRICTIVE CARDIOMYOPATHY AND HYPEREOSINOPHILIC HEART DISEASE

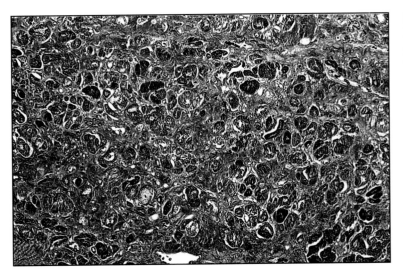

FIGURE 1-56.

Idiopathic restricted cardiomyopathy. Cross-sectional view of myocytes surrounded by fibrous tissue (Mallory-azan stain). Whereas severe interstitial fibrosis is seen here, fibrous tissue surrounds each myocyte (predominantly endomysial fibrosis). (*Courtesy of* Yuzo Hirota.)

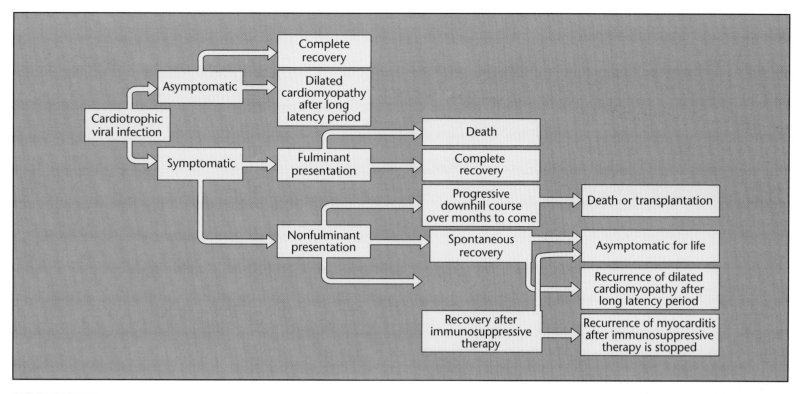

FIGURE 1-57.

The natural history of human myocarditis. Most patients with mild symptoms of acute myocarditis are not seen by cardiologists and most of these patients appear to recover fully. Of the patients with symptomatic heart disease typically seen by cardiologists, a small number have fulminant presentations and either die in the acute stage or appear to recover fully. Of the remaining patients with myocarditis, a few are characterized by a progressive downhill course over a period of months to years that ends in death from heart failure or intractable arrhythmias [56,57]. Some spontaneously recover and remain asymptomatic for life, and others have an asymptomatic period followed by development of dilated cardiomyopathy. The heterogeneity of clinical presentations and natural history in human myocarditis probably reflect the genetic predisposition of the individual, the virulence of the cardiotropic virus, and environmental factors. With the advent of molecular viral probes, it will be critical to relate the presence of persistent enterovirus RNA with the patterns of the natural history of myocarditis. (*Courtesy of Ahvie Herskowitz and Aftab A. Ansari.*)

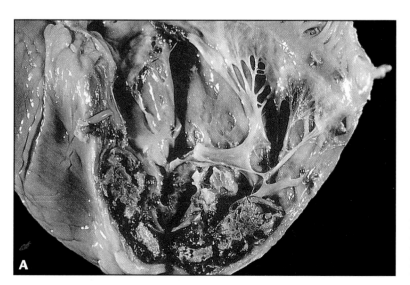

FIGURE 1-58.

A, Gross autopsy specimen of a heart with fulminant myocarditis. The right ventricle is cut along the long axis to demonstrate an apical mural thrombus. Fulminant myocarditis is characterized by a nonspecific, severe influenza-like illness and the distinct onset of cardiac involvement. The patient's condition deteriorates rapidly, and the disorder frequently results in profound hemodynamic compromise and multisystem failure. Endomyocardial biopsies from fulminant myocarditis patients demonstrate unequivocal active myocarditis and are particularly notable for very extensive inflammatory infiltrates and numerous foci of myocyte necrosis. Within 1 month, the patients usually recover left ventricular function completely or die [58]. In contrast, acute myocarditis describes the clinical spectrum of the largest group of patients with active or borderline myocarditis. These patients have minimally dilated, hypokinetic left ventricles on presentation.

(*Continued*)

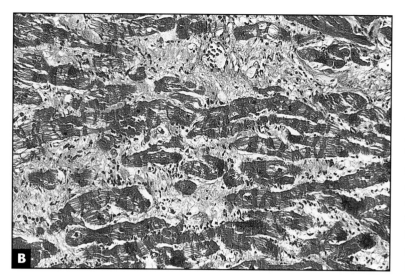

FIGURE 1-58. (*CONTINUED*)
The onset of cardiac symptoms is frequently indistinct, and some patients provide a vague history consistent with (but not diagnostic of) an antecedent viral illness. Active or borderline myocarditis is present on initial (but not subsequent) endomyocardial biopsies. Although some patients in this group appear to respond to immunosuppressive therapy [59], others experience either partial recovery of ventricular function or continue to deteriorate to end-stage dilated cardiomyopathy. **B,** Masson's trichrome (which stains collagen blue) of an endomyocardial biopsy of a patient with chronic active myocarditis. Note the extensive collagen deposition characteristically seen in end-stage dilated cardiomyopathy. Patients with chronic active myocarditis usually have a vague clinical presentation. Such patients have a slowly progressive course that inevitably deteriorates but may be punctuated by brief, often dramatic but unsustained responses to immunosuppressive therapy. Serial endomyocardial biopsies demonstrate ongoing myocarditis with the development of extensive interstitial fibrosis. Inflammatory infiltrates in this subgroup of myocarditis patients may contain multinucleated giant cells. (*Courtesy of* Ahvie Herskowitz and Aftab A. Ansari.)

PERICARDIAL DISEASE

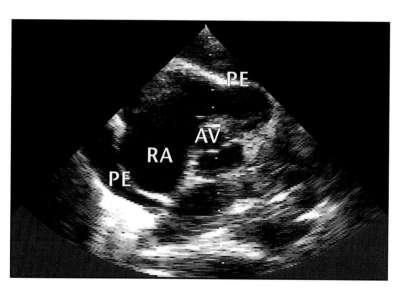

FIGURE 1-59.
Cardiac tamponade. Two-dimensional echocardiogram, parasternal short-axis view, showing right ventricular diastolic collapse (*arrow*) in a patient with a large pericardial effusion (PE) and cardiac tamponade. AV—aortic valve; RA—right atrium. (*Courtesy of* Brian Hoit.)

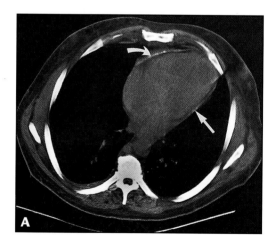
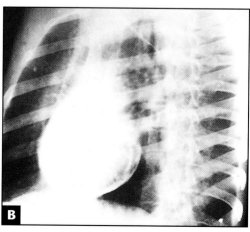

FIGURE 1-60.
Constrictive pericarditis. **A,** Computed tomography of the chest showing thickened pericardium and calcification (*arrows*) in a patient with constrictive pericarditis.
B, Extensive pericardial calcification may occur with chronic pericarditis without constriction. The typical hemodynamic pattern must also be present to make the diagnosis of constrictive pericarditis. (Panel A *from* Fowler [60]; with permission; panel B *courtesy of* Noble Fowler.)

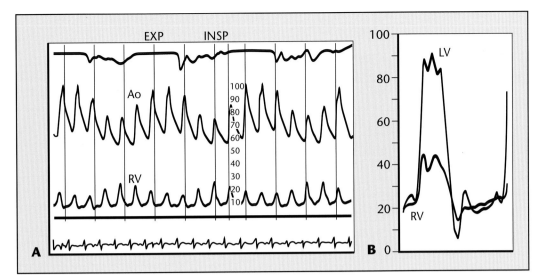

FIGURE 1-61.

Contrasting pattern of a ventricular pressure pulse recording in cardiac tamponade (**A**) and in constrictive pericarditis (**B**) [61]. In constrictive pericarditis, there is a dip and plateau pattern (square-root sign) in both ventricular pressure pulse tracings with equalization of right (RV) and left ventricular (LV) end-diastolic pressures. In cardiac tamponade, there is no pronounced diastolic dip in the RV pressure pulse. The patient with cardiac tamponade demonstrates a pronounced inspiratory decline of aortic pressure (Ao). Pressure scale is in mm Hg. EXP—expiration; INSP—inspiration. (*From* Shabetai *et al.* [61]; with permission.)

■ ARRHYTHMIAS

CONDUCTION AND EXCITATION: NORMAL PATHWAY OF ELECTRICAL CONDUCTION

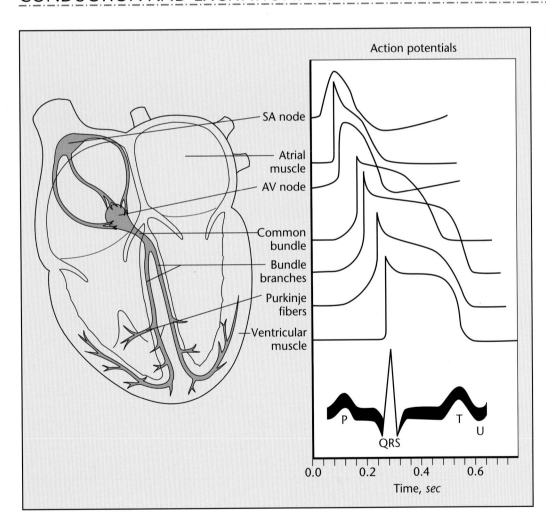

FIGURE 1-62.

Localized variations in the action potential of the heart's electrical system. Cardiac action potentials from different locations in the heart have different shapes, leading to different electrophysiologic properties. The SA node and AV node depolarize in response to the slow inward current of calcium and sodium. The two nodes differ in that the SA node possesses the property of automaticity and the AV node does not. All other cardiac cells depolarize in response to the rapid inward current of sodium ions. Note the progressive increase in the action potential duration beginning at the AV node and reaching its maximum in the Purkinje fiber. This results in the functional refractory period of the ventricular tissue being dependent on the effective refractory period of the Purkinje cell. Furthermore, specialized cells depolarize during phase 4, whereas atrial and ventricular muscle does not. (*Adapted from* CIBA Pharmaceutical Company Division of CIBA-GEIGY Co [62].)

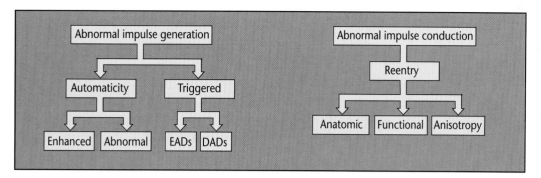

FIGURE 1-63.

Mechanism of arrhythmias. Mechanistically, arrhythmias can be separated into those due to abnormal impulse generation and those due to abnormal impulse conduction. EAD—early after-depolarization; DAD—delayed after-depolarization. (*Courtesy of* Randall J. Lee and Edmund C. Keung.)

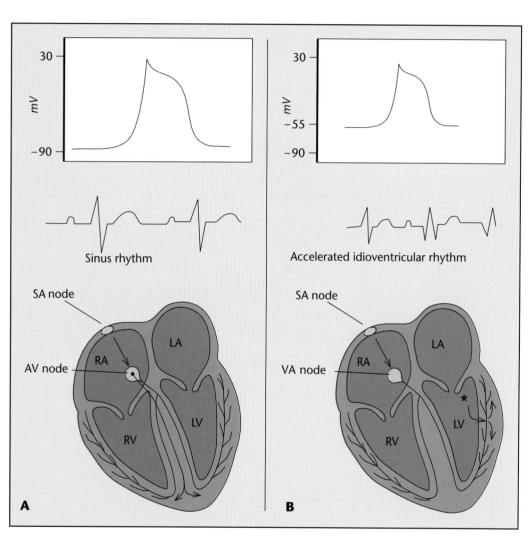

FIGURE 1-64.

Automaticity. Abnormal automaticity occurs when spontaneous depolarizations are generated in partially depolarized tissue (reduced maximum diastolic potential or resting membrane potential) as a result of some pathologic process such as ischemia. Arrhythmias that may arise because of abnormal automaticity are certain types of ectopic atrial tachycardias, accelerated idioventricular rhythms, and ventricular tachycardias (especially within the first 72 hours after a myocardial infarction). Compared are normal ventricular tissue (**A**) and ischemic ventricular tissue (*asterisk* in **B**). The action potentials and the possible conduction throughout the heart and the resultant rhythms are shown. LA—left atrium; LV—left ventricle; RA—right atrium; RV—right ventricle. (*Courtesy of* Randall J. Lee and Edmund C. Keung.)

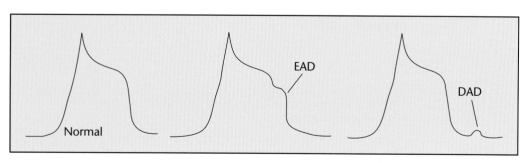

FIGURE 1-65.

Triggered arrhythmias. Triggered activity arises as a consequence of increased positive ions within the cardiac cell, leading to distortion of the action potential (after-depolarization). After-depolarizations can occur in the late phase 3 (early after-depolarization [EAD]) or early phase 4 (delayed after-depolarization [DAD]). (*Courtesy of* Randall J. Lee and Edmund C. Keung.)

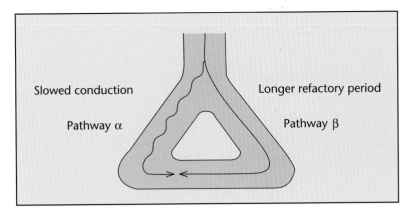

FIGURE 1-66.

Reentry. Prerequisites for reentry arrhythmias include: (1) an anatomic circuit with two pathways eventually joined by a common tissue, (2) the two pathways have different electrophysiologic properties, and (3) a section within the circuit (pathway β) has a longer refractory period than the pathway α, thus permitting unidirectional block. (*Courtesy of* Randall J. Lee and Edmund C. Keung.)

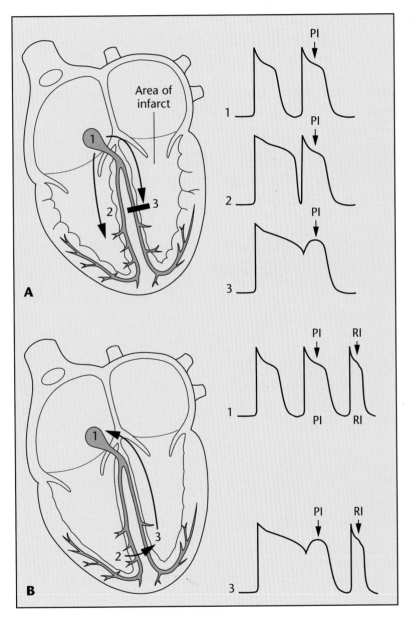

FIGURE 1-67.

Mechanism for reentry resulting from dispersion of refractoriness in the subendocardial Purkinje fiber network over an area of extensive myocardial infarction. This figure shows the endocardial surface of the left ventricular anterior papillary muscle. The color area in each diagram is the scar resulting from the myocardial infarct that is covered by a blanket of the surviving Purkinje fibers. As depicted, Purkinje fibers in different regions have markedly different action potentials with respect to duration and refractory periods. Action potentials are recorded from normal tissue (site 1) and from subendocardial Purkinje fibers with prolonged repolarization phases (sites 2 and 3), surviving in the infarct. In **A**, premature impulse (PI) occurs at the infarct border (site 1) and conducts into the infarcted regions as indicated by the *large arrows*. Note that the action potentials are prolonged. The action potential at site 3 is longer than at site 2 in the infarcted area. Consequently, premature impulses can excite cells at site 2, but conduction blocks at site 3. **B**, The continuation of these events after the premature impulse conducts through site 2 and activates the cells at site 3. As a reentering impulse (RI), it then proceeds to its site of origin (site 1), which also re-excites as a reentry impulse (RI). (*Adapted from* Wit *et al.* [63].)

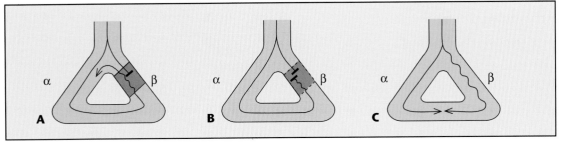

FIGURE 1-68.

Effect of antiarrhythmic drugs on reentry. The question of how antiarrhythmic drugs suppress arrhythmias must be addressed by considering arrhythmia mechanisms. Most arrhythmias based on abnormal conduction involve reentry circuits (**A**). The *shaded area* represents the depolarized tissue in which conduction block occurs, and retrograde conduction is slow enough to allow the cells in limb α to recover and propagate the reentrant impulse. Antiarrhythmic drugs can eliminate reentry tachyarrhythmias by impairing conduction sufficiently to cause interruption of conduction through the circuit (**B**) or by improving conduction in limb β, which prevents the development of conduction block (**C**). Class I drugs prevent reentry by causing a greater amount of slow conduction in depolarized tissue, thus producing conduction block in both the forward and reverse directions in limb β. (*Courtesy of* Randall J. Lee.)

Comparative Efficacy of Oral Antiarrhythmic Drugs

Drug	Premature Atrial Contractions	Atrial Fibrillation	Antegrade Slowing of AV Nodal Conduction	AV Node Re-entrant Tachycardia	Effects on Accessory Pathway Conduction	WPW- Paroxysmal Supraventricular Tachycardia	Sustained Ventricular Tachycardia/Ventricular Fibrillation PES, %
Quinidine	++	++	+/-	+	+	+	20–25
Procainamide	++	++	+/-	+	+	+	20–25
Disopyramide	++	++	+/-	+	++	++	20–25
Tocainide	0	0	0	0	+/-	0	10–15
Mexiletine	0	0	0	0	+/-	0	10–20
Moricizine	+	NE	0	NE	+	NE	20
Flecainide	++	++	+	++	+++	+++	20–25
Encainide	++	++	++	++	+++	+++	20–25
Propafenone	++	++	++	++	++	++	20–25
Recainam	+	++	+	++	++	++	20
β-Blockers	+*	+	++	+	0	+	5
Amiodarone	++	+++	++	++	+	++	20–60
Sotalol	+	++	++	++	+	+	30
Digoxin	0	+*	++	+	+/-	+	NA
Verapamil	0	+*	++	+	+/-	+	NA
Diltiazem	0	+*	++	+	+/-	+	NA

*Rate control data.

FIGURE 1-69.

Efficacy of antiarrhythmic drugs. This table compares the efficacy of a number of antiarrhythmic drugs on some of the more common types of arrhythmias. NA—not applicable; NE—not established; PES—programmed electrical stimulation. (*Courtesy of* Randall J. Lee.)

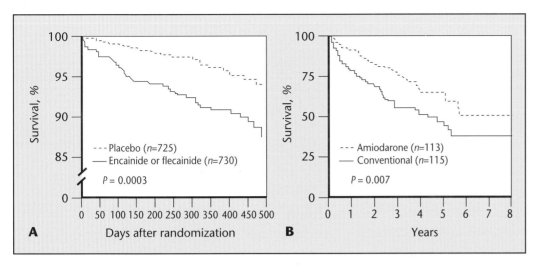

infarction survival) and provided a strong incentive for the development of alternatives to the use of class I drugs. The recent findings of the CASCADE (Cardiac Arrest in Seattle, Conventional versus Amiodarone Drug Evaluation) study [66] (**B**) and the ESVEM (Electrophysiologic Study Versus Electrocardiographic Monitoring) trial [67] demonstrated improved survival in patients with life-threatening ventricular arrhythmias, confirmed the usefulness of the class III agents and has led to their use as first line agents in ventricular arrhythmias. *Panel B* compares the cumulative cardiac survival of patients with aborted cardiac arrest treated with empiric amiodarone with that of conventional antiarrhythmic therapy, Class I agents. (Panel A *adapted from* CAST I [64] and CAST II [65]; panel B *adapted from* the CASCADE Investigators [66].)

FIGURE 1-70.

Comparison of antiarrhythmic drugs. The surprising results of CAST (Cardiac Arrhythmic Suppression Trial) I (**A**), which demonstrated an increase in mortality in post–myocardial infarction patients treated with the class Ic antiarrhythmic agents, encainide and flecainide, compared with placebo (CAST) [64]. These results were corroborated by CAST II [65] (comparison of moricizine, also a Class I agent, versus placebo for post–myocardial

SINUS NODE DISORDERS

Therapeutic Options for Sinus Node Disorders

Diagnosis	Therapy
Symptomatic sinus node dysfunction (bradycardia, chronotropic incompetence, sinus arrest, sinoatrial exit block)	AAIR pacing when no evidence of AV conduction disease DDDR pacing with evidence of AV conduction disease
Tachy-brady syndrome	Type I or III antiarrhythmics to treat atrial arrhythmias β-Blockers, calcium-channel blockers, or digoxin to control ventricular response VVI or DDD pacing for bradycardic episodes (drug used to treat atrial arrhythmia may worsen bradyarrhythmias and precipitate the need for cardiac pacing) AV junction ablation with DDDR or VVIR pacing in patients whose ventricular response is difficult to control
Sinus node reentry	β-Blockers, calcium-channel blockers Type I and III antiarrhythmics Catheter ablation (sinus node modification)
Inappropriate sinus tachycardia	β-Blockers, calcium-channel blockers Catheter ablation (sinus node ablation/modification) Pindolol, Norpace
Carotid sinus hypersensitivity	Cardiac pacing Avoidance of tight collars

FIGURE 1-71.

Therapeutic options for sinus node disorders. Pacing nodes are standard. AAIR—rate-responsive atrial pacing; AV—atrioventricular; DDD—dual chamber pacing; DDDR—rate-responsive dual chamber pacing; VVI—ventricular pacing; VVIR—rate-responsive ventricular pacing. (*Courtesy of* Laurence M. Epstein.)

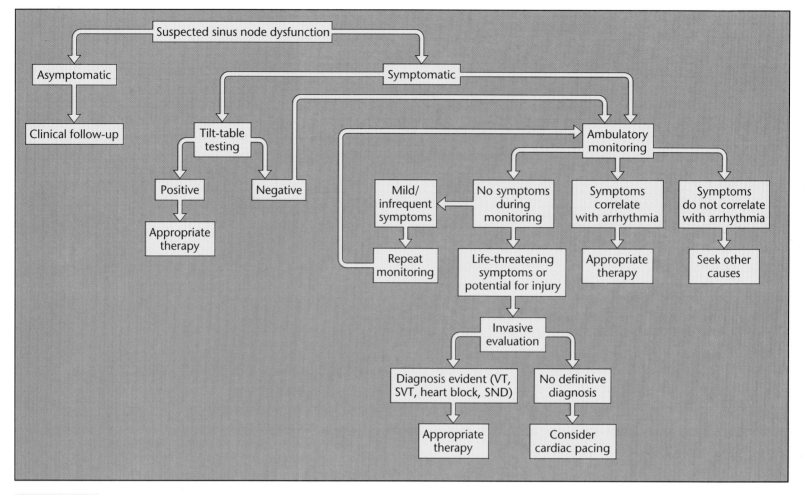

FIGURE 1-72.

The approach to diagnosing and treating sinus node dysfunction (SND). In patients with suspected SND, the correlation with symptoms is crucial. The presence of bradycardia alone is not an indication for treatment. In symptomatic patients, a careful history may reveal diagnostic clues. In patients with syncope or syncope associated with standing, a tilt-table test may be in order. In patients with frequent symptoms, 24-hour monitoring is often diagnostic. When symptoms are less frequent, an event-type recorder may be more useful. If symptoms do not correlate with cardiac arrhythmias, other causes (*ie*, neurologic) should be sought. If no symptoms occur during monitoring but the patient has recurrent syncope or has been injured during episodes, a more invasive evaluation is indicated. SVT—supraventricular tachycardia; VT—ventricular tachycardia. (*Adapted from* Gomes [68].)

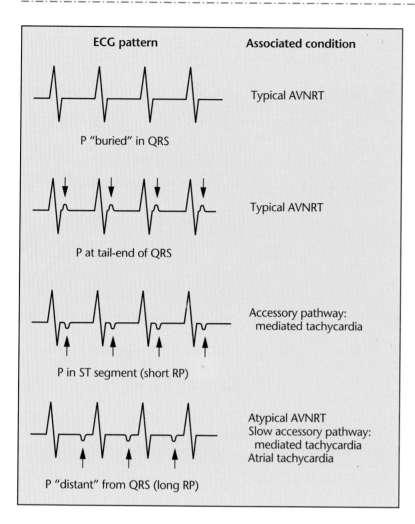

ECG pattern	Associated condition

P "buried" in QRS — Typical AVNRT

P at tail-end of QRS — Typical AVNRT

P in ST segment (short RP) — Accessory pathway: mediated tachycardia

P "distant" from QRS (long RP) — Atypical AVNRT / Slow accessory pathway: mediated tachycardia / Atrial tachycardia

FIGURE 1-73.

Electrocardiographic patterns of narrow complex tachycardias. The most important clue to the mechanism of a narrow complex tachycardia is the relationship of the P wave to the QRS complex. No visible P wave often means that the P wave is buried in the QRS complex. This is usually due to typical atrioventricular (AV) nodal reentry. With typical AV nodal reentry, the P wave may also be located just at the start or end of the QRS complex, giving a qRs or Rsr' pattern. When the P wave is located close to the previous QRS complex, it is identified as a short-RP tachycardia. This is often seen with accessory pathway–mediated tachycardia and is due to retrograde atrial activation over the accessory pathway. The P wave may also be far from the previous QRS complex and classified as a long-RP tachycardia. If the P wave is inverted, it may be the result of atypical AV node reentry, or it may be using a slowly conducting accessory pathway in the retrograde direction. AVNRT—atrioventricular nodal reentry tachycardia; ECG—electrocardiogram. (*Courtesy of* Harlan R. Grogin.)

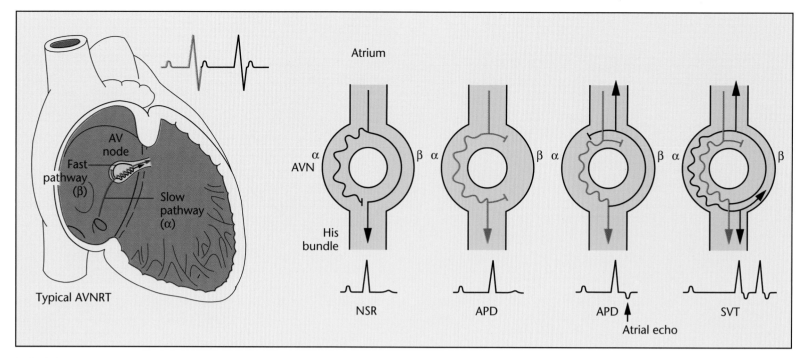

FIGURE 1-74.

Typical and atypical atrioventricular node reentrant tachycardia (AVNRT). Typical atrioventricular (AV) node reentry is shown in **A**. An impulse from the atrium enters the AV node and travels down both the slow and fast pathway. It quickly travels down the fast pathway resulting in activation of the ventricles with a short PR interval and results in the blocking of the impulse from the slow pathway when it reaches the terminal portion of the AV node since the tissue is still refractory. An atrial premature depolarization (APD) results in the conduction of the impulse down the slow pathway and thus longer PR interval. It blocks in the fast pathway since that tissue has a longer refractory period. If the tissue of the fast pathway regains conduction, the impulse after traveling down the slow pathway can return retrogradely back to the atrium via the fast pathway resulting in an atrial echo beat. A key component of the circuit is that the retrograde impulse finds the fast pathway no longer refractory. For this to occur, there must be a suitable delay in antegrade conduction over the slow pathway. The QRS complex is narrow because the ventricle is being activated via the normal HPS. Retrograde activation over the fast pathway happens quickly, and on the surface electrocardiogram, the retrograde P wave is usually "buried" or at the tail end of the QRS complex. This can give the appearance of a "pseudo" right bundle branch pattern in lead V_1. This is a short-RP tachycardia. α—slow pathway; β—fast pathway; NSR—normal sinus rhythm; SVT—supraventricular tachycardia. (*Courtesy of* Harlan R. Grogin.)

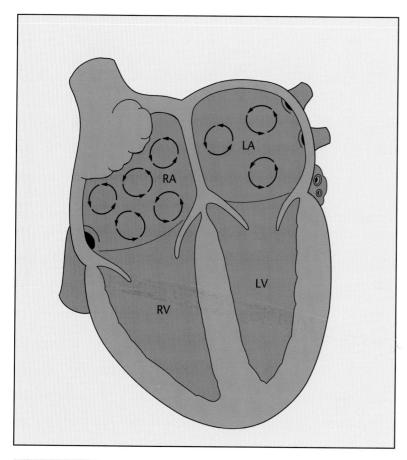

FIGURE 1-75.

Atrial fibrillation. Based on the work of Allessie *et al.* [69], atrial fibrillation (AF) is thought to be due to multiple wavelets of conduction produced by reentry. Perpetuation of AF depends on the relative dimensions of the atria and the size of the reentrant circuit. Compared with atrial flutter, in which there is one reentrant circuit and organized atrial activity, atrial fibrillation demonstrates no organized atrial contraction. This leads to blood stasis, the formation of clots, and the possibility of embolic events. Thus, most patients with chronic atrial fibrillation are given anticoagulants to reduce the risk of embolic events such as strokes. LA—left atrium; LV—left ventricle; RA—right atrium; RV—right ventricle. (*Courtesy of* Harlan R. Grogin.)

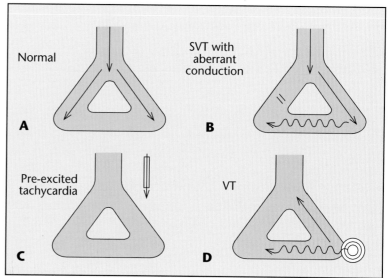

FIGURE 1-76.

Differential diagnosis of wide complex tachycardia (WCT). Normal QRS complexes are narrow because conduction proceeds over the His Purkinje system to rapidly activate the ventricles (**A**). A WCT can result from supraventricular tachycardia (SVT) with aberrant conduction (**B**), from an atrial or other supraventricular arrhythmia with rapid conduction over an accessory atrioventricular connection in a patient with Wolff-Parkinson-White syndrome (**C**), or from an origin in the ventricle itself (**D**). VT—ventricular tachycardia. (*Courtesy of* Michael D. Lesh.)

FIGURE 1-77.

Treatment options for patients with ventricular tachycardia (VT) or ventricular fibrillation (VF). The therapy recommended depends on presentation and substrate. ATP—antitachycardia pacing; RF—radiofrequency. (*Courtesy of* Michael D. Lesh.)

POLYMORPHIC VENTRICULAR TACHYCARDIA

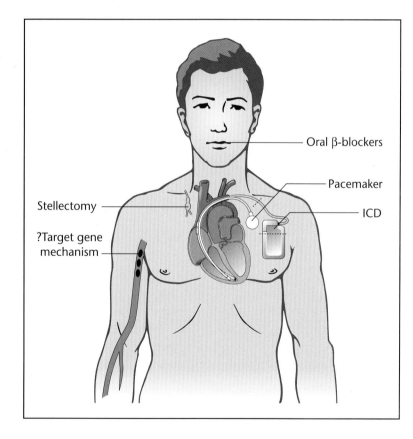

Stellectomy

?Target gene mechanism

Oral β-blockers

Pacemaker

ICD

FIGURE 1-78.

Treatment of congenital long QT syndrome (LQTS). Treatment for LQTS has evolved and changed as our understanding of the mechanism for the arrhythmia increases. Left cervicoganglion stellectomy was used early on, but this has been replaced by more effective methods of treatment, including implantable cardioverter defibrillators (ICDs) and the use of the combination of β blockade and permanent pacing [70,71]. The efficacy of β-blocker therapy has been demonstrated and remains the drug of first choice for patient management. Failing this therapy, other available options include a left cervicosympathectomy, cardiac pacing with full doses of β-blockers, or use of a defibrillator. The available data suggest that although symptoms are reduced, there is, nevertheless, a significant incidence of recurrent syncope (40%) or sudden cardiac death (8%) in patients undergoing cervicothoracic sympathectomy. The rationale for use of chronic cardiac pacing rests on the observations that in some patients with LQTS, polymorphic ventricular tachycardia may be triggered by pauses. The recurrence rate of syncope or torsade de pointes in patients treated with combined therapy is less than 10%. There is a growing experience in the use of defibrillator therapy for these patients, especially with the availability of smaller generators and transvenous insertions. Even in patients undergoing defibrillator treatment, adjunctive therapy with β-blockers and possibly cardiac pacing may be required to decrease the incidence of device discharges. As our understanding of genetic mechanisms for genes coding for abnormal proteins or receptors increases, it may be possible to prophylactically direct therapy at the underlying etiology rather than treating the resultant arrhythmia. (*Courtesy of* Harlan R. Grogin.)

THE CARDIAC PACING SYSTEM

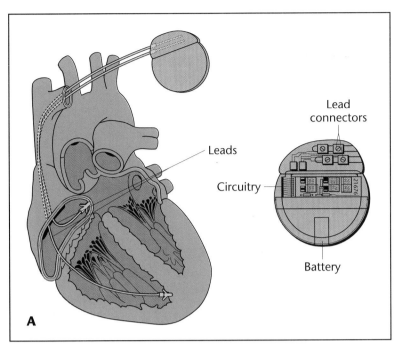

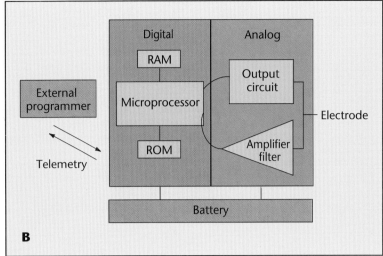

B

FIGURE 1-79.

The pulse generator design. Whereas early designs included a few hand-soldered transistors, resistors, and capacitors, the present devices include highly advanced, highly integrated microcircuits and microprocessors (**A**) resembling that found in personal computers. The microprocessor performs the logic chores of the pacemaker, including storage of programmable settings and interpretation and response to various sensed and paced cardiac electrical events, as well as the control of radiofrequency telemetry communications with external programmers. The microprocessor is dependent on a highly precise timer circuit based on a crystal oscillator.

Many devices (**B**) employ both "read only memory" (ROM), which contains the pacing algorithm, and "read and write memory" (RAM) for data, including programmed settings, device identification, and storage of a wide array of measured data values. Although the pacing algorithm and memory functions of the pacemaker represent the digital side of the device, certain analog elements, including filters and amplifiers for detecting intrinsic cardiac activity and controlling pacing output levels at appropriate intervals as instructed by the microprocessor, are necessary components as well.

All of these components are mounted on a circuit board and placed along with the battery within a hermetically sealed container, usually a titanium canister, for protection from the hostile environment of body fluids. (*Courtesy of* James L. Cockrell and Andreana Siu.)

SUDDEN CARDIAC DEATH AND THE USE OF INTERNAL DEFIBRILLATORS

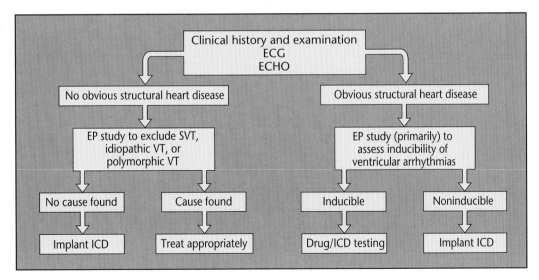

FIGURE 1-80.

Diagnostic work-up in patients with aborted sudden cardiac death. ECG—electrocardiogram; ECHO—echocardiogram; EP—electrophysiology; ICD—implantable cardioverter defibrillator; SVT—supraventricular tachycardia; VT—ventricular tachycardia. (*Courtesy of* Adam Fitzpatrick.)

■ HYPERTENSION

PATHOGENESIS OF HYPERTENSION

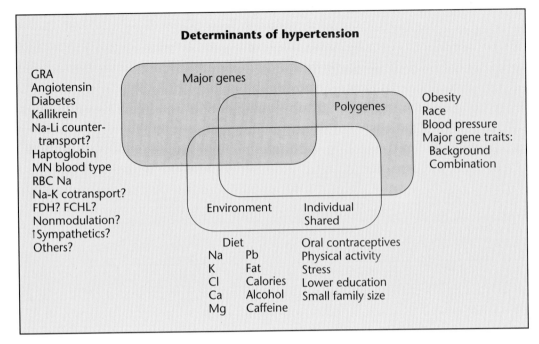

Determinants of hypertension

GRA
Angiotensin
Diabetes
Kallikrein
Na-Li counter-
   transport?
Haptoglobin
MN blood type
RBC Na
Na-K cotransport?
FDH? FCHL?
Nonmodulation?
↑Sympathetics?
Others?

Major genes

Polygenes

Obesity
Race
Blood pressure
Major gene traits:
   Background
   Combination

Environment   Individual
                Shared

Diet
Na   Pb
K   Fat
Cl   Calories
Ca   Alcohol
Mg   Caffeine

Oral contraceptives
Physical activity
Stress
Lower education
Small family size

FIGURE 1-81.

Genetic and environmental factors for hypertension. A model indicating the mechanisms by which essential hypertension could result from the combined effects of individual major genes that have a large impact on blood pressure, blended polygenes with small individual contributions, and environmental effects operating on individuals or within families. FCHL—familial combined hyperlipidemia; FDH—familial dyslipidemic hypertension; GRA—glucocorticoid-remediable aldosteronism. (*Courtesy of* Roger R. Williams.)

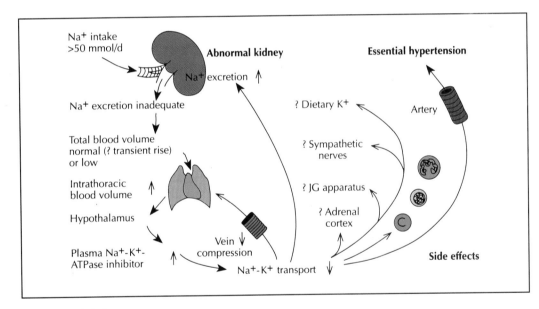

FIGURE 1-82.

Hypothetical sequence of events demonstrating the role of sodium retention in cases of hypertension. An underlying genetic lesion may be expressed as a deficiency of sodium excretion,

which becomes more apparent as sodium intake increases. The reduction in sodium excretion may initially cause a transient increase in total blood volume and a rise in intrathoracic blood volume. This change stimulates the hypothalamus to secrete a circulating sodium transport inhibitor, which adjusts renal sodium excretion, returning the sodium balance to normal. This balance is sustained only by a continuously high circulating sodium transport inhibitor, which raises the tone and reactivity of vascular smooth muscle. As a result, arterial pressure rises and venous compliance diminishes. Increased venous tone shifts blood from the periphery to the central vascular bed and thus raises intrathoracic pressure and perpetuates the stimulus for greater secretion of the sodium transport inhibitor. Total blood volume may be normal or low. (*Adapted from* de Wardener and MacGregor [72].)

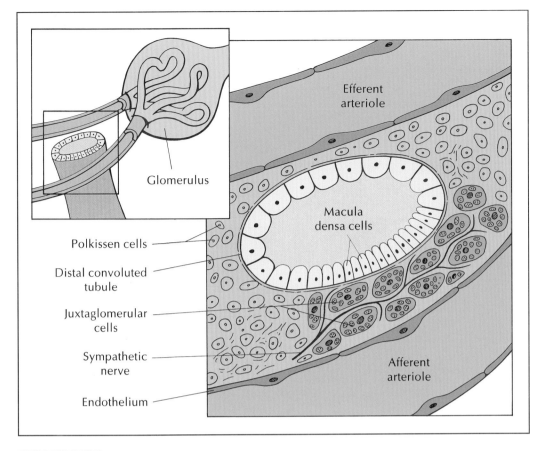

FIGURE 1-83.
The juxtaglomerular apparatus, illustrating tubular and vascular components. The tubular component consists of 1) a specialized region of the distal convoluted tubule, which bends between the afferent and efferent arterioles, and 2) the macula densa, which contains cells that are sensitive to sodium chloride flux and control renin secretion. The macula densa cells can be identified by the proximity of their nuclei to each other. The vascular component consists of the afferent and efferent arterioles as well as the extraglomerular mesangium. The extraglomerular mesangium is a collection of small cells with pale nuclei, called Polkissen cells, the function of which is unknown. The juxtaglomerular cells, in which renin is synthesized, stored, and secreted, are vascular smooth muscle cells modified by the presence of secretory and lysosomal granules; juxtaglomerular cells are absent from the efferent arteriole. The macula densa cells have no basement membrane, allowing intimate contact of the juxtaglomerular cells with tubular cells. Renin is stored in and secreted from the granules of the juxtaglomerular cells. The vascular and tubular components are innervated by sympathetic nerves. Renal nerve stimulation increases renin secretion by norepinephrine-induced stimulation of β-adrenergic receptors. Juxtaglomerular cells also have angiotensin II receptors, the stimulation of which leads to inhibition of renin secretion. (*Courtesy of* Helmy M. Siragy and Robert M. Carey.)

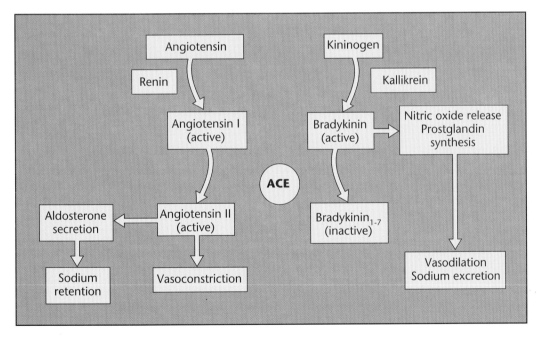

FIGURE 1-84.
The actions of angiotensin-converting enzyme (ACE). The left side of the figure demonstrates how the enzyme converts inactive angiotensin I to active angiotensin II. The right side depicts how ACE metabolizes bradykinin, an active vasodilator and natriuretic substance, to bradykinin$_{1-7}$, an inactive metabolite. ACE therefore increases production of a potent vasoconstrictor, angiotensin II, while promoting the degradation of a vasodilator, bradykinin. Both actions of ACE increase vasoconstriction, and inhibition of ACE leads to vasodilation and natriuresis. Bradykinin is formed by the action of the enzyme kallikrein on substrate kininogen. Bradykinin acts as a vasodilator and natriuretic substance by releasing nitric oxide (an endothelium-derived relaxing factor) and stimulating formation of prostaglandins E$_2$ and I$_2$. (*Courtesy of* Helmy M. Siragy and Robert M. Carey.)

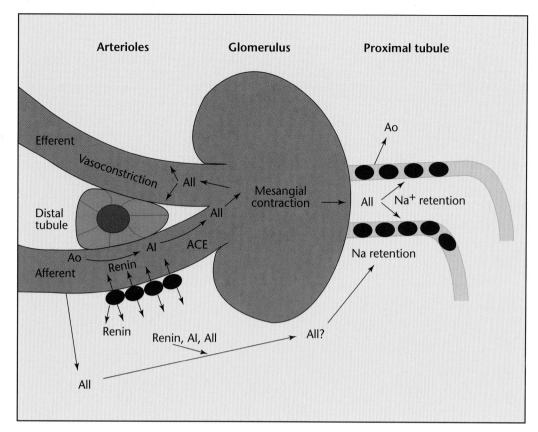

Arterioles　　　　**Glomerulus**　　　　**Proximal tubule**

Efferent

Vasoconstriction　　AII ←

Distal
tubule

Ao

Afferent　　AI　　ACE

Renin

Renin

Mesangial
contraction

AII

Ao

AII ⟨ Na⁺ retention

Na retention

Renin, AI, AII　　　　AII?

AII

FIGURE 1-85.

The cell-to-cell (*ie*, paracrine) effects of angiotensin II in the kidney. Angiotensinogen (Ao) either circulates to the kidney from the site of production in the liver or is synthesized in proximal tubular cells in the kidney. It is likely that renal interstitial angiotensinogen is derived predominantly from proximal tubular synthesis. Renin is synthesized and released from the juxtaglomerular cells into the afferent arteriolar lumen or into the renal interstitium. Angiotensin I (AI) is generated in the afferent arteriole and is converted to angiotensin II (AII) by angiotensin-converting enzyme (ACE). AII can cause mesangial cell contraction or efferent arteriolar constriction. AII can also be filtered at the glomerulus and may subsequently act at the proximal tubular cells to increase sodium reabsorption. In the renal interstitium, renin can cleave angiotensinogen to produce angiotensin peptides; these peptides may act at vascular and tubular structures. Angiotensin peptides may also be synthesized in and released from renal juxtaglomerular cells. Alternatively, the peptides may be taken up by renal cells from either interstitial fluid or the renal circulation. (*Courtesy of* Helmy M. Siragy and Robert M. Carey.)

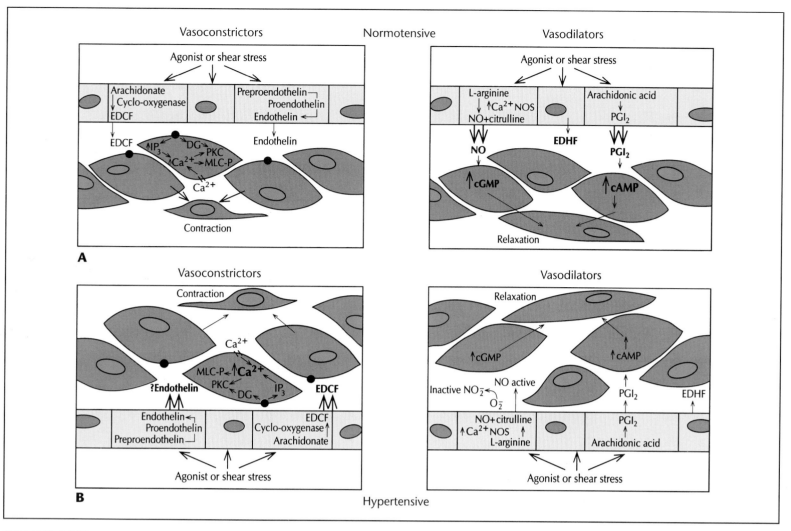

FIGURE 1-86.

Vascular mechanisms. Endothelium-dependent vasodilator and vasoconstrictor mechanisms: modification in hypertension. Normal endothelial cells secrete both vasodilators, the most prominent of which are nitric oxide (NO), prostacyclin (PGI_2), and endothelium-derived hyperpolarizing factor (EDHF), and vasoconstrictors, including endothelin and endothelium-derived contracting factor (EDCF) [73]. Vessel tone is dependent on the balance between these factors and on the ability of the smooth muscle cell to respond to them.

A, In normotensive vessels there is a predominance of vasodilator secretion. These substances may also contribute to the inhibition of smooth muscle cell growth or hypertrophy. The relative concentrations of the vasoconstricting/vasodilating agents are indicated by the relative sizes of the *arrows* and *bold type*.

B, In hypertension, release of vasoconstrictor substances may predominate [74]. In addition, vasodilator release may be decreased or, alternatively, the vasodilator itself may be inactivated by superoxide anion. Under certain circumstances, endothelin can also be growth-promoting, thereby contributing to smooth muscle

cell hypertrophy or hyperplasia and intimal thickening. The biochemical pathways activated by endothelial agonists and by contracting and relaxing factors acting on smooth muscle can also be affected in hypertension. NO, produced by the conversion of L-arginine to citrulline, traverses the endothelial cell membrane, and activates the smooth muscle cell guanylate cyclase to generate intracellular cGMP. PGI_2 and EDCF are produced via cyclo-oxygenase action on arachidonic acid. PGI_2 relaxes vessels by increasing smooth muscle cell cAMP; the mechanism of action of EDCF is unknown. Endothelin is made and modified by endothelium. It then stimulates the phospholipase C pathway in smooth muscle to produce the second messengers inositol triphosphate (IP_3) and diacylglycerol (DG), which in turn activate the Ca^{2+} and protein kinase C (PKC) signaling pathways. This leads to phosphorylation of the myosin light chain (MLC-P), causing contraction. Alterations of any of these signals could easily augment contraction or decrease the ability of the vessel to dilate. (*Courtesy of* R. Wayne Alexander, Randolph A. Hennigar, and Kathy K. Griendling.)

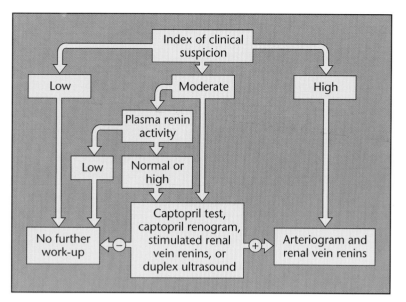

FIGURE 1-87.

Renovascular hypertension. The work-up for renovascular hypertension depends on the index of clinical suspicion. In the absence of suggestive signs it is likely that test results would be inconclusive; in such cases, no work-up is recommended. Patients with suggestive clinical clues have a 5% to 15% likelihood of having renovascular hypertension. Such patients can be screened with noninvasive studies and, if results are positive, confirmation of the diagnosis can be accomplished with renal arteriography and sampling of renin in the renal vein. If renovascular hypertension is strongly suggested, renal arteriography and sampling of renin in the renal vein are recommended, regardless of the results of noninvasive tests. (*Courtesy of* Helmy M. Siragy and Robert M. Carey.)

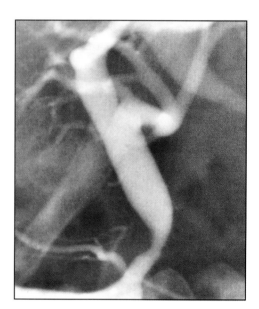

FIGURE 1-88.

Selective renal arteriogram of a 41-year-old nonsmoking white man with a 1-year history of hypertension. The arteriogram shows 80% stenosis of the left renal artery with poststenotic dilatation caused by atherosclerotic vascular disease. Transluminal angioplasty or surgery can be successful in opening the artery and abrogating or curing the hypertension. (*Courtesy of* Helmy M. Siragy and Robert M. Carey.)

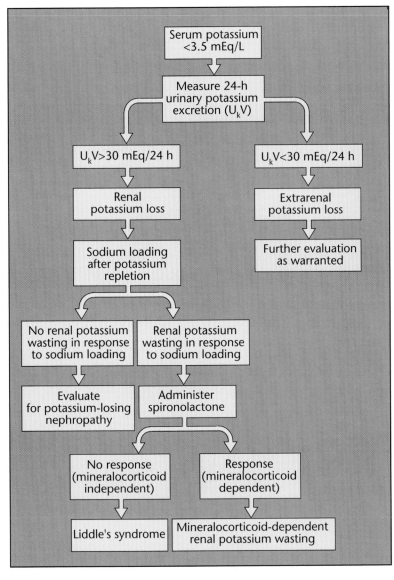

FIGURE 1-89.

Hypertensive syndromes secondary to the hypersecretion of aldosterone. Algorithmic approach to suspected mineralocorticoid-induced hypertension, which is usually associated with spontaneous hypokalemia. Although hypokalemia is often simply a side effect of diuretics, evaluation is recommended under the following circumstances: diuretic therapy results in serum potassium less than 3.0 mEq/L even if levels normalize when diuretics are withdrawn; oral potassium supplementation and potassium-sparing agents fail to maintain serum potassium values greater than 3.5 mEq/L in a patient on diuretics; or serum potassium levels fail to normalize after 4 weeks of diuretic abstinence.

The initial assessment and subsequent studies should be designed to answer three questions: Is potassium loss renal or extrarenal? If renal, is it steroid or nonsteroid-dependent? If steroid-dependent, what is its cause? A 24-hour urinary potassium excretion greater than 30 mEq/24 h when the serum potassium is equal to or less than 3.0 mEq/L usually reflects renal potassium wasting. Correction of hypokalemia, especially in the face of continued high dietary sodium, by short-term administration (3 to 5 days) of the specific aldosterone-receptor antagonist, spironolactone, indicates that the renal potassium wasting is steroid-dependent.

Specific diagnostic tests should then be performed to confirm the diagnosis. Serum potassium levels of 3.4 mEq/L or less associated with urinary potassium excretion greater than 30 mEq/24 h indicates renal wasting, and lower excretion rates suggest extrarenal loss caused by diarrhea, vomiting, or laxative abuse. Renal wasting should be investigated further after adequate repletion of total body potassium with oral chloride potassium supplementation. Salt-loading (oral sodium of 250 mEq/24 h for 5 to 7 days) that results in hypokalemia with renal potassium wasting suggests an exaggerated exchange mechanism of sodium for potassium at distal tubular sites mediated by inappropriate secretion of electrolyte-active steroids. An exception to this rule is Liddle's syndrome, a familial, nonsteroid-dependent renal potassium wasting disorder associated with hypokalemia and hypertension. Response to spironolactone (50 mg four times daily for 3 to 5 days) can demonstrate conclusively whether renal potassium wasting is truly mineralocorticoid-dependent. If spironolactone produces an elevation in the serum potassium level with concomitant reduction in urinary excretion, potassium wasting is probably mediated by electrolyte-active steroids.

The determination of dexamethasone responsiveness is the final step in the evaluation, to be undertaken if the physician suspects familial primary aldosteronism. This glucocorticoid-responsive aldosteronism should be suspected in patients with a family history of aldosteronism when imaging techniques fail to reveal anatomic abnormalities in the adrenal glands. Administration of dexamethasone, in doses of 0.5 mg four times daily, usually results in remission of hypertension and hypokalemia in 10 to 14 days. (*Adapted from* Bravo [75].)

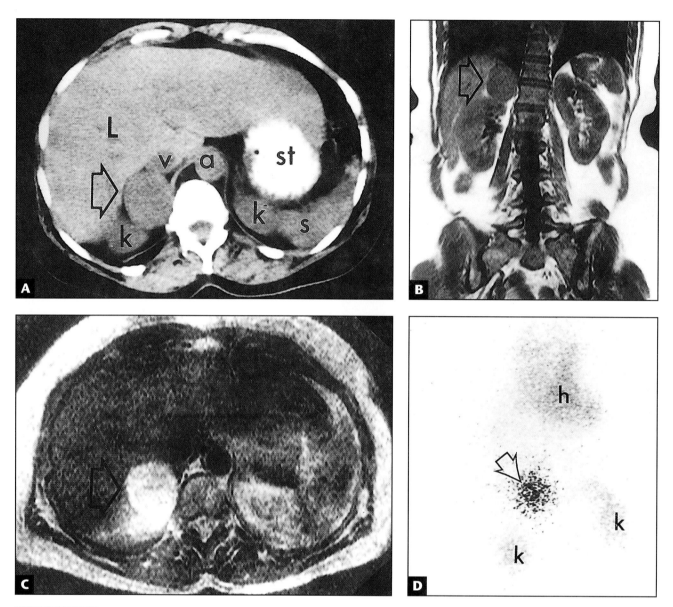

FIGURE 1-90.

Three modalities used to localize pheochromocytomas. Computed tomography (CT) can accurately detect tumors larger than 1.0 cm and has a localization precision of approximately 98%, although it is only 70% specific. CT is the most widely applied and accepted modality for the anatomic localization of pheochromocytomas. Magnetic resonance (MR) imaging is equally sensitive to CT and lends itself to *in vivo* tissue characterization, which is not possible with CT. MR imaging is nearly 100% sensitive but is only 67% specific. Scintigraphic localization with radioiodinated ^{131}I-meta-iodobenzylguanidine (MIBG) provides both anatomic and functional characterization. Although this modality is less sensitive than CT and MR imaging, it has a specificity of 100%. Ninety-seven percent of pheochromocytomas are found in the abdominal region, with most found in the adrenal glands. Less likely sites are the thorax (2% to 3%) and the neck (1%). Multiple tumors may arise in 10% of adults. Familial pheochromocytomas are frequently bilateral or arise from multiple sites. Pheochromocytomas occurring in children are more commonly bilateral and more frequently lie outside the adrenal glands than in adults. Tumor localization not only serves to confirm the diagnosis of pheochromocytoma but also assists the surgeon in planning the surgical strategy. Advances in noninvasive imaging techniques now provide safe and reliable means of localizing pheochromocytomas regardless of their location.

A, CT of the adrenal glands (*arrow*). **B** and **C**, Coronal and sagittal MR imaging sections of the abdomen, respectively. Pheochromocytomas demonstrate high signal intensity on a T_2-weighted image, unlike a benign tumor, which has a low signal intensity. **D**, Scintigraphic localization of a pheochromocytoma (*arrow*) with radioiodinated ^{131}I-MIBG. This modality provides both anatomic and functional characterization of a tumor. Because ^{131}I-MIBG is actively concentrated in sympathomedullary tissue through the catecholamine pump, the administration of drugs that block the reuptake mechanism (*eg*, tricyclic antidepressants, guanethidine, labetalol) may result in false-negative results. a—aorta; h—heart; k—kidney; L—liver; s—spleen; st—stomach; v—vena cava. (Panels A, C, and D *from* Bravo *et al.* [76]; with permission; panel B *from* Bravo [77]; with permission.)

NONPHARMACOLOGIC THERAPY FOR HYPERTENSION

Nonpharmacologic (Nutritional-Hygienic) Therapy

Advantages

May reduce blood pressure substantially without drugs

Enhances efficacy of drug therapy

May prevent or mitigate adverse drug effects (*eg*, hypokalemia, hyperlipidemia)

May regress left ventricular hypertrophy

Disadvantages

Labor-intensive, expensive

Requires high patient and provider motivation

Requires continuous monitoring and reinforcement

May not protect against coronary artery disease and cardiovascular disease, including stroke, as well as does the addition of drugs

FIGURE 1-91.

Nonpharmacologic (nutritional-hygienic) therapy is of great potential value. However, there are disadvantages to its use as well. (*Courtesy of* Barry J. Materson.)

PRINCIPLES OF PHARMACOLOGIC THERAPY FOR HYPERTENSION

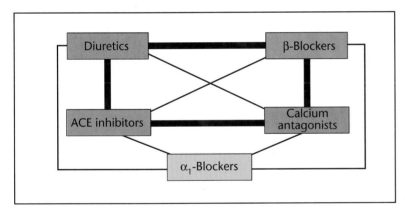

FIGURE 1-92.

First-line antihypertensive drugs. Different classes of antihypertensive agents are proposed as first-line treatment for hypertension, *ie*, diuretics, β- (and α-) adrenergic blockers, angiotensin-converting enzyme (ACE) inhibitors, and calcium antagonists [78,79]. These agents reduce blood pressure by various mechanisms. They are therefore more or less effective, depending on the prevailing pathogenic factors in a given hypertensive patient. There is no reliable way to predict a positive response (*ie*, normalized blood pressure) to a specific therapeutic approach. A patient may respond favorably to one class of drugs exclusively or to several types of antihypertensive agents. Some patients may remain hypertensive regardless of the drug used as monotherapy. When necessary, different types of antihypertensive agents can be combined. Some drug associations are particularly effective (*thick lines*) [80]. (*Courtesy of* Bernard Waeber and Hans R. Brunner.)

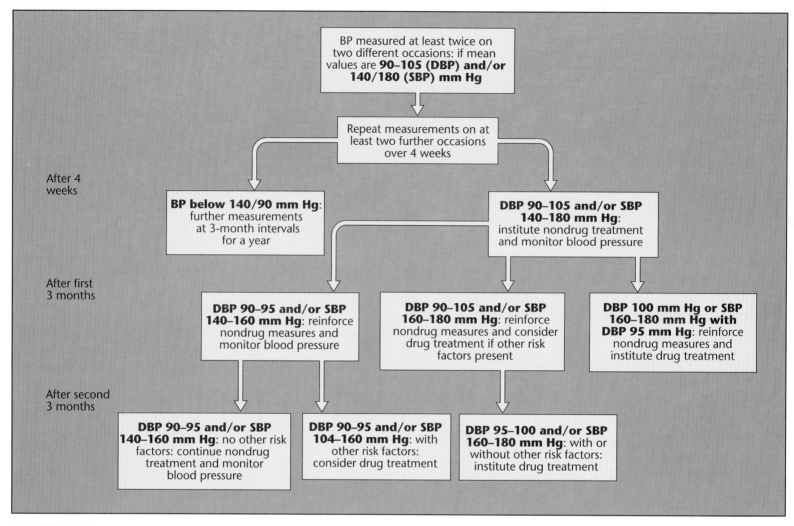

FIGURE 1-93.

Management of mild hypertension. *Mild hypertension* is defined as diastolic blood pressure (DBP) of 90 to 105 mm Hg or systolic blood pressure (SBP) of 140 to 180 mm Hg. Drug treatment should be instituted more promptly in patients with evidence of substantial risk of cardiovascular disease or in patients with blood pressure above the mild hypertension range. Although the World Health Organization and Joint National Committee disagree on the definition of "mild" hypertension, both groups recommend nondrug treatment for 3 months before initiating drug treatment in this group. Many experts are sanguine about patient compliance with nondrug treatment, however, and would disagree with this recommendation. Although weight loss will correct hypertension in many who are overweight, and reduction in salt or alcohol intake will help if these are employed to excess, the ability of physicians to persuade patients to change their behavior—unless they have a strong support group and show evidence of being prepared to change their behavior—remains ambiguous. (*Courtesy of* Norman K. Hollenberg.)

■ VALVULAR HEART DISEASE

MITRAL STENOSIS

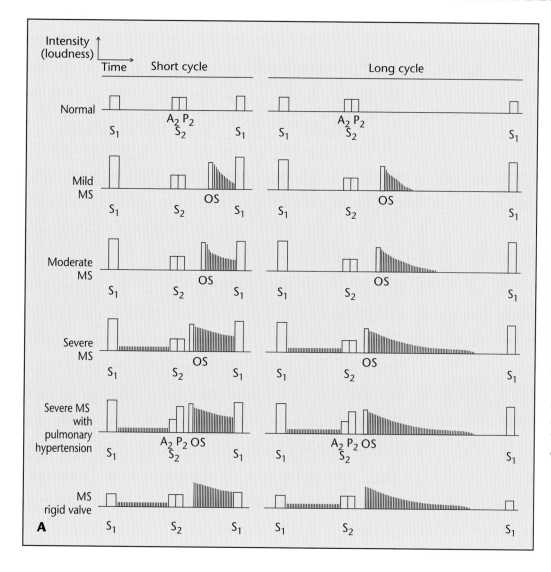

FIGURE 1-94.

Physical signs of mitral stenosis (MS). A, The classic auscultatory signs of MS in atrial fibrillation (AF). The auscultatory findings are much more variable on a beat-to-beat basis in AF. The presystolic murmur is usually absent. The loud S_1 and the opening snap (OS) are still heard. In the short cycles, the duration of diastole is short and the mid-diastolic rumble occupies the whole of diastole (*left*). In the long cycles (*right*) the duration of the mid-diastolic murmur is related to the severity of MS. As the MS becomes more severe, the length of this murmur is increased. In AF, with a slow ventricular response and very long R-R intervals, the diastolic rumble may not occupy the whole diastolic period and the presystolic murmur is absent. Thus, one may get the impression that the MS is moderate rather than severe. Increasing the heart rate, *eg*, with brief physical exertion, may produce more characteristic auscultatory findings. Alternatively, when the ventricular rate in AF is rapid or in short cycles, the auscultatory findings may suggest a more severe degree of MS than is really the case (*left*).

(*Continued*)

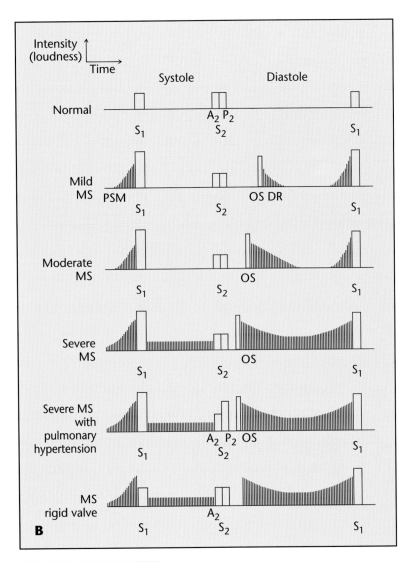

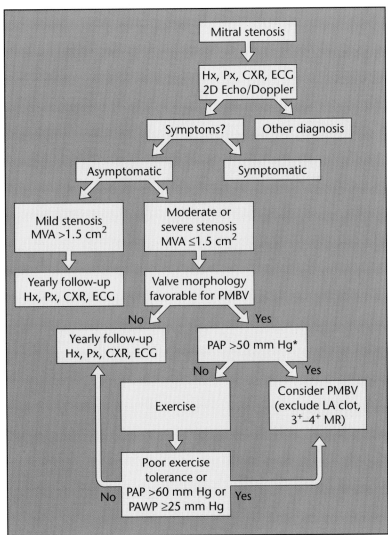

FIGURE 1-94. (CONTINUED)

B, The classic auscultatory signs of MS in patients in sinus rhythm. These include a presystolic murmur, a loud S_1, an opening snap (OS), and a mid-diastolic murmur (DR, low-pitched, decrescendo diastolic rumble). These signs may be accentuated or at times may only be heard by placing the patient in the left lateral decubitus position.

Importantly, these signs are helpful in assessing the severity of the MS; as the MS becomes more severe, the S_2–OS interval is shortened and the length of the mid-diastolic rumble is increased. In mild MS, the S_2–OS interval is long and the diastolic murmur is short. In moderate MS, the S_2–OS interval is shorter and although the diastolic murmur is longer at rest, there is usually a gap between the end of the murmur and the onset of the presystolic murmur. When the MS is severe, the S_2–OS interval is short (usually 0.04 second) and the diastolic murmur is a full-length murmur. With pulmonary arterial hypertension, P_2 is increased in intensity. In the presence of a rigid mitral valve (with or without calcification), S_1 is soft and the OS is usually not heard. With severe MS and also with a rigid valve, a holosystolic murmur of mitral regurgitation is often present. (*Courtesy of* David T. Kawanishi and Shahbudin H. Rahimtoola.)

FIGURE 1-95.

Management strategy for patients with mitral stenosis (MS). There is controversy as to whether patients with severe MS (mitral valve area [MVA] < 1.0 cm^2) and severe pulmonary hypertension (pulmonary artery pressure [PAP] > 60–80 mm Hg) should undergo mitral valve replacement (MVR) to prevent right ventricular failure [81,82]. CXR—chest x-ray; ECG—electrocardiogram; HX—history; LA—left atrial; PMBV—percutaneous mitral balloon valvotomy; PAWP—pulmonary artery wedge pressure; Px—physical examination. *Assuming no other cause for pulmonary hypertension is present. (*Adapted from* [82].)

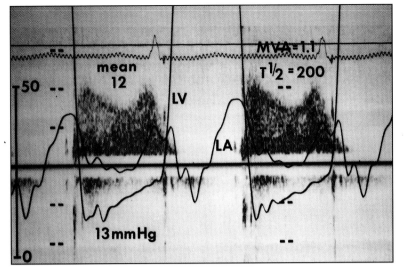

FIGURE 1-96.

Continuous-wave Doppler tracing in mitral stenosis (MS). The continuous-wave velocity curve across the mitral valve provides an accurate measurement of the mean mitral gradient in patients with MS [83]. As opposed to the measurement of a mean aortic valve gradient, the measurement of the mean mitral valve gradient by Doppler ultrasound is simple to obtain from a technical standpoint. Thus a Doppler-derived mitral gradient is reliable and actually provides a more accurate measurement than conventional cardiac catheterization using pulmonary capillary wedge pressure [84]. Shown are the simultaneous pressure curves from direct left atrial (LA) and left ventricular (LV) measurements and the simultaneous mitral flow velocity curve in a patient with MS. There is an excellent correlation between the catheter-derived mean gradient of 13 mm Hg and the Doppler-derived mean gradient of 12 mm Hg. The mitral valve area (MVA) of 1.1 cm^2 is calculated from the diastolic half time (t$_{1/2}$). Doppler ultrasound can also be used to assess pulmonary pressures and the presence of coexistent mitral regurgitation in the patient with MS. (*From* Nishimura and Tajik [84]; with permission.)

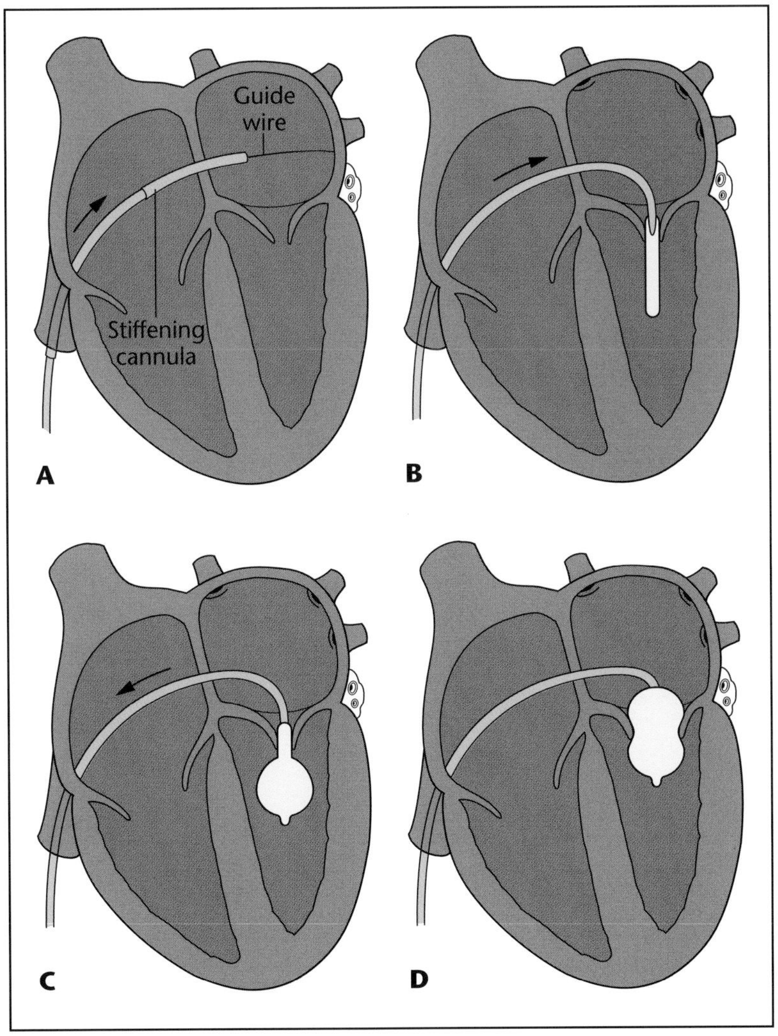

FIGURE 1-97.

Inoue balloon technique for catheter balloon commissurotomy [85]. A transseptal puncture is performed (**A**) and the deflated Inoue balloon catheter is placed across the mitral valve into the left ventricle (LV) (**B**). Stepwise inflation of first the front then the rear of the Inoue balloon is performed (**C**). Inflation of the middle of the Inoue balloon and final expansion at the "waist" (**D**) suggests that enlargement of the valve orifice has occurred. The staged inflation of the various parts of this balloon are depicted. (*Adapted from* Inoue *et al.* [85].)

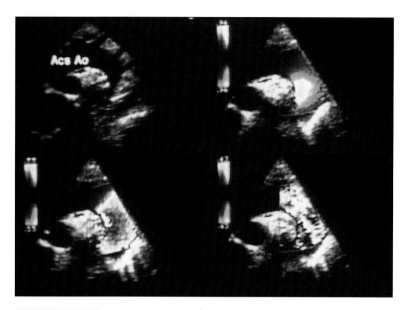

FIGURE 1-98.

Echocardiography for determination of severity of mitral regurgitation (MR). It is difficult to determine the exact severity of MR on echocardiography. Two-dimensional echocardiographic findings that suggest severe MR include a dilated hyperdynamic left ventricle or a flail mitral valve leaflet. Indirect clues to the severity of MR include the continuous-wave Doppler mitral regurgitation jet intensity, the initial mitral inflow velocity, the contour of the continuous-wave Doppler MR velocity curve, and interruption of pulmonary venous flow (vide infra). The area or extent of the jet into the left atrium on color-flow imaging was initially proposed as a method for determining the severity of MR [86]. However, subsequent reports showed that the color-flow jet area cannot be equated directly with the volume of regurgitation [87], because the jet area is also dependent on other physical factors such as the velocity of the jet. In addition, frequently eccentric jets impinge on adjacent structures, which will decrease the appearance of the jet on color-flow imaging [88]. Finally, the jet area appearance may change with instrument adjustments in pulse repetition frequency, transducer frequency, filter setting (shown here), color maps, and gain level. Thus, the severity of MR cannot be based on the color-flow area alone but must be a culmination of all information provided by the clinical setting, two-dimensional echocardiographic findings, the color-flow jet, and the indirect Doppler findings. In experienced laboratories, a regurgitant fraction or volume can be calculated from volumetric flow rates [89]. Newer techniques such as amplitude-weighted continuous-wave signal intensity [90] and proximal isovelocity surface areas [91] show promise as future methods of further quantitating the severity of MR. Asc Ao—ascending aorta. (*Courtesy of* Peter C. Nishan and Rick A. Nishimura.)

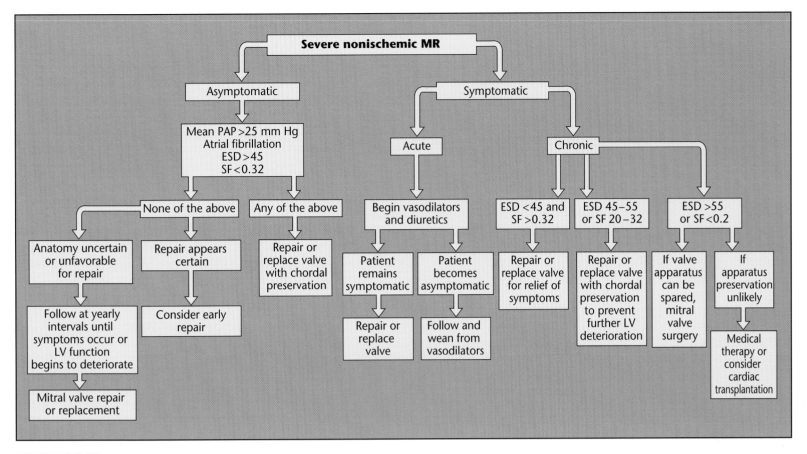

FIGURE 1-99.

Management of patients with severe, nonischemic mitral regurgitation (MR). It is likely that preservation of the chordae tendineae and their effects on contractile function [92] allowed the entire ventricle to decrease in size postoperatively, reducing the radius (r) term in the stress equation (stress = P x r/2h, where *P* = pressure and *h* = wall thickness). Thus, wall stress actually fell when the chordae were preserved. Chordae tendineae are an integral part of the left ventricle (LV) and its systolic function. When the chordae tendineae are severed, LV function worsens; this tendency is exaggerated if preoperative muscle dysfunction is already present. When the chordae tendineae are preserved, LV ejection fraction is maintained both because afterload is reduced and because ventricular

contractile performance is maintained at its preoperative level. These factors combined with a lower incidence of thromboembolism, the avoidance of anticoagulation, and a lower risk of late postoperative valve failure all lead to a reduced operative mortality rate and better long-term outcome for repair than for replacement with valve ablation.

It is important to note that not all valves can be repaired. Abnormalities involving the anterior leaflet of the mitral valve are more difficult to repair than those involving the posterior leaflet and severe rheumatic deformity may prevent an adequate repair. ESD—end-systolic dimension; PAP—pulmonary artery pressure; SF—shortening fraction. (*Courtesy of* Blase A. Carabello.)

MITRAL VALVE PROLAPSE

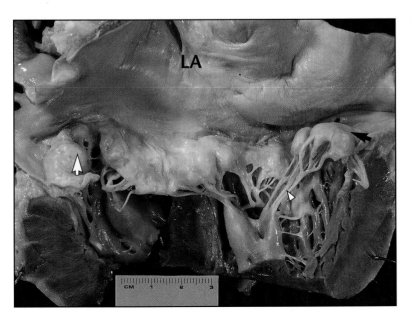

FIGURE 1-100.

Mitral valve prolapse (MVP). The incidence of MVP in the general population is 3% to 5% and is higher in women. The majority of patients are asymptomatic. Symptomatic mitral regurgitation (MR) occurs in 10% to 15% of patients and is more common in men older than 50 years [93]. A 54-year old white man died suddenly without previous cardiac history. Note the enlarged and billowing intermediate (*black arrow*) and medial (*white arrow*) scallop of the posterior mitral valve leaflet. *White arrowhead* denotes elongated chordal tendineae and *black arrowhead* denotes endocardial plaque. (*From* Farb *et al.* [93]; with permission.)

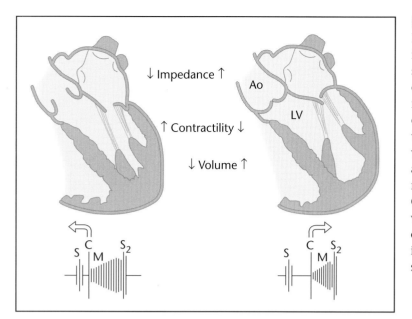

FIGURE 1-101.

Dynamic auscultation. Mid-systolic clicks (C) may be secondary to factors aside from MVP. These include extracardiac causes, atrial septal aneurysms, and pericarditis. The mid-systolic click of MVP can be reliably distinguished from these by its temporal response to maneuvers that alter hemodynamic conditions. Any maneuver that decreases left ventricular (LV) volume (*eg*, decreased venous return, tachycardia, decreased outflow impedance, increased contractility) will worsen the mismatch in size between the enlarged mitral valve and LV chamber, resulting in prolapse earlier in systole and movement of the click and murmur (M) toward the first heart sound (S_1). Conversely, maneuvers that increase LV volume (*eg*, increased venous return, bradycardia, increased outflow impedance, decreased contractility) will delay the occurrence of prolapse, resulting in movement of the click and murmur toward the second heart sound (S_2). Ao—aorta. (*Adapted from* O'Rourke and Crawford [94].)

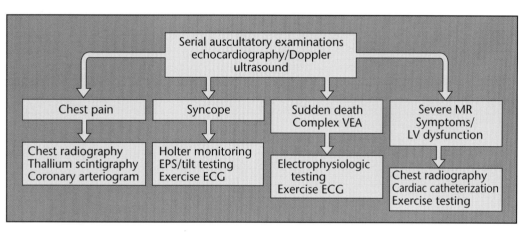

FIGURE 1-102.

Diagnostic testing in mitral valve prolapse (MVP). The diagnosis of MVP is based on the presence of typical auscultatory findings detected during carefully performed serial examinations. Echocardiography (M-mode, two-dimensional, and Doppler) is the single most useful test in the definition of MVP. It is used to assess natural history and prognosis, the presence of associated conditions (*eg*, atrial septal defect, hypertrophic cardiomyopathy), the need for antibiotic prophylaxis, and the degree of mitral regurgitation (MR). Echocardiography should *not* supplant the physical examination in the diagnosis of MVP; up to 10% of patients diagnosed with MVP by typical auscultatory findings will have a non-diagnostic two-dimensional echocardiogram [95]. Electrocardiography (ECG) is routinely performed to assess for ventricular preexcitation and resting ST- and T-wave abnormalities. The tests listed in the lowest level of the flow diagram are not required for the diagnosis of MVP, but they are useful in assessing certain symptoms and complications that can occur in this disorder. EPS—electrophysiology; LV—left ventricular; MR—mitral regurgitation; VEA—ventricular ectopic arrhythmia. (*Courtesy of* Sumanth D. Prabhu and Robert A. O'Rourke.)

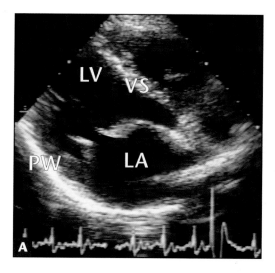

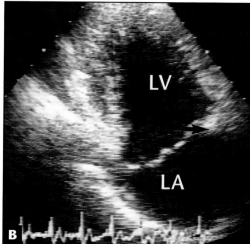

FIGURE 1-103.
Two-dimensional echocardiographic and Doppler ultrasound images from a 55-year-old man with classic mitral valve prolapse and associated tricuspid valve prolapse. **A,** The parasternal long axis view shows significant leaflet thickening of both mitral leaflets (*arrows*). **B,** The apical long axis view shows prolapse of both leaflets and the coaptation point beyond the annular plane (*arrow*). LA—left atrium; LV—left ventricle; PW—posterior wall; VS—ventricular septum. (*Courtesy of* Sumanth D. Prabhu and Robert A. O'Rourke.)

AORTIC STENOSIS

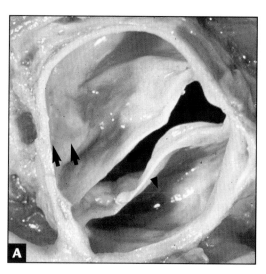

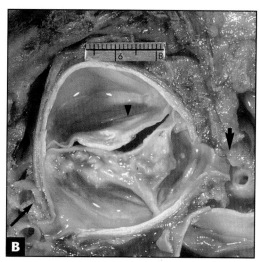

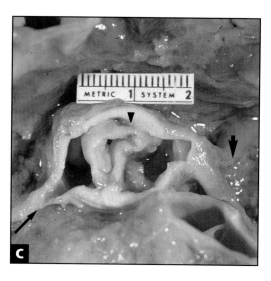

FIGURE 1-104.
Congenital aortic valve (AV) disease. **A,** A normally functioning bicuspid AV with two commissures and the two leaflets, which are almost equal in size in a 58-year-old man who died of metastatic lung carcinoma. The commissures are located right and left and both coronary ostia arise from the anterior aortic sinus. Note the absence of raphe in either leaflet. The right coronary artery is denoted by an *arrow*; the left coronary artery is denoted by an *arrowhead*.

B, A mildly calcified congenitally bicuspid AV in a 69-year-old man. Note a nonstenotic functionally normal bicuspid valve with mild calcification (*arrows*) and a raphe (*arrowhead*) in the anterior leaflet.

C, A bicuspid dysplastic and fibrotic AV (*arrowhead*) from a 24-year-old woman who had a commissurotomy 5 years before death. She was found dead in the hospital while awaiting repeat surgery. The commissures are located anterior and posterior and the leaflets are right and left with the right coronary artery (*long arrow*) and the left coronary artery (*short arrow*) arising from the right and left coronary sinuses. Whereas patients with dysplastic bicuspid valves usually become symptomatic early in life, those with calcified and fibrotic bicuspid valves usually present in the fifth to seventh decade. (*Courtesy of* Renu Virmani, Allen P. Burke, and Andrew Farb.)

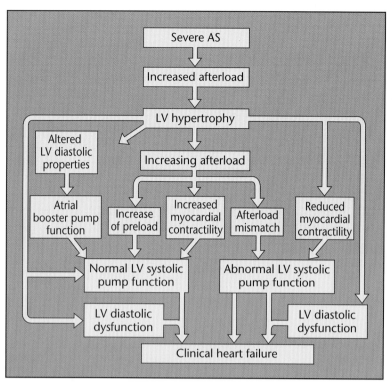

FIGURE 1-105.

Pathophysiology of aortic stenosis (AS). With reduction in the aortic valve area (AVA), energy is dissipated during the transport of blood from the left ventricle (LV) to the aorta. The AVA has to be reduced by 50% of normal before a measurable gradient can be demonstrated. When a pressure gradient develops between the LV and the ascending aorta, LV pressure rises and LV wall stress (afterload) increases. This could result in an impairment of LV function. The heart responds by becoming hypertrophied and myocardial stress remains normal. LV mass in patients with severe AS undergoing valve replacement averages 229 g/m^2 (normal mass, 105 g/m^2) [96]; at autopsy, LVs weighing as much as 1000 g have been reported. LV volume remains within the normal range; therefore, there is considerable thickening of the LV wall. As a result of the LV hypertrophy, LV systolic pump function remains normal. LV hypertrophy may alter the LV diastolic properties and there is increased resistance to LV filling. As a result, LV end-diastolic pressure is elevated; but this cannot be used as a measure of LV failure. Powerful atrial contraction produces the required LV filling [97,98] and fiber length (atrial booster pump function). Because atrial systole occupies only a small part of the cardiac cycle, there is only a transient increase in left atrial pressure; therefore, mean left atrial pressure remains in the normal range [97] or is only minimally increased.

As LV afterload continues to increase, the LV uses two additional compensatory mechanisms, namely, increase of preload and increase of myocardial contractility. Both of these help maintain normal LV systolic pump function. When the limit of the preload reserve has been reached (afterload mismatch) [99] or myocardial contractility is reduced, LV systolic pump function becomes abnormal. Clinical heart failure is usually a result of abnormal LV systolic pump function; diastolic dysfunction may also be present in some patients. Clinical heart failure in those with normal systolic pump function is a result of LV diastolic dysfunction. (© Copyright SH Rahimtoola, MB, FRCP, MACP.)

Indications for Surgery for Severe Aortic Stenosis

All Symptomatic Patients
LV function normal: as soon as possible
LV dysfunction: urgent
Heart failure: emergent

Asymptomatic Patients
All patients
Alternative strategy
  All patients with AVA ≤ 0.75 cm^2
  Patients with AVA 0.76–1.0 cm^2
    LV dysfunction
    Associated significantly obstructive CAD
    Patients ≥ 60–65 y
    Severe LV hypertrophy
    Painless ischemia
    Significant arrhythmias
    LV dysfunction on exercise

FIGURE 1-106.

Indications for surgery for severe aortic stenosis (AS). Symptomatic patients with severe AS should have aortic valve surgery (usually valve replacement) unless there is a specific contraindication to its performance. The urgency of surgery depends on the state of left ventricular (LV) function and the severity of the symptoms. For example, if there is LV dysfunction, the procedure is urgent; in the presence of heart failure or cardiogenic shock, it is usually an emergency.

Probably all asymptomatic patients with severe AS should have valve surgery. An alternative strategy is to perform surgery on all patients with aortic valve areas (AVAs) of 0.75 cm^2 or less. In patients with small or large body size an equivalent value after correcting for body size may need to be determined. For patients with valve areas of 0.76 to 1.0 cm^2 surgery is performed in those at "higher risk." These include patients with LV dysfunction, associated significantly obstructive coronary artery disease (CAD), age 60 to 65 years or older, severe LV hypertrophy, painless ischemia, significant arrhythmias, and significant LV dysfunction on exercise. (© Copyright SH Rahimtoola, MB, FRCP, MACP.)

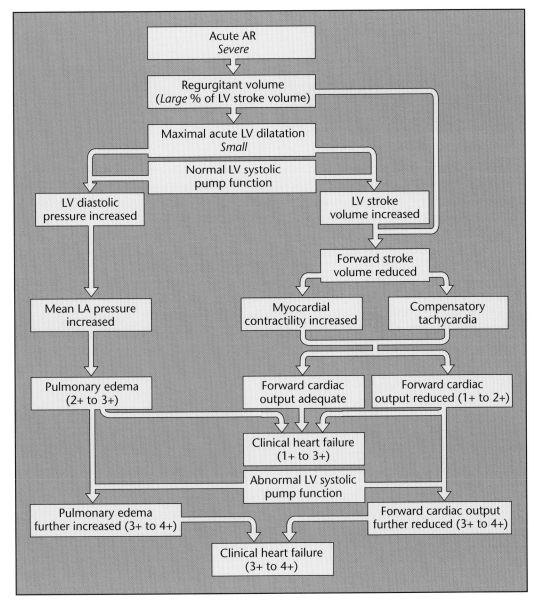

FIGURE 1-107.

Hemodynamic abnormalities in acute aortic regurgitation (AR). Mild acute AR (*eg*, when associated with systemic hypertension) produces little or no hemodynamic abnormality. Increasing severity of regurgitation produces greater degrees of hemodynamic abnormalities, and severe AR often produces the clinical picture of heart failure.

Severe acute AR results in a large volume of regurgitant blood in the left ventricle (LV) in diastole. In an acute situation, the LV end-diastolic volume can only increase mildly (no more than 20% to 30%) and the LV diastolic pressure-volume relationships are particularly important. The LV systolic pump function is initially normal. The increased LV diastolic pressure results in increases in mean left atrial (LA) and pulmonary venous pressures and produces varying degrees of pulmonary edema [100]. The normal LV systolic pump function in the presence of LV dilatation results in an increase in LV stroke volume. However, a large percentage of the LV stroke volume is returned to the LV in diastole; as a result, the forward stroke volume is reduced. The LV uses two mechanisms, an increase of myocardial contractility and, importantly, a compensatory tachycardia to maintain an adequate forward cardiac output. As a result, initially the forward cardiac output may be appropriate. However, if the compensatory mechanisms are inadequate, forward cardiac output is reduced. The pulmonary edema with or without an adequate cardiac output produces the picture of clinical heart failure. Subsequently, LV systolic pump function may become abnormal; when that occurs, the pulmonary edema is further increased and the forward cardiac output is further reduced, leading to more severe manifestations of clinical heart failure. (© Copyright SH Rahimtoola, MB, FRCP, MACP.)

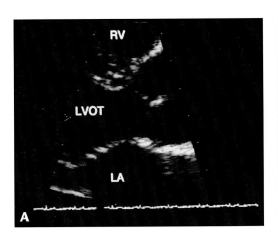

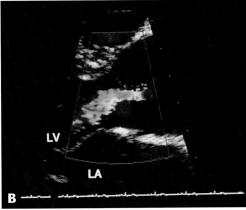

FIGURE 1-108.

Echocardiography for chronic aortic regurgitation. Doppler ultrasound imaging in the determination of the severity of aortic regurgitation (AR). The severity of AR can be assessed by several echocardiographic methods. The left ventricular (LV) size and function reflect the ventricular response to volume overload and should be considered when assessing the severity of the regurgitation. There are indirect Doppler findings, such as the diastolic half time, pulsed-wave Doppler interrogation of the descending aorta, LV outflow velocity, and mitral inflow velocity curve, which are useful in assessing the severity of regurgitation [101].

(Continued)

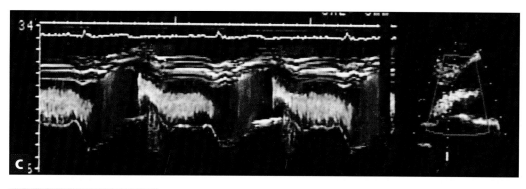

FIGURE 1-108. (*CONTINUED*)

In the absence of mitral regurgitation, quantitative Doppler ultrasound measurements of regurgitant volume and regurgitant fraction can be obtained by experienced laboratories [89]. Color-flow imaging, which superimposes a color-coded display of the intracardiac velocities directly on the real-time two-dimensional image, has been used as a semiquantitative approach for

determination of the severity of regurgitation in patients with central jets [102]. For AR, it is not the extent of the jet into the LV cavity but rather the width (or area) of the jet in the LV outflow tract (LVOT) that correlates with the severity of regurgitation.

A and **B**, mild-to-moderate AR with the regurgitant jet width occupying 30% of the LVOT on the parasternal long-axis view. A color M-mode can be placed through the jet to further define the width of the jet in relation to the width of the LVOT (**C**). This method cannot be used when there is an eccentric jet of AR. LA—left atrium; RV—right ventricle. (*Courtesy of* Peter C. Nishan and Rick A. Nishimura.)

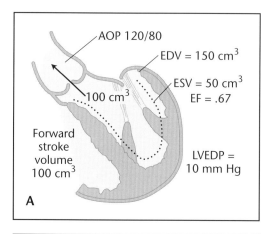

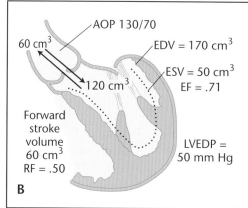

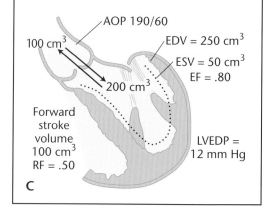

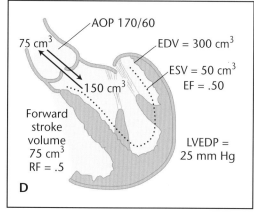

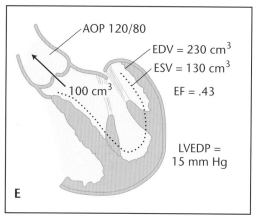

FIGURE 1-109.

Hemodynamics of aortic regurgitation. **A**, Normal conditions. **B**, Hemodynamic changes that occur in severe aortic regurgitation. Although total stroke volume is increased, forward stroke volume is reduced, and left ventricular end-diastolic pressure rises dramatically. **C**, Hemodynamic changes occurring in chronic compensated aortic regurgitation. Eccentric hypertrophy produces increased end-diastolic volume, which permits an increase in total as well as forward stroke volume. The volume overload is accommodated and left ventricular filling pressure is normalized. Ventricular emptying and

end-systolic volume remain normal. **D**, In chronic decompensated aortic regurgitation, impaired left ventricular emptying produces an increase in end-systolic volume and a fall in ejection fraction, total stroke volume, and forward stroke volume. There is further cardiac dilatation and re-elevation of left ventricular filling pressure. **E**, Immediately following valve replacement, preload estimated by end-diastolic volume decreases, as does filling pressure. End-systolic volume also is decreased, but to a lesser extent. The result is an initial fall in ejection fraction. Despite these changes, elimination of regurgitation leads to an increase in forward stroke volume [103]. AOP—aortic pressure; EDV—end-diastolic volume; ESV—end-systolic volume; EF—ejection fraction; LVEDP—left ventricular end-diastolic pressure; RF—regurgitant fraction. (*Adapted from* Carabello [103].)

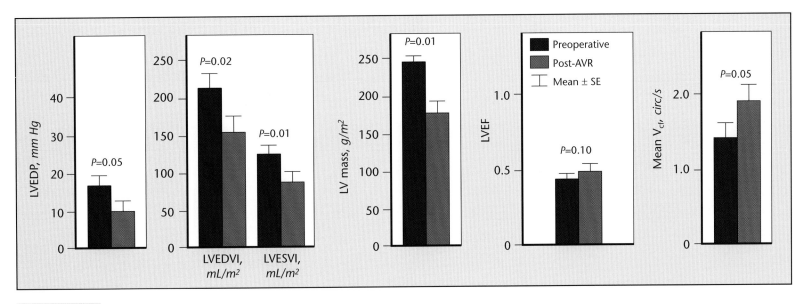

FIGURE 1-110.

Effects of aortic valve replacement (AVR) on severe aortic regurgitation (AR) and left ventricular (LV) dysfunction. Patients who have abnormal LV systolic pump function undergo important changes in LV size and function over a 1-year period [104]. These patients had significant reductions in LV end-diastolic pressure (LVEDP), LV end-diastolic and end-systolic volume indices (LVEDVI and LVESVI) and LV hypertrophy (mass). LV systolic pump function was improved as demonstrated by increases in mean velocity of circumferential fiber (V_{cf}) shortening; however, LV ejection fraction (LVEF) in this study increased mildly and this change was not statistically significant.

However, it appears that these patients have no further changes in LV size, hypertrophy [105], or LVEF, which is different from those who have normal LV systolic function preoperatively. circ—circumferences. (*Adapted from* Clark *et al.* [104].)

COR PULMONALE, PRIMARY PULMONARY HYPERTENSION, AND CARDIAC TUMORS

COR PULMONALE

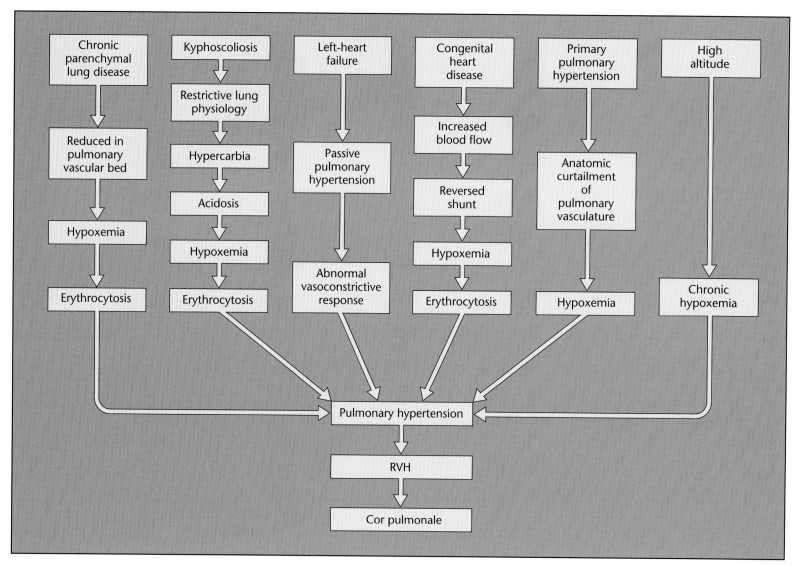

FIGURE 1-111.

Etiology and pathophysiology of cor pulmonale. General categories of disease states and the various pathophysiologic mechanisms that lead to development of the disorder are shown. Note that the final common pathway for the group of diseases that comprise cor pulmonale is advanced, long-standing pulmonary hypertension. RVH—right ventricular hypertrophy. (*Courtesy of* Evan Loh.)

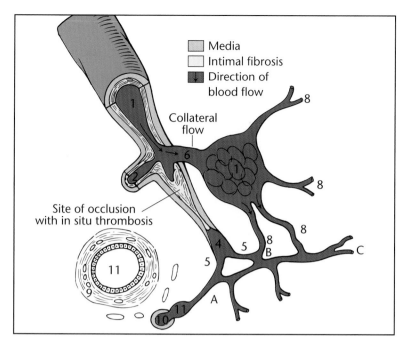

FIGURE 1-112.

The origin and probable connections of small, thin-walled collateral blood vessels in the lung in advanced cases of pulmonary hyperten-sion. Such connections create functional arteriovenous fistulae and right-to-left shunting that contribute to the hypoxemia observed in patients with advanced cor pulmonale. 1—Dilated muscular pul-monary artery with thin wall media and intimal fibrosis considered part of the generalized dilatation proximal to the site of vascular occlusion; 2—hypertrophied muscular pulmonary artery arising as a side branch of the muscular pulmonary artery with an accumula-tion of intimal fibrous tissue at the site of origin; 3—terminal mus-cular pulmonary artery occluded by fibrous tissue and/or thrombo-sis *in situ*; 4—terminal dilated pulmonary arteriole; 5—capillaries in alveolar walls arising from the pulmonary arteriole; 6—dilated, thin-walled, veinlike branch of hypertrophied parent muscular pul-monary artery; 7—localized angiomatoid lesion; 8—capillaries in alveolar walls arising from dilatation lesions; 9—dilated thin-walled vessels in submucosa of small bronchus with vascular smooth muscle proliferation; 10—small bronchial artery in fibrotic coat of a small bronchus giving rise to thin-walled branches; 11—cross-sec-tional view of the small bronchial artery with medial hyperplasia; A—bronchopulmonary anastomosis at capillary level; B—anasto-mosis between capillaries arising from parent muscular pulmonary artery and dilatation lesions; C—possible anastomosis between thin-walled vessels of the pulmonary artery and those of the pul-monary vein. (*Adapted from* Harris and Heath [106].)

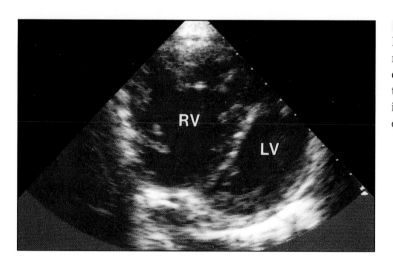

FIGURE 1-113.

Echocardiographic features of the heart in a patient with cor pul-monale. Shown here is a short-axis view demonstrating a markedly enlarged right ventricle (RV) with RV hypertrophy. Abnormal bowing of the interventricular septum into the left ventricle (LV) gives a character-istic *D* configuration of the LV, consistent with volume and pressure overload of the RV. (*Courtesy of* Evan Loh.)

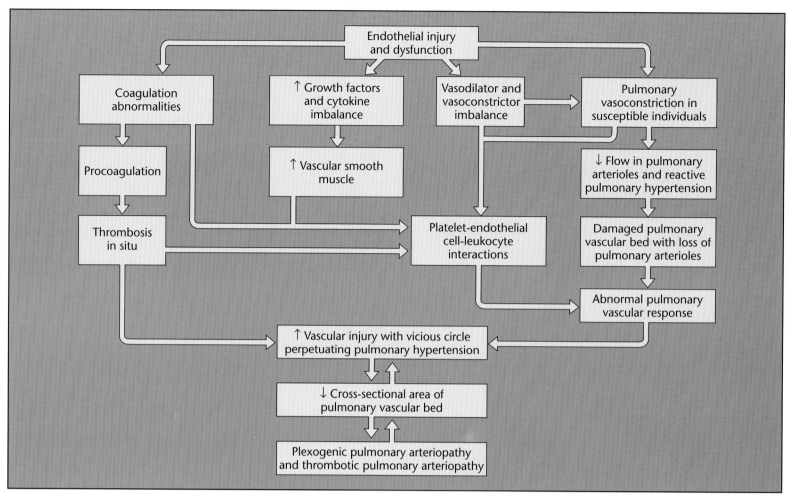

FIGURE 1-114.

Possible pathogenesis of primary pulmonary hypertension (PPH). Endothelial injury or dysfunction sets off a cascade of cellular events that lead to the abnormal pulmonary vascular response seen in PPH, and subsequently to a perpetuating circle promoting plexogenic and thrombotic pulmonary arteriopathy [107,108]. (*Adapted from* Rubin [108].)

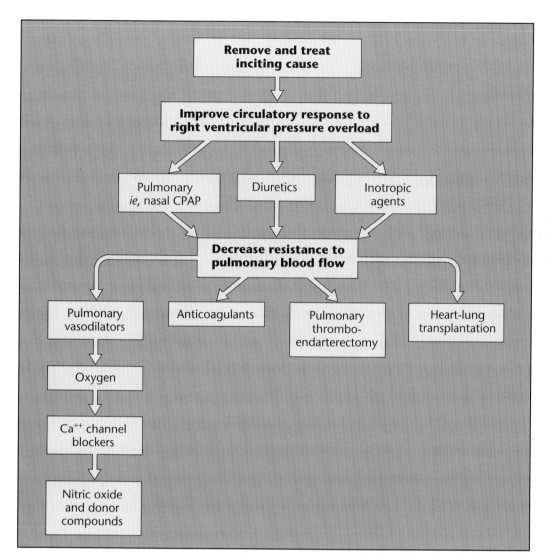

FIGURE 1-115.
Therapy for patients with advanced cor pulmonale. It is important to establish the underlying cause of the disease in order to direct therapy appropriately. General goals of therapy include improving the circulatory response to right ventricular overload and/or decreasing resistance to pulmonary blood flow by various means, such as the administration of pulmonary vasodilators, anticoagulation therapy, pulmonary thromboendarterectomy, and also heart-lung transplantation as indicated. CPAP—continuous positive airway pressure. (*Courtesy of Evan Loh.*)

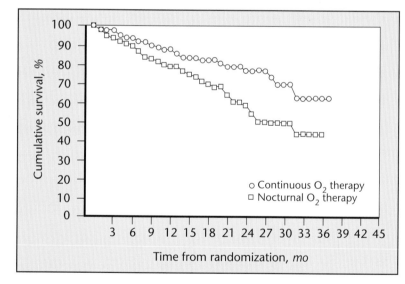

FIGURE 1-116.
Oxygen therapy for hypoxemic chronic obstructive lung disease. When chronic bronchitis or emphysema is complicated by hypoxic cor pulmonale, the prognosis for surviving several years is poor. Therefore, the Medical Research Council sponsored a controlled clinical trial of administering nocturnal oxygen at home (15 hours per night of nasal prong oxygen; usually 2 L/min) versus no oxygen to determine whether oxygen therapy reduced the 1-year mortality rate [109]. The annual mortality rate was 29% among controls compared with 12% among those who received oxygen ($P = 0.04$). Interestingly, no difference in the survival curves appeared until after approximately 500 days of oxygen therapy. It was not apparent whether continuous oxygen therapy would be superior to nocturnal oxygen. Therefore, the National Heart, Lung and Blood Institute initiated a trial at six centers in which 203 patients with hypoxemic chronic obstructive lung disease were allocated randomly either to continuous oxygen therapy or 11-hour nocturnal oxygen therapy and followed up for an average of 19 months [110]. The mortality rate was almost halved among patients who received continuous oxygen. The mechanism for this beneficial effect is not clear. Continuous oxygen reduced pulmonary vascular resistance more than nocturnal oxygen at 6 months after entry into the study; however, patients with larger decreases in pulmonary vascular resistance ($<$ dynes/s X cm^5) paradoxically tended to have a greater mortality rate than patients with smaller decreases. Whereas patients receiving continuous oxygen therapy had an average decrement of 11% in pulmonary vascular resistance, patients receiving nocturnal oxygen therapy had an average increase of 6% in pulmonary vascular resistance ($P = 0.04$). Thus, these data suggest that although continuous O_2 therapy reduced both mortality and pulmonary vascular resistance, the two phenomena appeared unrelated. (*Adapted from* Nocturnal Oxygen Therapy Trial Group [110].)

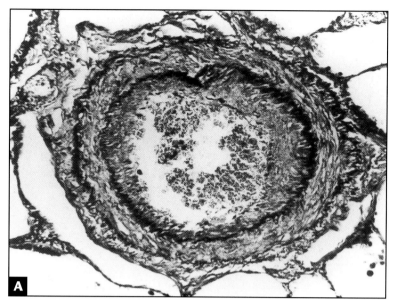

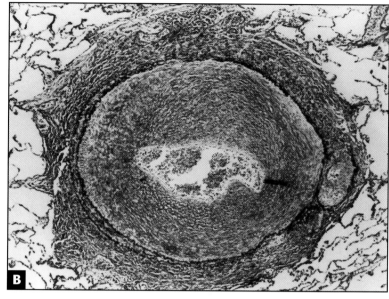

FIGURE 1-117.

Histopathologic features of primary pulmonary hypertension (PPH). Several lesions have been identified in patients with PPH. **A**, Hypertrophy of the medial layer of muscular arteries is seen to some degree in virtually all cases of PPH. Medial hypertrophy is present in all forms of pulmonary hypertension and probably correlates with the degree of pulmonary arterial pressure elevation.

Medial hypertrophy is generally considered a reversible lesion. **B**, Cellular proliferation and concentric fibrosis in the intima. Intimal proliferation may be a primary process or secondary to endothelial cell damage and release of growth factors. Intimal fibrosis may lead to complete obliteration of the vessel lumen. (*Courtesy of* Richard N. Channick.)

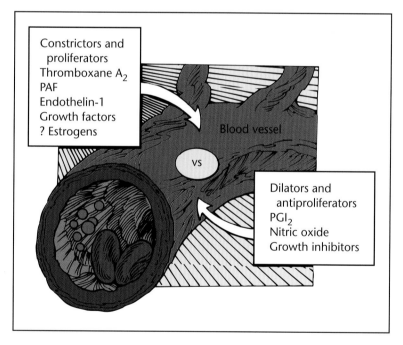

FIGURE 1-118.

Potential mediators involved in the pathogenesis and maintenance of primary pulmonary hypertension (PPH). In the normal, high-flow, low-resistance pulmonary vascular bed, a favorable balance exists between endogenous vasodilators (*eg*, PGI_2 [111], nitric oxide [112]) and vasoconstrictors (*eg*, endothelin [113], thromboxane A_2, platelet activating factor [PAF] [114]), and antiproliferators (*eg*, heparin-like substances, nitric oxide) and proliferators (*eg*, platelet-derived growth factor). In response to some insult such as endothelial damage, the balance may change to favor vasoconstriction and cell proliferation. This results in further endothelial damage, thrombosis, and self-perpetuation of the proliferative, constrictive, fibrotic, and thrombotic process and, thus, the clinical syndrome of PPH. Individual susceptibility also likely plays some role in the development of PPH. (*Courtesy of* Richard N. Channick.)

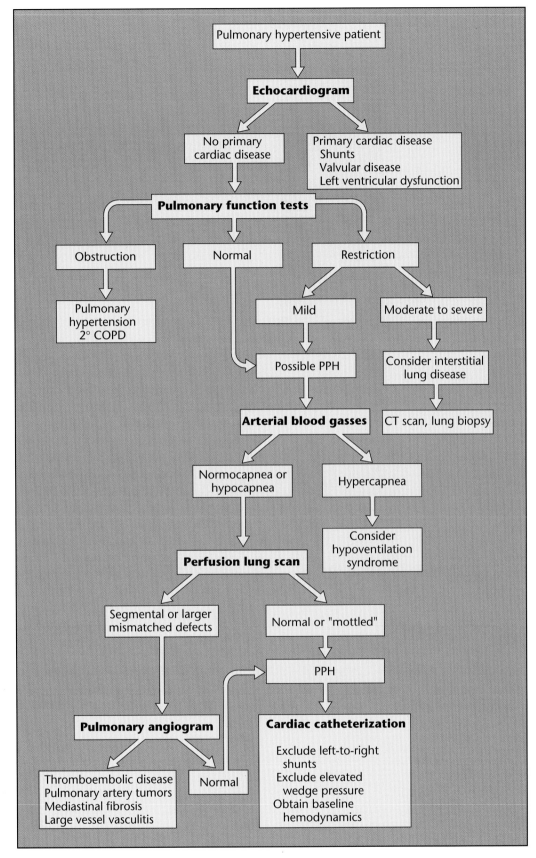

FIGURE 1-119.
Diagnostic approach. An orderly approach with the stepwise elimination of possible secondary causes can yield the diagnosis of primary pulmonary hypertension (PPH) with a high degree of accuracy. Important diagnostic points include the following. 1) Interstitial lung disease does not lead to significant pulmonary hypertension unless quite severe (lung volumes < 50%); therefore, mild restriction should not lead the clinician to attribute the pulmonary hypertension to interstitial lung disease. In the National Institutes of Health Registry of PPH, in fact, a mild restrictive defect was common, with an average total lung capacity of 80% of predicted in these individuals. 2) Although perfusion lung scans may underestimate the degree of obstruction in chronic thromboembolic pulmonary hypertension [115], the absence of *any* segmental or larger defects is highly accurate in distinguishing PPH from chronic thromboembolic pulmonary hypertension [116]. 3) In a small number of cases, uncertainty will remain, even following pulmonary angiography. In these instances, we have found pulmonary angioscopy to be useful in assessing the proximal vascular bed. COPD—chronic obstructive pulmonary disease; CT—computed tomography. (*Courtesy of* Richard N. Channick.)

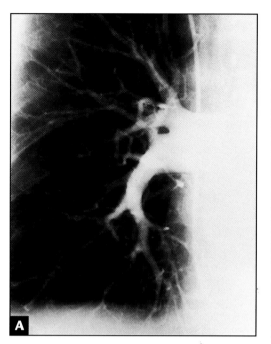
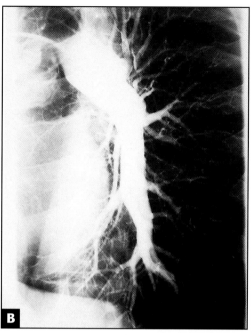

FIGURE 1-120.
Pulmonary angiograms. **A**, The normal angiogram demonstrates a diffuse branching pattern with smoothly tapering vessels and branches leading to the periphery of the lung. **B**, In primary pulmonary hypertension, pulmonary angiography demonstrates marked "pruning" of small vessels with absent peripheral flow. No segmental or larger vascular abnormalities are noted. (*Courtesy of* Richard N. Channick.)

CARDIAC TUMORS

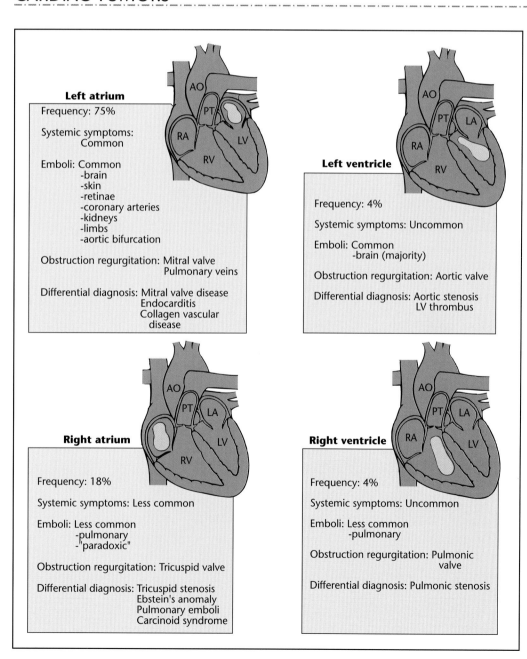

Left atrium

Frequency: 75%

Systemic symptoms:
Common

Emboli: Common
-brain
-skin
-retinae
-coronary arteries
-kidneys
-limbs
-aortic bifurcation

Obstruction regurgitation: Mitral valve
Pulmonary veins

Differential diagnosis: Mitral valve disease
Endocarditis
Collagen vascular
disease

Left ventricle

Frequency: 4%

Systemic symptoms: Uncommon

Emboli: Common
-brain (majority)

Obstruction regurgitation: Aortic valve

Differential diagnosis: Aortic stenosis
LV thrombus

Right atrium

Frequency: 18%

Systemic symptoms: Less common

Emboli: Less common
-pulmonary
-"paradoxic"

Obstruction regurgitation: Tricuspid valve

Differential diagnosis: Tricuspid stenosis
Ebstein's anomaly
Pulmonary emboli
Carcinoid syndrome

Right ventricle

Frequency: 4%

Systemic symptoms: Uncommon

Emboli: Less common
-pulmonary

Obstruction regurgitation: Pulmonic
valve

Differential diagnosis: Pulmonic stenosis

FIGURE 1-121.
Clinical manifestations of cardiac myxomas according to chamber involvement. Most myxomas occur sporadically [117]. Patients are predominantly female and middle-aged, although children and the elderly may also be affected. Myxomas may be familial, occurring more often in young patients, and are often multiple, involving more than one cardiac chamber at the time of presentation (*ie*, synchronous) [117]. Systemic symptoms may include fever, weight loss, fatigue, anemia (possibly hemolytic), increased immunoglobulin levels, leukocytosis, thrombocytopenia, erythrocytosis, Raynaud's phenomenon, and clubbing; breast fibroadenomas may also be found [118]. Ao—aorta; LA—left atrium; LV—left ventricle; PT—pulmonary trunk; RA—right atrium; RV—right ventricle. (*Adapted from* Hall and Cooley [119].)

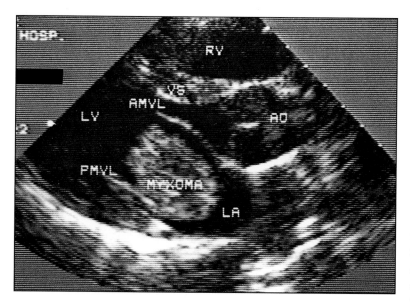

FIGURE 1-122.

Transthoracic two-dimensional echocardiogram of left atrial myxoma. Typically, left atrial (LA) myxomas attach to the fossa ovalis; although myxomas are rarely located posteriorly, a mass in this location should arouse suspicion of malignancy. During diastole, an atrial myxoma is visualized on M-mode echocardiography as multiple echoes behind the AMVL on the left and the tricuspid valve on the right. M-mode echocardiography is most useful for intracavitary, pedunculated masses of the LA; however, it is less effective for visualizing tumors during systole and immobile tumors. Although ventricular myxomas can be seen as multiple intracavitary echoes, they are less frequently detected by this method. Two-dimensional echocardiography provides sufficient information (*ie*, size, attachment, and mobility) for surgical treatment. This imaging modality reveals intracavitary masses with alternating areas of echodensity and lucency and is useful for visualizing small, ventricular, and nonprolapsed tumors. Two-dimensional echocardiography also allows recognition of multiple masses. LV—left ventricle; LVOT—left ventricular outflow tract; PMVL—posterior leaflet of mitral valve; RV—right ventricle; VS—ventricular septum. (*Courtesy of* CR Thompson.)

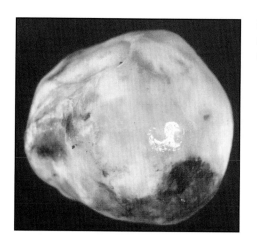

FIGURE 1-123.

Calcified myxoma. Gross photograph of an operatively excised myxoma from a 71-year-old woman. (*Courtesy of* J. Radio.)

■ REFERENCES

1. Ross R: The pathogenesis of atherosclerosis: a perspective for the 1990s. *Nature* 1993, 362:801–809.

2. Richardson PD, Davies MS, Born GVR: Influence of plaque configuration and stress distribution on fissuring of coronary atherosclerotic plaques. *Lancet* 1989, 2:941–944.

3. Bini A, Fenoglio JJ Jr, Mesa-Tejada R, *et al.*: Identification and distribution of fibrinogen, fibrin and fibrin(ogen) degradation products in atherosclerosis: use of monoclonal antibodies. *Arteriosclerosis* 1989, 9:109–121.

4. Menotti A, Keys A, Aravanis C, *et al.*: Seven Countries Study. First 20-year mortality data in 12 cohorts of six countries. *Ann Med* 1989, 21:175–179.

5. Keys A: High density lipoprotein cholesterol and longevity. *J Epidemiol Community Health* 1987, 42:60–65.

6. Castelli WP, Garrison RJ, Wilson PWF, *et al.*: Incidence of coronary heart disease and lipoprotein cholesterol levels. The Framingham study. *JAMA* 1986, 256:2835–2838.

7. Ginsberg HN: Lipoprotein metabolism and its relationship to atherosclerosis. *Med Clin North Am* 1994, 78:1–20.

8. Grundy SM: HMG-CoA reductase inhibitors for treatment of hypercholesterolemia. *N Engl J Med* 1988, 319:24–33.

9. Bilheimer DW, Grundy SM, Brown MS, *et al.*: Mevinolin and colestipol stimulate receptor-mediated clearance of low density lipoprotein from plasma in familiar hypercholesterolemia heterozygoses. *Proc Natl Acad Sci USA* 1983, 80:4124–4128.

10. National Cholesterol Education Program: Second report of the National Cholesterol Education Program (NCEP) expert panel on detection, evaluation, and treatment of high blood cholesterol in adults (adult treatment panel II). *Circulation* 1994, 89:1329–1445.

11. Muller JE, Tofler GH, Stone PH: Circadian variation and triggers of onset of acute cardiovascular disease. *Circulation* 1989, 79:733–743.

12. Falk E, Andersen HR: Pathology of atherosclerotic plaque: stable, unstable, and infarctional. In *Interventional Cardiovascular Medicine: Principles and Practice*. Edited by Roubin GS, Califf RM, O'Neill WW, *et al*. New York: Churchill Livingstone; 1994:57–68.

13. Falk E: Coronary thrombosis: pathogenesis and clinical manifestations. *Am J Cardiol* 1991, 68(suppl B):28–35.

14. Lau J, Antman E, Jimenez-Silva J, *et al.*: Cumulative meta-analysis of therapeutic trials for myocardial infarction. *N Engl J Med* 1992, 327:248–254.

15. Braunwald E, Antman EM, Beasley JW, *et al.*: ACC/AHA guidelines for the management of patients with unstable angina and non–ST-segment elevation and myocardial infarction: executive summary and recommendations. *Circulation* 2000, 102:1193–1209.

16. Cannon CP, Braunwald E: Unstable angina. In *Heart Disease* edn 6. Edited by Braunwald E, Zipes DP, Libby P. Philadelphia: WB Saunders; 2001:1232–1263.

17. Braunwald E: Unstable angina: an etiologic approach to management. *Circulation* 1998, 98:2219–2222.

18. Hamm CW, Braunwald E: A classification of unstable angina revisited.*Circulation* 2000, 102:118–122.

19. ISIS-4 (Fourth International Study of Infarct Survival) Collaborative Group: A randomised factorial trial assessing early oral captopril, oral mononitrate, and intravenous magnesium sulphate in 5850 patients with suspected acute myocardial infarction. *Lancet* 1995, 345:669–685.

20. Gruppo Intaliano per lo Studio del Sopravvivenza nell'Infarto Miocardico: GISSI-3: effects of lisinopril and transdermal glyceryl trinitrate single and together on 6-week mortality and ventricular function after acute myocardial infarction. *Lancet* 1994, 343:1115–1122.

21. Smith PP, Arnesen H, Holme I: The effect of warfarin on mortality and reinfarction after myocardial infarction. *N Engl J Med* 1990, 323:147–152.

22. ISIS-2 (Second International Study of Infarct Survival) Collaborative Group: Randomised trial of intravenous streptokinase, oral aspirin, both, or neither among 17,187 cases of suspected acute myocardial infarctions: ISIS-2. *Lancet* 1988, ii:349–360.

23. Gruppo Italiano per lo Studio della Streptochinasi nell'Infarto Miocardico (GISSI): Effectiveness of intravenous thrombolytic treatment in acute myocardial infarction. *Lancet* 1986, i:397–402.

24. The GUSTO Investigators: An international randomized trial comparing four thrombolytic strategies for acute myocardial infarction. *N Engl J Med* 1993, 329:673–682.

25. Friedman M, Van den Bovenkamp GJ: The pathogenesis of a coronary thrombus. *Am J Pathol* 1966, 48:19–44.

26. Epstein S, Talbot T: Dynamic coronary tone in precipitation, exacerbation and relief of angina pectoris. *Am J Cardiol* 1981, 48:797–803.

27. Kaul S, Lilly D, Gascho J, *et al.*: Prognostic utility of the exercise thallium-201 test in ambulatory patients with chest pain: comparison with cardiac catheterization. *Circulation* 1988, 4:745.

28. Muhlbaier LH, Pryor DB, Rankin JS, *et al.*: Observational comparison of event-free survival with medical and surgical therapy in patients with coronary artery disease: 20 years of follow-up. *Circulation* 1992, 86(suppl II):198–204.

29. Califf RM, Harrell FE Jr, Lee KL, *et al.*: The evolution of medical and surgical therapy for coronary artery disease: a 15-year perspective. *JAMA* 1989, 261:2077–2086.

30. Katz AM: Congestive heart failure: role of altered myocardial cellular control. *N Engl J Med* 1975, 293:1184–1191.

31. Braunwald E: Myocardial reperfusion, limitation of infarct size, reduction of left ventricular dysfunction, and improved survival: should the paradigm by expanded? *Circulation* 1989, 79:441–444.

32. Kim C, Braunwald E: Potential benefits of late reperfusion of infarcted myocardium: the open artery hypothesis. *Circulation* 1993, 88:2426–2436.

33. Paganelli WC, Creager MA, Dzau VJ: Cardiac regulation of renal function. In *The International Textbook of Cardiology*. Edited by Cheng TO. New York: Pergammon Press; 1986:1010–1020.

34. Underwood RD, Chan DP, Burnett JC: Endothelin: an endothelium derived vasoconstrictor peptide and its role in congestive heart failure. *Heart Failure* 1991, 7:50–58.

35. Ho KKL, Pinsky JL, Kannel WB, *et al.*: The epidemiology of heart failure: the Framingham Study. *J Am Coll Cardiol* 1993, 22(suppl A):6–13.

36. Colucci WS, Braunwald E: Pathophysiology of heart failure. In *Heart Disease* edn 6. Edited by Braunwald E, Zipes DP, Libby P. Philadelphia: WB Saunders; 2001:503–533.

37. Hunter JJ, Chien KR: Signaling pathways for cardiac hypertrophy and failure. *N Engl J Med* 1999, 341:1276–1283.

38. Sawyer DB, Colucci WS: Molecular and cellular events in myocardial hypertrophy and failure. In *Atlas of Heart Diseases* vol IV. Philadelphia: Current Medicine; 1999:4.2.

39. Katz AM: *Heart Failure*. Philadelphia: Lippincott Williams & Wilkins; 2000:38.

40. CONSENSUS Trial Study Group: Effects of enalapril on mortality in severe congestive heart failure. *N Engl J Med* 1987, 316:1429–1435.

41. The SOLVD Investigators: Effect of enalapril on survival in patients with reduced left ventricular ejection fractions and congestive heart failure. *N Engl J Med* 1991, 325:293–302.

42. McKay RG, Pfeffer MA, Pasternal RC, *et al.*: Left ventricular remodeling after myocardial infarction: a corollary to infarct expansion. *Circulation* 1986, 74:693–702.

43. Ganz P, Ganz W: Coronary blood flow and myocardial ischemia. In *Heart Disease* edn 6. Edited by Braunwald E, Zipes DP, Libby P. Philadelphia: WB Saunders; 2001:1087–1113.

44. Pitt B, Zannad F, Remme WJ, *et al.*: The effect of spironolactone on morbidity and mortality in patients with severe heart failure. Randomized Aldactone Evaluation Study Investigators. *N Engl J Med 1999*, 341:709–717.

45. CIBIS II Investigators and Committees: The Cardiac Insufficiency Bisoprolol Study [CIBIS] II: A randomised trial. *Lancet* 1999, 353:9–13.

46. Stevenson LW, Miller L: Cardiac transplantation as therapy for heart failure. *Curr Prob Cardiol* 1991, 16:4:219–305.

47. Mudge GH, Goldstein S, Addonizio LJ, *et al.*: Bethesda Conference on Transplantation Task Force 3: recipient guidelines/prioritization. *J Am Coll Cardiol* 1993, 22:21–31.

48. Kaye MP: Registry of the International Society for Heart and Lung Transplantation: Tenth Official Report—1993. *J Heart Lung Transplant* 1993, 12:541–548.

49. Grattan MT, Moreno-Cabral CE, Starnes VA, *et al.*: Eight-year results of cyclosporine-treated patients with cardiac transplants. *J Thorac Cardiovasc Surg* 1990, 99:500–509.

50. Sharples LD, Caine N, Mullins P, *et al.*: Risk facto analysis for the major haxards following heart transplantation: refection, infection, and coronary occlusive disease. *Transplantation* 1991, 52:244–252.

51. Wigle ED, Sasson Z, Henderson MA, *et al.*: Hypertrophic cardiomyopathy. The importance of the site and the extent of hypertrophy: a review. *Prog Cardiovasc Dis* 1985, 28:1–85.

52. Shah PM, Taylor RD, Wong M: Abnormal mitral valve coaptation in hypertrophic obstructive cardiomyopathy: proposed role in systolic anterior motion of mitral valve. *Am J Cardiol* 1981, 48:258–262.

53. Grigg LE, Wigle ED, Williams WG, *et al.*: Transesophageal Doppler echocardiography in obstructive hypertrophic cardiomyopathy: clarification of pathophysiology and importance in intraoperative decision making. *J Am Coll Cardiol* 1992, 20:42–52.

54. Roberts WC, McAlister HA, Ferrano VJ: Sarcoidosis of the heart. *Am J Med* 1977, 63:86–108.

55. Klein AL, Hatle LK, Burstow DJ, *et al.*: Doppler characterization of left ventricular diastolic function in cardiac amyloidosis. *J Am Coll Cardiol* 1989, 13:1017–1026.

56. Strain JE, Grose RM, Factor SM, *et al.*: Results of endomyocardial biopsy in patients with spontaneous ventricular tachycardia but without apparent structural heart disease. *Circulation* 1983, 68:1171–1181.

57. Smith WG: Coxsackie B myopericarditis in adults. *Am Heart J* 1980, 80:34–36.

58. Rockman HA, Adamson RM, Dembitsky WP, *et al.*: Acute fulminant myocarditis: long-term follow-up after circulatory support with left ventricular assist device. *Am Heart J* 1991, 121:922–926.

59. Jones SR, Herskowitz A, Hutchins GM, *et al.*: Effects of immunosuppressive therapy in biopsy-proved myocarditis and borderline myocarditis on left ventricular function. *Am J Cardiol* 1991, 68:370–376.

60. Fowler NO: Pericardial disease. *Heart Dis Stroke* 1992, 1:85–94.

61. Shabetai R, Fowler NO, Guntheroth WG: The hemodynamics of cardiac tamponade and constrictive pericarditis. *Am J Cardiol* 1970, 26:480–489.

62. CIBA Pharmaceutical Company Division of CIBA-GEIGY Corporation: The CIBA Collection of Medical Illustrations by Frank H. Netter, MD, 1969.

63. Wit AL, Rosen MR, Hoffman BF: Electrophysiology and pharmacology of cardiac arrhythmias. II: Relationship of normal and abnormal electrical activity of cardiac fibers to the genesis of arrhythmias. B. Reentry. *Am Heart J* 1974, 88:799.

64. The Cardiac Arrhythmia Suppression Trial (CAST) Investigators: Preliminary report: effect of encainide and flecainide on mortality in a randomized trial of arrhythmia suppression after myocardial infarction. *N Engl J Med* 1989, 321:406–412.

65. The Cardiac Arrhythmia Suppression Trial (CAST) II Investigators: Effect of the antiarrhythmic agent moricizine on survival after myocardial infarction. *N Engl J Med* 1992, 327:227–233.

66. The Cardiac Arrest in Seattle, Conventional Versus Amiodarone Drug Evaluation (CASCADE) investigators: Randomized antiarrhythmic drug therapy in survivors of cardiac arrests (the CASCADE study). *Am J Cardiol* 1993, 72:280–287.

67. Mason JW: A comparison of seven antiarrhythmic drugs in patients with ventricular tachyarrhythmias. Electrophysiologic Study versus Electrocardiographic Monitoring Investigators. *N Engl J Med* 1993, 329(7):452–458.

68. Gomes JA: The sick sinus syndrome and evaluation of the patient with sinus node disorders. In *Cardiology*. Edited by Parmley W, Chatterjee K. Philadelphia: J.B. Lippincott Co; 1988:1–16.

69. Allessie MA, Lammers WJEP, Bonke FIM, Hollen J: Experimental evaluation of Moe's multiple wavelet hypothesis of atrial fibrillation. In *Cardiac Electrophysiology and Arrhythmias*. Edited by Zipes DP, Jalife J. Orlando: Grune and Stratton; 1985:265–275.

70. Eldar M, Griffin JC, Abbott JA, Scheinman MM: Permanent cardiac pacing in patients with the long QT syndrome. *J Am Coll Cardiol* 1987, 10:600.

71. Moss AJ, Liu JE, Gottlieb S, et al.: Efficacy of permanent pacing in the management of high-risk patients with long QT syndrome. Circulation 1991, 84:1524.

72. de Wardener HE, MacGregor GA: Natriuretic hormone and essential hypertension as an endocrine disease. In Essential Hypertension as an Endocrine Disease. Edited by Edwards CRW, Carey RM. London: Butterworths; 1985:132–157.

73. Griendling KK, Alexander RW: Cellular biology of blood vessels. In Hurst's The Heart. Edited by Schlant RC, Alexander RW, O'Rourke R, et al.: New York: McGraw-Hill; 1994:31–45.

74. Lüscher TF, Vanhoutte PM: Endothelium-dependent contraction to acetylcholine in the aorta of the spontaneously hypertensive rat. Hypertension 1986, 8:344–348.

75. Bravo EL: What to do when potassium is low or high. Diagnosis 1988, 10:1–6.

76. Bravo EL, Gifford RW, Manger WM: Adrenal medullary tumors: pheochromocytoma. In Endocrine Tumors. Edited by Mazzaferri EL, Samaan NA. Boston: Blackwell Scientific Publications; 1993:426–447.

77. Bravo EL: Evolving concepts in the pathophysiology, diagnosis, and treatment of pheochromocytoma. Endocrinology 1993, 15:426.

78. The Fifth Report of the Joint National Committee on Detection, Evaluation, and Treatment of High Blood Pressure. Arch Intern Med 1993, 153:154–182.

79. 1993 Guidelines for the Management of Mild Hypertension. Memorandum from a World Health Organization/International Society of Hypertension meeting. Hypertension 1993, 22:392–403.

80. Chalmers J: The place of combination therapy in the treatment of hypertension in 1993. Clin Exp Hypertens 1993, 15:1299–1313.

81. Braunwald E: In Heart Disease edn 6. Edited by Braunwald E, Zipes DP, Libby P. Philadelphia: WB Saunders; 2001:1643–1722.

82. Task Force on Practice Guidelines (Committee on Management of Patients with Valvular Heart Disease). ACC/AHA guidelines for the management of patients with valvular heart disease. J Am Coll Cardiol 1998, 32:1486–1588.

83. Holen J, Aaslid R, Landmark K, et al.: Determination of pressure gradient in mitral stenosis with a noninvasive ultrasound Doppler technique. Acta Med Scand 1976, 199:455–460.

84. Nishimura RA, Tajik AJ: Quanititative hemodynamics by Doppler echocardiography: a noninvasive alternative to cardiac catheterization. Prog Cardiovasc Dis 1994, 36:309–342.

85. Inoue K, Owaki T, Nakamura T, et al.: Clinical application of transvenous mitral commissurotomy by a new balloon catheter. J Thorac Cardiovasc Surg 1984, 87:394–402.

86. Helmcke F, Nanda N, Ming H, et al.: Color Doppler assessment of mitral regurgitation with orthogonal planes. Circulation 1987, 75:175–183.

87. Spain M, Smith M, Grayburn P, et al.: Quantitative assessment of mitral regurgitation by Doppler color-flow imaging: angiographic and hemodynamic correlations. J Am Coll Cardiol 1989, 13:585–590.

88. Cape E, Yoganathan P, Weyman A, et al.: Adjacent solid boundaries alter the size of regurgitant jets on Doppler color-flow maps. J Am Coll Cardiol 1991, 17:1094–1102.

89. Enriquez-Sarano M, Bailey KR, Seward JB, et al.: Quantitative Doppler assessment of valvular regurgitation. Circulation 1993, 87:841–848.

90. Jenni R, Ritter M, Eberli F, et al.: Quantification of mitral regurgitation with amplitude-weighted mean velocity. Circulation 1989, 79:1294–1299.

91. Bargiggia G, Tronconi L, Sahn D, et al.: A new method for quantification of mitral regurgitation based on color-flow Doppler imaging of flow convergence proximal to regurgitant orifice. Circulation 1991, 84:1481–1489.

92. Straub U, Feindt P, Huwer, et al.: Mitral valve replacement with preservation of the subvalvular structures where possible: an echocardiographic and clinical comparison with cases where preservation was not possible. Thorac Cardiovasc Surg 1994, 42:2–8.

93. Farb A, Tang AL, Atkinson JB, et al.: Comparison of cardiac findings in patients with mitral valve prolapse who die suddenly to those who have congestive heart failure from mitral regurgitation and to those with fatal noncardiac conditions. Am J Cardiol 1992, 70:234–239.

94. O'Rourke RA, Carwford MH: The systolic click-murmur syndrome: clinical recognition and management. Curr Probl Cardiol 1976, 1:9–60.

95. Alpert MA, Cardney RJ, Flaker GC, et al.: Sensitivity and specificity of two-dimensional echocardiographic signs of mitral valve prolapse. Am J Cardiol 1984, 54:792–796.

96. Plantely G, Morton MJ, Rahimtoola SH: Effects of successful, uncomplicated valve replacement on ventricular hypertrophy, volume, and performance in aortic stenosis and aortic incompetence. J Thorac Cardiovasc Surg 1978, 75:383–391.

97. Braunwald E, Frahm CJ: Studies on the Starling's law of the heart. IV. Observations on the hemodynamic functions of the left atrium in man. Circulation 1961, 24:633–642.

98. Stott DK, Marpole DGF, Bristow JD, et al.: The role of left atrial transport in aortic and mitral stenosis. Circulation 1970, 41:1031–1041.

99. Ross J Jr: Afterload mismatch and preload reserve: a conceptual framework for the analysis of ventricular function. Prog Cardiovasc Dis 1976, 18:255–264.

100. DeMots H, Rahimtoola SH, McAnulty JH, Murphy ES: Pulmonary edema. In Cardiac Emergencies. Edited by Mason DT. Baltimore: Williams & Wilkins; 1978:173–223.

101. Nishimura RA, Vonk GD, Rumberger JA, et al.: Semiquantitation of aortic regurgitation by different Doppler echocardiographic techniques and comparison with ultrafast- computed tomography. Am Heart J 1992, 124:995–1001.

102. Perry G, Helmcke F, Nanda N, et al.: Evaluation of aortic insufficiency by Doppler color-flow mapping. J Am Coll Cardiol 1987, 9:952–959.

103. Carabello BA: Aortic regurgitation: hemodynamic determinants of prognosis. In Aortic Regurgitation: Medical and Surgical Management. Edited by Cohn LH, DiSesa V. New York: Marcel Dekker; 1986.

104. Clark DG, McAnulty JH, Rahimtoola SH: Valve replacement in aortic insufficiency with left ventricular dysfunction. Circulation 1980, 61:411–421.

105. Bonow RO, Dodd JT, Maron BJ, et al.: Long-term serial changes in left ventricular function and reversal of ventricular dilatation after valve replacement for chronic aortic regurgitation. Circulation 1988, 78:1108–1120.

106. Harris P, Heath D: Unexplained pulmonary hypertension. In The Human Pulmonary Circulation, ed 2. Edited by Harris P, Heath D. Edinburgh: Churchill-Livingston; 1977:418–440.

107. Rich S: Pulmonary hypertension. In Heart Disease edn 6. Edited by Braunwald E, Zipes DP, Libby P. Philadelphia: WB Saunders; 2001:1908–1935.

108. Rubin LJ: Primary pulmonary hypertension. Chest 1993, 104:236–250.

109. Report of the Medical Research Council Working Party: Long term domiciliary oxygen therapy in chronic hypoxic cor pulmonale complicating chronic bronchitis and emphysema. Lancet 1981,1:681–686.

110. Nocturnal Oxygen Therapy Trial Group: Continuous or nocturnal oxygen therapy in hypoxemic chronic obstructive lung disease: a clinical trial. Ann Intern Med 1980, 93:391–398.

111. Christman BW, McPherson CD, Newman JH, et al.: An imbalance between the excretion of thromboxane and prostacyclin metabolites in pulmonary hypertension. N Engl J Med 1992, 327:70–75.

112. Dinh-Xuan AT, Higenbottam TW, Clelland CA, et al.: Impairment of endothelium-dependent pulmonary-artery relaxation in chronic obstruction lung disease. N Engl J Med 1991, 324:1539–1547.

113. Stewart DJ, Levy RD, Cernacek P, Langleben D: Increased plasma endothelin-1 in pulmonary hypertension: marker or mediator of disease? Ann Intern Med 1991, 114:464–469.

114. Ohar JA, Waller KS, Dahms TE: Platelet-activating factor induces selective pulmonary arterial hyperreactivity in isolated perfused rabbit lungs. Am Rev Respir Dis 1993, 148:158–163.

115. Ryan KL, Fedullo PF, Davis GB, et al.: Perfusion scan findings understate the severity of angiographic and hemodynamic compromise in chronic thromboembolic pulmonary hypertension. Chest 1988, 98:1180–1185.

116. Fedullo PF, Fishmann AJ, Moser KM: Pulmonary perfusion scans in primary pulmonary hypertension. Chest 1983, 127:82–86.

117. Carney JA: Differences between nonfamilial and familial cardiac myxoma. Am J Surg Pathol 1985, 9:53–55.

118. Peters MN, Hall RJ, Cooley DA, et al.: The clinical syndrome of atrial myxoma. JAMA 1974, 230:694.

119. Hall RJ, Cooley DA: Neoplastic diseases of the heart. In Hurst's The Heart ed 5. Edited by Logue RB, Rackley CE, Schlant RC, et al. New York: McGraw-Hill; 1982:1403–1421.

Pulmonary and Critical Care Medicine

D. KEITH PAYNE

Pulmonary and critical care medicine continues to be a diverse, demanding, and fascinating discipline. Many systemic diseases have pulmonary manifestations, and critical care medicine involves diseases and disorders of many organ systems. As a result, the practice of pulmonary and critical care medicine remains closely linked with its internal medicine roots. General internists frequently encounter patients with pulmonary complaints such as cough and dyspnea. Disease processes such as asthma, chronic bronchitis, and COPD are more frequently treated in the internist's office than in the office of a subspecialist. Many internists may therefore find a work such as this useful in their day-to-day practice.

The content of this chapter has been gleaned from the published and personal collections of a number of experts in the field of pulmonary and critical care medicine. Topics include obstructive lung diseases, lung neoplasms, infections of the lung, venous thromboembolism, interstitial lung diseases, pleural diseases, and critical care. The goal of this chapter is to present in succinct, graphic format commonly encountered diseases of the respiratory system that internists may expect to encounter with some frequency. The drawings, radiographs, tables, algorithms, and histopathology are accompanied by brief legends which provide a "quick take" on these disorders. For the curious reader interested in learning more about a particular subject, carefully selected, current references are provided.

■ OBSTRUCTIVE LUNG DISEASES

CHRONIC OBSTRUCTIVE PULMONARY DISEASE (COPD)

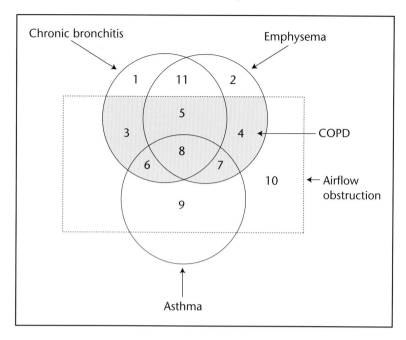

FIGURE 2-1.

Nonproportional Venn diagram showing subsets of patients with bronchitis, emphysema, asthma, and combinations of these components of chronic obstructive pulmonary disease (COPD). The subsets comprising COPD are shaded. Patients with reversible asthma (subset 9) do not have COPD, whereas patients with emphysema and/or bronchitis (subsets 6, 7, and 8) are considered to have "asthmatic bronchitis." Most patients with COPD have chronic bronchitis and emphysema (subset 5). (*Adapted from* Celli *et al.* [1].)

Clinical Characteristics of Emphysema and Chronic Bronchitis

Feature	"Pink Puffer" (Emphysematous)	"Blue Bloater" (Bronchitic)
Onset	Age 40–50 y	Age 30–40 y; disability in middle age
Etiology	Smoking; genetic predisposition; unknown factors; air pollution	Smoking; unknown factors; air pollution
Sputum	Minimal	Copious
Dyspnea	Relatively early onset	Relatively late onset
$\dot{V}/\dot{Q}$ ratio	Minimal imbalance	Marked imbalance
Anteroposterior diameter of chest	"Barrel chest" common	Not increased
Pathologic lung anatomy	Centrilobular emphysema	Mucus gland hypertrophy
Pulmonary function tests	Low FEV_1, marked increase in total lung capacity and residual volume, low D_{LCO}	Low FEV_1; moderate increase in residual volume, normal D_{LCO}
$PaCO_2$	Normal or low	Elevated
$SaCO_2$	Normal	Decreased
Hematocrit	Normal	Elevated
Cyanosis	Rare	Common
Cor pulmonale	Rare, except terminally	Frequent

D_{LCO}–diffusing capacity of lung for carbon monoxide; FEV_1–forced expiratory volume in 1 s; $\dot{V}/\dot{Q}$–ventilation perfusion.

FIGURE 2-2.

Characteristics of emphysema and chronic bronchitis. Differences between the clinical findings in emphysema and chronic obstructive bronchitis were first recognized many years ago by clinicians who noted that some patients with chronic obstructive pulmonary disease (COPD) were "pink puffers" (emphysematous), whereas others were "blue bloaters" (chronic bronchitic). These represent the extremes of a wide clinical spectrum. Most patients with COPD fall somewhere between these two extremes and demonstrate some characteristics of both. Although emphysema and chronic bronchitis are characterized by an imbalance between ventilation and perfusion, chronic bronchitis results in more shunting of arterial blood through unventilated alveoli and therefore results in more severe hypoxemia and cor pulmonale. However, emphysema is associated with more air-trapping, hyperinflation, and dyspnea than would be expected for a given degree of hypoxemia. (*Adapted from* Owens [2].)

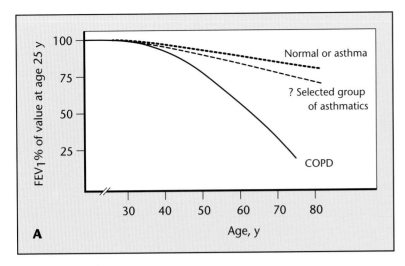

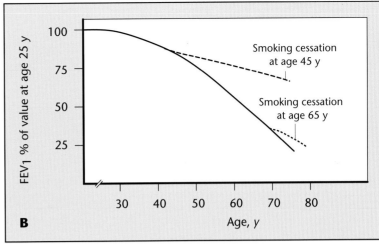

A

B

FIGURE 2-3.

Clinical course of airway function in asthma, chronic obstructive pulmonary disease (COPD), smoking, and after smoking cessation. **A,** Long-term clinical course of patients with asthma and COPD. It is generally thought that patients with asthma have a change in pulmonary function with aging that is comparable to that of normal nonsmoking individuals. Questions have been raised whether a select group of asthmatics have decreases in pulmonary function

that are excessive for their age. However, patients with COPD have a much more dramatic decline in pulmonary function over time. **B,** Effect of smoking cessation at 45 and 65 years of age. It is generally thought that the decline in pulmonary function seen in patients after smoking cessation is the same as that seen in nonsmokers, although smokers may start from a lower baseline. FEV_1—forced expiratory volume in 1 second. (*Courtesy of* Gregory R. Owens.)

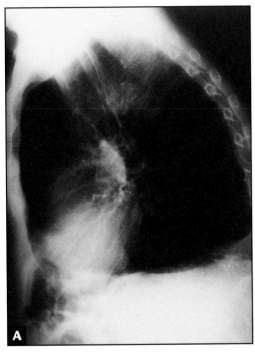

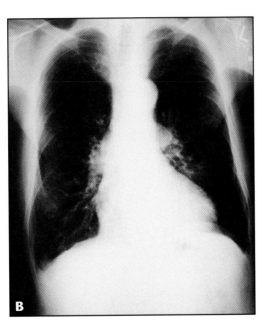

A

B

FIGURE 2-4.

Chest radiograph in obstructive lung disease. Posteroanterior (**A**) and lateral (**B**) chest radiographs demonstrating many of the radiographic features of obstructive lung disease. The posteroanterior radiograph shows hyperlucent lung fields and vascular crowding with a curvilinear pattern. The lateral radiograph demonstrates significantly increased anteroposterior diameter, flattening of the diaphragms, and an increased retrosternal air space. Again, note the hyperlucent lung fields on the lateral view. (*Courtesy of* Charles J. Grodzin.)

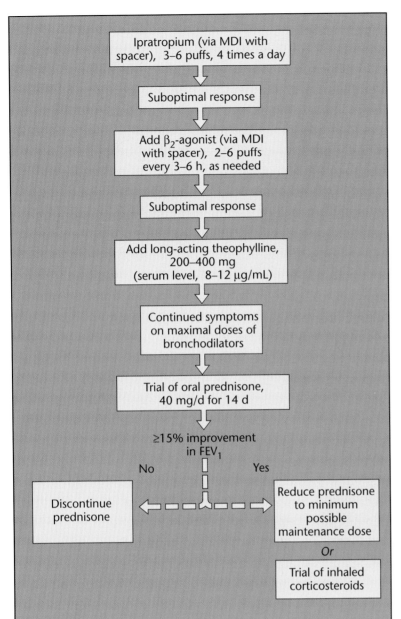

FIGURE 2-5.

Proposed algorithm for the pharmacologic management of stable chronic obstructive pulmonary disease. Inhaled ipratropium bromide is recommended as first-line bronchodilator therapy because of its relatively long duration of action and lack of side effects. The package insert recommends a dose of two puffs four times daily via metered-dose inhaler (MDI); however, some experts recommend much higher doses, up to a total dosage of 24 puffs per day. If patients complain of bouts of dyspnea during ipratropium therapy, an inhaled $\beta2$-agonist should be added at 3- to 6-hour intervals as needed. The as-needed administration of a β-agonist decreases the likelihood of tolerance, and the number of puffs required may be used as a measure of symptoms. If patients are still symptomatic, long-acting oral theophylline may be administered at bedtime, with dosage adjusted to maintain a peak serum level of 8 to 12 µg/mL. Alternatively, for nocturnal dyspnea, a very long-acting β-agonist, such as salmeterol, may be administered at bedtime. If symptoms persist on maximum bronchodilator therapy, a trial of oral prednisone is justified. An improvement of 15% or more in forced expiratory volume in 1 second (FEV_1) on corticosteroid therapy is an indication for long-term maintenance, preferably via inhaled corticosteroids. Long-term, low-dose oral prednisone is an alternative to inhaled corticosteroid therapy; however, it is associated with a marked increase in side effects. (*Adapted from* Ferguson and Cherniack [3].)

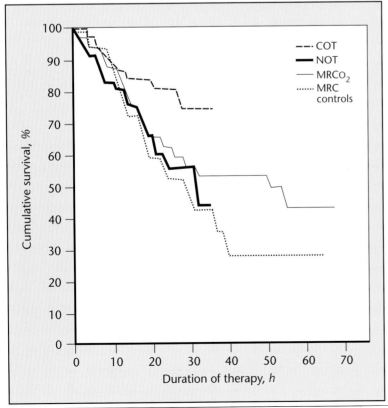

FIGURE 2-6.

Survival of men younger than 70 years of age with hypoxemic chronic obstructive pulmonary disease receiving long-term oxygen therapy versus survival of control subjects who did not receive oxygen. The data summarized in the figure were obtained from the Medical Research Council (MRC; limited oxygen therapy) and the Nocturnal Oxygen Therapy (NOT) trials, whose subjects received varying amounts of oxygen throughout the day. Survival of men in the control group who received no oxygen was the worst, but survival of men in the NOT group who received oxygen for 12 hours per 24-hour day was similar to that of men in the MRC group who received 15 hours of oxygen per day ($MRCO_2$). The best survival was in the continuous oxygen therapy (COT) group, whose members received oxygen for more than 19 hours per day. (*Adapted from* Flenley [4].)

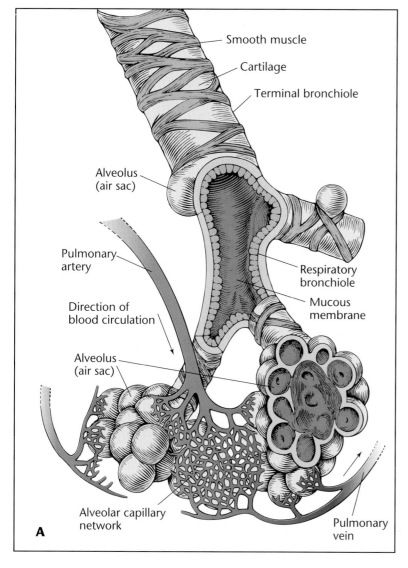

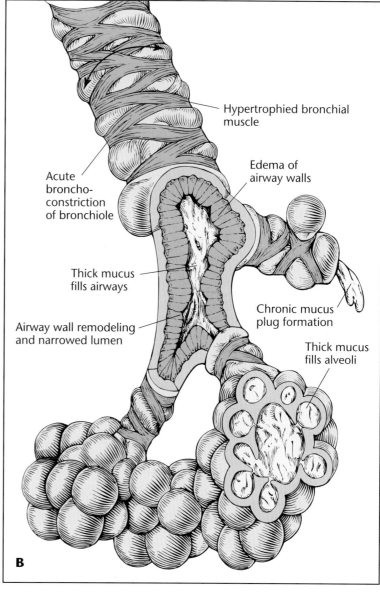

FIGURE 2-7.

A, Normal anatomy of lung near the terminal bronchiole demonstrating the efficiency with which normal gas exchange occurs. B, Same region during acute asthmatic episode, demonstrating airflow obstruction I asthma. Smooth muscle along airway walls is constricted and hypertrophied. Along with extensive plugging of the airways by mucus, airway walls are thickened and edematous as a result of inflammatory changes. Eventually, airway walls may be remodeled, leading to fixed obstruction in some patients. Unchecked airway inflammation resulting in such extensive pathologic changes may cause severe hypoxemia from ventilation-perfusion mismatches and even intrapulmonary shunting.

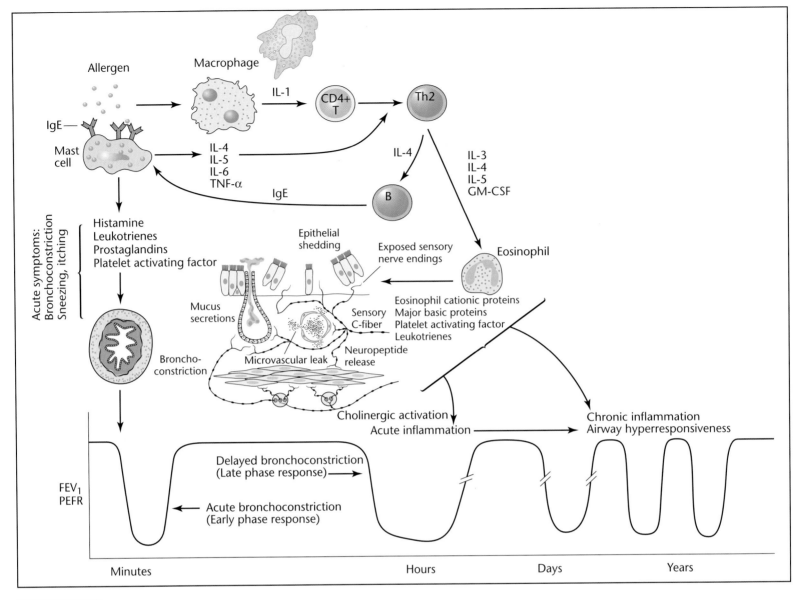

FIGURE 2-8.

Mechanisms of airway inflammation in asthma. Allergen exposure initiates a complex, self-amplifying interplay among cells, cytokines, and neurogenic components resulting in chronic, symptomatic inflammation with bronchial hyperresponsiveness. Mast cells in the bronchial lumen and epithelium and within the bronchial wall may become activated by allergen exposure, releasing a variety of mediators. These mediators initiate an acute phase reaction (within minutes), including bronchospasm, thus resulting in airflow obstruction. Quiescent CD4+ T-helper (Th2) lymphocytes may also become activated by cytokines secreted by allergen-stimulated cells such as macrophages, initiating a more chronic inflammatory process. Activated Th2 lymphocytes secrete various cytokines that attract other cells, such as eosinophils, which in turn release potent epithelial-disrupting agents. Exposed epithelial sensory nerve endings may contribute to ongoing inflammation by releasing neuropeptides and by initiating reflex arcs involving cholinergic pathways. Th2-secreted interleukin-4 (IL-4) initiates B-lymphocyte IgE release, which in turn amplifies mast cell–mediated events. Some evidence exists that mast cells also produce cytokines, such as IL-4, which may be important in chronic inflammation [5–7]. FEV_1—forced expiratory volume in 1 second; GM-CSF—granulocyte-macrophage colony-stimulating factor; PEFR—peak expiratory flow rate; TNF—tumor necrosis factor. (*Adapted from* Barnes [7] and Freitag and Newhouse [8].)

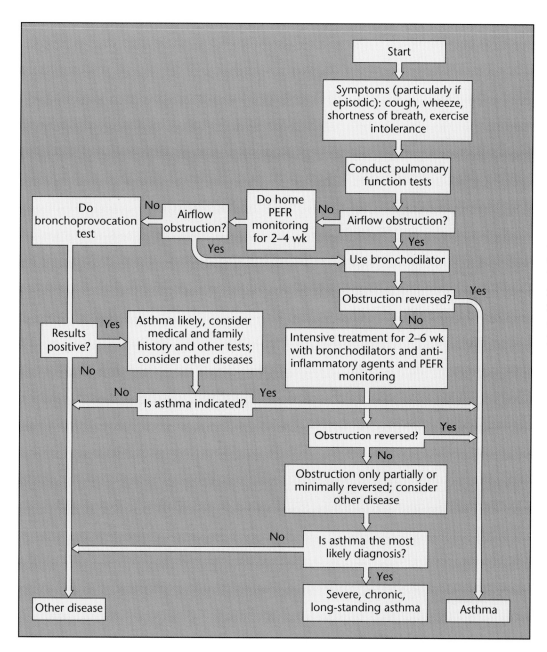

FIGURE 2-9.

Algorithm for the diagnosis of asthma. This diagnosis may be relatively simple, or it may be complicated by other diseases. Symptomatic patients may be tested for the presence of reversible airway obstruction. If none is present on initial testing, repeated testing or the use of home peak flow meters may increase the likelihood of documenting an obstructive episode. In symptomatic patients with no obstruction, bronchoprovocation testing may be useful. In a few patients, long-standing airway inflammation may result in minimally reversible airflow obstruction. If compatible symptoms are present and no other explanation is likely, a diagnosis of asthma may be made. PEFR—peak expiratory flow rate. (*Adapted from* the National Asthma Education Program [9].)

Goals of Asthma Therapy

Maintain (near) normal pulmonary function
Maintain normal activity levels
Prevent chronic and troublesome symptoms
Prevent recurrent exacerbations of asthma
Avoid adverse effects of asthma medications
Satisfy patient's and family's expectations for asthma care

FIGURE 2-10.

Goals of asthma therapy. Because asthma is a chronic disease with episodic exacerbations, the patient and physician must recognize the importance of adhering to general principles of therapy. The National Asthma Education Program Expert Panel Report II set forth six distinct goals for the effective, long-term treatment of asthma [10].

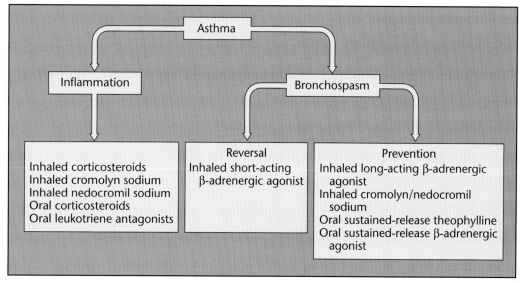

FIGURE 2-11.

Drug treatment for asthma. Overall pharmacologic therapy for asthma consists of drugs to control inflammation and bronchospasm. Drugs used to control bronchospasm may be subdivided into short-acting agents designed to reverse bronchospasm (rescue therapy) and agents designed to prevent bronchospasm. Anti-inflammatory agents such as cromolyn and nedocromil sodium may also be used to prevent exercise-induced bronchospasm. (*Adapted from* Kamada and Szefler [11].)

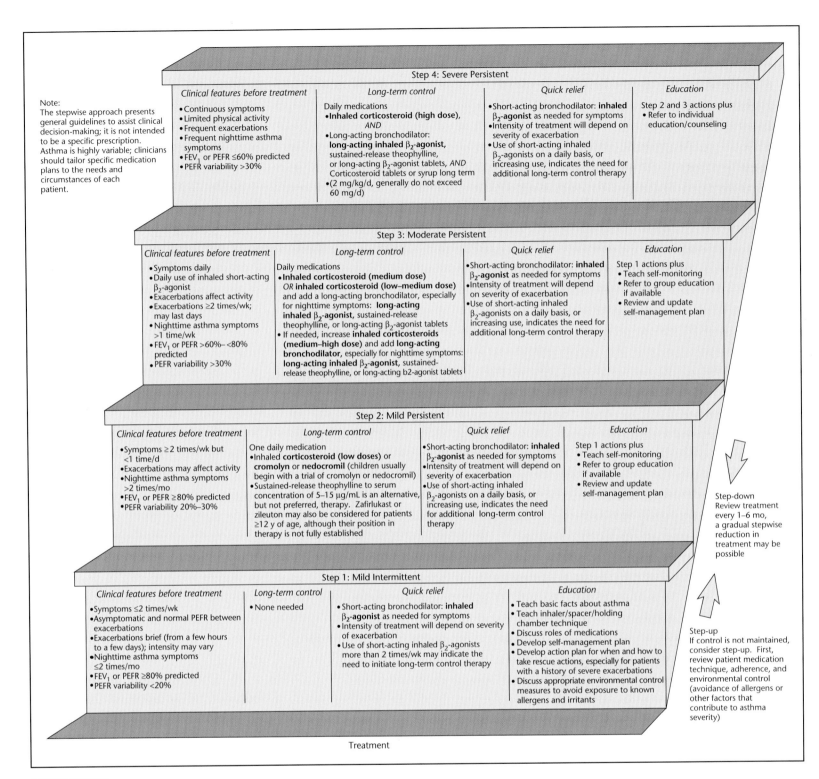

FIGURE 2-12.

Stepwise approach for managing asthma in adults and children older than 5 years of age. The presence of one of the features of severity is sufficient to place a patient in that category. An individual should be assigned to the most severe grade in which any feature occurs. The characteristics noted in this figure are general and may overlap because asthma is highly variable; furthermore, an individual's classification may change over time. Patients at any level of severity can have mild, moderate, or severe exacerbations. Some patients with intermittent asthma experience severe and life-threatening exacerbations separated by long periods of normal lung function and no symptoms. The physician should gain control as quickly as possible, then decrease treatment to the least medication necessary to maintain control. Gaining control may be accom-plished by either starting treatment at the step most appropriate to the initial severity of the condition or starting at a higher level of therapy. A rescue course of systemic corticosteroids may be needed at any time and at any step. At each step, patients should control their environment to avoid or control factors that make their asthma worse (*eg*, allergens, irritants); this requires specific diagnosis and education. Referral to an asthma specialist for consultation or comanagement is recommended if there are difficulties achieving or maintaining control of asthma or if the patient requires step 4 care. Referral may be considered if the patient requires step 3 care. Preferred treatments are in bold print. FEV$_1$—forced expiratory volume in 1 second; PEFR—peak expiratory flow rate. (*Adapted from the National Heart, Lung, and Blood Institute [10].*)

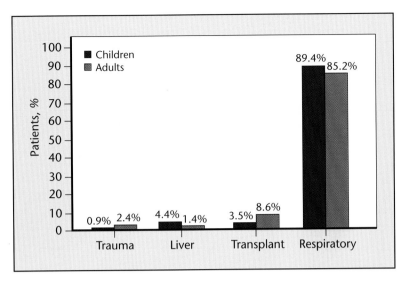

FIGURE 2-14.

Incidence of cystic fibrosis. Cystic fibrosis, also known as "mucovisci-dosis" (especially in some European countries), occurs equally in both sexes. Although it appears in virtually every race, it is most common among whites. (*Courtesy of* Stanley B. Fiel and Daniel V. Schidlow.)

FIGURE 2-13.

Primary cause of death in adult and pediatric cystic fibrosis populations, 1994. Although the manifestations of cystic fibrosis can be widespread, the primary cause of morbidity and mortality in patients with cystic fibrosis is lung disease. Respiratory disease—bronchiectasis and obstruc-tive pulmonary disease—accounts for nearly 90% of deaths in children and adults. (*Adapted from* the New Insights Editorial Board [12].)

FIGURE 2-15.

Predicting the structure of the cystic fibrosis transmembrane con-ductance regulator (CFTR) protein. The CFTR gene, located on chro-mosome 7, was first cloned and sequenced in 1989 [13–15]. The gene contains 27 exons and is flanked by genetic markers KM-19 and J3-11. The messenger RNA (mRNA) is 6129 bp in length, including two hydrophobic transmembrane domains, two nucleotide-binding sites, and a highly charged regulatory (R) domain. The diagram of protein folding is hypothetical. The CFTR protein plays a critical role in electrolyte transport, serving not only as a chloride channel [16], but also as a "switch" that regulates other transepithelial ion channels [17]. (*Adapted from* Ramsey [18].)

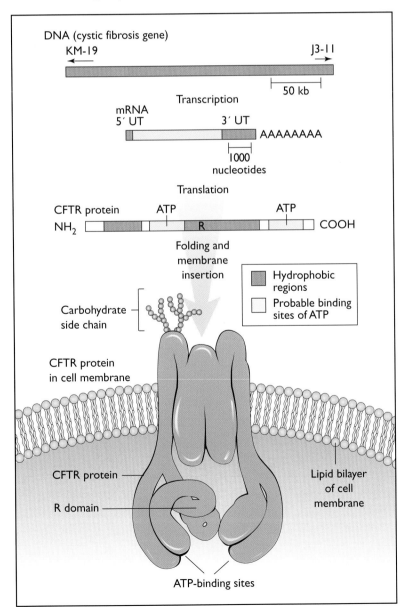

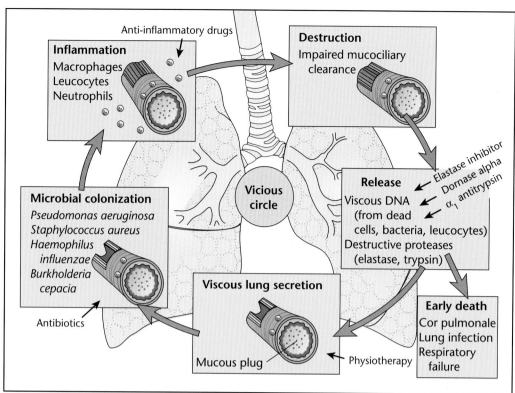

The "vicious circle" of lung disease in cystic fibrosis. Pulmonary disease associated with cystic fibrosis is characterized by a "vicious circle" of obstruction, infection, and inflammation that impairs local host-defense mechanisms, produces progressive bronchiectasis and, ultimately, causes respiratory failure. Although much has been learned about the effect of CFTR on the cell, investigators are still trying to understand how defective transepithelial electrolyte transport leads to the devastating consequences seen throughout the airways. The pathophysiology of airway obstruction, infection, and inflammation is being actively studied. *Courtesy of* Stanley B. Fiel and Daniel V. Schidlow.)

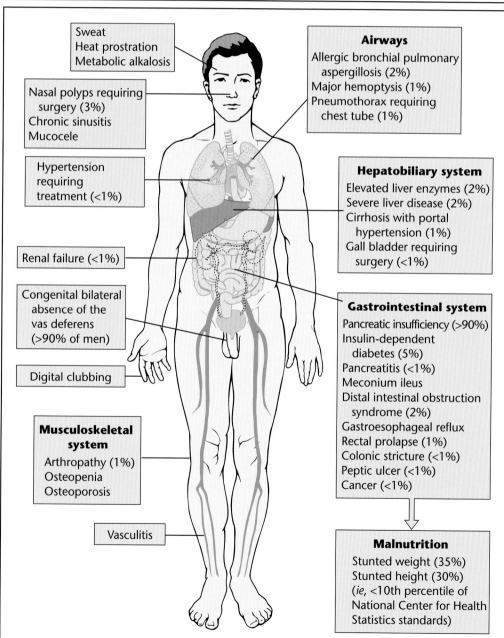

Clinical manifestations and co-morbidity of cystic fibrosis. Cystic fibrosis is associated with numerous complications and co-morbid conditions. As indicated in the figure, almost every patient with cystic fibrosis who lives long enough will eventually develop pulmonary symptoms. However, the age of onset, the rate at which cystic fibrosis progresses, and the incidence of co-morbid conditions are extremely variable. The 1999 incidence of some of these manifestations and co-morbid conditions, obtained from the Cystic Fibrosis Foundation Registry, are provided in parentheses. It is important to note that the incidence of most of these conditions increases significantly with age and disease progression. Thus, the prevalence of some conditions (*eg*, liver disease and diabetes mellitus) in a clinical setting that includes adolescents and young adults can be significantly higher than these figures suggest. (*Courtesy of* Stanley B. Fiel and Daniel V. Schidlow.)

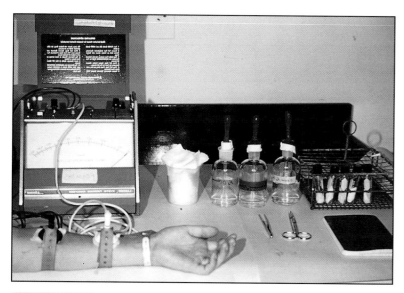

FIGURE 2-18.

The sweat test. Sweat testing, genotyping, and measurement of nasal potential difference (nasal PD) are available to confirm or

exclude the diagnosis of cystic fibrosis. Other specialized diagnostic capabilities include electron microscopic examination of bronchial biopsies for the immotile cilia syndromes and immunologic evaluation for various immune deficiencies that predispose patients to respiratory infections. The sweat test remains one of the cornerstones of the diagnosis and characterization of the cystic fibrosis (CF) syndrome, and it is helpful in confirming the diagnosis in patients with a suspicious clinical picture. Quantitative determinations of chloride in sweat obtained by the Gibson and Cooke iontophoresis method [19] are highly reliable; errors are usually a consequence of sample contamination and technical inexperience. Subcutaneous edema and severe malnutrition can cause false-negative results. False-negative results are associated with hypothyroidism, hypoparathyroidism, and other rare metabolic disorders. Sweat test administration. Indications for a sweat test include a history of CF in the immediate family, chronic pulmonary disease, or pancreatic insufficiency. Other indicators include nasal polyposis, cirrhosis in childhood, and clinical signs or symptoms suggesting a diagnosis. (*Courtesy of* Stanley B. Fiel and Daniel V. Schidlow.)

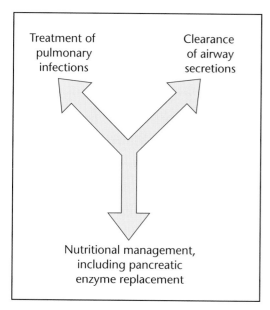

FIGURE 2-19.

Cornerstones of pulmonary therapy for cystic fibrosis. Treatment of cystic fibrosis is directed toward alleviating symptoms and correcting organ dysfunction. Shown here are the three cornerstones of conventional treatment. (*Courtesy of* Stanley B. Fiel and Daniel V. Schidlow.)

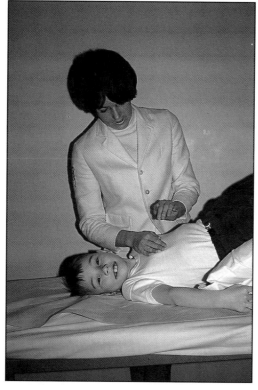

FIGURE 2-20.

Postural drainage and percussion with vibration. For more than 50 years, this technique has been the primary nonpharmacologic strategy for mobilizing viscous secretions and clearing them from the airways [20]. Postural drainage percussion with vibration is still considered by many the gold standard of

therapy, although several alternative airway clearance techniques (ACTs) exist, including 1) autogenic drainage, which can be performed independently by adolescents and adults; 2) positive expiratory pressure, which involves exhaling against expiratory resistance applied through a mask; and 3) active cycle of breathing technique, an independently performed breathing exercise. These three techniques are less demanding than postural drainage and percussion with vibration and can be performed independently; thus, they are often preferred by patients. Newer ACTs (*eg*, high-frequency chest percussors and oral oscillators) are less time-consuming and promote independence; however, their effects on patient compliance have not been determined. Although the short-term effect of ACTs on lung function seems limited, lung function appears to deteriorate when they are discontinued. Exercise is considered an important adjunct to ACT, not a replacement. Patients should be encouraged to incorporate ACTs and exercise into their life styles from the time cystic fibrosis is first diagnosed, even when they are asymptomatic. Clinical judgment is the best guide to selecting a regimen that will be most suitable for a particular patient of a given age and circumstance [20]. (*Courtesy of* Stanley B. Fiel and Daniel V. Schidlow.)

MAJOR TYPES OF LUNG CANCER

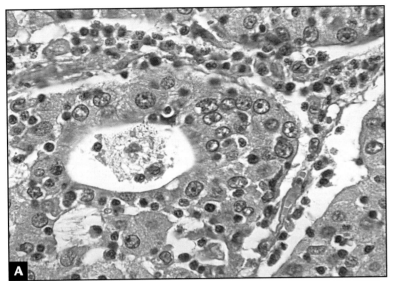

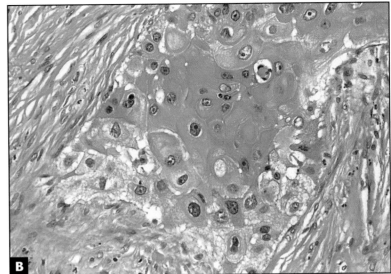

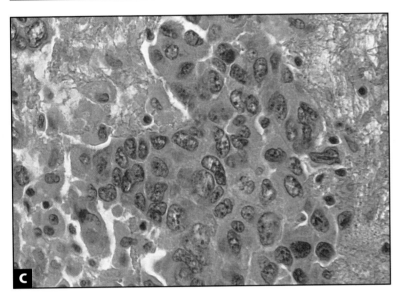

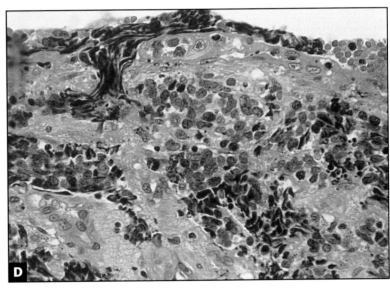

FIGURE 2-21.

Major types of lung cancer. Ninety percent to 95% of all lung cancers can be classified under the four major histologic cell types:
A, Adenocarcinoma accounts for 33% to 35% of all cases.
B, Squamous cell carcinoma accounts for 30% to 32% of all cases.
C, Large cell carcinoma accounts for 15% to 20% of all cases.
D, Small cell carcinoma accounts for 20% to 25% of all cases.
E, Bronchioloalveolar cell carcinoma, a subtype of adenocarcinoma, is less common. (*Courtesy of* Dessmon Y.H. Tai, Raed A. Dweik, Atul C. Mehta, and Muzaffar Ahmad.)

CLINICAL PRESENTATION OF LUNG CANCER

Presentation of Lung Cancer

Local				
Central	**Peripheral**	**Regional**	**Distant**	**Systemic**
Cough	Cough	Horner's syndrome	Bone pain	Weight loss
Hemoptysis	Pain	Pancoast's syndrome	Headache	Anorexia
Pain	Dyspnea	Superior vena cava obstruction	Stroke	Fatigue
Dyspnea		Pleural effusion	Confusion	Fever
Wheezing		Chest pain	Pericardial effusion	
Stridor		Dysphagia	Jaundice	
Pneumonia		Hoarseness (recurrent laryngeal nerve paralysis)	Ascites	
		Elevated hemidiaphragm (phrenic nerve paralysis)	Abdominal pain	
			Hepatomegaly	
			Lymphadenopathy	
			Skin nodules	
			Pulmonary embolism	

FIGURE 2-22.
Clinical presentation of lung cancer. Patients with lung cancer may have local, regional, or metastatic disease. Only 10% to 25% are asymptomatic at the time of diagnosis, when incidental abnormalities are found on chest radiograph. (*Courtesy of* Dessmon Y.H. Tai, Raed A. Dweik, Atul C. Mehta, and Muzaffar Ahmad.)

DIAGNOSIS OF LUNG CANCER

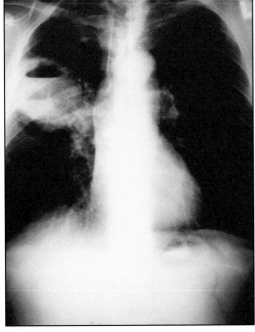

FIGURE 2-23.
Squamous cell lung cancer. Chest radiograph demonstrating two cavitating lesions of squamous cell lung cancer. Squamous cell carcinoma makes up approximately 30% of primary lung tumors. They are usually central, cause partial or complete bronchial obstruction, are usually visualized endoscopically, and may be diagnosed by sputum cytology. The 5-year survival rate is approximately 35%. (*Courtesy of* Charles J. Grodzin.)

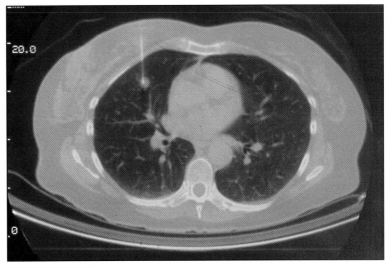

FIGURE 2-24.
Percutaneous transthoracic needle aspiration (TTNA) using computed tomographic guidance. In peripheral lesions, percutaneous TTNA is reported to have twice the diagnostic yield of bronchoscopy, independent of the size of the lesion [21]. Unfortunately, it is also associated with a higher incidence of adverse events. For example, the incidence of pneumothorax with TTNA is 32% to 36% compared with less than 1% with bronchoscopy. The incidence of bleeding is also greater with TTNA (3.5%) than with bronchoscopy (>1%). (*Courtesy of* Dessmon Y.H. Tai, Raed A. Dweik, Atul C. Mehta, and Muzaffar Ahmad.)

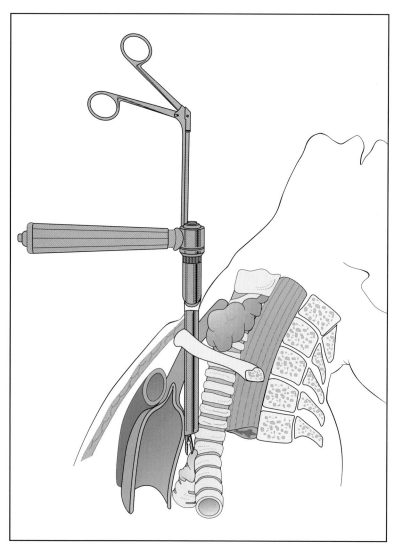

FIGURE 2-25.
Mediastinoscopy and mediastinotomy. Mediastinoscopy is an invasive, yet safe, procedure that can be used to identify malignant
lymph nodes in the superior mediastinum. Mediastinal lymph node
metastasis usually denotes unresectability. (*Courtesy of* Dessmon
Y.H. Tai, Raed A. Dweik, Atul C. Mehta, and Muzaffar Ahmad.)

STAGING OF LUNG CANCER

Stages of Bronchogenic Carcinoma

Stage	Tumor Location	5-y Survival
I	Confined to lung	40% to 80%, with surgical resection
II	Hilar involvement	10% to 20%, with surgical resection
IIIA	Locally extensive intrathoracic involvement	10%, with surgical resection
IIIB	Locally extensive intrathoracic involvement	5%, no surgical resection indicated
IV	Metastases to other organs	1%, no surgical resection indicated

FIGURE 2-26.
Stages of non–small cell bronchogenic carcinoma. Staging provides a guide to available therapeutic options and prognostic information. In most cases, the tumor is incurable at the
time that it is diagnosed. Although the 5-
year survival rate with therapy is only 10%
to 15% overall, it may be as high as 70% to
80% in tumors presenting as a small solitary
pulmonary nodule that are treated promptly.
Early recognition of such cases mainly
depends on the vigilance and timely intervention by the primary care physician. In
general, whereas small cell carcinoma is more
sensitive to radiation or chemotherapy,
non–small cell tumors are treated surgically
when possible due to decreased sensitivity to
radiation or chemotherapy. (*Courtesy of*
Samuel Louie and Glen Lillington.)

Staging of Small Cell Lung Cancer

Limited disease (30%–40%)
Primary tumor confined to one hemithorax
Ipsilateral hilar lymph nodes
Ipsilateral and contralateral supraclavicular lymph nodes
Ipsilateral and contralateral mediastinal lymph nodes
Ipsilateral pleural effusion, independent of cytology
Extensive disease (60%–70%)
Metastatic lesions in the contralateral lung
Distant metastatic involvement (*eg*, brain, bone, liver)

FIGURE 2-27.
Staging and therapy in small cell lung cancer (SCLC). The extent of disease affects chemotherapeutic and radiation therapy options and is helpful when estimating survival time. From time of diagnosis, median survival range for limited disease is 14 to 20 months. For extensive disease, it is 8 to 13 months. (*Courtesy of* Dessmon Y.H. Tai, Raed A. Dweik, Atul C. Mehta, and Muzaffar Ahmad.)

TREATMENT OF LUNG CANCER

Contraindications for Pneumonectomy or Lobectomy

Predicted postoperative FEV_1 <40%, or 0.8 L
$PaCO_2$ >45 mm Hg
PaO_2 <50 mm Hg
Pulmonary hypertension (mean pulmonary artery pressure > 30 mm Hg)
Cor pulmonale
Maximum oxygen consumption <10 mL/kg/min
Intractable congestive cardiac heart failure
Intractable ventricular arrhythmia
Recent myocardial infarction (<3 mo)

FEV_1–forced expiratory volume in 1 s.

FIGURE 2-28.
Treatment of non–small cell lung cancer (NSCLC). Surgery is the primary curative therapy for stage I and II NSCLC and is being used increasingly as a component of multimodality in locally advanced disease (stage IIIa and IIIb). Contraindications for surgery are listed in the figure. (*Courtesy of* Dessmon Y.H. Tai, Raed A. Dweik, Atul C. Mehta, and Muzaffar Ahmad.)

■ INFECTIOUS DISEASES OF THE LUNG

COMMUNITY ACQUIRED AND NOSOCOMIAL PNEUMONIAS

Diagnostic Evaluation

Chest radiograph
Sputum Gram stain/culture
Blood cultures
Serology
Sputum direct fluorescent antibody/urinary antigen for *Legionella pneumophila*

FIGURE 2-29.
Diagnostic evaluation for pneumonia. The usual diagnostic work-up for pneumonia includes a chest radiograph. Although useful in determining if pneumonia is present, the chest radiograph offers little information on the causative pathogen. Sputum cultures are often obtained, but their usefulness is a subject of a great deal of debate [22, 23]. False-positive and false-negative results are common for *Streptococcus pneumoniae* and *Haemophilus influenzae*. A sputum Gram stain actually provides more information than a sputum culture when pneumococcus is the causative organism [24]. Serology is rarely useful and, therefore, is usually not indicated in the typical case of community-acquired pneumonia [23]. Urinary *Legionella* antigen is very sensitive and specific for *Legionella pneumophila* serotype I. A direct fluorescent antibody text on sputum for *Legionella* has a sensitivity of only about 50% [23]. Blood cultures should be obtained in every patient admitted to the hospital, because bacteremia occurs in 20% to 30% of patients with pneumococcal pneumonia. (*Courtesy of* John Segreti.)

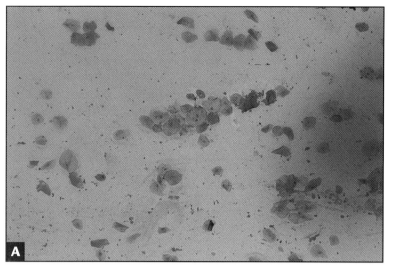

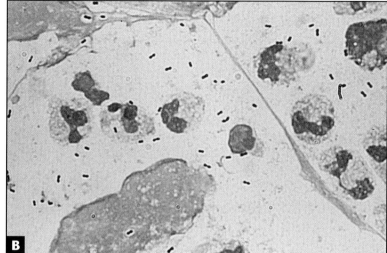

FIGURE 2-30.

Examples of inappropriate and appropriate sputum samples. **A,** Sputum should not be cultured if more than 25 epithelial cells per low-powered field are seen. **B,** A sputum Gram stain showing many white cells and gram-positive diplococci is more sensitive and specific for pneumococcal infecton than a sputum culture [24]. (*Courtesy of* John Segreti.)

A. Community-acquired Pneumonia Pathogens* in Hospitalized Patients

Not Maximally Severe Pneumonia
Streptococcus pneumoniae
Haemophilus influenzae
Polymicrobial (including anaerobes)
Aerobic gram-negative bacilli
Legionella spp.
Staphylococcus aureus
Chlamydia pneumoniae
Respiratory tract viruses
Other: *Mycoplasma pneumoniae, Moraxella catarrhalis*
Unusual organisms: *Mycobacterium tuberculosis*, endemic fungi,
    Pneumocystis carinii

Severe Pneumonia (often treated in the intensive care unit)
S. pneumoniae
Legionella spp.
Aerobic gram-negative bacilli (including *Pseudomonas aeruginosa*)
M. pneumoniae
Respiratory tract viruses
Others: *H. influenzae*
Unusual organisms: *M. tuberculosis*, endemic fungi, *P. carinii*

*Pathogens are listed in descending order of frequency.

B. Pathogens* in Community-acquired, Mild Pneumonia in Outpatient Therapy

Patient Younger Than 60 Years of Age with No Comorbidity
Streptococcus pneumoniae
Mycoplasma pneumoniae
Respiratory tract viruses
Chlamydia pneumoniae
Haemophilus influenzae (especially in smokers)
Others: *Legionella* spp., *Staphylococcus aureus, Pneumocystis
    carinii*, gram-negative bacilli
Unusual organisms: *Mycobacterium tuberculosis*, endemic fungi

Patient Older Than 60 Years of Age with or without Comorbid Illness
S. pneumoniae
H. influenzae
Aerobic gram-negative bacilli
Oropharyngeal anaerobes
S. aureus
Respiratory tract viruses
Others: *Legionella* spp., *Moraxella catarrhalis*
Unusual organisms: *M. tuberculosis*, endemic fungi, *P. carinii*

*Pathogens are listed in descending order of frequency.

FIGURE 2-31.

Pathogens in community-acquired, mild pneumonia in hospitalized (**A**) and non-hospitalized (**B**) patients. In 50% of cases of pneumonia, an infectious isolate may not be found. In all categories, *Streptococcus pneumoniae* is the most common organism. Host risk factors include patient age, presence of comorbidities, severity of illness, recent antibiotic therapy, acquired or congenital immunosuppression, and presence of structural lung disease (*eg*, bronchiectasis). Risk factors for mortality in community-acquired pneumonia include a respiratory rate greater than 30 breaths per minute, a diastolic blood pressure less than 60 mm Hg, and evidence of dehydration with a blood urea nitrogen level greater than 20 mg/dL. Nosocomial pneumonia is the most common hospital acquired infection to lead to patient mortality. (*Courtesy of* Michael S. Niederman.)

A. Empirical Therapy of Patients with Community-acquired Pneumonia

Outpatient Therapy

Patient younger than age 60 years with no comorbidity
Erythromycin
or New macrolides: clarithromycin, azithromycin
or Tetracyclines*
Patient older than age 60 years with or without comorbid illness
Second- or third-generation cephalosporin
or β-Lactam/β-lactamase inhibitor combination
or Newer quinolones: levofloxacin, sparfloxacin

Inpatient Therapy

Not maximally severe pneumonia
Second- or third-generation (cefotaxime, ceftriaxone) cephalosporin
or β-Lactam/β-lactamase inhibitor combination
± Macrolide
or Levofloxacin
Severe pneumonia
Macrolide ± Rifampin (if *Legionella* spp. likely)
PLUS:†
Third- or fourth-generation cephalosporin with anti-Pseudomonal activity (ceftazidime, cefepime)
or Meropenem
or Imipenem/cilastatin
or Ciprofloxacin
or Mevopenem

*Many *Streptococcus pneumoniae* are resistant, and this antimicrobial should only be used if the patient is allergic to or intolerant of macrolides.
†Consider initial dual anti-Pseudomonal therapy.

B. Antibiotic Therapy of Nosocomial Pneumonia

Treatment of the Core Pathogens
"Core antibiotics"

Second-generation or non-Pseudomonal third-generation cephalosporin
β-Lactam/β-lactamase inhibitor combination
Fluoroquinolone (ciprofloxacin or ofloxacin)*
Aztreonam and clindamycin*

Treatment of Core Pathogens Plus Specific Organisms Dictated by Risk Factors

Aspiration, recent abdominal surgery (anaerobes): Core antibiotic plus clindamycin or β-lactam/β-lactamase inhibitor alone
Coma, head trauma, diabetes, renal failure (*S. aureus*): Use core antibiotic active against *S. aureus*, consider adding vancomycin
Corticosteroids (*Legionella*): core antibiotic plus erythromycin
Prolonged stay in hospital or intensive care unit, recent antibiotics: treat as severe pneumonia

Treatment of Severe Pneumonia

Aminoglycoside or ciprofloxacin **plus one of the following:**
Anti-pseudomonal penicillin (piperacillin)
Anti-pseudomonal cephalosporin (ceftazidime, cefepime)
Imipenem or meropenem
Aztreonam
Anti-pseudomonal β-lactam/β-lactamase inhibitor combination (ticarcillin/ clavulanate, piperacillin/tazobactam)

PLUS:
Consider vancomycin if methicillin-resistant *S. aureus* is likely

*For use in patients allergic to penicillin.

FIGURE 2-32.

Empiric therapy of patients with community-acquired (**A**) and nosocomial (**B**) pneumonia. The bacteriology of early-onset and late-onset nosocomial pneumonia differs. Resistant Gram-negative organisms are a particular concern for late-onset pneumonia. Therapy can be directed by sputum Gram stain and culture or may be empiric. Empiric therapy is necessary because many episodes of infectious pneumonia remain undiagnosed. Most patients should be treated for a duration of 10 to 14 days. Clinical improvement may not be seen for 48 to 72 hours, and radiographic resolution may not be evident for weeks to months. Lack of clinical response should prompt several considerations: sensitivity of the organism to the antibiotic used, the identity of the suspected organism, development of a super infection, presence of a second organism, presence of a non-infectious process, and the possibility of a complicating circumstance, such as bronchial obstruction or empyema. (*Courtesy of Michael S. Niederman.*)

A. Presentation of Mycobacterium Tuberculosis Infection Versus Acute Disease

Criteria	Infection	Disease
PPD+	Yes	Yes
Symptoms	No	Yes
Chest radiograph	Normal (patients may have an abnormal chest radiograph)	Abnormal
Communicable	Abnormal	Yes
	Yes	

PPD+ — positive PPD+ - positive purified protein derivative (skin test for tuberculosis)

B. Factors Leading to Disease Progression

HIV
Substance abuse
Diabetes mellitus
Silicosis
Cancer
Chemotherapy
Malnutrition

FIGURE 2-33.

A, Presentation of *Mycobacterium tuberculosis* infection versus active disease. After exposure to *M. tuberculosis* and the development of an immune response (positive tuberculin skin test), patients have a 5% chance of developing active disease in the next 2 years. Over the rest of their lifetime, there is an additional 5% risk of disease.

B, In the presence of any of the risk factors listed in this figure, the odds of developing active disease are much higher. A person infected with HIV exposed to *M. tuberculosis* has a 10% chance per year of developing active disease, unless adequate prophylactic measures are taken. (*Courtesy of* Joseph H. Bates.)

Risk Factors Associated with Latent Tuberculosis Infection

>5 mm Induration	>10 mm Induration	>15 mm Induration
Contacts with patients with tuberculosis	Residents of countries with high prevalence rates	No risk factors
HIV infection and other forms of immunosuppression	Residents of prisons, nursing homes, and homeless shelters	
Abnormal chest radiograph results	Intravenous drug use	
	Some low-income populations	
	Medical risk factors (*eg.*, diabetes, renal failure, steroids, malignancies, transplantation, malnutrition, silicosis)	
	Locally defined high-risk populations	
	Children in close contact with persons with active disease	

PPD–purified protein derivative.

FIGURE 2-34.

Approximately 75% of newly diagnosed cases of tuberculosis are tuberculin skin test (TST) positive when first diagnosed, although almost all cases become TST-positive after approximately 2 months of successful chemotherapy. Vaccination with bacille Calmette-Guerin (BCG) produces a positive TST in most subjects, but this reaction tends to wane over time. After 10 years, most subjects are TST-negative unless they have inhaled viable *M. tuberculosis* in the interim. For those at high risk of becoming infected with *M. tuberculosis*, such as some health care workers, prison employees, workers in homeless shelters, and those visiting countries that have a high prevalence of tuberculosis, annual TSTs are advised. For these patients, the initial skin test should be repeated in 2 to 4 weeks if the first reading shows less than 10 mm induration. The second TST may elicit a "booster reaction," giving a larger degree of induration on the second test; the second test reading should be recorded as the baseline measure of the skin test [25]. (*Courtesy of* Joseph H. Bates.)

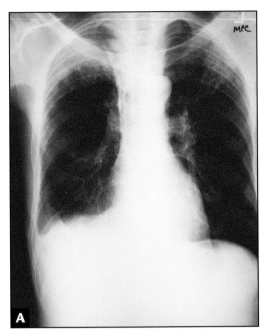
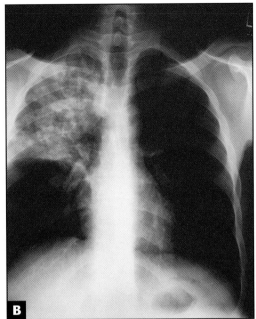
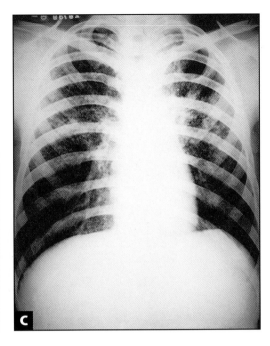

FIGURE 2-35.

Tuberculosis. **A** and **B**, Radiographs demonstrating two patterns of apical opacification, each proven to be due to *Mycobacterium tuberculosis* infection. Note that the opacification in **B** delineates the minor fissure on the *right*, which means that the anterior segment of the right upper lobe is also involved. **C**, Radiograph demonstrating a miliary pattern in *M. tuberculosis* infection.

First-line Antituberculosis Agents

Drug	Dosage Form	Daily Dose	Twice-weekly Dosage	Adverse Reactions	Drug Interactions
Isoniazid	Oral, intramuscular	5 mg/kg, up to 300 mg	15 mg/kg, up to 900 mg	Hepatic enzyme elevation, hepatitis, peripheral neuropathy, hypersensitivity	Phenytoin, disulfiram, corticosteroids
Rifampin	Oral	10 mg/kg, up to 600 mg	10 mg/kg, up to 600 mg	Orange discoloration of body fluids, nausea, vomiting, hepatits, febrile reaction, purpura	Warfarin, nortriptyline, barbituates, benzodiazepines, oral contraceptives, corticosteroids, digitalis, halothane, oral hypoglycemics, quinidine
Pyrazinamide	Oral	15–30 mg/kg, up to 2 g	15–70 mg/kg, up to 4 g	Hepatoxicity, hyperuricemia, arthralgia, rash, gastrointestinal upset	Allopurinol; diuretics may amplify uricemia
Ethambutol	Oral	15–25 mg/kg	50 mg/kg	Optic neuritis (decreased red-green color discrimination, decreased visual acuity), rash	Aluminum salts
Streptomycin	Intramuscular	15 mg/kg, up to 1 g in persons age < y; 10 mg/kg up to 750 mg in persons > 60 y	25–30 mg/kg, up to 1.5 g	Ototoxicity, nephrotoxicity	Furosemide, ethacrynic acid, mannitol, cisplatin, indomethacin, acyclovir, amphotericin B, capreomycin, bacitracin, polymyxin B, vancomycin, aminoglycosides

FIGURE 2-36.

Treatment of active tuberculosis requires the use of at least two potent antituberculosis drugs to which the infecting isolate is sensitive. When there is a slight possibility of a resistant strain, three drugs are advised when therapy is begun. The most common combination used in the United States is isoniazid, rifampin, and pyrazinamide. When this combination is given and ingested in the proper doses, the cure rate can be as high as 98% for those who complete a full course of treatment lasting from 6 to 9 months. If drug resistance is unlikely, as is the case for some patients in select geographic areas of the United States, isoniazid and rifampin alone may be given as the initial regimen for newly diagnosed patients older than 60 years. When drug resistance is a possibility, four or more drugs should be selected for the initial regimen, with adjustments in the treatment regimen planned after results of drug susceptibility are reported. (*Courtesy of* Joseph H. Bates.)

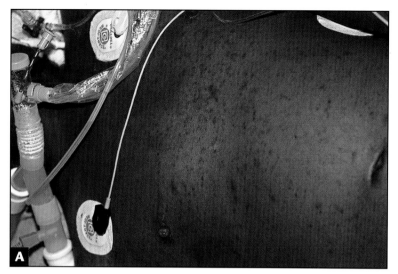

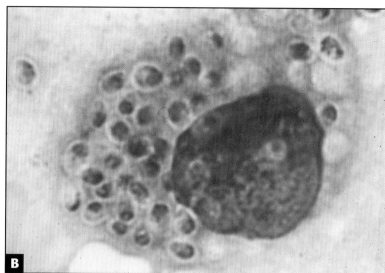

FIGURE 2-37.

Progressive disseminated histoplasmosis [26]. In Southeast Asia, patients infected with HIV have an illness caused by *Penicillium marnefeii,* which resembles histoplasmosis. Itraconazole is effective in this condition as it is in histoplasmosis. **A,** Patient with HIV and cutaneous manifestations of progressive disseminated histoplasmosis. **B,** Organisms of *Histoplasma capsulatum* inside human macrophage. (*Courtesy of* Robert W. Bradsher.)

Guidelines for Management of Patients with Histoplasmosis, 2000

	Severe	Moderate
Acute pulmonary	AmB, steroids, then itra	None, itra if symptomatic 4 wk
Chronic pulmonary	AmB, then itra 12–24 mo	Itra 12–24 mo
Disseminated non-HIV	AmB, then itra 6–8 mo	Itra 6–18 mo
Disseminated AIDS	AmB, then itra life	Itra life
Meningitis	AmB 3 mo, then flucon 1 y	Same, because of poor prognosis
Granulomatous mediastinitis	AmB, then itra 6–12 mo	Itra 6–12 mo
Fibrosing mediastinitis	Itra 3 mo	Itra 3 mo
Pericarditis	Steroids	NSAIDS
Rheumatologic	NSAIDS	NSAIDS

FIGURE 2-38.

Guidelines for management of patients with histoplasmosis, 2000. AmB—amphotericin B; Flucon—fluconazole; Itra—itraconzaole; NSAID—nonsteroidal anti-inflammatory drug. (*Adapted from* Wheat *et al.* [27].)

VENOUS THROMBOEMBOLISM

Risk Factors for Venous Thromboembolic Disease

Stasis of Blood Flow
Prolonged bedrest or immobility
Congestive heart failure
Paralytic stroke

Intimal Injury
Prior thromboembolism
Trauma (especially to lower extremities, pelvis, and spinal cord)
Major surgery (especially involving lower extremity, abdomen, and pelvis)

Hypercoagulable States
Primary
Antithrombin III deficiency
Protein C deficiency
Protein S deficiency
Factor V Leiden mutation
Dysfibrinogenemia
Homocystinuria
Increased factor VIII levels
Secondary
Malignancy
Pregnancy (especially in the puerperium)
Trauma/major surgery
Oral contraceptives
Nephrotic syndrome
Myeloproliferative syndromes
Lupus anticoagulant/antiphospholipid syndrome
High-dose chemotherapy
Heparin-induced thrombocytopenia and thrombosis
Obesity
Age >40 y

FIGURE 2-39.

Risk factors associated with venous thromboembolism (VTE). The great 19th century German pathologist Rudolph Virchow proposed three basic factors leading to thrombus formation. Today, "Virchow's triad"—stasis of blood flow, intimal injury, and hypercoagulability—still provides the basis for our understanding of clinically apparent risk factors for VTE. VTE is unusual in patients who do not have at least one risk factor. As the number of risk factors increases, the degree of risk also increases.

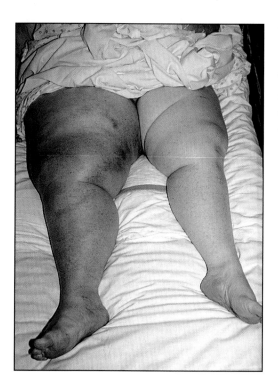

FIGURE 2-40.

Deep vein thrombosis (DVT). A 35-year-old woman with slightly prolonged activated partial thromboplastin time had a massively swollen leg. DVT was confirmed by noninvasive testing. The patient was also found to have a lupus anticoagulant. Several other disease processes may mimic DVT, and the clinical examination is less than 50% accurate. In symptomatic individuals, noninvasive tests such as impedance plethysmography or ultrasonography are extremely accurate (above the knees) and are usually sufficient to make the diagnosis.

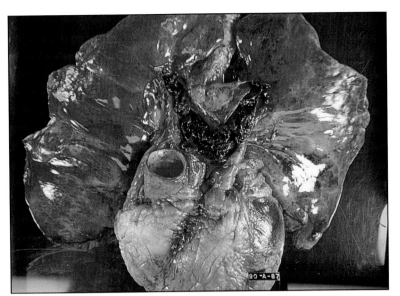

FIGURE 2-41.
Autopsy specimen showing saddle pulmonary embolism. *Saddle embolism* is a term used to describe embolic obstruction at the bifurcation of the main trunk of the pulmonary artery. This massive embolus resulted in acute right-sided heart failure, cardiogenic shock, and death. Appropriate prophylaxis therapy may prevent such a catastrophic sequela of deep vein thrombosis.

CLINICAL FEATURES

Signs or Symptoms Observed in Patients with Thromboembolism

		Study	
		Stein *et al.* [28], % (*n* = 117)	Anderson *et al.* [29], % (*n* =131)
Pulmonary embolism	Dyspnea	73	77
	Tachypnea	70	70
	Chest pain	66	55
	Cough	37	—
	Tachycardia	30	43
	Cyanosis	1	18
	Hemoptysis	13	13
	Wheezing	9	—
	Hypotension	—	10
	Syncope	—	10
	Elevated jugular venous pulse	—	8
	Temperature >38.5°C	7	—
	S-3 gallop	3	5
	Pleural friction rub	3	2
Deep vein thrombosis	Swelling	28	88*
	Pain	26	56
	Tenderness	—	55
	Warmth	—	42
	Redness	—	34
	Homan's sign	4	13
	Palpable cord	—	6

*n = 274.

FIGURE 2-42.
Signs and symptoms associated with acute thromboembolism. The study by Stein *et al.* [28] consisted of patients from the Prospective Investigation of Pulmonary Embolism Diagnosis (PIOPED) trial and was screened to exclude patients with preexisting cardiac or pulmonary disease. In contrast, almost one third of patients in the retrospective study by Anderson *et al.* [29] had evidence of chronic obstructive pulmonary disease and congestive heart failure. Although individual signs and symptoms are not sensitive or specific, Stein's group reported that 91% of patients with proven pulmonary embolism were found to have dyspnea, hemoptysis, or pleuritic chest pain.

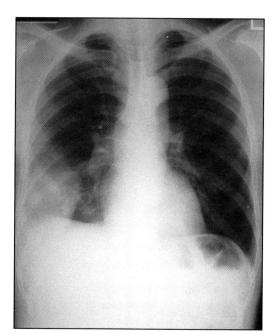

FIGURE 2-43.

Chest radiograph showing pulmonary infarct in the right lower lobe. This patient had low-grade fever, hemoptysis, and pleuritic chest pain. The ventilation-perfusion scan was read as high probability for pulmonary embolism. A pleural-based density in the lower lobe with the convexity directed toward the hilum signifies pulmonary infarction. This sign is also known as "Hampton's hump."

DIAGNOSIS OF VENOUS THROMBOEMBOLISM

Tests Used in Diagnosis of Deep Vein Thrombosis

Test	Description
Contrast venography	Diagnostic gold standard and the only accurate method for determining the presence or absence of DVT in asymptomatic individuals. The test is difficult to perform and many patients experience discomfort from the procedure. Approx 1-2 percent of patients and up to 10% of test results may be uninterpretable due to inadequate examinations or interobserver variability [30].
IPG	Inflation and deflation of a thigh cuff causes changes in electrical impedance, which are attenuated by presence of thrombus. The negative predictive value of IPG and ultrasonography are identical. Serial negative IPG or ultrasonography is comparable in accuracy to negative venography in patients with suspected DVT [31, 32].
Compression ultrasound	In many centers, this is the diagnostic modality of choice. The sensitivity and specificity approach 97%–98% for symptomatic patients. The sensitivity for high-risk asymptomatic individuals is only 50%–60% [31].
Magnetic resonance imaging	Preliminary studies indicate very high sensitivity and specificity. Useful for accurate imaging of clots in all areas. Although noninvasive, the test is expensive and experience is limited [33].
D-Dimer	Recent studies indicate that low levels of plasma D-dimer (<500 ng/mL) by ELISA technique may have a high negative predictive value when used in patients with suspected venous thromboembolism. The sensitivity is reported to be 95%–98% and the specificity below 50% [34]. A whole blood agglutination assay has also been reported to have a sensitivity of 97.5%. The result of a D-dimer assay in addition to noninvasive imaging may be useful in excluding thromboembolic disease with more confidence [35].

DVT—deep vein thrombosis; ELISA—enzyme-linked immunosorbent assay; IPG—impedance plethysmography.

FIGURE 2-44.

Tests used in the diagnosis of deep vein thrombosis. The various tests used to diagnose thrombosis in proximal thigh veins are summarized in the figure. The reliable diagnosis of calf vein thrombi is possible only with contrast venography or magnetic resonance imaging. The clinical significance of these thrombi is debatable because less than 20% migrate proximally. If calf thrombi are diagnosed, serial noninvasive testing to observe for proximal migration is prudent.

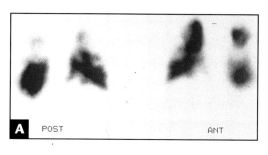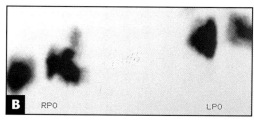

FIGURE 2-45.

High-probability ventialtion-perfusion scan. The ventilation-perfusion lung scan is frequently the first diagnostic test ordered in patients suspected of having a pulmonary embolism. **A** and **B**, Multiple large segmental and subsegmental perfusion defects are seen bilaterally.

(Continued)

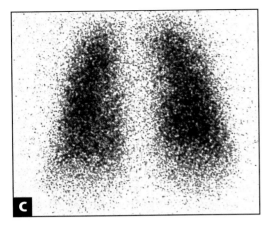

FIGURE 2-45. *(CONTINUED)*
C, The corresponding ventilation image was normal. The patient was treated for pulmonary embolism.

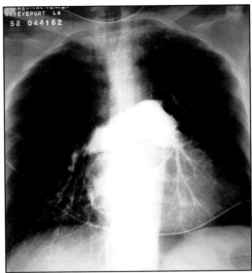

FIGURE 2-46.
Pulmonary angiogram showing pulmonary embolism. Pulmonary angiography remains the diagnostic gold standard for pulmonary embolism. Access to the pulmonary artery is obtained via transvenous catheter placement. The diagnosis is confirmed by persistent filling defect or abrupt cut-off of flow. Abrupt cut-off of flow to the right and left upper lobe vessels is seen in this patient.

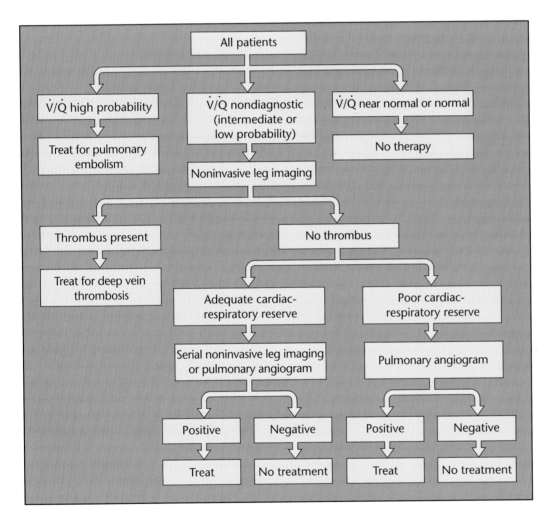

FIGURE 2-47.
Suggested diagnostic strategy for venous thromboembolism. The PIOPED study revealed that results of ventilation-perfusion (V̇/Q̇) scans are nondiagnostic in more than 70% of the cases. The diagnostic strategy proposed in the figure provides a rational approach to work up patients with suspected thromboembolic disease. The role of spiral CT scan in the diagnosis of pulmonary embolism remains controversial with a wide range of reported sensitivities (53%–100%) and specificities (81%–100%) [36]. (*Adapted from* Stein *et al.* [37].)

Recommendations for the Prevention of Venous Thromboembolism

Nature of Illness/Surgery	Grade/Level of Evidence	Recommendation
Low-risk general surgical patients undergoing minor surgery; age <40 y, no specific risk factors	Grade C/level 3 data	Early ambulation
Moderate-risk general surgical patients undergoing major operations; age >40 y, no specific risk factors	Grade A/level 1 data	Elastic stockings; IPC, LDUH every 12 h
High-risk patients undergoing major general surgical procedures; age > 40 y, other risk factors present	Grade A/level 1 data	LDUH every 8 or LMWH IPC would be a good choice if high-risk for wound hematoma
Very high-risk general surgical patients with multiple risk factors	Grade B/level 2 data	LDUH or LMWH or dextran plus IPC; start heparin preoperatively Dextran and IPC can be used intraoperatively
Hip replacement	Grade A/level 1 data	LMWH or warfarin (INR 2.0–3.0) or adjusted-dose heparin Start preoperatively or immediately postoperatively IPC and elastic stockings plus anticoagulants have added benefit
Knee replacement	Grade A/level 1 data	LMWH or IPC
Hip fracture	Grade A/level 1 data	LMWH or warfarin
Intracranial neurosurgery	Grade A/level 1 data	IPC and/or elastic stockings; LDUH acceptable; IPC plus LDUH are more effacious and should be considered in high-risk patients.
Spinal cord injury and paralysis	Grade B/level 2 data Grade C/level 4 Grade B/level 2	Adjusted-dose heparin or LMWH Warfarin (INR 2.0–3.0) LDUH, elastic stockings, and IPC used alone are ineffective; they may be useful in combination
Multiple trauma	Grade C/level 3, 4	IPC/LMWH warfarin when feasible Consider inferior vena caval filter, serial duplex/IPG
Myocardial infarction	Grade A/level 1 Grade C/level 4	LDUH or full-dose anticoagulation IPC/elastic stockings if heparin contraindicated
Ischemic stroke; lower extremity paralysis	Grade A/level 1 data Grade C/level 4	LDUH or LMWH IPC/elastic stockings
General medical patients/congestive heart failure/chest infection	Grade A/level 1 data	LDUH or LMWH
Long-term central vein catheter	Grade A/level 1 data	Coumadin 1 mg daily

FIGURE 2-48.

Recommendations for prevention of venous thromboembolism (VTE). Recommendations based on level 1 or level 2 evidence are supported by findings in randomized controlled trials of meta-analysis. Despite widespread recognition of the risks of VTE in selected patient groups with known risk factors, prophylaxis remains underused. Effective methods of prevention are more practical and cost effective than intensive surveillance. Because VTE may be clinically silent (and suddenly fatal), it is unwise to rely on the development of compatible signs and symptoms. (*Adapted from* Clagget *et al.* [38].)

Dosage and Monitoring of Anticoagulant Therapy

After initiating heparin therapy, repeat APTT every 6 h for first 24 h and then every 24 h when therapeutic APTT is achieved

Warfarin 5 mg/d can be started on day 1 of therapy; there is no benefit from higher starting doses

Platelet count should be monitored at least every 3 d during initial heparin therapy

Therapeutic APTT should correspond to plasma heparin level of 0.2–0.4 IU/mL

Heparin is usually continued for 5–7 d

Heparin can be stopped after 4–5 d of warfarin therapy when INR is in 2.0–3.0 range

APTT—activated partial thromboplastin time; INR—International Normalized Ratio.

FIGURE 2-49.

Dosage and monitoring of anticoagulant therapy [39,40]. An activated partial thromboplastin time ratio of 1.5 to 2.5 has traditionally been used to define the boundaries of therapeutic heparin effects. The actual therapeutic range may vary according to the thromboplastin reagent used by a particular laboratory. Warfarin acts by inhibiting the synthesis of vitamin K-dependent coagulation factors in the liver (II, VII, IX, and X). The half-lives of these factors are relatively long (60, 6, 24, and 40 hours, respectively), thus the onset of action of warfarin is slow—3 or more days may be required to achieve a therapeutic response. Traditionally, warfarin therapy has been monitored by measuring the prothrombin time (PT). To standardize the monitoring of therapy, the INR is used by many laboratories. The PT of the patient is compared with a normal control PT value; this ratio is then plotted against the International Sensitivity Index (ISI) to calculate the INR (INR = PT ratio^{isi}). The ISI is obtained by comparing the local thromboplastin reagent used for testing with a standardized international reagent [41].

Low–molecular-weight Heparin Preparations

Product Name (Trade Name)	Type of Use	Indications	Dosage	Pregnancy Category	FDA Approval Date
Ardeparin (Normiflo; Wyeth-Ayerst, Philadelphia, PA)	Prophylaxis	Knee replacement	50 units/kg SC q 12 h	C	January 1998
Dalteparin (Fragmin; Pharmacia & Upjohn, Peapack, NJ)	Prophylaxis	Abdominal surgery	2500 units SC QD	B	December 1994
		Orthopedic surgery/high-risk patient	5000 Units SC QD		
	Treatment	DVT and/or PE	200 units/kg SC QD up to 18,000 units SC QD		
Enoxaparin (Lovenox; Aventis, Parsippany, NJ)	Prophylaxis	Knee replacement/hip replacement	30 units SC q 12 h	B	March 1993
		Abdominal surgery/hip replacement/very high risk patient	40 units SC QD		
Tinzaparin (Innohep; DuPont, Wilmington, DE)	Treatment	DVT and/or PE	1 mg/kg SC q 12 h	B	July 2000
	Treatment	DVT and/or PE	175 units/kg SC QD		

FIGURE 2-50.

Low–molecular-weight heparin preparations. Ardeparin, dalteparin, enoxaparin, and tinzaparin are low-molecular-weight heparins approved for use in the United States. This group of agents acts by inhibition of factor Xa more than thrombin (IIa), thus they have much less effect on the activated partial thromboplastin time than unfractionated heparin. They have a longer half-life and the convenience of once or twice daily dosing. However, they are 10 to 20 times more expensive than unfractionated heparin [42].

Outpatient Therapy of DVT with Low Molecular Weight Heparin

Confirmed diagnosis by objective criteria (Doppler ultrasonography or venography)

Obtain complete blood count with platelets, PT, and PTT; initiate any further work-up for underlying cause of thrombosis

Patient (or family member/caretaker) must demonstrate ability to give subcutaneous injections

First dose of LMWH administered at health facility

Begin oral anticoagulant

Arrange outpatient laboratory twice weekly (PT, INR, and complete blood count)

Follow up with full clinical visit within 7 days of initiating therapy, discontinue LMWH when INR ranges from 2.0 to 3.0

Consider in-patient therapy when:

    Signs or symptoms of pulmonary embolism, or confirmed PE

    Comorbid condition prompting admission

    History of heparin-induced thrombocytopenia

    History of nonadherence with medical regimen

    Inaccessible to close follow-up

    High risk for complications and bleeding

        Elderly or high risk for falls

        Low hemoglobin at diagnosis

        Active bleeding (ie, heme-positive stool)

        History of CVA within 6 weeks

        History of major surgery within 2 weeks

        Thrombocytopenia

        Any other medical condition with increased risk of bleeding

        Patients on hemodialysis

FIGURE 2-51.

Outpatient therapy of DVT with low molecular weight heparin (LMWH). Studies have shown that outpatient treatment of DVT with LMWH has comparable efficacy and safety compared to inpatient treatment with heparin and/or coumadin [43–45]. LMWH has made outpatient treatment of thromboembolic disease feasible because of its ease of administration, safety, and reduced need for laboratory monitoring, as well as decreased health care costs and improved patient satisfaction. However, because of the longer half-life of LMWH, patients at high risk for bleeding may benefit from UFH, which allows for quicker reversal of anticoagulation in the event of bleeding. Careful selection of patients who are good candidates for outpatient treatment will help lessen complications [46]. These are general recommendations only. The decision to admit or discharge early must be individualized. The outpatient treatment of patients with documented pulmonary embolism is being investigated, and studies have been promising in those with hemodynamically stable pulmonary embolism [47,48].

Complications of Anticoagulation

	Complications	Management
Heparin	Bleeding	Stop heparin infusion. For severe bleeding, the anticoagulant effect of heparin can be reversed with intravenous protamine sulfate 1 mg/100 units of heparin bolus or 0.5 mg for the number of units given by constant infusion over the past hour; provide supportive care including transfusion and clot evacuation from closed body cavities as needed.
	Heparin-induced thrombocytopenia and thrombosis	Carefully monitor platelet count during therapy. Stop heparin for platelet counts <75,000. Replace heparin with direct inhibitors of thrombin-like desirudin if necessary. These agents do not cause heparin-induced thrombocytopenia. Avoid platelet transfusion because of the risk of thrombosis.
	Heparin-induced osteoporosis (therapy >1 mo)	LMWHs may have lower propensity to cause osteoporosis as compared with unfractionated heparin; consider LMWH if prolonged heparin therapy is necessary.
Warfarin	Bleeding	Stop therapy. Administer vitamin K and fresh-frozen plasma for severe bleeding; provide supportive care including transfusion and clot evacuation from closed body cavities as needed.
	Skin necrosis (rare)	Supportive care.
	Teratogenicity	Do not use in pregnancy or in patients planning to become pregnant.

FIGURE 2-52.

Complications of anticoagulation. Major bleeding episodes with the use of heparin are much more likely to occur in patients with identifiable risks for bleeding rather than an excessively long activated partial thromboplastin time per se low molecular weight heparin (LMWH) does not affect the APTT to a significant degree; therefore, the APTT need not be routinely measured. Many factors influence the prothrombin time during warfarin therapy. Weekly or biweekly measurements are necessary until the prothrombin time stabilizes. Thereafter, monthly measurements of the prothrombin time may be sufficient.

Approved Thrombolytics for Pulmonary Embolism

Streptokinase
  250,000 IU as loading dose over 30 min, followed by 100,000 U/h for 24 h

Urokinase
  4400 IU/kg as a loading dose over 10 min, followed by 4400 IU/kg/h for 12–24 h

Recombinant tissue-plasminogen activator
  100 mg as a continuous peripheral intravenous infusion administered over 2 h

FIGURE 2-53.

Approved thrombolytics for pulmonary embolism. All three US Food and Drug Administration–approved regimens used fixed or weight-adjusted doses. No further dosage adjustments are made. Heparin is resumed after the thrombolytic infusion when the activated partial thromboplastin time is less than 2.5 × control.

Indications and Contraindications for Thrombolytic Therapy in Pulmonary Embolism

Indications
Hemodynamic instability
Hypoxia on 100% oxygen
Right ventricular dysfunction by echocardiography [49]

Contraindications [50]
Relative
  Recent surgery within last 10 d
  Neurosurgery within 6 mo
  Ophthalmologic surgery within 6 wk
  Hypertension <200 mm Hg systolic or 110 mm Hg diastolic
  Hypertensive retinopathy with hemorrhages or exudates
  Cerebrovascular disease
  Major internal bleeding within the last 6 mo
  Infectious endocarditis
  Pericarditis
Absolute
  Active internal bleeding
  Previous arterial punctures within 10 d
  Bleeding disorder (thrombocytopenia, renal failure, liver failure)
  Placement of central venous catheter within 48 h
  Intracerebral aneurysm or malignancy
  Cardiopulmonary resuscitation within 2 wk
  Pregnancy and the first 10 d postpartum
  Severe trauma within 2 mo

FIGURE 2-54.

Indications and contraindications for thrombolytic therapy in pulmonary embolism. Thrombolytics may also be used to treat extensive ileofemoral venous thrombosis in selected patients with a low risk of bleeding. Some evidence exists that the incidence of post-thrombotic syndrome is reduced if complete thrombolysis is achieved. Often the decision to administer thrombolytic therapy has to be individualized after careful review of potential risks and benefits.

■ INTERSTITIAL LUNG DISEASE

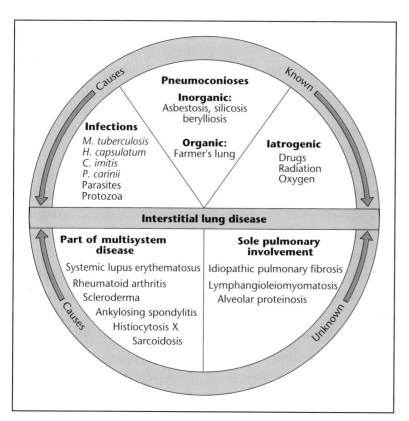

FIGURE 2-55.
Causes of interstitial lung disease (ILD): a clinical classification. The main pathology of ILD is seen in the alveolar walls and interstitium. The natural history spans the range of benign and self-limiting to progressive and irreversible. For many of these diseases, the clinical, radiologic, and physiologic profiles are similar. Dyspnea and dry cough are the most common symptoms. The presence of finger clubbing and end-inspiratory rales suggests idiopathic pulmonary fibrosis. Evidence of multisystem involvement suggests that the underlying etiology is either a collagen vascular disease, sarcoidosis, or a vasculitis. Lung biopsy is usually necessary for definitive diagnosis and should be carried out prior to development of end-stage disease. The chief categories of therapy are corticosteroids, cytotoxic agents, and, ultimately, lung transplantation. (*Courtesy of* Om P. Sharma and Takateru Izumi.)

Diagnostic Evaluation of Interstitial Lung Disease

Careful, occupational, exposure, drug, and family histories, and risk factors
Conventional chest radiographs (compare with old films)
Pulmonary function tests
  Spirometry, flow-volume loop, lung volumes, D_{LCO}, oximetry (rest, exercise)
  Formal cardiopulmonary exercise tests (arterial cannulation) for selected patients
Serologies for selected patients (*eg*, collagen vascular disease profile, complement fixation
  for fungi, serum angiotensin-converting enzyme, hypersensitivity pneumonitis screen)
High-resolution thin-section computed tomographic scan
Lung biopsy for selected patients
  Fiberoptic bronchoscopy with transbronchial lung biopsies and bronchoalveolar lavage
  Video-assisted thoracoscopic lung biopsy (when fiberoptic bronchoscopy is
  nondiagnostic and no contraindications to surgical biopsy exist)

D_{LCO}–diffusing capacity of lung for carbon monoxide.

FIGURE 2-56.
Diagnostic evaluation of interstitial lung disease. Idiopathic pulmonary fibrosis, a chronic lung disorder primarily affecting older adults, is characterized by cough, dyspnea, end-inspiratory velcro rales, diffuse parenchymal infiltrates on chest radiographs, hypoxemia, and a restrictive ventilatory defect on pulmonary function tests [51–54]. The need for lung biopsy depends on extent, severity, chronicity, and nature of the disease. The risks and benefits of biopsy and the therapeutic options available must be assessed carefully. In most patients, transbronchial lung biopsies and bronchoalveolar lavage are performed before considering video-assisted thoracoscopic surgery because a specific diagnosis can sometimes be made by transbronchial biopsies (*eg*, sarcoidosis, pulmonary alveolar proteinosis, malignancy, granulomatous infections), averting the need for surgical biopsies. (*Courtesy of* Joseph P. Lynch III and Jeffrey L. Myers.)

Differential Diagnosis of Diffuse Interstitial Lung Disease

Disease	History	Clinical Features	Laboratory Test	Chest Radiographic Features	Lung Histology
Sarcoidosis	Multisystem involvement	Dyspnea; red-eye, erythema nodosum	Hypercalcemia, Kveim test positive hyperglobulinemia, high SACE	Bilateral hilar adenopathy with or without pulmonary infiltrate	Noncaseating granuloma
Extrinsic allergic alveolitis	Exposure to an organic dust	Fever, cough, chest tightness	Precipitin antibodies in serum	Upper lung fields commonly affected	Cellular infiltration, granulomas
Rheumatoid disease	Arthritis, morning stiffness	Multisystem involvement, dyspnea	Rheumatoid factor positive	Diffuse lung involvement, pleural effusion	Necrobiotic nodules, vasculitis
Progressive systemic sclerosis	Raynaud's phenomenon, dysphagia	Progressive dyspnea		Lower lung fields	Fibrosis
Systemic lupus erythematosus	Multisystemic involvement	Dyspnea, cough, hemoptysis	Lupus erythematous cells and antinuclear antibodies	Bibasilar linear shadows, vanishing lungs	Vasculitis
Drug-induced lung disease	Relevant drug intake	Fever, chest tightness, dyspnea	Eosinophilia in some cases	Diffuse infiltration	Cellular infiltrate, granulomas, vasculitis
Pneumoconiosis	Exposure to dust (silica, asbestos, beryllium)	Dyspnea; may be asymptomatic	Not helpful	Upper lung fields commonly affected in silicosis, eggshell calcification; diffuse reticulonodular infiltrates in asbestosis, pleural calcification; diffuse interstitial infiltrate	Asbestos bodies; beryllium in tissue
Miliary tuberculosis	History of tuberculosis contact	Fever, weight loss, cough	Tuberculin test may be positive; sputum, urine, and bone marrow cultures may show acid-fast bacilli	Miliary nodular infiltrate	Caseating granulomas, acid-fast bacilli present
Lymphangitic carcinoma	Smoking history	Dyspnea, fever, weight loss	Sputum, transbronchial lung biopsy	Diffuse interstitial infiltration	Carcinoma
Histiocytosis X	Smoking, dyspnea	None	Langerhans' cells in bronchoalveolar lavage	Honeycombing, pneumothorax	Histiocytosis X bodies
Idiopathic pulmonary fibrosis History	Flu-like illness	Dyspnea, finger clubbing, basilar rales	Lung biopsy	Diffuse interstitial infiltrate, honeycombing	Cellular infiltration, fibrosis

SACE—serum angiotensin-converting enzyme.

FIGURE 2-57.

Differential diagnosis of diffuse interstitial lung disease. Diagnosis of interstitial lung disease requires thorough collection of data. The chief sources of information include the patient's history, the clinical features, laboratory tests, radiographic features, and lung histology. (*Courtesy of* Om P. Sharma and Takateru Izumi.)

High-Resolution Computed Tomographic Features of Idiopathic Pulmonary Fibrosis

Typical Findings

Predilection for the basilar and subpleural regions

Patchy involvement, with areas of intervening normal lung

Honeycomb cysts (4–20 mm in diameter)

Coarse reticular (linear) opacities; thick septal lines

Patchy ground glass opacities

Possible coexisting zones of emphysema in smokers

Late Findings

Anatomic distortion, severe volume loss

Traction bronchiectasis or bronchiolectasis

Dilated pulmonary arteries

FIGURE 2-58.

High-resolution computed tomographic (HRCT) features of idiopathic pulmonary fibrosis. HRCT scans are superior to conventional chest radiographs in depicting the salient parenchymal aberrations (*eg*, honeycomb cysts, alveolar or reticular opacities, distortion) and demarcating the extent and distribution of the disease [55–60]. Salient HRCT features of idiopathic pulmonary fibrosis (usual interstitial pneumonia variant) are outlined here. (*Courtesy of* Joseph P. Lynch III and Jeffrey L. Myers.)

Prognostic Value of HRCT Pattern in Idiopathic Pulmonary Fibrosis

Pattern of HRCT Scans

Ground glass (alveolar) opacities

    Usually associated with alveolitis and a favorable response to therapy

    In some cases, ground glass opacities represent irreversible fibrosis involving intralobular and alveolar septae

Reticular pattern (intersecting fine or coarse lines)

    May reflect fibrosis or inflammation

    The prognosis of reticular or mixed ground glass/reticular patterns is less favorable than predominant ground glass patterns

    Regression occurs with therapy in some patients

Honeycomb cysts

    Indicates end-stage, irreversible fibrosis

    Traction bronchiolectasis, and distortion also indicate irreversible fibrosis

Extent of Abnormality of HRCT Scans

Quantitative scoring systems assessing the *extent* and *pattern* of HRCT have prognostic value

HRCT—high-resolution computed tomography.

FIGURE 2-59.

Prognostic value of high-resolution computed tomographic (HRCT) patterns in idiopathic pulmonary fibrosis. The extent of disease on HRCT correlates roughly with severity of functional impairment [53,60]. Specific HRCT patterns may discriminate early alveolar inflammation (alveolitis) from fibrosis and have prognostic value [53,59–61]. (*Courtesy of* Joseph P. Lynch III and Jeffrey L. Myers.)

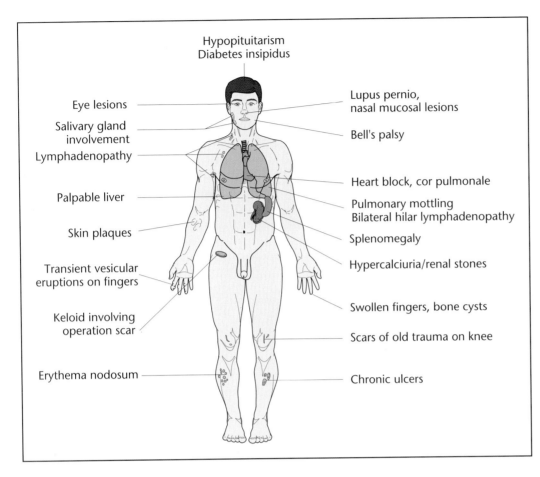

Hypopituitarism
Diabetes insipidus

Eye lesions

Salivary gland involvement

Lymphadenopathy

Palpable liver

Skin plaques

Transient vesicular eruptions on fingers

Keloid involving operation scar

Erythema nodosum

Lupus pernio, nasal mucosal lesions

Bell's palsy

Heart block, cor pulmonale

Pulmonary mottling Bilateral hilar lymphadenopathy

Splenomegaly

Hypercalciuria/renal stones

Swollen fingers, bone cysts

Scars of old trauma on knee

Chronic ulcers

FIGURE 2-60.

Multisystem involvement in sarcoidosis. Sarcoidosis is a multisystem granulomatous disorder of unknown etiology that most commonly affects young adults. The lungs are the most commonly involved organ. In 20% to 50% of patients, symptoms of cough, dyspnea, and chest discomfort may be present. The combination of ocular involvement, parotid enlargement, and cranial nerve palsy is known as *Heerfordt's syndrome*. Granulomas feature densely packed epithelioid cells and giant cells and few lymphocytes. The natural history may either be progressive and destructive or may feature periods of remission. The presence of erythema nodosum portends a favorable course. Accepted indications for treatment with corticosteroids include involvement of the lung with a decrease in pulmonary function, ocular involvement, myocardial disease, central nervous system disease, hypersplenism, or the presence of disfiguring skin lesions. Other treatment options include chloroquine, immunosuppressive drugs, and radiation. (*Courtesy of* Om P. Sharma and Takateru Izumi.)

Sarcoidosis Resolution Within 2 Years of Diagnosis*

Sarcoidosis Involvement	Number[†]	Resolution, %
Erythema nodosum	210/251	84
Acute arthritis	148/178	83
Hilar adenopathy	334/458	73
Nodes plus infiltrate	77/150	51
Ocular	105/224	47
Heart	3/9	33
Central nervous system	19/77	25
Lupus pernio	5/33	15
SURT	3/21	14
Cor pulmonale	0/18	0

*n=818 patients.
[†]Number resolving/number with condition.
SURT—sarcoidosis of upper respiratory tract.

FIGURE 2-61.

The manifestations of sarcoidosis. The rates of resolution of some symptoms of the disease within 2 years of diagnosis are shown [62]. Disease that is present longer than 2 years is considered chronic; patients with chronic disease may require long-term therapy. (*Courtesy of* Robert P. Baughman.)

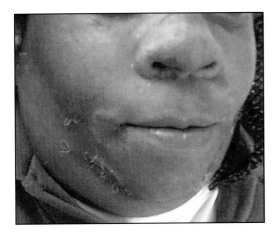

FIGURE 2-62.
Lupus pernio. The macular lesions also occur on the eyelids and spread across the bridge of the nose. This form of the disease is usually chronic. (*Courtesy of* Robert P. Baughman.)

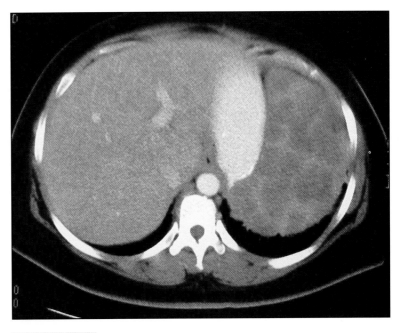

FIGURE 2-63.
Computed tomographic scan of the spleen of a patient with sarcoidosis. Liver and spleen abnormalities are often found in sarcoidosis. Increased liver function tests usually include increased alkaline phosphatase levels, but almost any abnormality can be seen [63,64]. The computed tomographic scan demonstrates the multiple defects in the spleen, which can be seen in sarcoidosis [65]. (*Courtesy of* Robert P. Baughman.)

Trials of Corticosteroids for Pulmonary Sarcoidosis

Study	Study Design	Patients, *n*	Duration of Therapy, *mo*	Duration of Observation, *y*	Outcome
Israel *et al.* [66]	Randomized, double-blinded	90	3	5.2	No difference
Selroos and Sellegren [67]	Randomized	39	7	4	Steroids helped only during treatment
Zaki *et al.* [68]	Randomized block, blind	183	24	3	No difference
Harkleroad *et al.* [69]	Randomized, double-blind	25	6	2,15	No difference
Gibson *et al.* [70]	Randomized, double-blind	58	18	5	Steroids helpful
Emirgil *et al.* [71]	Nonrandomized	38	24	12	Corticosteroids helpful
Johns *et al.* [72]	Single-arm	153	>9	10	Steroids helpful
Stone and Schwartz [73]	Single-arm	37	3–9	6	No benefit from steroids
Sharma *et al.* [74]	Nonrandomized	43	12–36	6	No difference

FIGURE 2-64.
Effects of corticosteroids in patients with pulmonary sarcoidosis. The use of corticosteroids remains controversial in patients with sarcoidosis. A summary of several trials comparing steroids to placebo is shown. With the exception of one study [70], the double-blind randomized trials did not demonstrate a difference between the placebo and steroid treatment. Many open-label studies did find benefits for treated patients. (*Adapted from* Baughman *et al.* [75].)

Occupational Exposure Causing Pneumoconioses

Type of Pneumoconiosis	Exposure Settings
Asbestosis	Construction
	Insulators
	Sheet-metal workers
	Boilermakers
	Factory workers
	Textiles
	Friction products
	Shipyard workers
Silicosis	Underground mines
	Foundries
	Factories
	Pottery
	Enamel
	Bricks
	Sand-blasting
	Glass-making
Coal-workers' pneumoconiosis	Underground coal mines
	Drillers
	Continuous miner-operators
	Roof bolters
	Surface coal mines
	Drillers
Hard metal disease	Tungsten carbide production
	Manufacture
	Fabrication
	Finishing
Berylliosis	Beryllium production
	Processing
	Fabrication

FIGURE 2-65.

Occupational exposure causing pneumoconiosis. The chronic inhalation of inorganic dusts, most commonly in an industrial setting, may cause a form of interstitial lung disease known as a *pneumoconiosis.* The necessary exposure period is 20 to 30 years, and the latency period to the presentation of disease is often 20 to 30 years. Exposure to beryllium compounds may lead to earlier disease. To enter the lower respiratory tract, particles must be on the order of 0.2 to 10 μm in diameter. Asbestos fibers, although up to 150 μm in length, have aerodynamic qualities that allow deeper penetration into the lower respiratory tract. Due to the introduction of greater safety precautions, asbestosis and silicosis are seen less often. Asbestos exposure can also cause pleural effusion or plaques, rounded atelectasis, and mesothelioma, and, synergistically with smoking, it heightens the risk for developing lung cancer. (*Courtesy of* Guillermo A. do Pico and Keith C. Meyer.)

Differential Diagnosis of Selected Pneumoconioses

Observation	Asbestosis	Silicosis	Berylliosis
History	Exposure	Exposure	Exposure
Physical examination	Rales	No rales	No or few rales
	Clubbing		
Radiology			
Radiography	Small irregular opacities	Well-circumscribed nodules	Miliary pattern
	Lower lung field	Upper lung field	Upper- or mid-lung field
	Pleural plaques	Massive fibrosis	Hilar adenopathy
Computed tomography	Subpleural lines	Dense nodules	Ill-defined nodules
	Pleural plaques		Adenopathy
Pulmonary function	Restriction	Restriction	Restriction
	Late obstruction		Late obstruction

FIGURE 2-66.

Differential diagnosis of selected pneumoconiosis. A complete environmental and occupational exposure history is key to making the diagnosis of the offending agent. Clues found on history and physical examination are the presence of progressive dyspnea, adventitial lung sounds, or finger clubbing, and a restrictive pattern of pulmonary function testing. Chest radiography may reveal a nodular or reticulonodular pattern chiefly in the lower lobes. (*Courtesy of* Guillermo A. do Pico and Keith C. Meyer.)

Drugs and Agents that Cause Lung Disease

Antibiotics	Cardiac Medications	Chemotherapeutic Drugs
Nitrofurantoin	Amiodarone	Bleomycin
Sulfonamides	Procainamide	Busulfan
Penicillins	Tocainide	Mitomycin C
Cephalosporins	Propranolol	Nitrosourea carmustine
Isoniazid	Hydralazine	Methotrexate
Tetracycline	Illicit drugs	Cyclophosphamide
Hydrochlorothiazide	Heroin	Chlorambucil
Anti-inflammatory agents	Methadone	Melphalan
Aspirin	Propoxyphene	Vinblastine
Nonsteroidal anti-	Toxic gases	Azathioprine
inflammatory agents	O_2	Miscellaneous agents
Penicillamine	SO_2	Radiation
Gold	NO_2	Talc
Corticosteroids		Tryptophan
		Tocolytics
		Diphenylhydantoin
		Methysergide
		Lymphangiography dye

FIGURE 2-67.

Drugs and agents that cause lung disease. Since the clinical profile of drug-induced interstitial lung disease (ILD) is the same as that of other ILD, the history harbors key information to support a drug-induced lung disease. However, lung biopsy should be carried out to rule out other causes, since patients often have a complex clinical picture. For many of these agents (eg, bleomycin) subsequent administration of high concentrations of oxygen can activate lung disease, even when the drug was taken in the past. Methotrexate can be responsible for acute respiratory distress syndrome, even when administered intrathecally. (*Courtesy of* Om P. Sharma and Takateru Izumi.)

■ CRITICAL CARE

ACUTE RESPIRATORY FAILURE

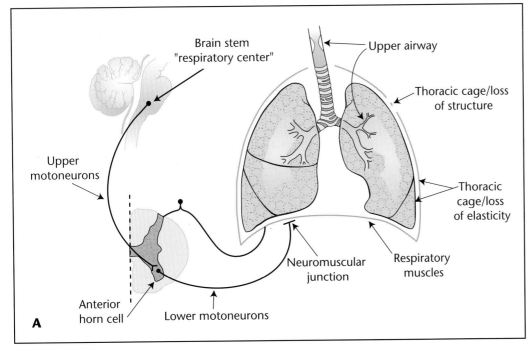

A

B. Hypercarbic Respiratory Failure ("Pump Failure")

Features
Disease involving the extrapulmonary compartment
Impaired alveolar ventilation
Associated respiratory acidosis

Gas Exchange Abnormalities
Hypercarbia predominance
± Hypoxemia

Malfunctioning Component–Ventilatory Pump
Brain stem "respiratory center" (*eg*, narcotic overdose)
Upper motoneurons (*eg*, cervical spine trauma)
Anterior horn cell (*eg*, poliomyelitis)
Lower motoneurons (*eg*, ascending polyradiculopathy)
Neuromuscular junction (*eg*, myasthenia gravis)
Respiratory muscles (*eg*, myopathy)
Thoracic cage/loss of elasticity (*eg*, kyphoscoliosis)
Thoracic cage/loss of structure (*eg*, "flail" chest wall)
Upper airway (*eg*, laryngospasm)

FIGURE 2-68.

A and B, Hypercarbic respiratory failure ("pump failure"). The pathophysiology of respiratory failure may be approached in terms of the component of the system that is malfunctioning—the "ventilatory pump" or the lung parenchyma, although components of both may be evident in a single patient. Hypercarbic respiratory failure is primarily failure to provide adequate alveolar ventilation. (*Adapted from* Nunn [76].) (*Courtesy of* David Leasa and Frank Rutledge.)

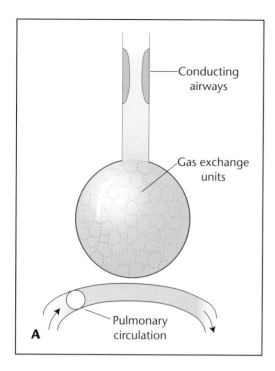

Conducting airways

Gas exchange units

Pulmonary circulation

A

FIGURE 2-69.

A and B, Hypoxemic respiratory failure ("lung failure"). Hypoxemic respiratory failure is primarily failure to adequately oxygenate the blood. (*Courtesy of* David Leasa and Frank Rutledge.)

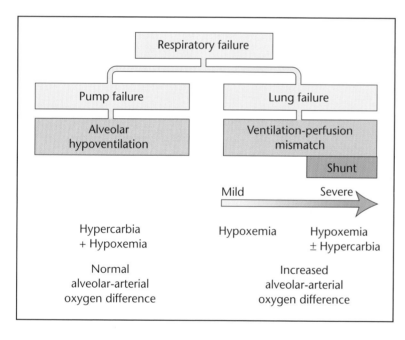

FIGURE 2-70.

Lung and pump failure and their effect on gas exchange. Hypercarbic respiratory failure results from disease states causing a decrease in minute ventilation or an increase in physiologic dead space, such that alveolar ventilation is inadequate to meet metabolic demands. Acute hypercarbic respiratory failure is considered present when $PaCO_2$ is at least 50 mm Hg and the arterial pH is less than 7.30. Chronic hypercarbic respiratory failure is characterized by $PaCO_2 \geq 50$ mm Hg, but with an arterial pH ≥ 7.30. The degree of hypoxemia associated with pure hypoventilation can be estimated from the alveolar gas equation, assuming that the alveolar-arterial difference for the PO_2 will be minimal or normal. Hypoxemic respiratory failure most commonly results from pulmonary conditions that cause ventilation/perfusion mismatch. Mild to moderate ventilation/perfusion mismatch results in hypoxemia, with a low or normal $PaCO_2$. Severe ventilation/perfusion mismatch results in hypoxemia and hypercarbia, as the increased ventilatory demand cannot be met. Shunting might be viewed as an extreme ventilation/perfusion abnormality, in which lung units are perfused but not ventilated. Hypoxemic respiratory failure is considered present when arterial oxygen saturations of less than 90% are observed, despite an inspired oxygen fraction above 0.60. (*Courtesy of* David Leasa and Frank Rutledge.)

FIGURE 2-71.
A and B, Hypoxemia responsive to O_2 (*panel A*) and poorly responsive to O_2 (*panel B*) in the absence of parenchymal disease on chest radiograph. A differential diagnosis for hypoxemia, in the absence of evidence of parenchymal disease on chest radiograph, can be generated through the understanding of gas exchange pathophysiology. (*Courtesy of* David Leasa and Frank Rutledge.)

A. Hypoxemia Responsive to O_2 in the Absence of Parenchymal Disease on Chest Radiograph

	$\dot{V}/\dot{Q}$ Mismatch	Diffusion-perfusion Defect
Example	Obstructive disease of the lung	Pulmonary vascular dilations of HPS*
	Thromboembolic disease	
	Spirometry with obstructive pattern	Low D_{LCO}
	$\dot{V}/\dot{Q}$ scan	Orthodeoxia
	Pulmonary angiogram	"Bubble" echocardiography†

*May also act like arteriovenous shunting if hepatocellular dysfunction is severe.
†Echocardiography with bubble study demonstrating delayed microbubble opacification of the left atrium.
D_{LCO}—diffusing capacity of the lungs for carbon monoxide; HPS—hepatopulmonary syndrome; $\dot{V}/\dot{Q}$—ventilation-perfusion.

B. Hypoxemia Poorly Responsive to O_2 in the Absence of Parenchymal Disease on Chest Radiograph

	Intrapulmonary Shunt			Intracardiac Shunt
	Arteriovenous Shunt	Inapparent Airspace Disease	Inapparent Dependent Atelectasis	
Example	HHT	Early PCP	After surgery	ASD
Diagnostic tests	"Bubble" echocardiography*	HRCT of the lungs	CT scan of the lungs	"Bubble" echocardiography†
	HRCT of the lungs with contrast			Cardiac catheterization
	Pulmonary angiogram			

*Echocardiography with bubble study demonstrating delayed microbubble opacification of the left atrium.
†Echocardiography with bubble study demonstrating immediate microbubble opacification of the left atrium.
ASD—atrial septal defect; HHT—hereditary hemorrhage telangiectasia; HRCT—high-resolution computerized tomography; PCP—*Pneumocystis carinii* pneumonia.

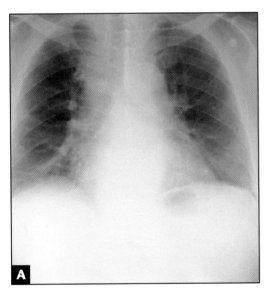
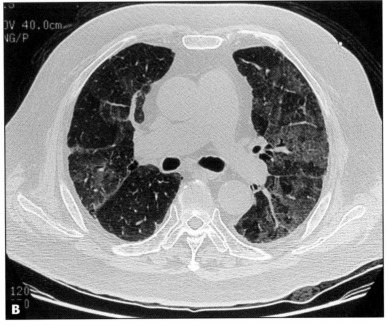

FIGURE 2-72.
A and B, Chest radiographs without apparent parenchymal disease to account for severe hypoxemia in an immunocompromised patient. High-resolution computed tomography of the lungs reveals extensive "ground glass" changes (alveolitis). Lung biopsy allowed a diagnosis of *Pneumocystis carinii* pneumonia. (*Courtesy of* David Leasa and Frank Rutledge.)

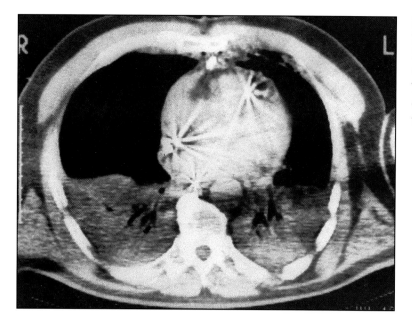

FIGURE 2-73.

Thoracic computed tomographic scan identifying the cause of hypoxemia. In patients requiring mechanical ventilation, the dependent (dorsal) lung regions bear a greater degree of atelectasis. This patient developed acute hypoxemic respiratory failure after cardiac surgery, and a conventional supine chest radiograph failed to explain the cause. (*From* Brussel *et al.* [77]; with permission.)

ACUTE RESPIRATORY DISTRESS SYNDROME

The Definition of ALI and ARDS

	Timing	Oxygenation	Chest Radiograph	Pulmonary Artery Wedge Pressure
ALI criteria	Acute onset	Pao$_2$ ≤300 mm Hg (regardless of PEEP level)	Bilateral infiltrates (seen on frontal chest radiograph)	≤18 mm Hg when measured (or no clinical evidence of left atrial hypertension)
ARDS criteria	Acute onset	Pao$_2$/Fio$_2$ ≤200 mm Hg (regardless of PEEP level)	Bilateral infiltrates (seen on frontal chest radiograph)	≤18 mm Hg when measured (or no clinical evidence of left atrial hypertension)

ALI—acute lung injury; ARDS—acute respiratory distress syndrome; Fio$_2$—fractional inspired oxygen; PEEP—positive end-expiratory pressure.

FIGURE 2-74.

The definition of acute lung injury (ALI) and ARDS, according to the American-European Consensus Conference on ARDS. Acute lung injury is defined as a syndrome of acute and persistent inflammation of the lung with increased permeability that is associated with a characteristic constellation of clinical, radiologic, and physiologic abnormalities. ARDS represents the most severe end of this spectrum. (*Adapted from* Bernard *et al.* [78].)

Etiology of Acute Lung Injury and Acute Respiratory Distress Syndrome

Direct Lung Injury

Aspiration pneumonitis

Other causes of pneumonitis: oxygen, smoke inhalation, radiation, bleomycin

Infectious pneumonia: community-acquired, nosocomial opportunistic

Trauma: lung contusion, penetrating chest injury

Near-drowning

Fat embolism

After relief of upper airway obstruction

After bone marrow and lung transplantation

After lung re-expansion

Distant Injury

Tissue inflammation, necrosis, infection ("sepsis syndrome")

Multiple trauma, major burns

Shock, hypoperfusion

Acute pancreatitis

Transfusion-associated lung injury

After cardiopulmonary bypass

Drug overdose: tricyclic antidepressants, cocaine

Neurogenic: intracerebral bleed, seizure

FIGURE 2-75.

The etiologies of acute lung injury and acute respiratory distress syndrome. To date, more than 60 distinct causes have been identified. (*Adapted from* Bigatello and Zapol [79].)

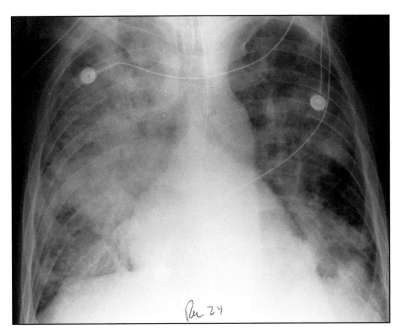

FIGURE 2-76.

An anteroposterior chest radiograph (supine) of a 60-year-old man with urosepsis and acute respiratory distress syndrome. The patchy, widespread opacities reflect diffuse air space disease and edema. (*Courtesy of* David Leasa and Frank Rutledge.)

Ventilator Management of Acute Respiratory Distress Syndrome

Strategy	Recommended	Grade
Volume-cycled, assist-control mode using low-stretch ventilation (tidal volumes ≤6 mL/kg predicted body weight; plateau pressures ≤30 cm H$_2$O)	yes	B
Lateral decubitus positioning in unilateral lung disease for persistent hypoxemia	Yes	C
PEEP to maintain Sao$_2$ 88% to 95% and Fio$_2$ ≤0.60	Yes	C
Open-lung approach (higher levels of PEEP and lung recruitment maneuvers)	?*†‡	B
Pressure-control inverse-ratio ventilation	?*†	C
High frequency jet ventilation	No	B
High frequency oscillatory ventilation	?*†	C
Prone position ventilation	?*†‡	C
Extracorporeal membrane oxygenation (ECMO)	No†	B
Extracorporeal carbon dioxide removal (ECCO$_2$-R)	No†	B
Partial liquid ventilation	?*	C
Airway pressure-release ventilation	?*	C
Tracheal gas insufflation (washes out dead space)	?*†	C
Prophylactic PEEP (>5 H$_2$O)	No	B
Noninvasive mask positive pressure ventilation (NIPPV)	Yes (in selected cases)	B

*Inconclusive, needs further study.

†May be considered a rescue therapy (for inadequate oxygenation, severe hypercarbia, or high airway pressures)

‡Large level 1 study being conducted.

Fio$_2$–fractional inspired oxygen; PEEP–positive end-expiratory pressure; Sao$_2$–arterial oxygen percent saturation.

FIGURE 2-77.

Ventilator management of acute respiratory distress syndrome. Mechanical ventilation is supportive in acute respiratory distress syndrome, maintaining acceptable gas exchange until lung recovery can occur. Conventional strategies have combined volume-cycled mechanical ventilation, to achieve a normal alveolar minute ventilation, with the addition of positive end-expiratory pressure, to ensure arterial oxygenation with minimal oxygen toxicity. (*Adapted from* Kollef and Schuster [80–82].)

Pharmacologic Management of ARDS

Treatment	Class	Proposed Mechanism of Action	Recommended	Grade
Early fluid restriction/diuresis	S	Reduce the amount of extravascular lung water and alveolar flooding	Yes	B
Surfactant replacement therapy	S	Replace dysfunctional surfactant; improve alveolar stability	No*	B**
Early corticosteroids	MI	Alter early host inflammatory cascade	No	A
Late corticosteroids	MI	Alter late host fibroproliferative response to injury	No*	C
N-acetylcysteine	MI	Scavenger of oxygen-free radicals	No†	B
Ketoconazole	MI	Inhibitor of thromboxane and leukotriene synthesis	No‡	B
Ibuprofen	MI	Inhibitor of prostaglandin pathways	No	D
Alprostadil (prostaglandin E_1)	MI	Blocks platelet aggregation, modulates inflammation, vasodilator	No	B
Lisofylline	MI	Phosphodiesterase inhibitor; inhibits chemotaxis/activation of PMNs	No	B
Antiendotoxins and anticytokines	MI	Antagonists of the mediators of sepsis	No	D
Selective digestive decontamination	MI	Reduce risk of nosocomial infection	No	D
Inhaled nitric oxide	S	Modulation of hypoxic pulmonary vasoconstriction	No†	B
Supernormal oxygen transport	S	Oxygen consumption supply dependency in ARDS	No	D
Almitrine	S	Physiologic improvement in oxygenation	?§	C
Recombinant human activated protein C	MI	Antithrombotic, anti-inflammatory, profibrinolytic	Yes¶	D

*Large level 1 study being conducted.
†May be considered a rescue therapy (nonresolving ARDS or inadequate oxygenation).
‡Use for prophylaxis to be determined.
§Inconclusive, needs further study.
¶In ARDS caused by sepsis.
**Lack of efficacy in level 1 study, but dose, delivery methodology, and choice of surfactant questioned.
ARDS—acute respiratory distress syndrome; MI—modulator of inflammation; PMNs—polymorphonuclear leukocytes; S—supportive therapy.

FIGURE 2-78.

Pharmacologic management of acute respiratory distress syndrome (ARDS). Pharmacologic modalities in patients with ARDS can be considered supportive therapies or modulators of inflammation. Unfortunately, anti-inflammatory therapies, to date, have been discouraging in disease prevention and in survival improvement. (*Data from* Kolleff and Schuster [80,81], Hudson [82], and Ware and Matthay [83].) (*Courtesy of* David Leasa and Frank Rutledge.)

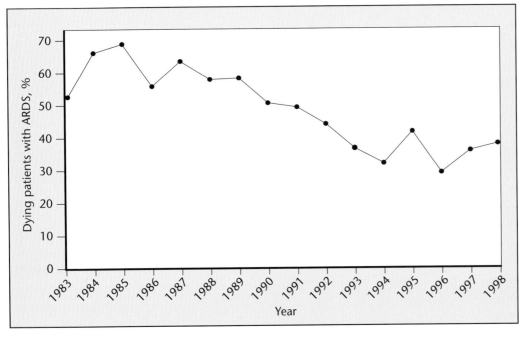

FIGURE 2-79.

Survival of patients with acute respiratory distress syndrome (ARDS). There is evidence that mechanical ventilation strategies and better supportive care may reduce ARDS mortality, at least in one center, from 60% in the 1980s to between 30% and 40% in the mid-1990s. Lung-protective ventilatory strategies aim to avoid the consequence of volutrauma and barotrauma that may amplify the injury to the alveolar-apillary membrane [84–86].

■ REFERENCES

1. Celli BR, Snider GL, Heffner J, *et al.* for the American Thoracic Society: Standards for the diagnosis and care of patients with chronic obstructive pulmonary disease. *Am J Respir Crit Care Med* 1995, 152:S77–S121.

2. Owens GR: Chronic obstructive pulmonary disease: asthma, emphysema, chronic bronchitis, bronchiectasis, and related conditions. In *Pulmonary and Critical Care Medicine.* Edited by Bone RC, Dantzker DR, George RB *et al.* St. Louis: Mosby; 1993:G3–G5.

3. Ferguson GT, Cherniack RM: Management of chronic obstructive pulmonary disease. *N Engl J Med* 1993, 328:1017–1022.

4. Flenley DC: Oxygen therapy in the treatment of COPD. In *Chronic Obstructive Pulmonary Disease* edn 1. Edited by Cherniack NS. Philadelphia: WB Saunders; 1991:468–476.

5. Shelhamer JH, Levine SJ, Wu T, *et al.*: Airway Inflammation. *Ann Intern Med* 1995, 123:288–304.

6. Horwitz RJ, Busse WW: Inflammation and asthma. In *Clinics in Chest Medicine.* Edited by Martin RJ. Philadelphia: WB Saunders; 1995:583–602.

7. Barnes PJ: Inflammatory mediators and neural mechanisms in severe asthma. In *Severe Asthma: Pathogenesis and Clinical Management.* Edited by Szefler SJ, Leung DYM. New York: Marcel Dekker; 1996:129–163.

8. Freitag A, Newhouse MT: Management of asthma in the 1990s. *Curr Pulmonol* 1994, 15:19–74.

9. National Asthma Education Program: Guidelines for the Diagnosis and Management of Asthma: Expert Panel Report. Bethesda, MD: National Heart, Lung, and Blood Institute; 1991. [DHHS publication no. (PHS) 91-3042A.]

10. National Heart, Lung, and Blood Institute: Expert Panel Report II: Guidelines for the Diagnosis and Management of Asthma. Bethesda, MD: National Institutes of Health: 1997. [NIH publication no. 97-4051.]

11. Kamada AK, Szefler SJ: Pharmacological management of severe asthma. In *Severe Asthma: Pathogenesis and Clinical Management.* Edited by Szefler SJ, Leung DYM. New York: Marcel Dekker; 1996:165–205.

12. New Insights Editorial Board: A look at the national CF patient registry. *New Insights Into Cystic Fibrosis* 1996, 3:1–6.

13. Kerem BS, Rommens JM, Buchanan JA, *et al.*: Identification of the cystic fibrosis gene: genetic analysis. *Science* 1989, 245:1073–1080.

14. Riordan JR, Rommens JM, Kerem B-S, *et al.*: Identification of the cystic fibrosis gene: cloning and characterization of complementary DNA. *Science* 1989, 245:1066–1073.

15. Rommens JM, Iannuzzi MC, Kerem B-S, *et al.*: Identification of the cystic fibrosis gene: chromosome walking and jumping. *Science* 1989, 245:1059–1065.

16. Anderson M, Gregory RJ, Thompson S, *et al.*: Demonstration that CFTR is a chloride channel by alteration of its anion selectivity. *Science* 1991, 53:202–205.

17. Stutts MJ, Canessa JC, Olsen M, *et al.*: CFTR as a cAMP-dependent regulator of sodium channels. *Science* 1995, 269:847–850.

18. Ramsey BW: Management of pulmonary disease in patients with cystic fibrosis. *N Engl J Med* 1996, 335:179–188.

19. Gibson LE, Cooke RE: A test for concentration of electrolytes in sweat in cystic fibrosis of the pancreas. *Pediatrics* 1959, 23:545–549.

20. Davidson G, McIlwaine M: Airway clearance techniques in cystic fibrosis. New Insights into Cystic Fibrosis 1995, 3:6–11.

21. Swensen SJ, Brown LR: Conventional radiography of hilum and mediastinum in bronchogenic carcinoma. *Radiol Clin North Am* 1990, 28:521–538.

22. Bartlett JG, Mundy LM: Community-acquired pneumonia. *N Engl J Med* 1995, 333:1618–1624.

23. Niederman MS, Bass JB Jr., Campbell GD, *et al.*: Guidelines for the initial management of adults with community-acquired pneumonia: diagnosis, assessment of severity, and initial antimicrobial therapy. *Am Rev Respir Dis* 1993, 148:1418–1426.

24. Rein MF, Gwaltney JM, O'Brien WM, *et al.*: Accuracy of Gram's stain in identifying pneumococci in sputum. *JAMA* 1978, 239:2671–2673.

25. Center for Disease Control and Prevention: Essential components of a tuberculosis prevention and control program. *MMWR* 1995, 44(RR-II):1–34.

26. Bradsher RW: Histoplasmosis and blastomycosis. *Clin Infect Dis* 1996, 22 (suppl 2):S102–S111.

27. Wheat J, Sarosi G, McKinsey D, *et al.*: Practice guidelines for the management of patients with histoplasmosis. Infectious Diseases Society of America. *Clin Infect Dis* 2000, 30:688–695.

28. Stein PD, Terrin ML, Hales CA, *et al.*: Clinical, laboratory, roentgenographic, and electrocardiographic findings in patients with acute pulmonary embolism and no pre-existing cardiac or pulmonary disease. *Chest* 1991, 100:598–603.

29. Anderson FA Jr., Wheeler HB, Goldberg RJ, *et al.*: A population-based perspective on the hospital incidence and case fatality rates of deep vein thrombosis and pulmonary embolism: the Worcester DVT study. *Arch Intern Med* 1991, 151:933–938.

30. Burke B, Sostman HD, Carrol BA, Witty LA: The diagnostic approach to deep venous thrombosis. *Clin Chest Med* 1995, 16:253–268.

31. Heijboer H, Buller HR, Lensing AWA, *et al.*: A comparison of real time ultrasonography with impedance plethysmography for the diagnosis of deep vein thrombosis in symptomatic outpatients. *N EngL J Med* 1993, 329:1365–1369.

32. Huisman MV, Buller HR, ten Cate JW, *et al.*: Management of clinically suspected acute venous thrombosis in outpatients with serial impedance plethysmography in a community hospital setting. *Arch Intern Med* 1989, 149:511–513.

33. Meaney JFM, Weg JG, Chenevert TL, *et al.*: Diagnosis of pulmonary embolism with magnetic resonance angiography. *N Engl J Med* 1997, 336:1422–1427.

34. Bounameaux H, Moerloose P, Perrier A, Reber G: Plasma measurement of D-dimer as diagnostic aid in suspected venous thromboembolism: an overview. *Thromb Haemost* 1994, 71:1–6.

35. Ginsberg JS, Kearon C, Douketis J, *et al.*: The use of D-dimer testing and impedance plethysmographic examination in patients with clinical indications of deep vein thrombosis. *Arch Intern Med* 1997, 157:1077–1081.

36. Rathbun SW, Raskob GE, Whitsett TL: Sensitivity and specificity of helical computed tomography in the diagnosis of pulmonary embolism: a systematic review. *Ann Intern Med* 2000, 132:227–232.

37. Stein PD, Hull RD, Pineo G: Strategy that includes serial non-invasive leg tests for diagnosis of thromboembolic disease in patients with suspected acute pulmonary embolism based on data from PIOPED—Prospective Investigation of Pulmonary Embolism Diagnosis. *Arch Intern Med* 1995, 155:2101–2104.

38. Clagett GP, Anderson FA, Heit J, *et al.*: Prevention of venous thromboembolism. *Chest* 1995, 108:312S–334S.

39. Hull RD, Raskob GE, Lemaire J, *et al.*: Optimal therapeutic level of heparin therapy in patients with venous thrombosis. *Arch Intern Med* 1992, 152:1589–1595.

40. Harrison L, Johnston M, Massicotte MP, *et al.*: Comparison of 5 mg and 10 mg loading doses in initiation of warfarin therapy. *Ann Intern Med* 1997, 126:133–136.

41. Hirsh J, Dalen JE, Deykin D, *et al.*: Oral anticoagulants: mechanism of action, clinical effectiveness and optimal therapeutic range. *Chest* 1995, 108:231S–246S.

42. Weitz JI: Low molecular weight heparins. *N Engl J Med* 1997, 337:688–698.

43. Koopman MMW, Prandoni P, Piovella F, *et al.*: Treatment of venous thrombosis with intravenous unfractionated heparin administered in the hospital as compared with subcutaneous low-molecular-weight heparin administered at home. *N Engl J Med* 1996, 334:682.

44. Levine M, Gent M, Hirsh J, *et al.*: A comparison of low-molecular-weight heparin administered primarily at home with unfractionated heparin administered in the hospital. *N Engl J Med* 1996, 334:677.

45. Boccalon H: Clinical outcome and cost of hospital vs. home treatment of proximal deep vein thrombosis with a low-molecular-weight heparin: the Vascular Midi-Pyrenees Study. *Arch Intern Med* 2000, 160:1769–1773.

46. Yusen R: Criteria for outpatient management of proximal lower extremity deep venous thrombosis. *Chest* 1999, 115:972–979.

47. Kovacs MJ, Anderson D, Morrow B, *et al.*: Outpatient treatment of pulmonary embolism with dalteparin. *ThromB Haemost* 2000, 83(2):209–211.

48. Well PS, Kovacs MJ, Bormanis J, *et al.*: Expanding eligibility for outpatient treatment of deep venous thrombosis and pulmonary embolism with low-molecular-weight heparin. *Arch Intern Med* 1998, 158:1809–1812.

49. Goldhaber SZ, Haire WD, Feldstein ML, *et al.*: Alteplase versus heparin in acute pulmonary embolism: randomized trial assessing right-ventricular function and pulmonary perfusion. *Lancet* 1993, 341:507–511.

50. A collaborative study by the PIOPED investigators: Tissue plasminogen activator for the treatment of acute pulmonary embolism. *Chest* 1990, 97:528–533.

51. American Thoracic Society and European Respiratory Society: Idiopathic pulmonary fibrosis: diagnosis and treatment. International Consensus Statement. *Am J Respir Crit Care Med* 2000, 161:646–664.

52. Lynch JP III, Toews GB: Idiopathic pulmonary fibrosis. In *Textbook of Pulmonary Diseases and Disorders* edn 3. *Edited by Fishman A. New York: McGraw-Hill; 1997:1193–1210.*

53. Wells AU: Clinical usefulness of high resolution computed tomography in cryptogenic fibrosing alveolitis. *Thorax* 1998, 53:1080–1087.

54. Douglas WW, Rhy JH, Schroeder DR: Idiopathic pulmonary fibrosis: impact of oxygen and colchicine, prednisone, or no therapy on survival. *Am J Resp Crit Care Med* 2000, 161:1172–1178.

55. Colby TV, Swensen SJ: Anatomic distribution and histopathologic patterns in diffuse lung disease: correlation with HRCT. *J Thorac Imaging* 1996, 11:1–26.

56. Grenier P, Chevret S, Beigelman C, *et al.*: Chronic diffuse infiltrative lung disease: determination of the diagnostic value of clinical data, chest radiography, and CT with Bayesian analysis. *Radiology* 1994, 191:383–390.

57. Raghu G: Interstitial lung disease, a diagnostic approach: Are CT scan and lung biopsy indicated in every patient? *Am J Respir Crit Care Med* 1995, 151:909–914.

58. Johkoh T, Muller NL, Cartier Y, *et al.*: Idiopathic interstitial pneumonias: diagnostic accuracy of thin-section CT in 129 patients. *Radiology* 1999, 211:555–560.

59. Gay SE, Kazerooni EA, Toews GB, *et al.*: Idiopathic pulmonary fibrosis: predicting response to therapy and survival. *Am J Respir Crit Care Med* 1998, 157:1063–1072.

60. Wells AU, King AD, Rubens MB, *et al.*: Lone cryptogenic fibrosing alveolitis: a functional-morphologic correlation based on extent of disease on thin section computed tomography. *Am J Respir Crit Care Med* 1997, 155:1367–1375.

61. Hartman TE, Primack SL, Swensen SJ, Hansell D: Desquamative interstitial pneumonia: thin-section CT findings in 22 patients. *Radiology* 1993, 787–790.

62. Neville E, Walker AN, James DG: Prognostic factors predicting the outcome of sarcoidosis: an analysis of 818 patients. *QJ Med* 1983, 208:525–533.

63. Lower EE, Baughman RP: Prolonged use of methotrexate for sarcoidosis. *Arch Intern Med* 1995, 155:846–851.

64. Maddrey WC, Johns CJ, Boitnott JK, Iber FL: Sarcoidosis and chronic hepatic disease: a clinical and pathologic study of 20 patients. *Medicine* 1970, 49:375–395.

65. Warshauer DM, Molina PL, Hamman SM, *et al.*: Nodular sarcoidosis of the liver and spleen: analysis of 32 cases. *Radiology* 1995, 195:757–762.

66. Israel HL, Fouts DW, Beggs RA: A controlled trial of prednisone treatment of sarcoidosis. *Am Rev Respir Dis* 1973, 107:609–614.

67. Selroos O, Sellergren TL: Corticosteroid therapy of pulmonary sarcoidosis. *Scand J Resp Dis* 1979, 60:212–215.

68. Zaki MH, Lyons HA, Leilop L, Huang CT: Corticosteroid therapy in sarcoidosis: a five year controlled follow-up. *NY State J Med* 1987, 87:496–499.

69. Harkelroad LE, Young RL, Savage PJ, *et al.*: Pulmonary sarcoidosis: long-term follow-up of the effects of steroid therapy. *Chest* 1982, 82:84–87.

70. Gibson GJ, Prescott RJ, Muers MF, *et al.*: British Thoracic Society Sarcoidosis Study: effects of long term corticosteroid treatment. *Thorax* 1996, 51:238–247.

71. Emirgil C, Sobol BJ, Williams MHJ: Long-term study of pulmonary sarcoidosis: the effect of steroid therapy as evaluated by pulmonary function studies. *J Chronic Dis* 1969, 22:69–86.

72. Johns CJ, Zachary JB, Ball WC: A ten-year study of corticosteroid treatment of pulmonary sarcoidosis. *Johns Hopkins Med* 1974, 134:271–283.

73. Stone DJ, Schwartz A: A long-term study of sarcoid and its modification by steroid therapy: lung function and other factors in prognosis. *Am J Med* 1966, 41:528–540.

74. Sharma OP, Colp C, Williams MHJ: Course of pulmonary sarcoidosis with and without corticosteroid therapy as determined by pulmonary function studies. *Am J Med* 1966, 41:541–551.

75. Baughman RP, Lower EE, Lynch JP: Treatment modalities for sarcoidosis. *Clin Pulm Med* 1994, 1:223–231.

76. Nunn JF: Causes of failure of ventilation. In *Applied Respiratory Physiology.* London: Butterworth & Co.; 1987:381.

77. Brussel T, Hachenberg T, Roos N, *et al.*: Mechanical ventilation in the prone position for acute respiratory failure after cardiac surgery. *J Cardiothorac Vasc Anesth* 1993, 7:541–546.

78. Bernard GR, Artigas A, Brigham KL, *et al.*: The American-European Consensus Conference on ARDS: definitions, mechanisms, relevant outcomes, and clinical trial coordination. *Am J Respir Crit Care Med* 1994, 149:818–824.

79. Bigatello LM, Zapol WM: New approaches to acute lung injury. *Br J Anaesth* 1996, 77:99–109.

80. Kollef MH, Schuster DP: The acute respiratory distress syndrome. *N Engl J Med* 1995, 332:27–37.

81. Kollef MH, Schuster DP: Acute respiratory distress syndrome. *Dis Mon* 1996, 5:275–326.

82. Hudson LD: New therapies for ARDS. *Chest* 1995, 108:795–915.

83. Ware LB, Matthay MA: The acute respiratory distress syndrome. *N Engl J Med* 2000, 342:1334–1349.

84. Sessler CN, Bloomfield GL, Fowler AA: Current concepts of sepsis and acute lung injury. *Clin Chest Med* 1996, 17:213–235.

85. Milberg JA, Davis DR, Steinberg KP, Hudson LD: Improved survival of patients with ARDS: 1983-1993. *J Am Med Assoc* 1995, 273:306–309.

86. Steinberg KP, Hudson MA: Acute lung injury and acute respiratory distress syndrome. The clinical syndrome. *Clin Chest Med* 2000, 21:401–417.

Endocrinology

STANLEY G. KORENMAN

Hormones are molecules that convey information about the state of the body to individual cells via complex regulated systems that have been subjected to scientific study for over 100 years. As a result of this body of research results, we possess a relatively complete understanding of the regulatory feedback mechanisms controlling the release of hormones, their modes of circulation, and the processes by which they act and are metabolized. This in turn has led endocrinologists to develop effective diagnostic and therapeutic approaches to virtually all endocrine disorders. This is not to deny that new hormones (like leptin) and regulated processes are still being discovered. Specifically, studies of tissue specificity of hormone production and action, and extensive paracrine and autocrine regulation of cellular processes have been delineated. Furthermore, the complex genetic basis of common endocrine disorders offers not only much more precise diagnostic information but great opportunities for entirely new treatments.

The high degree of awareness by physicians of the classical presentations of endocrine disorders has led to consideration of these diagnoses at much less advanced stages of disease, when the physical findings may be quite subtle. Biochemical testing using regulatory manipulations has become necessary to establish the presence of endocrine conditions prior to treatment.

Therefore, this chapter focuses not on pictures of classical presentations but rather on diagnosis and differential diagnosis of endocrine conditions relying on algorithms that hopefully lead to unequivocal diagnoses and sensitive specific tests that have evolved from our understanding of endocrine pathophysiology. These include assessments for hyponatremias, acromegaly, Cushing's syndromes, euestrogenic amenorrhea, and hypoglycemia. Detailed algorithms for the differential diagnosis of hypo- and hyperthyroidism, thyroid masses, endocrine hypertension, and hypogonadism are also given. Together these give the clinician the opportunity to understand the reasoning by which specialists reach a diagnosis and therapeutic approach in endocrinology and metabolism and the wherewithal to undertake efficient diagnostic testing when they suspect an endocrine condition.

■ REGULATION OF THYROID HORMONE SYNTHESIS AND RELEASE

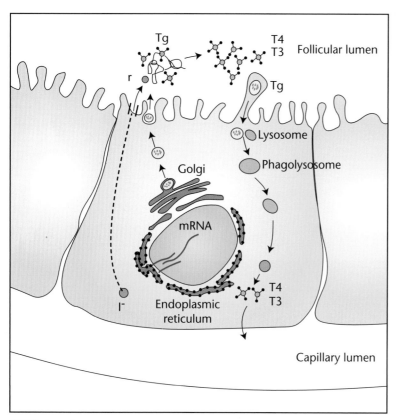

FIGURE 3-1.

Thyroid hormone production, storage, and release. Synthesis of thyroid hormones by thyroid follicular cells requires thyroglobu-

lin (Tg) and transport of iodine into the thyroid cell. Tg is a high molecular weight glycoprotein in the matrix of which thyroid hormones are synthesized. The protein components of Tg are synthesized on polyribosomes of the endoplasmic reticulum, and its glycosylation occurs within the reticular lumen before its movement to the Golgi apparatus. Additional processing of the carbohydrate components of Tg occurs within the Golgi apparatus. Transport of Tg from the Golgi to the apical plasma membrane occurs in membrane vesicles that fuse with the apical membrane, resulting in exocytosis of the thyroglobulin into the follicular lumen as colloid. Iodide is concentrated by the thyroid from plasma against a 30/1 gradient. It is oxidized by the peroxidase enzyme and bound to tyrosine residues in Tg to form monoiodotyrosine (MIT) and diiodotyrosine (DIT). Peroxidase-catalyzed iodination of tyrosine residues and coupling of two DITs to form T4 and one DIT and one MIT to form T3 occur within the Tg molecules in the follicular lumen, immediately adjacent to the apical plasma membrane.

The initial step of thyroid hormone release is the uptake of colloid by the follicular cell by pinocytosis at the apical cell membrane. Colloid droplets that enter the cytoplasm fuse with lysosomes, the Tg in the colloid is degraded by lysosomal enzymes, and the thyroid hormones are released and transported to the capillaries adjacent to the basal cell membrane. Thyroid hormones circulate bound to plasma proteins by noncovalent bonds; their unbound (free) fraction enters the cells of the body and exerts characteristic effects of thyroid hormones on cell metabolism.

A. Conditions Associated with Deranged Thyroid-Stimulating Hormone Regulation

Type of Derangement	Clinical Status	Serum TSH	Serum Free Thyroxine
Long-term derangements:			
Hypothalamic failure or tumor	Hypothyroid	Usually normal	Decreased
Pituitary failure or tumor	Hypothyroid	Usually normal	Decreased
Resistance to thyroid hormone	Variable	Usually normal	Increased
Resistance to thyroid-stimulating hormone (TSH)	Euthyroid	Increased	Normal
Treated primary congenital hypothyroidism	Euthyroid	Increased	Normal
TSH-secreting pituitary tumors	Hyperthyroid	Increased	Increased
Transient derangements:			
Serious organic nonthyroidal illnesses	Euthyroid	Variable	Normal or increased
Acute psychiatric disorders	Euthyroid	Normal	Normal or increased
Recovery from recent hyperthyroidism	Hypothyroid or euthyroid	Decreased	Decreased or normal
TSH suppression, dopamine	Euthyroid	Decreased	Usually normal
TSH suppression, glucocorticoids	Euthyroid	Normal or decreased	Usually normal
Non-steady state thyroxine administration	Variable	Variable	Variable
Treated primary congenital hypothyroidism	Euthyroid	Increased	Normal
Acute salsalate/salicylate loading	Euthyroid	Decreased then increased	Increased then normal

FIGURE 3-2.

Relationships between serum thyroid-stimulating hormone (TSH) levels and free-thyroxine (T4) levels in health and disease.
A, Conditions associated with deranged thyroid-stimulating hormone regulation. A negative log-linear relationship exists between serum TSH levels and free-T4 levels in persons with intact hypothalamic-

pituitary-thyroid-peripheral tissue axis under steady-state conditions. When this axis is intact, serum TSH concentrations provide an endogenous bioassay of thyroid hormone status. In a number of circumstances the hypothalamic-pituitary-thyroid-peripheral tissue negative-feedback axis is deranged [1,2]. *(Continued)*

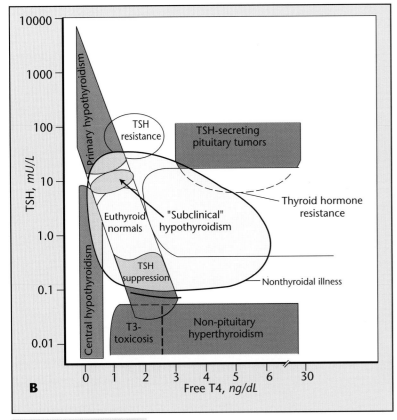

FIGURE 3-2. (CONTINUED)
Such derangements may either be long term or transient. **B,** Serum
TSH concentrations obtained using a third-generation assay with a
functional sensitivity of 0.0l mU/L (interassay coefficient of variation
of 14%; normal range, 0.4–4.2 mU/L) and serum free-T4 measurements
obtained with a direct equilibrium dialysis method, which has a functional sensitivity of 0.2 ng/dL (normal range, 0.8–2.7 ng/dL).

Patients with overt primary hypothyroidism have elevated TSH
levels with reduced free-T4 levels. Patients with overt nonpituitary
hyperthyroidism have suppressed TSH levels with elevated free-T4
levels, elevated free-triiodothyronine (T3) levels, or both. Patients
with "subclinical hypothyroidism" have elevated TSH levels with
free-T4 levels in the normal range. Patients with TSH suppression
have free-T4 and free-T3 concentrations in the normal range.

In patients with hypothalamic or pituitary gland failure (central
hypothyroidism), free-T4 values are decreased in association with
reduced, normal, or even slightly elevated TSH levels. With pituitary suppression by pharmacologic doses of dopamine or glucocorticoids, TSH levels and free-T4 levels may be reduced in the absence
of T3 toxicosis. A similar pattern occurs after recent thyroid
hormone withdrawal and may persist for 1 to 2 years after treatment of severe primary hyperthyroidism. In patients with hyperthyroidism caused by excessive TSH production, resulting from TSH
secreting tumors or thyroid hormone resistance states, both serum
TSH and free-T4 concentrations may be elevated. In thyroid
hormone resistance, which is due to loss-of-function mutations in
T4 receptor genes, free-T4 concentrations are paradoxically high for
the concentrations of TSH; when free-T4 concentrations are
returned to normal by misguided thyroid ablation, TSH concentrations increase to very high levels. In the resistance to TSH syndrome caused by a loss-of-function mutation in the human TSH
receptor gene, serum TSH concentrations are markedly elevated,
whereas free-T4 and free-T3 levels are normal and patients are clinically euthyroid. Some patients with congenital primary hypothyroidism treated with L-T4 do not recover normal TSH regulation for
months or years. In these persons the deranged TSH regulation is
evidenced by paradoxical TSH elevations when free T4 levels are
normal, or paradoxical free-T4 elevations when TSH levels are
normal. In euthyroid patients with acute critical nonthyroidal illnesses, serum TSH values may decrease transiently, but rarely to
below 0.01 mU/L, in association with elevated, normal, or reduced
free-T4 concentrations (direct equilibrium dialysis). In some
patients with nonthyroidal illnesses, TSH levels may transiently
increase, occasionally into the hypothyroid range during recovery,
in the presence of normal or somewhat elevated free-T4 concentrations. Disparities between TSH immunoreactivity and bioactivity
caused by an altered carbohydrate content of TSH molecules also
can result in apparently paradoxical TSH free-T4 relationships [3].
In all of these instances, accurate measurements of free-T4 concentrations in conjunction with appropriately sensitive TSH measurements can identify derangements of the hypothalamic-pituitary-
thyroid-peripheral tissue axis. (Panel A *adapted from* Kaptein [1] and
Nelson and Wilcox [2]; panel B *adapted from* Kaptein [1].)

■ THYROID FUNCTION TESTING

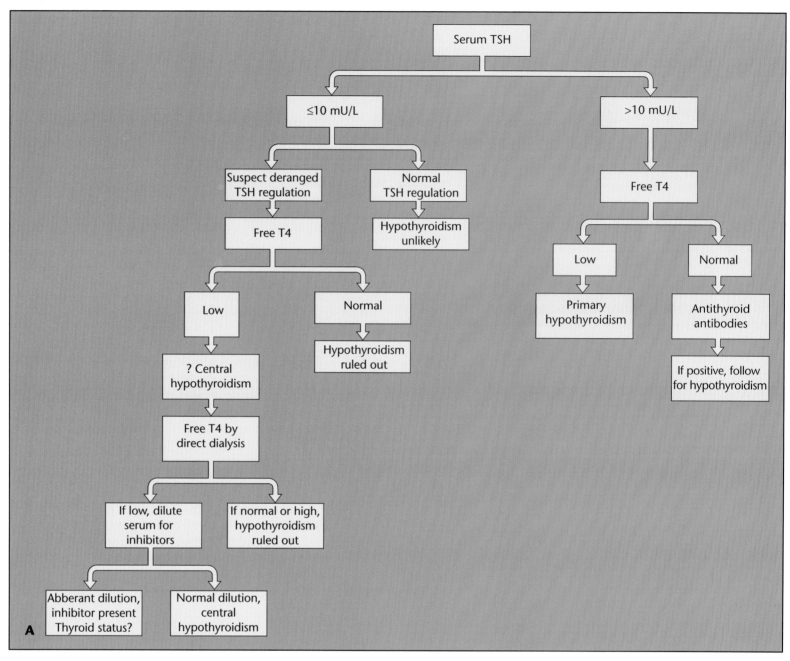

FIGURE 3-3.

Laboratory evaluation for hypothyroidism. Strategies for thyroid function testing depend on whether the hypothalamic-pituitary-thyroid-peripheral tissue axis is intact or deranged. When this axis is intact, serum thyroid-stimulating hormone (TSH) measurements (using appropriate methods) accurately reflect free-hormone status. In these instances, serum TSH values are suppressed with free-T4 or free-T3 excess and elevated with free-T4 deficiency. When the hypothalamic-pituitary-thyroid-peripheral tissue axis is functionally deranged [1,2], serum TSH relationships to free-hormone status are paradoxical, which can only be identified by determination of free-hormone and TSH levels. Because serum TSH normal ranges are calculated to include 95% of TSH values from healthy persons, 5% of healthy persons have TSH values outside normal ranges. Because these TSH values are regarded as abnormal, they are false-positive TSH values and overlap true-positive values.

A, Diagnosing hypothyroidism. When hypothyroidism is clinically suspected in patients presumed to have intact hypothalamus and pituitary, serum TSH is the most reasonable first-line thyroid

function test because of its diagnostic sensitivity [1]. When TSH concentration is elevated and free-T4 concentration is reduced, overt primary hypothyroidism is present. When TSH concentration is elevated and free-T4 concentration is normal, other evidence of thyroid disease should be sought. Previously unrecognized autoimmune thyroiditis can be identified by elevated antithyroid antibodies (thyroid peroxidase or thyroglobulin antibodies).

In patients with concurrent nonthyroidal illnesses, or patients with deranged hypothalamic or pituitary function, a serum TSH less than 10 mU/L does not necessarily exclude hypothyroidism. Spuriously low free-T4 measurements are common in patients with nonthyroidal illness and with use of any of a number of pharmacologic agents [1,2,4–7]. When thyroid status is not readily apparent, measurement of free T4 levels by direct dialysis can be useful. When free-T4 concentrations by this method are normal or slightly elevated, euthyroid nonthyroidal illness is most likely [1,4,6,7]. When free-T4 measurement is reduced, a circulating inhibitor of T4 binding may cause spuriously low values. This result is most likely in patients receiving

(Continued)

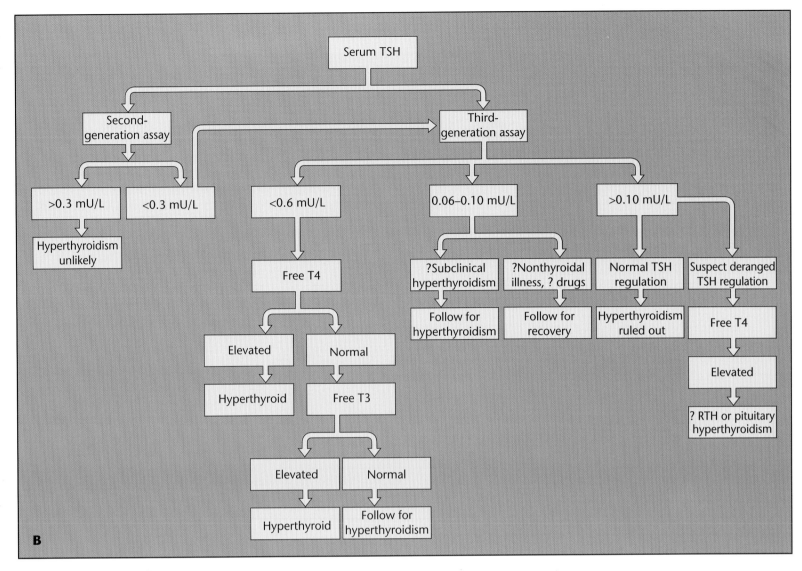

FIGURE 3-3. (CONTINUED)

nonsteroidal anti-inflammatory drugs, anticonvulsants, or parenteral high-dose furosemide, which can interfere with the binding of thyroid hormone to proteins; and in severe nonthyroidal illnesses, particularly uremia [5,8,9]. In these instances, free-T4 levels can be measured by direct dialysis after serial serum dilutions [10]. Reduced free-T4 concentrations that remain unchanged with serial dilutions are characteristic of hypothyroidism. Free-T4 concentrations that decrease progressively with serial dilutions are characteristic of interfering inhibitors of T4 binding. Their presence does not allow accurate free-T4 measurement by available clinical laboratory methods.

In nonthyroidal illnesses, the measurement of serum reverse T3 (rT3) concentrations has not proved to be efficacious in differentiating hypothyroidism from euthyroidism [11]. Patients with hypothyroidism plus nonthyroidal illness, as well as those with nonthyroidal illness alone, may have either low or normal reverse T3 concentrations [11].

B, Diagnosing hyperthyroidism. When hyperthyroidism is suspected in patients presumed to have an intact pituitary and hypothalamus, serum TSH measurements by second-generation assays with values above 0.3 mU/L (three times the level of functional sensitivity) usually exclude hyperthyroidism. Values of 0.3 mU/L or less are consistent with primary hyperthyroidism (values will vary between laboratories). Repeating these measurements with a third-generation assay helps differentiate patients with hyperthyroidism from those without it who have TSH suppression for other reasons. When serum TSH measurements in a third-generation TSH assay are 0.06 mU/L or less (values will vary among laboratories), a high probability of hyperthyroidism exists. Free-T4 levels should then be measured. When the serum TSH

level is less than 0.06 mU/L and the free-T4 level is elevated, hyperthyroidism is almost certainly present. When the free-T4 concentration is normal, T3-toxicosis should be considered. The free T3 level should then be measured. When both free T4 and free T3 levels are normal, "subclinical" hyperthyroidism may be present. Serum TSH levels should then be monitored at 3- to 6-month intervals. Serum TSH concentrations between 0.06 and 0.10 mU/L usually normalize at follow-up and may be the consequence of remitting subclinical hyperthyroidism, nonthyroidal illnesses, or drug effects [5]. When subclinical hyperthyroidism is suspected, TSH levels should be monitored at 3- to 6-month intervals until normalized or hyperthyroidism confirmed.

Patients with nonthyroidal illnesses (in the absence of hyperthyroidism) who have serum TSH concentrations less than 0.1 mU/L by second-generation assay only occasionally have TSH levels below 0.01 mU/L by third-generation assay [1]. In addition, severely ill patients with primary hyperthyroidism may have misleadingly normal or low free-T4 levels, depending on the method used [1,6,12] thus masking the typical findings of hyperthyroidism. Free-T4 measurements by direct dialysis typically are elevated in these patients [1]. If hyperthyroidism is clinically suspected in patients with serum TSH concentrations of 0.1 mU/L or greater, resistance to thyroid hormone (RTH) or central hyperthyroidism should be considered and further evaluated [1,2].

Therapy for hyperthyroidism should be aimed at normalizing both free-T4 and free-T3 concentrations before attempting to normalize TSH concentrations because TSH may remain low for a prolonged time despite response to therapy. (*Adapted from* Kaptein [5].)

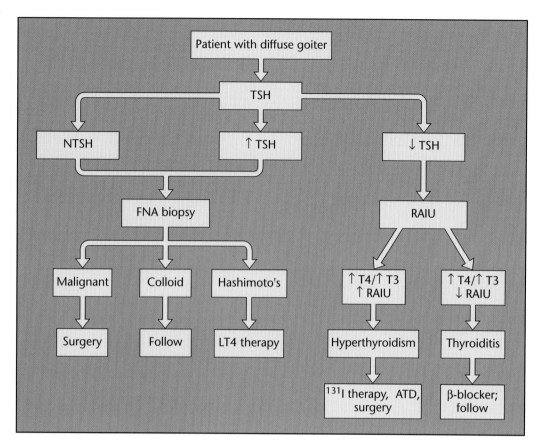

FIGURE 3-4.

Work-up for a patient with a diffuse goiter. Serum thyrotropin (TSH) measurement determines whether the patient is euthyroid or hyperthyroid. A suppressed TSH value suggests hyperthyroidism, which is then further evaluated by radioactive iodine uptake (RAIU). Increased RAIU with increased thyroid hormone levels is consistent with hyperthyroidism, whereas suppressed RAIU suggests thyroiditis. In most patients, serum TSH level is normal (NTSH) or slightly increased. In either case, fine-needle aspiration (FNA) biopsy determines the type of goiter present. Alternatively, antithyroid antibody measurement can be helpful, because when antibodies are present, the diagnosis is Hashimoto's thyroiditis, whereas if antibodies are negative, FNA is informative. If the goiter is malignant, surgical treatment is recommended. However, most goiters prove to be colloid and can be either observed or treated with levothyroxine (LT4). In the event that diffuse goiter is due to Hashimoto's thyroiditis, LT4 treatment (Rx) usually is recommended. ATD—antithyroid drugs; T3—triiodothyronine; T4—thyroxine.

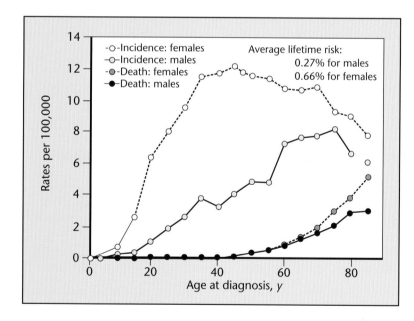

FIGURE 3-5.

Incidence of thyroid cancer. The incidence of thyroid carcinoma of all types varies with gender and age. It is highest in women between the ages of 30 and 70 years, reaching a peak incidence of 13.2 per 100,000 per year between 50 and 54 years of age [13]. The annual incidence is lower in men and peaks later in life, between the ages of 60 and 70 years, when it is 9.6 per 100,000. In the latest Surveillance, Epidemiology, and End Result (SEER) report, the average lifetime risk over a 95-year life span after having been diagnosed with some form of thyroid cancer is about 2.5 times higher in women than in men [13]. According to American Cancer Society estimates, about 17,200 new cases of thyroid cancer of all types will be diagnosed in 1998. This statistic ranks the United States 17th in incidence among the various forms of cancer and accounts for only about 1.4% of all cancers diagnosed [14]. Most of these are papillary (over 80%) or follicular thyroid cancers (5% to 10%), which have a good prognosis [15]. Thus, only about 1200 deaths resulting from thyroid carcinoma are anticipated during 1998, accounting for only about 0.2% of all cancer deaths and ranking it 37th among all cancer deaths.

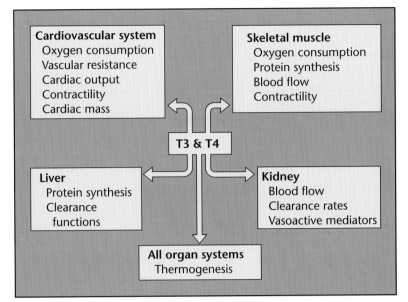

FIGURE 3-6.

Effects of thyroid hormone in various tissues. The clinical consequences of thyrotoxicosis reflect the end result of effects of excessive amounts of the thyroid hormones thyroxine (T4) and triiodothyronine (T3) on virtually all tissues and organs. Thus, increased cellular metabolism leads to energy production and increased thermogenesis, with the clinical manifestations of heat intolerance, increased sweating, and warm, moist skin. Increased oxygen consumption with hypermetabolism leads to weight loss and accumulation of waste byproducts, and muscle dysfunction ensues, with easy fatigue and muscle weakness. Increased levels of thyroid hormones lead to increased cardiac inotropy and contractility, increased heart rate, and reduced peripheral vascular resistance, all leading to an increase in cardiac output. With prolonged and more severe hyperthyroidism, these changes can culminate in a dilated cardiomyopathy with congestive heart failure.

Distinction Between Elevated Serum T4 of Thyrotoxicosis and Euthyroid Hyperthyroxinemia

Increased binding proteins

Estrogen

Infectious hepatitis

Opiates

Genetic

Anti-thyroxine antibodies

Thyroid hormone resistance

Amiodarone

Porphyria

Hyperemesis gravidarum*

Acute psychiatric disorders[†]

*Hyperemesis gravidarum may be associated with high levels of hCG, a weak but effective thyroid stimulator that may cause thyrotoxicosis.

[†]Some acute psychiatric disorders are associated with suppressed levels of TSH and blunted TSH responses to TRH, implying acute thyroid hyperfunction. These abnormalities usually are transient, with recovery to normal thyroid function tests resulting from therapy of the psychiatric disorder.

FIGURE 3-7.

Differential diagnosis of elevated total serum thyroxine. There are many causes for an increased level of circulating thyroxine (T4) that do not reflect a state of actual increased production and secretion of T4 from the thyroid gland. Because T4 and triiodothyronine (T3) are over 99% bound to circulating binding proteins, any cause of increased binding protein or binding protein capacity results in an increase in measurable total T4. The prototypic model for this is pregnancy, birth control pills, or estrogen replacement therapy, in which there is an increase in thyroxine-binding globulin (TBG). TBG is an inter-alpha globulin, and some disorders that are associated with increased globulin production (eg, hepatitis, biliary cirrhosis, porphyria) also may result in nonspecific increases in TBG production and release. The hyperthyroxinemia of hyperemesis gravidarum probably relates to increased production of human chorionic gonadotropin (hCG), because hCG is a weak thyroid stimulator. This disorder may be more accurately categorized as a form of mild hyperthyroidism, therefore, and not as euthyroid hyperthyroxinemia. Antithyroxine antibodies (as well as anti-T3 antibodies) are distinct from antithyroglobulin or antiperoxidase antibodies that are common in Hashimoto's disease, but these anti-T4 or anti-T3 antibodies do occur in patients with Hashimoto's disease and are a rare cause of hyperthyroxinemia. Clues that antibodies may be present include the presence of goiter, family history of autoimmune thyroid disease, and the concomitant finding of a marginally to frankly elevated serum thyrotropin (TSH).

Common Symptoms of Graves' Thyrotoxicosis

Symptom	Frequency, %
Nervousness, jitteriness, irritability	99
Increased perspiration	91
Easy fatigability	88
Heat intolerance	89
Weight loss	85
Tachycardia	82
Muscle weakness	70
Insomnia	65
Increased appetite	65
Reduced job performance; marital discord	58
Eye complaints	54
Hyperdefecation	33
Anorexia	9*
Constipation	4*

*May be due to associated hypercalcemia.

FIGURE 3-8.

Common symptoms of hyperthyroidism resulting from Graves' disease. The effects of thyroid hormone on virtually all tissues (see Fig. 3-6) are translated into many of the symptoms listed here. This is particularly true of patients in their second through fifth decades, whereas older patients may have masked symptoms (apathetic thyrotoxicosis). When present, anorexia and constipation (rather than the more common hyperphagia and hyperdefecation) may signal the presence of hypercalcemia of either or both total and ionized calcium, abnormalities that may be present in 20% to 35% of thyrotoxic patients. (*Adapted from* Larsen and Ingban [16].)

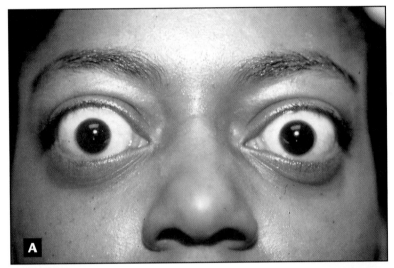

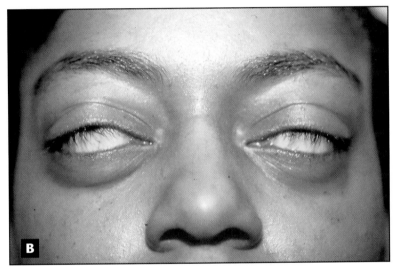

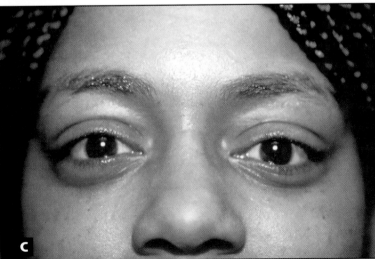

FIGURE 3-9.

A, Bilateral proptosis and eyelid retraction in a patient with Graves' ophthalmopathy. B, Bilateral lagophthalmos where the eyelids do not close normally, leaving patients susceptible to chronic ocular dryness. Bilateral lagophthalmos is a manifestation of Graves' disease. C, The same patient after bony orbital decompression and bilateral upper lid surgical reconstruction.

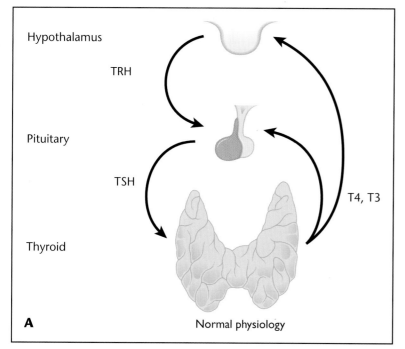

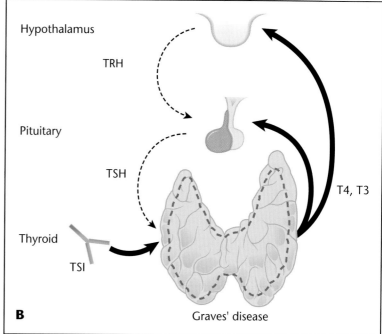

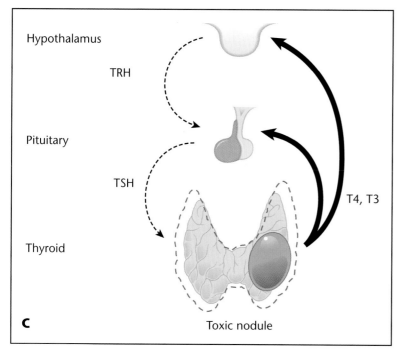

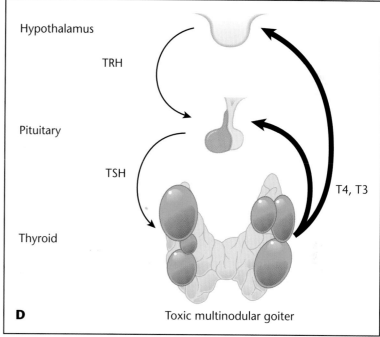

FIGURE 3-10.

Hypothalamic-pituitary-thyroid axis. **A,** Normal physiology in which thyroid function is controlled by pituitary thyroid-stimulating hormone (TSH) secretion, which in turn is influenced by hypothalamic thyroid-releasing hormone (TRH) stimulation. Negative feedback is exerted at the level of both the hypothalamus and pituitary by circulating thyroid hormones. **B,** Graves' disease in which thyroid function is increased and autonomous because of the presence of thyroid-stimulating antibodies (TSI) that mimic the effects of TSH on the TSH receptor. The gland is diffusely enlarged because of the trophic effects of the autoantibodies, TSH secretion is suppressed by negative feedback on the pituitary and hypothalamus, and circulating TSH concentrations become undetectable. **C,** Autonomously functioning thyroid nodule (AFTN). The thyroid gland contains a solitary, autonomous, hyperfunctioning nodule that suppresses TSH secretion by the pituitary because of its excessive secretion of thyroid hormones, and thereby reduces function of the "normal" thyroid tissue. **D,** Multiple, bilateral, hyperfunctioning nodules are seen in toxic multinodular goiter (TMNG). Although the biochemical effect is the same for TMNG and AFTN, the character of the goiter and physical examination are very distinct. T3—triiodothyronine; T4—thyroxine.

Causes of Transient or Permanent Hypothyroidism

Destructive
Postoperative
Radioactive iodine
External radiation to neck
Infiltrative disease (*eg*, sarcoidosis, amyloidosis, lymphoma, metastatic carcinoma)
Autoimmune
Hashimoto's disease
Following Graves' disease
Thyroiditis
Subacute (*eg*, viral)
Silent
Postpartum
Drug-induced
Iodides
Lithium
Thionamides
Hereditary or congenital
Enzyme deficiency affecting thyroid hormone biosynthesis
Agenesis
Hormone resistance
Endemic cretinism
Hypothalamic-pituitary disorders
Thyrotropin-releasing hormone deficiency
Thyroid-stimulating hormone deficiency
Idiopathic
Goitrous and nongoitrous primary hypothyroidism with negative anti-thyroid antibodies

FIGURE 3-11.

Causes of transient or permanent hypothyroidism. Adults with hypothyroidism often are diagnosed and managed in a uniform manner with little regard for the cause of their thyroid gland failure. It is important, however, for the cause of hypothyroidism to be considered in each case. By considering these differential diagnoses, it is possible to identify the rare but important patient with transient hypothyroidism or secondary hypothyroidism and treat him or her appropriately. (*Adapted from* Shapiro and Surks [17].)

Clinical Presentation of Thyroid Hormone Deficiency

Symptoms	Signs
General	
Cold intolerance	Hypothermia
Fatigue	Mild obesity
Mild weight gain	
Hoarse voice	
Nervous system	
Lethargy	Somnolence
Memory defects	Slow speech
Poor attention span	Myxedema wit
Personality change	Psychopathology: myxedema madness
	Diminished hearing and taste
	Cerebellar ataxia
	Delayed relaxation of deep tendon reflexes
	Carpal tunnel syndrome
Musculoskeletal	
Weakness	Normal strength
Muscle cramps	Normal joint examination
Joint pain	
Gastrointestinal system	
Nausea	Large tongue
Constipation	Ascites
Cardiorespiratory system	
Decreased exercise tolerance	Bradycardia
	Mild hypertension
	Pericardial effusion
	Pleural effusion
Reproductive system	
Decreased libido	Normal secondary sex characteristics
Decreased fertility	
Menstrual disorders	
Skin and appendages	
Dry, rough skin	Nonpitting edema of hands, face, and ankles
Puffy facies	
Hair loss	Periorbital swelling
Brittle nails	Pallor
	Yellowish skin (due to carotenemia)
	Coarse hair
	Dry axillae

FIGURE 3-12.

Clinical presentation of thyroid hormone deficiency. The symptoms and signs of hypothyroidism vary with the degree and duration of the hormone deficit. In mild hypothyroidism, laboratory testing may confirm a diagnosis in the absence of clinical disease. However, severe hypothyroidism affects virtually all organ systems. This table lists the symptoms and signs of severe thyroid hormone deficiency. (*Adapted from* Shapiro and Surks [17].)

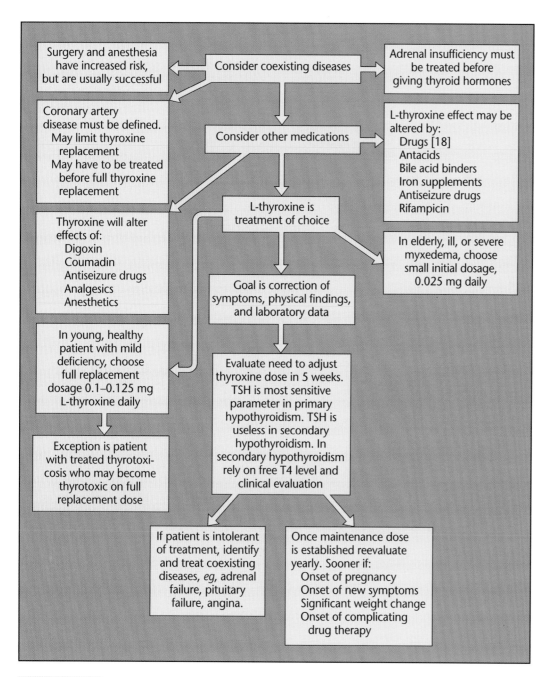

FIGURE 3-13.

Treatment of hypothyroidism. The treatment of hypothyroidism follows careful assessment of the cause of the disease and the clinical status of the patient. Coexisting diseases and current medications must be considered. The choice of initial dosage varies. The treatment goal in a patient with primary hypothyroidism without indication for suppression of thyrotropin (TSH), such as would exist in cases of large goiter or treated thyroid cancer, is normalization of TSH. In patients with secondary hypothyroidism, treatment is guided by clinical evaluation and serum free thyroxine (T4). Once optimum therapy is achieved, the dosage of T4 should be routinely checked at periods ranging from several weeks in patients on medications that are known to affect T4 levels to a year in otherwise healthy patients. Patients should be educated to return for evaluation earlier if symptoms of hormone excess or deficiency occur or if there is any significant change in their clinical status.

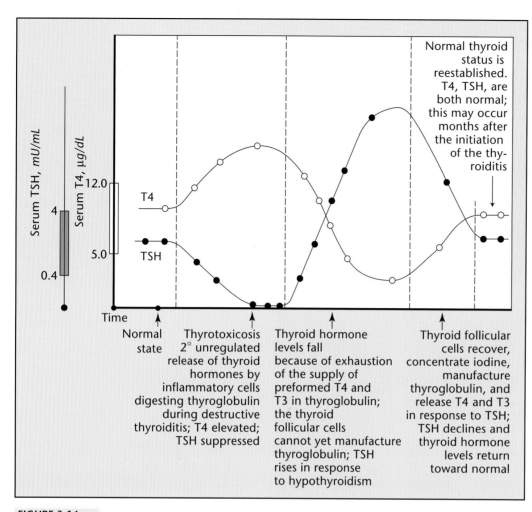

Serum TSH, mU/mL

Serum T4, µg/dL

12.0

5.0

0.4

4

0.4

T4

TSH

Normal thyroid status is reestablished. T4, TSH, are both normal; this may occur months after the initiation of the thyroiditis

Time

Normal state

Thyrotoxicosis 2° unregulated release of thyroid hormones by inflammatory cells digesting thyroglobulin during destructive thyroiditis; T4 elevated; TSH suppressed

Thyroid hormone levels fall because of exhaustion of the supply of preformed T4 and T3 in thyroglobulin; the thyroid follicular cells cannot yet manufacture thyroglobulin; TSH rises in response to hypothyroidism

Thyroid follicular cells recover, concentrate iodine, manufacture thyroglobulin, and release T4 and T3 in response to TSH; TSH declines and thyroid hormone levels return toward normal

FIGURE 3-14.

Serum concentrations of thyroid hormones during thyroiditis and recovery. When thyroiditis disrupts the thyroid follicle, the excessive release of thyroxine independent of

hypothalamic-pituitary regulation is detected by elevated serum thyroid hormone levels; however, not all patients experience clinical evidence of thyrotoxicosis. Because the affected thyroid does not trap iodine or synthesize thyroglobulin, the amount of thyroxine released during an episode of thyroiditis is limited by the amount of thyroglobulin that was present in the affected thyroid follicles at disease onset. The thyrotoxic phase therefore is self-limiting, and the patient is restored to euthyroidism. In classic descriptions of this illness, a hypothyroid phase follows when the preformed thyroxine (T4) and triiodothyronine (T3) contained in thyroglobulin has been exhausted and the thyroid follicular epithelial cells have not yet recovered sufficiently from the inflammatory insult to regain their capacity to synthesize thyroglobulin. During this hypothyroid phase, patients may exhibit symptoms and signs of thyroid hormone deficiency and will manifest laboratory measurements that typify this state. The duration of each phase is highly variable. Although current research has pointed to the presence of persistent thyroid abnormalities after recovery, this occurrence is not of clinical significance. Patients regain a state of normal thyroid function. TSH—thyroid-stimulating hormone.

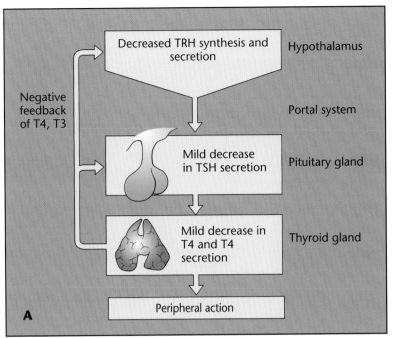

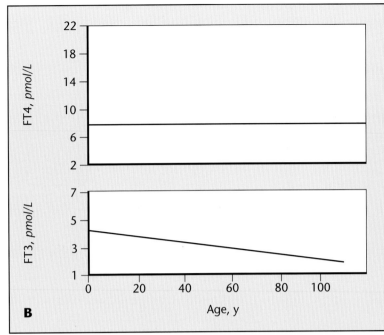

FIGURE 3-15.

Thyroid function alterations with normal aging. **A,** Hypothalamic-pituitary-thyroid axis. There are very mild decreases in the secretion of thyrotropin-releasing hormone (TRH), thyrotropin (TSH), and thyroid hormone with aging, especially in the very elderly. Conventional thyroid function tests, such as serum TSH and free thyroxine (FT4) measurements, remain normal, however, and therefore are not useful in assessing the presence and degree of thyroid dysfunction, as they are in younger individuals. **B,** Age-dependent changes in free thyroxine (T4) (*top panel*) and free triiodothyronine (T3) (*bottom panel*). Note that serum FT4 levels do not change with advancing age, despite a mild decrease in T4 secretion. This may be explained by a decrease in T4 clearance. Serum T3 and FT3 concentrations decrease with age, most likely due to less conversion of T4 to T3 from a reduced hepatic 59-deiodinase activity. Not shown here are TSH levels, which remain normal or may decrease slightly with aging as a result of a mild decrease in TRH secretion. The changes shown in this figure are considered to be normal changes of aging. (*Adapted from* Mariotti *et al.* [19].)

■ DIABETES

REGULATION OF INSULIN SECRETION AND ISLET CELL FUNCTION

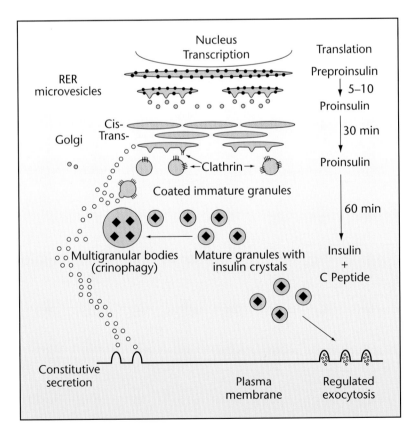

FIGURE 3-16.

Pathways of insulin biosynthesis. Glucose stimulates the production of preproinsulin through effects on transcription and even stronger influences on translation. Shortly after its inception preproinsdulin is cleaved to proinsulin which is then transported through the Golgi and packaged unto clathrin-coated immature granules, where proinsulin is further processed to proinsulin-like peptides, insulin and c-peptide. Granules containing crystallized insulin can either remain in a storage compartment, be absorbed into multigranular bodies where they are degraded by the process of crinophagy, or be secreted via the regulated pathway of secretion with its final event of exocytosis. Although the vast majority of insulin is secreted through the regulated pathway, a small amount can be released from microvesicles through the pathway of constitutive secretion. (See references 20 and 21 for more details.)

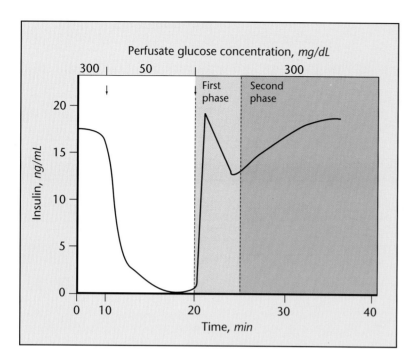

FIGURE 3-17.

Glucose stimulation of insulin secretion. Insulin secretion from the isolated perfused rat pancreas. At glucose concentrations at 50 mg/dL or below, insulin secretory rates are very low. Challenge with a high concentration of glucose provokes a biphasic pattern of insulin response [22]. (*Adapted from* Leahy *et al.* [23].)

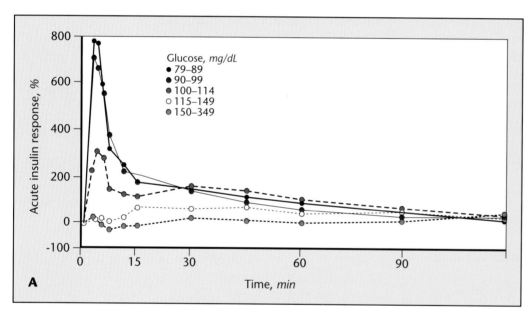

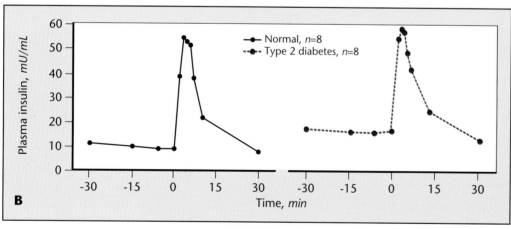

FIGURE 3-18.

Insulin secretory characteristics in type 2 diabetes. **A**, Loss of early insulin secretory response to an intravenous glucose challenge as fasting plasma glucose rises in subjects progressing from the normal state towards Type 2 diabetes [24]. It should be noted that impaired insulin responses to glucoses can even be seen before glucose levels rise to levels required for the diagnosis of impaired glucose tolerance (fasting glucose levels 110 mg/dL or above).

B, Preservation of acute insulin secretion in response to an intravenous pulse of arginine in Type 2 diabetes [25]. The acute insulin responses to glucose were lost in these subjects. Insulin responses can also be preserved when using a variety of other secretagogues including isoproterenol, sulfonylureas, and the gut hormones glucagon-like peptide 1 and GIP.

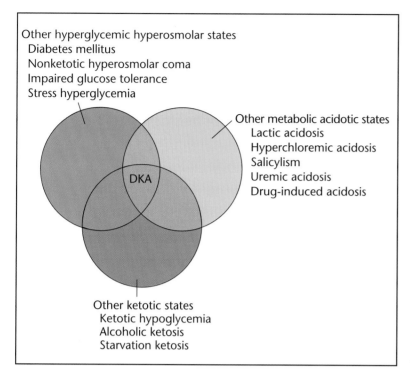

Other hyperglycemic hyperosmolar states
  Diabetes mellitus
  Nonketotic hyperosmolar coma
  Impaired glucose tolerance
  Stress hyperglycemia

Other metabolic acidotic states
  Lactic acidosis
  Hyperchloremic acidosis
  Salicylism
  Uremic acidosis
  Drug-induced acidosis

DKA

Other ketotic states
  Ketotic hypoglycemia
  Alcoholic ketosis
  Starvation ketosis

FIGURE 3-19.

Other conditions in which the components of the diagnostic triad for DKA (hyperglycemia, ketosis, and acidosis) may be found. (*Adapted from* Kitabchi and Wall [26].)

Diagnostic Criteria and Typical Total Body Deficits of Water and Electrolytes in DKA and HHS

Factor Studied	DKA			HHS
	Mild	Moderate	Severe	
Diagnostic Criteria and Classification				
Plasma glucose, *mg/dL*	> 250	> 250	> 250	> 600
Arterial pH	7.25–7.30	7.00–<7.24	< 7.00	> 7.30
Serum bicarbonate, *mEq/L*	15–18	10–<15	< 10	> 15
Urine ketone*	Positive	Positive	Positive	Small
Serum ketone*	Positive	Positive	Positive	Small
Effective serum osmolality†	Variable	Variable	Variable	> 320 mOsm/kg
Anion gap‡	Wide (> 14)	Wide (> 14)	Wide (> 14)	Normal to slightly wide (< 14)
Alteration in sensorium or mental obtundation	Alert	Alert/drowsy	Stupor/coma	Stupor/coma
Typical Deficit				
Total water, *L*		6		9
Water, *mL/kg*§		100		100–200
Na+, *mEq/kg*		7–10		5–13
Cl-, *mEq/kg*		3–5		5–15
K+, *mEq/kg*		3–5		4–6
PO$_4$, *mmol/kg*		5–7		3–7
Mg++, *mEq/kg*		1–2		1–2
Ca++, *mEq/kg*		1–2		1–2

*Nitroprusside reaction method.
†Calculation: Effective serum osmolality: 2[measure Na (mEq/L)] + glucose (mg/dL)/18.
‡Calculation: Anion gap: (Na+) - (Cl- - HCO3-) (mEq/L).
§Per kg of body weight.

FIGURE 3-20.

Diagnostic criteria and typical total body deficits of water and electrolytes in diabetic ketoacidosis (DKA) and hyperglycemic hyperosmolar syndrome (HHS). (*Adapted from* Kitabchi *et al.* [27].)

Laboratory Evaluation of Metabolic Causes of Acidosis and Coma

Factor Studied	Starvation of High Fat Intake	DKA	Lactic acidosis	Uremic Acidosis	Alcoholic Ketosis (Starvation)	Salicylate Intoxication	Methanol or Ethylene Glycol Intoxication	Hyperosmolar Coma	Hypoglycemic Coma	Rhabdomyolysis
pH	Normal	↓	↓	Mild ↓	↓↑	↓↑	↓	Normal	Normal	Mild ↓ may be ↓↓
Plasma glucose	Normal	↑	Normal	Normal	↓ or normal	Normal or ↓	Normal	↑↑ 500 mg/dL	↓↓ < 30 mg/dL	Normal
Glycosuria	Negative	++	Negative	Negative	Negative	Negative†	Negative	++	Negative	Negative
Total plasma ketones†	Slight ↑	↑↑	Normal	Normal	Slight to moderate	Normal	Normal	Normal or slight	Normal	Normal
Anion gap	Slight ↑	↑	↑	Slight ↑	↑	↑	↑	↑	Normal	↑↑
Osmolality	Normal	↑	Normal	↑ or	↑	Normal	↑↑	Normal ↑↑ > 330 mOsm /kg	Normal	
Uric acid	Mild (starvation)	↑	Normal	Normal ↑	Normal	Normal	Normal	Normal	Normal	Normal or slight ↑↑
Miscellaneous		May give false positive for ethylene glycol [28]	Serum lactate > 7 mM	BUN > 200 ↑ mg/dL		Serum salicylate +	Serum levels positive			Myoglobinuria, hemoglobinuria

*Acetest and Ketostix measure acetoacetic acid only. Thus, misleading low values may be obtained because the majority of "ketone bodies" are β-hydroxybutyrate.
†Respiratory alkalosis/metabolic acidosis.
‡May get false-positive or false-negative urinary glucose caused by the presence of salicylate or its metabolites.

FIGURE 3-21.

Laboratory evaluation of metabolic causes of acidosis and coma. (*Adapted from* Morris and Kitabchi [29].)

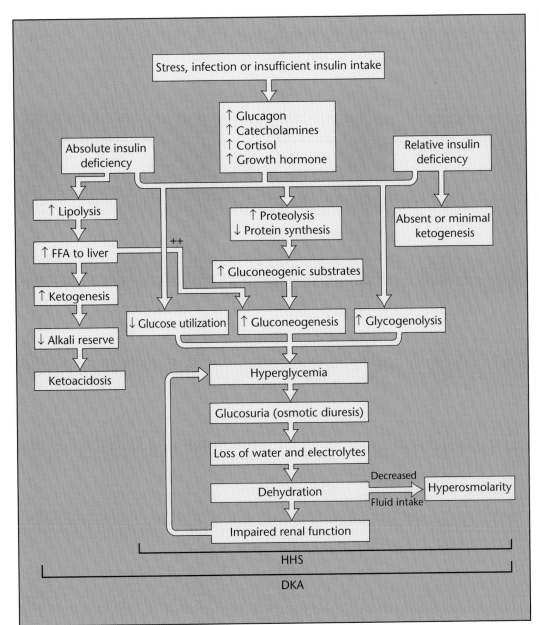

FIGURE 3-22.

Pathogenesis of DKA and HHS. Alteration of fat, protein and carbohydrate metabolism leads to metabolic changes toward catabolic states and symptoms of polyuria, polydipsia, polyphagia, osmotic diuresis, severe hydration and, if not treated, coma and death. The hallmark of these events is the insulin deficient state and increased counterregulatory hormones. In HHS, in addition to the relative insulin deficiency and greater dehydration, there is also a greater amount of hyperglycemia (secondary to lower intake of fluid) than in DKA. Although the mechanism for the lack of a significant amount of ketosis and acidemia in HHS (as compared with DKA) is not entirely clear, in one study the level of C-peptide (as an indication of pancreatic insulin reserve) was shown to be five- to ten-fold lower in DKA than in HHS [30]. This has been offered as a part of the explanation for the lack of ketonemia in HHS. Since the required amount of insulin for its antilipolytic action is about five- to ten-fold lower than for the glucose transport action [31], it follows that the larger amount of residual insulin (C-peptide) in HHS is sufficient to prevent lipolysis (thus no ketogenesis in HHS), but this amount of insulin is not enough to promote glucose transport and its metabolism, thus resulting in the hyperglycemia that one notes in HHS without severe ketonemia. (*Adapted from* Kitabchi *et al.* [27].)

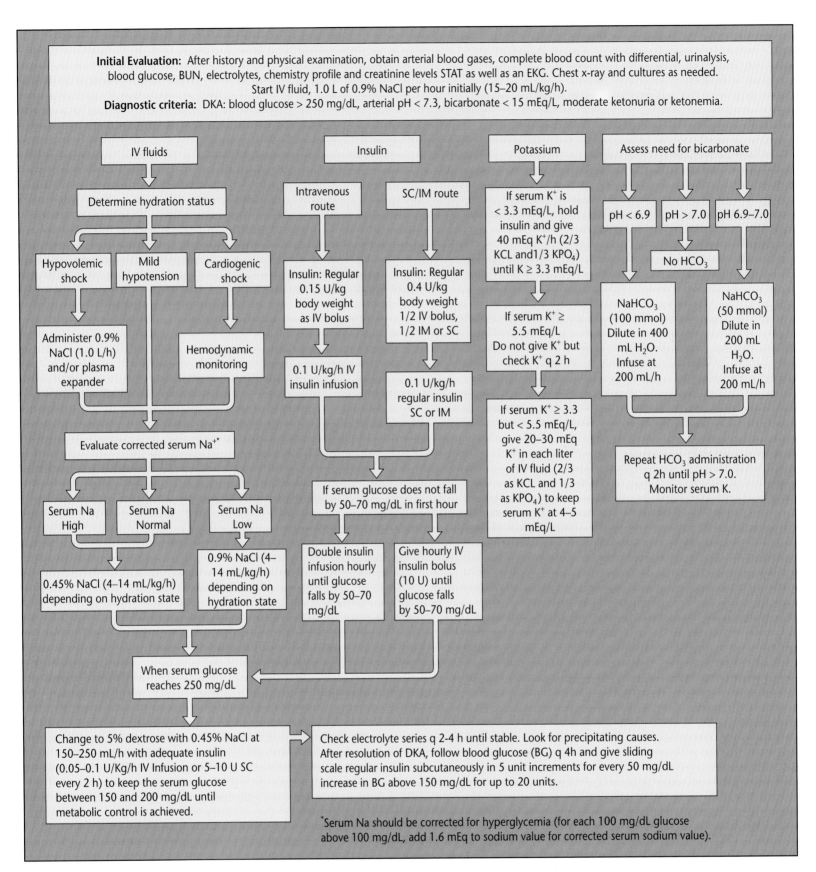

Initial Evaluation: After history and physical examination, obtain arterial blood gases, complete blood count with differential, urinalysis, blood glucose, BUN, electrolytes, chemistry profile and creatinine levels STAT as well as an EKG. Chest x-ray and cultures as needed. Start IV fluid, 1.0 L of 0.9% NaCl per hour initially (15–20 mL/kg/h).

Diagnostic criteria: DKA: blood glucose > 250 mg/dL, arterial pH < 7.3, bicarbonate < 15 mEq/L, moderate ketonuria or ketonemia.

IV fluids

Determine hydration status

Hypovolemic shock | Mild hypotension | Cardiogenic shock

Administer 0.9% NaCl (1.0 L/h) and/or plasma expander

Hemodynamic monitoring

Evaluate corrected serum Na⁺

Serum Na High | Serum Na Normal | Serum Na Low

0.45% NaCl (4–14 mL/kg/h) depending on hydration state

0.9% NaCl (4–14 mL/kg/h) depending on hydration state

Insulin

Intravenous route | SC/IM route

Insulin: Regular 0.15 U/kg body weight as IV bolus

Insulin: Regular 0.4 U/kg body weight 1/2 IV bolus, 1/2 IM or SC

0.1 U/kg/h IV insulin infusion

0.1 U/kg/h regular insulin SC or IM

If serum glucose does not fall by 50–70 mg/dL in first hour

Double insulin infusion hourly until glucose falls by 50–70 mg/dL

Give hourly IV insulin bolus (10 U) until glucose falls by 50–70 mg/dL

Potassium

If serum K⁺ is < 3.3 mEq/L, hold insulin and give 40 mEq K⁺/h (2/3 KCL and1/3 KPO₄) until K ≥ 3.3 mEq/L

If serum K⁺ ≥ 5.5 mEq/L Do not give K⁺ but check K⁺ q 2 h

If serum K⁺ ≥ 3.3 but < 5.5 mEq/L, give 20–30 mEq K⁺ in each liter of IV fluid (2/3 as KCL and 1/3 as KPO₄) to keep serum K⁺ at 4–5 mEq/L

Assess need for bicarbonate

pH < 6.9 | pH > 7.0 | pH 6.9–7.0

No HCO₃

NaHCO₃ (100 mmol) Dilute in 400 mL H₂O. Infuse at 200 mL/h

NaHCO₃ (50 mmol) Dilute in 200 mL H₂O. Infuse at 200 mL/h

Repeat HCO₃ administration q 2h until pH > 7.0. Monitor serum K.

When serum glucose reaches 250 mg/dL

Change to 5% dextrose with 0.45% NaCl at 150–250 mL/h with adequate insulin (0.05–0.1 U/Kg/h IV Infusion or 5–10 U SC every 2 h) to keep the serum glucose between 150 and 200 mg/dL until metabolic control is achieved.

Check electrolyte series q 2-4 h until stable. Look for precipitating causes. After resolution of DKA, follow blood glucose (BG) q 4h and give sliding scale regular insulin subcutaneously in 5 unit increments for every 50 mg/dL increase in BG above 150 mg/dL for up to 20 units.

*Serum Na should be corrected for hyperglycemia (for each 100 mg/dL glucose above 100 mg/dL, add 1.6 mEq to sodium value for corrected serum sodium value).

FIGURE 3-23.

Protocol for management of patients with diabetic ketoacidosis (DKA). This figure provides step by step methods for therapeutic management of patients with DKA. Important steps besides use of insulin are hydration and frequent monitoring of such patients [26,27,32]. (*Adapted from* Kitabchi *et al.* [33].)

Forms of Modified Insulin

Insulin Form	Modification	Onset of Action	Duration of Activity
Very rapid-acting			
Lispro*	B-chain proline (amino acid 28) and lysine (amino acid 29) reversed	10–15 min	2–3 h
Rapid-acting			
Crystalline zinc insulin (CZI)†	Zinc	30–45 min	4–6 h
Intermediate-acting			
Neutral protamine Hagedorn (NPH)†	Protamine	1–2 h	6–12 h
Lente†	Zinc	1–2 h	6–12 h
Long-acting			
Ultralente*	Zinc	6–8 h	18 h
Premixed combinations:			
70/30*	70% NPH and 30% CZI	30–45 min	6–12 h
50/50*	50% NPH and 50% CZI	30–45 min	6–12 h

*Available only as recombinant human insulin.
†Available as human, beef and pork, and pure pork. Effective January 1999, animal species insulin to be eliminated.

FIGURE 3-24.

The available forms of modified insulin provide a spectrum of action that facilitates near normalization of glucose levels when used in conjunction with frequent monitoring of glucose levels. Selection of dose size and timing of administration are dependent on an understanding of the impact of exercise and meal size and composition on glucose fluctuations. Even with these tools, intensive therapy is imperfect. True normalization of glucose levels rarely, if ever, is achieved. Realistically, hemoglobin A1c levels can be maintained at 4 to 5 standard deviations above the mean nondiabetic level, and then only with a substantial frequency of hypoglycemic reactions.

Long-term Complications of Type 1 Diabetes and the Risk of Developing Clinical Manifestations of Specified Complications

Cataract: 25% to 30% lifetime risk with 3% to 5% requiring cataract extraction

Glaucoma (open angle): 10% risk after 30 years

Retinopathy: 90% develop some degree over lifetime; 40% to 50% require laser and 3% to 5% blind after 30 years' duration

Adhesive capsulitis: frozen shoulder, prevalence 10%

CAD: major cause of mortality

Gastroparesis: 1% to 5% develop symptoms (lifetime risk)

Carpal tunnel syndrome: 30% with electrophysiologic evidence, 9% with symptoms (prevalence)

Nephropathy: 35% develop end-stage renal disease over lifetime

Trigger finger, DuPuytren's contractures: 10% prevalence

Autonomic neuropathy (prevalence): bladder, 1% to 5% with dysfunction; impotence, 10% to 40%; diarrhea, 1%

Peripheral vascular disease

Peripheral neuropathy: 54% lifetime risk; 2% to 3% foot ulcers/y

FIGURE 3-25.

Long-term complications of type 1 diabetes and the risks of developing clinical manifestations of specified complications. Data for some complications are sparse. The estimates provided reflect the era before the Diabetes Control and Complications Trial (DCCT). Intensive therapy of type 2 diabetes is anticipated to reduce the lifelong development of retinopathy, nephropathy, and neuropathy by 50% to 80%. The overall effect of diabetic complications results in a substantial 15-year reduction in life span, predominantly owing to the development of nephropathy and cardiovascular disease.

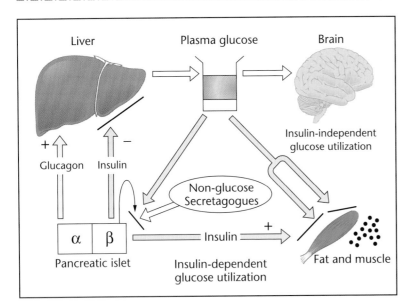

FIGURE 3-26.

Regulation of glucose homeostasis. The blood glucose level is a balance between glucose production by the liver and glucose utilization by insulin-independent tissues (such as the brain, kidney, and erythrocytes) and insulin-dependent tissues (such as fat and muscle). This balance is orchestrated by hormones of the endocrine pancreas: insulin from the beta cell and glucagon from the alpha cell. In type 2 diabetes, there is insulin resistance in the liver, muscle, and fat and a decrease in the ability of the beta cell to sense glucose and increase insulin levels appropriately. This figure also shows the defects in insulin action on the liver, muscle, and fat and defects in glucose sensing by the beta cell in type 2 diabetes. Recent evidence suggests that insulin action at the beta cell may be important in glucose sensing and that this is another site of insulin resistance in type 2 diabetes [34].

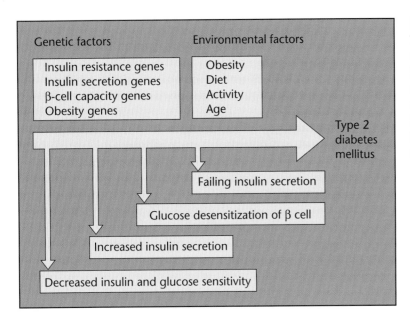

FIGURE 3-27.

The progressive pathogenesis of type 2 diabetes. The pathogenesis of the disease develops over many years. The earliest detectable lesion is insulin resistance. Initially, increased insulin secretion compensates for this defect. Eventually, the beta cell becomes desensitized to the glucose stimulus and insulin levels decrease, leading to clinically overt diabetes. Both the insulin resistance and beta-cell failure are genetically programmed and influenced by environmental factors, such as diet, activity, and aging.

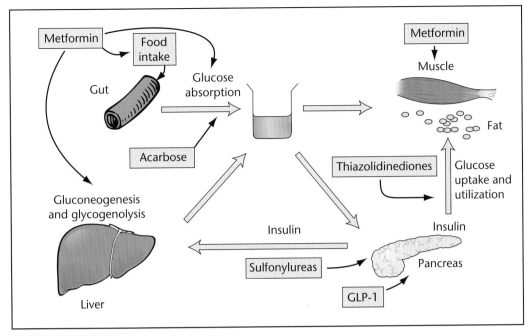

FIGURE 3-28.

Sites of action of drugs used to treat type 2 diabetes. Diet and exercise are directed at improving insulin sensitivity by reducing the effects of obesity and sedentary lifestyle. Different oral hypoglycemic agents have different sites of action. Sulfonylureas act on a receptor on the pancreatic beta cell to stimulate insulin secretion, thus bypassing the glucose-sensing apparatus [35]. Most studies suggest that the major site of action of metformin is the liver and an inhibition of hepatic glucose output [36,37]. The thiazolidine-diones improve insulin sensitivity in muscle and fat [37,38]. This occurs via interaction

with a nuclear receptor PPARg2, which also serves as the initial regulator of fat cell differentiation. Activation of this nuclear receptor increases the level of gene expression of many proteins involved in insulin action and insulin sensitivity. An interesting group of obese patients were recently described with activating mutations in PPARg; the phenotype of these patients includes massive obesity but relatively normal insulin sensitivity [39]. There are several thiazolidinediones, including troglitazone, rosiglitazone, pioglitazone, and englitazone. About one-third of patients with type 2 diabetes cannot be managed with the combination of lifestyle modification and oral agents and must be treated with insulin. Although there has been concern about the use of insulin in patients with type 2 diabetes because hyperinsulinemia has been associated with increased cardiovascular morbidity in several population studies [40], the United Kingdom Prospective Diabetes Study has definitively demonstrated that patients with type 2 diabetes receiving insulin have improved outcomes compared with less aggressively treated patients not receiving insulin (see Fig. 3-29).

UKPDS: Effects of Intensive Treatment of Type 2 Diabetes

Reduced HbA1c by 11% with intensive Rx (7.9 vs. 7.0%)
This leads to

    12% decrease in any diabetes-related endpoint
    25% decrease in microvascular endpoints
    21% decrease in retinopathy at 12 years
    33% decrease in microalbuminuria at 12 years
    24% decrease in cataract
    16% decrease in myocardial infarction (ns)
    5% decrease in stroke (ns)

FIGURE 3-29.

Results of the United Kingdom Prospective Diabetes Study (UKPDS) showed an unequivocal effect of intensive insulin therapy on long-term complications of diabetes and mortality [41,42]. HbA1c—glycated hemoglobin; ns–not significant; Rx—therapy.

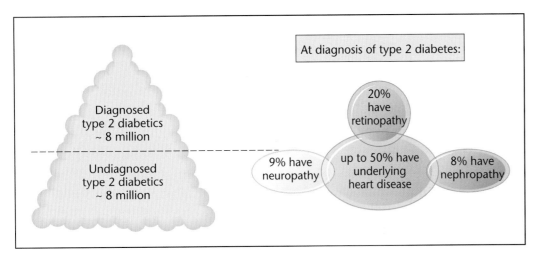

FIGURE 3-30.
The epidemiology of diabetes and its complications. Diabetes mellitus is an important clinical and public health problem in the United States. Nearly 8 million adults have been diagnosed with diabetes, 90% to 95% of whom have type 2 diabetes. In addition, it is estimated that a further 8 million persons who meet the diagnostic criteria for diabetes remain undiagnosed. It has been estimated that among patients in the United States, type 2 diabetes may have been present for up to 12 years before clinical diagnosis. During this period of undiagnosed and untreated diabetes, both micro- and macrovascular disease progress. By the time of diagnosis, 20% of patients have retinopathy, 8% have nephropathy, 9% have neuropathy, and up to 50% have cardiovascular disease [43–45].

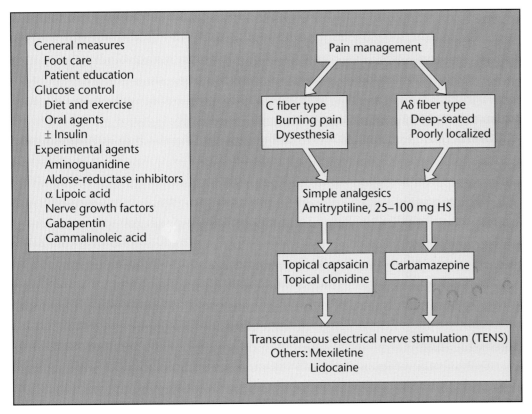

FIGURE 3-31.
Management of peripheral diabetic neuropathy. The pathophysiologic mechanisms underlying decreased nerve function and nerve fiber loss in diabetics still are not fully understood but may include formation of sorbitol by aldose reductase and the formation of advanced glycation end products (AGEs) [46]. Like other diabetic complications, the progression of neuropathy is related to glycemic control. Chronic sensory neuropathy with moderate or severe sensory loss involving large-fiber sensation (touch, vibration, and joint position sense) or small-fiber sensation (pain and temperature sense) is associated with a high risk of ulceration. Current approaches to prevention and treatment of diabetic neuropathy include measures to optimize glucose control, various symptomatic measures for pain control, and use of aldose reductase inhibitors, which appear to slow the progression of neuropathy rather than provide symptomatic relief [47].

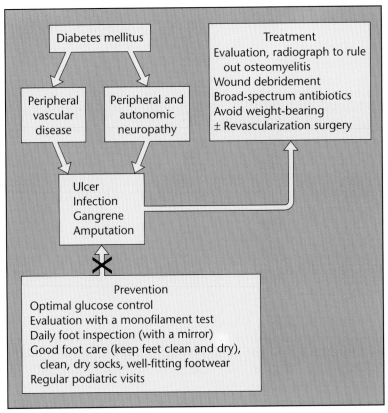

FIGURE 3-32.
Clinical features and management of diabetic foot disease. Diabetic foot lesions are a major cause of hospitalization, with approximately

20% of all diabetics entering the hospital because of foot problems. Nearly 55,000 lower extremity amputations are performed each year on diabetics, accounting for 50% of all nontraumatic amputations [48]. Diabetic foot lesions are the result of a combination of peripheral and autonomic neuropathy and peripheral vascular disease (ischemia). The cascade of events begins with foot ulcers, infection, and gangrene, and ultimately results in amputation. Management of diabetic foot ulcers should be aggressive, and should include detailed evaluation of the ulcer and the foot, radiography to exclude osteomyelitis, broad-spectrum antibiotics, wound debridement (if indicated), and avoidance of weight bearing. Topical application of antibacterial agents and platelet-derived growth factors may be useful adjunctive measures. Preventive measures include optimal glycemic control, daily foot inspections (with the aid of a mirror), good foot care (keeping feet clean and dry), wearing clean socks and appropriate, well-fitting shoes, and regular podiatric visits. Good patient education and a team approach are the keys to the prevention and treatment of diabetic foot disease.

Diabetics are particularly prone to foot deformities and the development of cocked-up toes, which results in pressure at the tips of the toes and under the first metatarsal head, leading to ulceration and infection. The ideal treatment is prophylactic surgery to straighten the toes. If this is not feasible, special shoes with a cushioned insole to protect the toes and metatarsal head should be worn.

All diabetics should have the protective sensory function in their feet evaluated with a 10-g Semmestel-Weinstein monofilament. If a patient cannot consistently feel a 10-g monofilament, protective sensory function has been lost, and the patient is at high risk of developing foot ulcers [49].

FIGURE 3-33.
Cardiovascular disease is the major cause of mortality in type 2 diabetics. **A**, Comparison of data from the Joslin Study and the Framingham Study shows that the mortality rate due to coronary artery disease is doubled in men with diabetes and nearly quadrupled in women with diabetes, as compared to the nondiabetic population [50]. Moreover, within the diabetic population, glucose control is an important predictor of coronary artery disease (CAD) mortality and all CAD events. **B**, In the Finnish population, the mortality rate in elderly diabetics (65 to 74 years old at baseline) with poor glycemic control (HbA$_{1C}$ > 7.9%) was more than three times that of those with good glycemic control (HbA$_{1C}$ < 6%) [51]. (Part A *adapted from* Krolewski *et al.* [50]; part B *adapted from* Kuusisto *et al.* [51].)

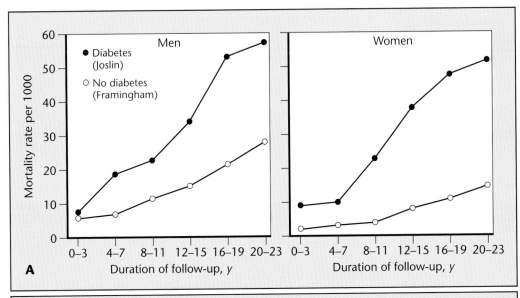

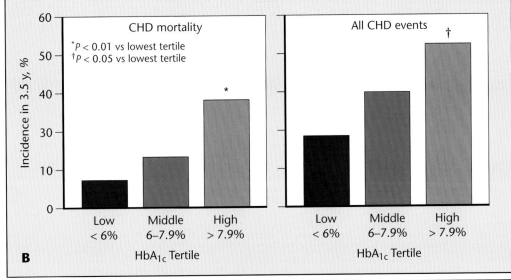

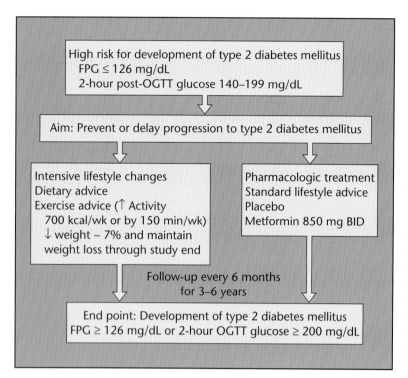

High risk for development of type 2 diabetes mellitus
FPG ≤ 126 mg/dL
2-hour post-OGTT glucose 140–199 mg/dL

Aim: Prevent or delay progression to type 2 diabetes mellitus

Intensive lifestyle changes
Dietary advice
Exercise advice (↑ Activity
700 kcal/wk or by 150 min/wk)
↓ weight ~ 7% and maintain
weight loss through study end

Pharmacologic treatment
Standard lifestyle advice
Placebo
Metformin 850 mg BID

Follow-up every 6 months
for 3–6 years

End point: Development of type 2 diabetes mellitus
FPG ≥ 126 mg/dL or 2-hour OGTT glucose ≥ 200 mg/dL

FIGURE 3-34.

National Institutes of Health (NIH) type 2 diabetes prevention program. It is now clear that type 2 diabetes is not a milder form of diabetes. Its complications can be the same as or more severe than those in type 1 diabetes. Moreover, these complications occur early during the natural course of the disease, even before clinical onset. At the time of diagnosis of type 2 diabetes, 20% of patients have retinopathy, 8% have nephropathy, 9% have neuropathy [44], and up to 50% have underlying coronary artery disease (CAD) [45]. Treatment of hyperglycemia, hypertension, and hyperlipidemia may prevent or retard the progression of diabetic complications. However, even with early intervention and intensive treatment, there are significant morbidity and high costs. Preventing or delaying the onset of diabetes may be more cost-effective [44]. Impaired glucose tolerance (IGT with FPG: 110–125 mg/dL, or 2-hour post-OGTT glucose 140–199 mg/dL) has been shown to be a strong risk factor for development of type 2 diabetes and a possible risk factor for CAD. There are data to suggest that at this stage of IGT, patients are at high risk for diabetes and CAD, but have not yet developed end-organ disease. The Diabetes Prevention Program (DPP) supported by the NIH will determine if it is possible to prevent or delay the progression to type 2 diabetes in patients who have IGT. Possible treatment options include intensive lifestyle measures (diet and exercise) or pharmacologic means (metformin). The study, which commenced in 1996, will be completed in 2002. FPG—fasting plasma glucose; OGTT—oral glucose tolerance test.

INSULIN RESISTANCE

Native and Experimental Insulin Resistance

Physiologic
  Puberty
  Pregnancy
  Bed rest
  Contraceptives
  High-fat diet
Metabolic
  Type 2 diabetes
  Uncontrolled type 1 diabetes
  Diabetic ketoacidosis
  Obesity
  Severe malnutrition
  Hyperuricemia
  Insulin-induced hypoglycemia
  Excessive alcohol consumption
Endocrine
  Thryotoxicosis
  Hypothyroidism
  Cushing syndrome
  Pheochromocytoma
  Acromegaly

Nonendocrine
  Essential hypertension
  Chronic uremia
  Liver cirrhosis
  Rheumatoid arthritis
  Acanthosis nigricans
  Chronic heart failure
  Myotonic dystrophia
  Trauma, burns, sepsis
  Surgery
  Neoplastic cachexia
Experimental
  Short-term hyperglycemia
  Short-term hypoglycemia
  Short-term hyperinsulinemia
  Short-term hypoinsulinemia
  Fat infusion
  Amino acid infusion
  Infusion of counterregulatory hormones
  Acidosis

FIGURE 3-35.

Native and experimental insulin resistance. This table lists conditions that have been found to be associated with insulin resistance or under which insulin resistance can be produced experimentally.

Clinical Presentations of Diabetic Eye Complications

Diabetes-Associated Pathology	Clinical Symptoms
Palsy of cranial nerves III, IV, VI	Diplopia: binocular
	Ptosis
	Anisocoria
	"Blurred vision": binocular
Reduced corneal sensitivity or corneal erosions or corneal infections	Ocular pain
	Ocular discharage
	Corneal opacification
	Decreased vision
Hyphema	Decreased vision
	Blood layering in anterior chamber
Angle closure glaucoma	Ocular pain
	Halos around lights
	Decreased vision
Iris neovascularization	Ocular pain
	Decreased vision
	Blood layering in anterior chamber
Cataract	Decreased vision
	Glare with bright lights
Vitreous hemorrhage	"Spots," "cobwebs," "lines" in vision (floaters)
	Decreased vision
Macular edema	Moderately decreased vision
	Image distortion
Proliferative diabetic retinopathy	Symptoms associated with vitreous hemorrhage and macular edema
Retina detachment	Photopsia
	Floaters
	Scotoma
	Decreased vision
	Image distortion
Diabetic papillopathy	Visual field change

FIGURE 3-36.
Clinical presentations associated with diabetic eye complications. Each of the numerous diabetes-associated ocular pathologies can present with a diverse array of symptoms. Only a partial list is presented here. It is important to realize that serious diabetic eye disease may exist without any discernible symptoms. This fact underscores the essential need for regular, routine, life-long follow-up regardless of the presence or absence of visual symptoms.

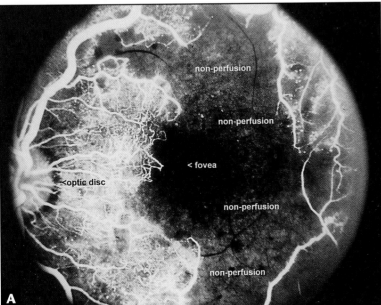

FIGURE 3-37.
Ophthalmic complications associated with visual loss in diabetic retinopathy. Visual loss associated with diabetic retinopathy can arise from multiple complications of the disease. If the characteristic progressive capillary loss eventually involves a large portion of the central macula, then visual acuity is compromised.

A, Fluorescein angiogram showing extensive macular capillary nonperfusion. Fluorescent dye (fluorescein) was injected into the patient's antecubital vein, and photographs were taken of the retina as the dye was passing through the retinal vessels. This technique, called fluorescein angiography, allows excellent visualization of the retinal vasculature. In this instance, the dye in the retinal vessels appears white, and the photograph shows nearly complete loss of the retinal vasculature perfusion in the macular region. These anatomic changes and their visual sequelae are irreversible. *(Continued)*

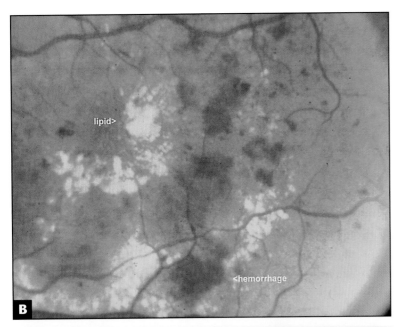

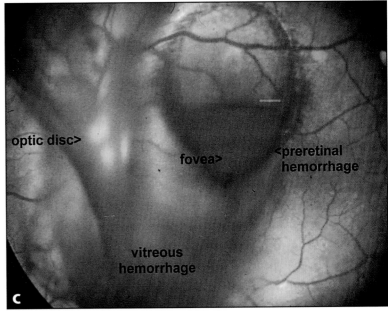

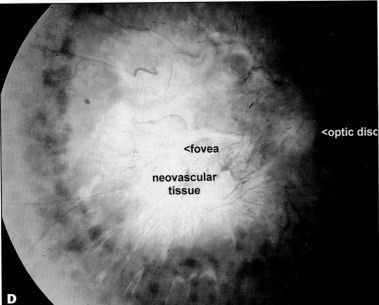

FIGURE 3-37. (*CONTINUED*)

B, Extensive retinal vascular leakage into the macular region with retinal thickening, lipid deposits, and retinal hemorrhage. This patient has severe macular edema, with associated visual loss.

C, Blood in the vitreous, a condition termed vitreous hemorrhage or preretinal hemorrhage. Preretinal hemorrhage refers specifically to blood immediately in front of the retina, whereas vitreous hemorrhage may be anywhere in the vitreous cavity. Vitreous hemorrhages are common in diabetic retinopathy owing to the fragility of new vessels and traction often exerted on these vessels by progressive retinal fibrosis. Although the hemorrhages usually clear spontaneously, surgical intervention may be required if they persist. Not only can vitreous hemorrhage obscure the patient's vision but also the ophthalmologist's view of the retina, which may necessitate evaluation of the retinal anatomy using ultrasonography if the hemorrhage is severe. **D**, A rare form of visual loss in diabetes in which a sheet of neovascular tissue obscures the visual axis. Removal of the tissue by vitrectomy surgery often can restore useful vision. (*Courtesy of* The Wilmer Ophthalmological Institute.)

DIABETES AND THE KIDNEY

Microalbuminuria and Macroalbuminuria

Definition of microalbuminuria
  < 30 mg/24 h or > 20 µg/min
  Albumin/creatinine ratio of > 30 mg/g
Definition of frank albuminuria or macroalbuminuria
  > 300 mg/24 h or > 200 µg/min
Common causes of transient increases in albuminuria
Exercise
Pregnancy
Poor glycemic control
Congestive heart failure
Hypertension
Urinary tract infection

FIGURE 3-38.
Detection of microalbuminuria. Microalbuminuria is the hallmark of early diabetic nephropathy, so all diabetic patients should be routinely screened for the presence of microalbuminuria. Although a timed urine collection is a very effective way to determine albumin excretion accurately, it is neither convenient nor cost-effective. Recent studies have shown that the albumin/creatinine ratio, obtained by measuring a spot urine sample for albumin and creatinine, is a highly accurate method for screening and following patients with diabetes mellitus [52]. The dipsticks used for the determination of protein in the urine are not sensitive enough to measure protein excretion less than 300 mg per 24 hours, however, so direct laboratory measurement of albumin is required to detect microalbuminuria. A spot measurement of albumin alone is affected by the urine volume, but normalizing to the amount of creatinine in the urine eliminates this concern. As shown, a value of 30 mg/g is suggestive of the presence of microalbuminuria. A number of studies have shown that the albumin/creatinine ratio is a highly accurate and effective test for the detection and following of patients with diabetes mellitus.

In determining the presence of microalbuminuria, causes of transient increases in albuminuria must be considered. Macroalbuminuria reflects progressive diabetic nephropathy. Increased attention to treatment should be given. Thus, repeat measurements of albumin excretion are recommended before labeling a patient with a diagnosis of early diabetic nephropathy.

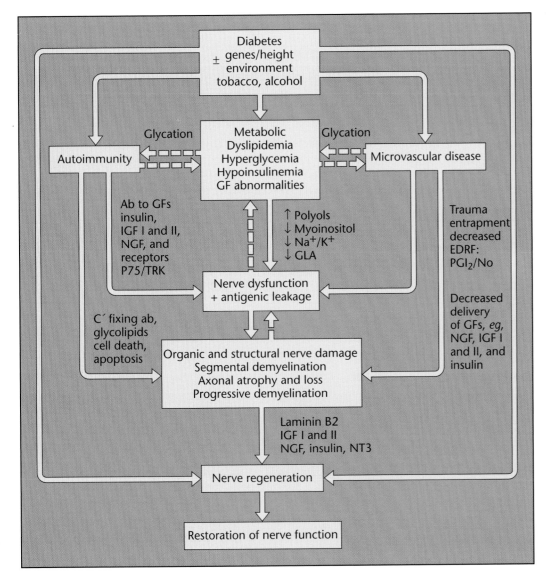

FIGURE 3-39.
Current view on the pathogenesis of diabetic neuropathy. The figure depicts multiple causes, as discussed above, including metabolic, vascular, autoimmune, and neurohormonal growth factor deficiency. Although there is increasing evidence that the pathogenesis of diabetic neuropathy comprises several mechanisms, the prevailing theory implicates persistent hyperglycemia as the primary factor within the metabolic hypothesis [53,54]. Persistent hyperglycemia increases polyol pathway activity with accumulation of sorbitol and fructose in nerves, damaging them by an as yet unknown mechanism. This is accompanied by decreased myoinositol uptake and inhibition of the sodium-potassium ion adenosine triphosphatase pathway, resulting in sodium retention, edema, myelin swelling, axoglial disjunction and nerve degeneration. Deficiency of dihomo g linoleic acid (GLA) as well as N acetyl L carnitine also have been implicated [55]. Metabolic factors cannot account for all forms of neuropathy nor for the heterogeneity of the clinical syndromes. In a subpopulation of patients with neuropathy, immune mechanisms may be responsible for the clinical syndrome, especially in patients with the proximal variety of neuropathy and those with a more marked motor component to their neuropathy. Our data support the hypothesis that circulating antineuronal antibodies are present in diabetic serum, at least in some patients. The circulating autoanti-

bodies directed against motor and sensory nerve structures have been detected by indirect immunofluorescence, and antibody and complement deposits in various components of sural nerves have been shown [56–58].

Microvascular insufficiency has been proposed by a number of investigators as a possible cause of diabetic neuropathy [59–61]. The interest in microvascular derangement in patients with diabetic neuropathy has arisen from studies, suggesting that absolute or relative ischemia may exist in the nerves of patients with diabetes owing to altered function of the endoneurial or epineurial blood vessels, or both. Histopathologic studies show the presence of different degrees of endoneurial and epineurial microvasculopathy, mainly thickening of blood vessel wall or occlusion [62,63]. A number of functional disturbances have also been demonstrated in the microvasculature of the nerves of patients with diabetes. Studies have demonstrated decreased neural blood flow, increased vascular resistance, decreased oxygen pressure and altered vascular permeability characteristics such as a loss of the anionic charge barrier and decreased charge selectivity [64,65]. It also has been shown that abnormalities of cutaneous blood flow correlate with neuropathy [66].

Apart from the metabolic, immunologic and vascular factors involved in the pathogenesis of neuropathy, data exist to support a role for growth factor deficiency. Many of the neuronal changes characteristic of diabetic neuropathy are similar to those observed following either removal of target-derived growth factors by axotomy or depletion of endogenous growth factors by experimental induction of growth factor autoimmunity. Because neuronal growth factors can promote the survival, maintenance, and regeneration of neurons subject to the noxious effects of diabetes, the success of patients with diabetes in maintaining normal nerve morphology and function may ultimately depend on the expression and efficacy of these factors [67]. Ab—antibody; EDRF—endothelium-derived relaxing factor; GF—growth factor; IGF—insulin-like growth factor; NGF—neuronal growth factor; NO—nitric oxide; NT3—neurotropin 3; PGI2—prostaglandin I2.

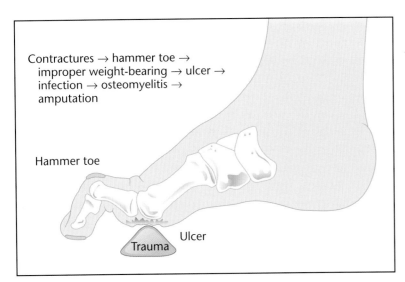

FIGURE 3-40.

Management of small fiber neuropathies. In the United States, 65,000 amputations are performed each year. Half of these are attributable to diabetes and small fiber neuropathy is implicated in 87% of cases. The combination of decreased pain perception with decreased warm thermal perception and the resulting hammer toe deformity that follows intrinsic minus feet leads to blisters on the top of the knuckles of the toes or ulcers over the heads of the metatarsals. These high-pressure points are easily recognized by forced gate analysis (F) scans of the feet. With correct shoes, padded socks and orthotics, the likelihood of amputation can be reduced by half. Patients should be instructed to protect their feet with padded socks, wear shoes that have adequate support, regularly inspect their feet and shoes, be careful of exposure to heat, and to use emollient creams for sympathetic dysfunction.

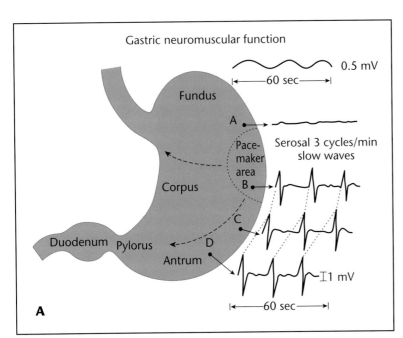

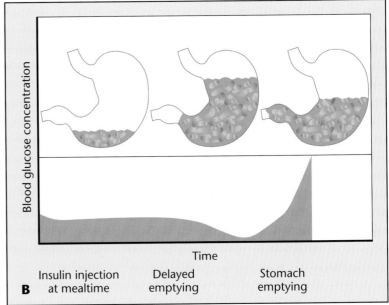

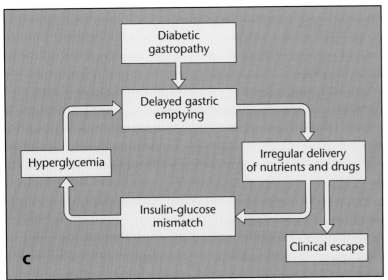

FIGURE 3-41.

Gastropathy. **A** and **B**, Gastric neuromuscular function. The stomach is a complex neuromuscular organ. It has a pacemaker that discharges rhythmic electrical impulses that intitiate propulsive contractions. It is sensitive to volume, viscosity, osmolarity, caloric density, and the nature of the fuel within. Functional disturbances may occur such as arrhythmias, tachygastria and bradygastria, pylorospasm, and hypomotility. Organic lesions include gastroparesis, antral dilation

and obstruction, inflammation, ulceration, and bezoar formation. Gastric dysfunction should be suspected in patients with type 1 and type 2 diabetes; who have had diabetes for over 20 years; who display evidence of distal symmetric polyneuropathy and autonomic neuropathy; observations of brittle diabetes in patients with previously well-controlled symptoms; and symptoms of early satiety, bloating, with a succussion splash. Anorexia, nausea, vomiting, and dyspepsia are nonspecific and herald other conditions.

C, Clinical presentation of gastropathy. Many more people with gastropathy present with brittle diabetes than do those who present with gastric symptoms. In fact, it has been shown that many of the gastrointestinal symptoms of gastropathy can be nonspecific and do not reflect an abnormality in gastric emptying. The most fertile soil for discovery of those with gastric dysfunction consists of patients with "difficult to control diabetes." The stomach can be regarded as the coarse regulator of blood glucose concentrations, releasing fuel to the small bowel at its own predetermined rate. Any dysfunction in the bowel therefore would result in a mismatch of fuel delivery and either endogenous or exogenous insulin, thereby creating the apparent pattern of insulin resistance or brittle diabetes. Of interest is that the irregular pattern of delivery applies to drugs used in treatment of diabetes and may confound the problem. Similar concern applies to other drugs that may fail to reach their absorptive site in the small bowel leading to clinical escape from the condition being treated. Overzealous adjustment of the insulin dose may result because the real cause may be easily overlooked.

Clinical Classification of Hypoglycemic Disorders

Patient Appears Healthy*

No coexistent disease
    Drugs
        Ethanol
        Salicylates
        Quinine
        Haloperidol
Insulinoma
Insulin or sulfonylurea factitial hypoglycemia
Severe exercise
Ketotic hypoglycemia

Compensated coexistent disease
    Drugs
        Dispensing error
        Disopyramide
        Beta-adrenergic blocking agents
        Sulfhydryl- or thiol-containing drugs with autoimmune insulin syndrome
        Unripe ackee fruit and undernutrition

Patient Appears Ill

Drugs
    Pentamidine and *Pneumocystis carinii* pneumonia
    Trimethoprim–sulfamethoxazole and renal failure
    Propoxyphene and renal failure
    Quinine and cerebral malaria
    Quinine and malaria
    Topical salicylates and renal failure

Predisposing illness
    Children
        Small-for-gestational-age infant
        Beckwith-Wiedemann syndrome
        Erythroblastosis fetalis
        Infant of diabetic mother
        Glycogen storage disease
        Defects in amino acid and fatty acid metabolism
        Reye's syndrome
        Cyanotic congenital heart disease
        Hypopituitarism
        Isolated growth hormone deficiency
        Isolated adrenocorticotropic hormone deficiency
        Addison's disease
        Galactosemia
        Hereditary fructose intolerance
        Carnitine deficiency
        Defective type 1 glucose transporter in the brain
    Adults
        Acquired severe liver disease
        Large non–β-cell tumor
        Sepsis
        Renal failure
        Congestive heart failure
        Lactic acidosis
        Starvation
        Anorexia nervosa
        Following removal of pheochromocytoma
        Insulin receptor antibody hypoglycemia
        Mutations in the β-cell sulfonylurea receptor gene
        Glutamate dehydrogenase gene
        Glucokinase gene

Hospitalized patient
    Diseases predisposing to hypoglycemia
    Total parenteral nutrition and insulin therapy
    Questran interference with glucocorticoid absorption
Shock

*Mutations in the β-cell sulfonylurea receptor gene, glutamate dehydrogenase gene, and glucokinase gene are rare causes of hyperinsulinemic hypoglycemia usually manifested in infancy or childhood.

FIGURE 3-42.

Clinical classification of hypoglycemic disorders.

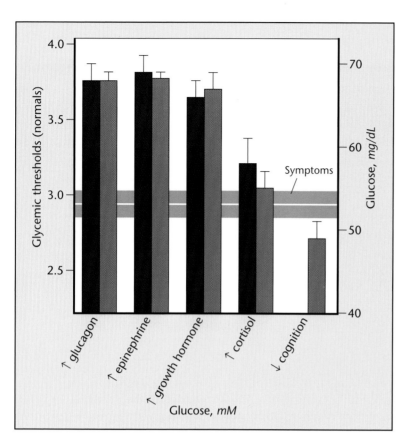

FIGURE 3-43.

Mean arterialized venous glycemic thresholds of increments in plasma levels of glucagon, epinephrine, growth hormone, and cortisol for symptoms of hypoglycemia and for impairment of cognitive function during decrements in plasma glucose levels in normal humans from two independent studies. Light blue bars represent data from a report by Service in 1995 [68]; dark blue bars represent data from a chapter by Service in 1989 [69]). Error bars are the upper bound of the standard error. (*Adapted from* Cryer [70].)

■ OSTEOPOROSIS

THE NATURE OF OSTEOPOROSIS

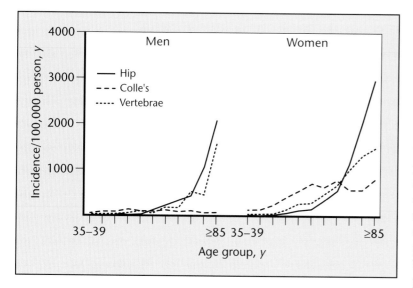

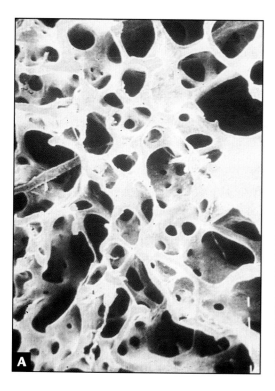 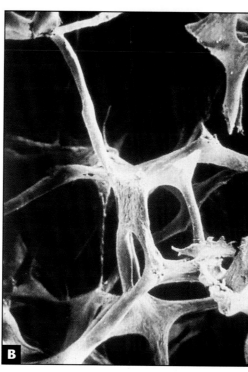

FIGURE 3-44.

Incidence of osteoporotic fractures. The clinical consequence of bone fragility is fracture. Shown here are curves representing the age-related incidences of vertebral, forearm, and hip fractures in North American men and women. The incidence of fractures is about twice as great in women as it is in men. However, osteoporosis is not a disorder exclusive to women. The incidence of hip fracture is increasing most rapidly in men over 70 years of age. One third of vertebral fractures result in pain sufficient to cause the patient to seek medical attention; however, many occur without obvious symptoms, becoming apparent only as a loss of height or development of curvature. Wrist fractures typically occur at an earlier age than do hip fractures. This fact is explained by differences in the types of falls that occur. Wrist fractures occur when a person standing upright falls forward and attempts to break the fall by arm extension. Hip fractures are more likely to occur when a person attempts to rise from a seated position but fails to generate adequate momentum to elevate the center of gravity to a stable position. A backward fall results, with direct impact on the femoral trochanter. Thus, the occurrence of fracture in patients with osteoporosis is a function not only of intrinsic bone strength but also of factors conducive to falls. (*Adapted from* Cooper and Melton [71].)

FIGURE 3-45.

Scanning electron micrograph of normal (**A**) and osteoporotic (**B**) trabecular structures. In osteoporosis, the platelike normal trabeculae have been replaced by thin rods, and trabecular perforation has disrupted trabecular continuity. (*Courtesy of* J. Kosek.)

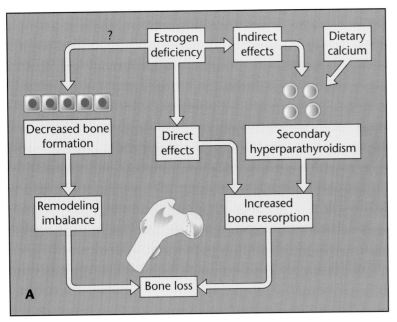

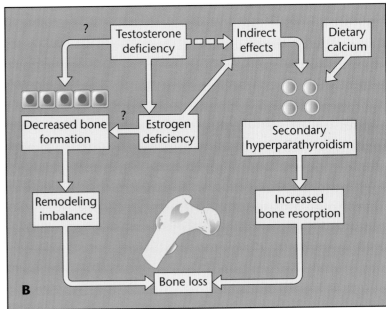

FIGURE 3-46.

A, Unitary model for bone loss in postmenopausal women. Based on recent studies of the relation between sex hormones and bone metabolism, an essential role for estrogen has emerged in involutional bone loss in both men and women. In this new unitary model proposed by Riggs *et al.* [72], estrogen deficiency plays a central role in the pathophysiology of both phases of involutional bone loss in women and plays a major contributory role in the continuous phase of bone loss in men. At menopause, the acute loss of the restraining effects of estrogen on bone cell activity leads to an accelerated phase of loss of predominantly cancellous bone lasting up to 20 years. The slow phase of bone loss, which also begins at menopause, then becomes dominant, involves loss of both cancellous and cortical bone, and continues throughout the remainder of life. The effects of loss of estrogen on extraskeletal calcium homeostasis lead to decreased intestinal calcium absorption, increased calcium wasting,

effects on vitamin D metabolism, and loss of a direct effect on the parathyroid gland that ordinarily decreases parathyroid hormone secretion. The resulting increase in parathyroid hormone causes increased bone resorption and bone loss. Estrogen deficiency also may cause an impairment in bone formation by the loss of estrogen-stimulated synthesis of bone matrix proteins by osteoblasts, although the evidence for this is lacking. B, Unitary model for bone loss in aging men. Recent data in men suggest that estrogen regulates bone metabolism as much or more than does testosterone. Elderly men have low levels of serum bioavailable estrogen, and thus estrogen may contribute to bone loss in men. This gradual induction of estrogen deficiency in aging men leads to bone loss by mechanisms similar to those in women (*Panel A*). In men, testosterone itself may exert effects on the skeleton directly or indirectly through conversion to estrogen. (*Adapted from* Riggs et al. [72].)

FIGURE 3-47.

Risk factors for osteoporosis. (*Adapted from* Wasnish [73].)

Risk Factors for Osteoporosis

Age or age-related
    Each decade associated with 1.4–1.8-fold increased risk
Genetic
    Ethnicity: whites and Asians > blacks
    Gender female > male
    Family history
Environmental
    Nutrition: calcium deficiency, vitamin D deficiency, excess dietary protein
    Physical activity and mechanical loading
    Medications, *eg*, corticosteroids
    Smoking
    Alcohol
    Falls (trauma)
Endogenous hormones and chronic diseases
    Estrogen deficiency
    Androgen deficiency
    Chronic conditions, *eg*, hyperthyroidism, gastrectomy, cirrhosis, hypercortisolism
Physical characteristics of bone
    Density (mass)
    Size and geometry
    Microarchitecture
    Composition

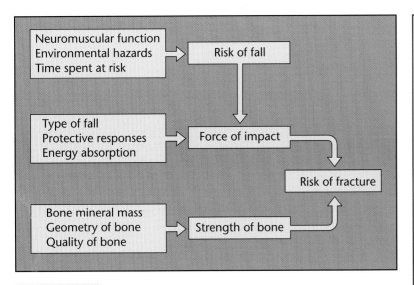

FIGURE 3-48.

Determinants of fracture risk. (*Adapted from* Kanis and McCloskey [74].)

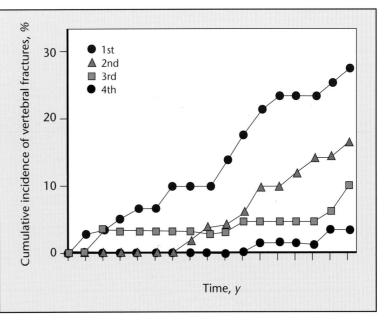

FIGURE 3-49.

Relationship between cumulative incidences of vertebral fractures vs. lumbar spine BMD. The fracture prevalence at eight years is six times greater in women with the lowest BMD (*ie*, 1st quartile) compared with those with the highest BMD (4th quartile). For every one standard deviation below age-predicted mean values that an individual's BMD falls, there is at least a doubling of fracture rate. Fractures are very uncommon at BMD values above 1.20 g/cm², but this should not be construed as evidence for a "fracture threshold." Whether a person fractures or not will always reflect a composite effect of the bone itself (as reflected in BMD) and the force that is applied to it (such as a fall). (*Adapted from* Melton *et al.* [75].)

ESTROGEN-DEPENDENT BONE LOSS AND OSTEOPOROSIS

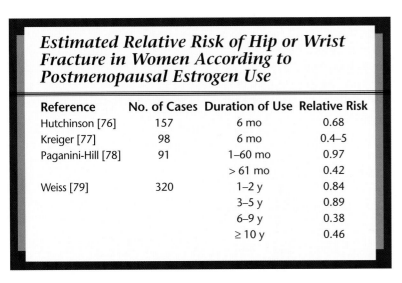

Estimated Relative Risk of Hip or Wrist Fracture in Women According to Postmenopausal Estrogen Use

Reference	No. of Cases	Duration of Use	Relative Risk
Hutchinson [76]	157	6 mo	0.68
Kreiger [77]	98	6 mo	0.4–5
Paganini-Hill [78]	91	1–60 mo	0.97
		> 61 mo	0.42
Weiss [79]	320	1–2 y	0.84
		3–5 y	0.89
		6–9 y	0.38
		≥ 10 y	0.46

FIGURE 3-50.

Estrogen replacement therapy (ERT) confers protection against forearm and hip fracture in postmenopausal women. The epidemiologic evidence that ERT reduces the risk of fracture is shown. Continuous ERT for 5 years or longer was associated with a reduction in fracture by about 60%. (*Adapted from* Weiss *et al.* [79].)

OSTEOPOROSIS IN MEN

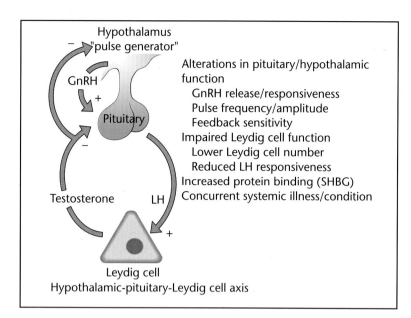

Hypothalamus
"pulse generator"

GnRH

Pituitary

Alterations in pituitary/hypothalamic function
    GnRH release/responsiveness
    Pulse frequency/amplitude
    Feedback sensitivity
Impaired Leydig cell function
    Lower Leydig cell number
    Reduced LH responsiveness
Increased protein binding (SHBG)
Concurrent systemic illness/condition

Testosterone   LH

Leydig cell
Hypothalamic-pituitary-Leydig cell axis

FIGURE 3-51.

Causes of the decrease in testosterone concentrations in aging men. Primary testicular factors (*eg*, impaired testicular perfusion and decreased Leydig cell number) undoubtedly play a major role in the age-dependent decrease in plasma testosterone levels. However, perturbations in central mechanisms also contribute. In elderly men with clinical and biochemical signs of hypoandrogenism, the expected increase in luteinizing hormone (LH) levels is much less pronounced than that observed in younger men with hypogonadism. The mechanism for the blunted response to diminshed androgen feedback inhibition in older men is unknown; however, alterations at the hypothalamic or pituitary level are presumed. *Plus signs* indicate positive influence; *minus signs* indicate negative influence. GNRH—gonadotropin-releasing hormone.

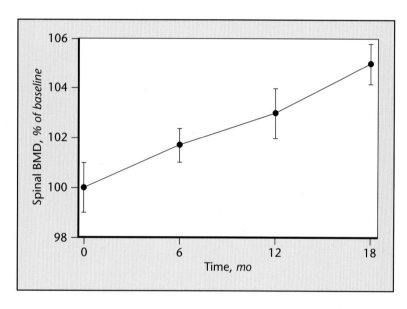

FIGURE 3-52.

Impact of testosterone replacement therapy on bone density. The effectiveness of androgen replacement therapy in men with hypogonadism is unclear. Several reports have suggested that androgen replacement therapy may have beneficial effects on bone mass, at least in the short term. For example, in the study shown here, mean spinal bone mineral density (BMD) increased by 5% (P < 0.001) in a group of 36 men with acquired hypogonadism [80]. However, it is not certain that all men respond or whether other factors (*eg*, age and duration of hypogonadism) influence the success of treatment. Moreover, all studies that suggest a beneficial effect of androgen therapy are of short duration (1–5 y), and it is uncertain whether a sustained increase in bone mass occurs with therapy or whether bone mass ever reaches eugonadal levels. In addition, the minimal effective dose of androgen is not known. Of great importance is that the potential risks of androgen replacement therapy, particularly in the elderly, are uncertain in relation to the possible skeletal benefits to be gained. Nevertheless, the concern of bone loss and fractures should represent one of the indications for androgen therapy in gonadal failure.

GLUCOCORTICOID-INDUCED OSTEOPOROSIS

Epidemiology of Glucocorticoid-induced Osteoporosis

Incidence estimated at 30% to 50% [81,82]

Studies limited because of confounding variables (*eg*, additional immunosuppressive therapy, altered drug clearance rates, autoimmune disease, or changing doses of glucocorticoids)

Bone loss is greatest in first 6 to 12 months of therapy [83–85]

Bone loss is related to duration and total cumulative dose [86,87]

FIGURE 3-53.

Epidemiology of glucocorticoid-induced osteoporosis.

FIGURE 3-54.
Risk factors for glucocorticoid-induced
osteoporosis.

Risk Factors for Glucocorticoid-induced Osteoporosis

Age < 15 years or > 50 years of age associated with risk for severe osteoporosis [88,89]
Postmenopausal women are at higher risk
High total cumulative dose of glucocosteroids
Low body mass index [86]
Secondary risk factors
Duration of therapy
Disorders associated with interleukin-1 production, such as rheumatoid arthritis
General osteoporosis risk factors (age, race, sex, body habitus, immobilization, genetics)
Relative risk of each factor remains unknown, although certain factors are associated with an acceleration of glucocorticoid-induced bone loss

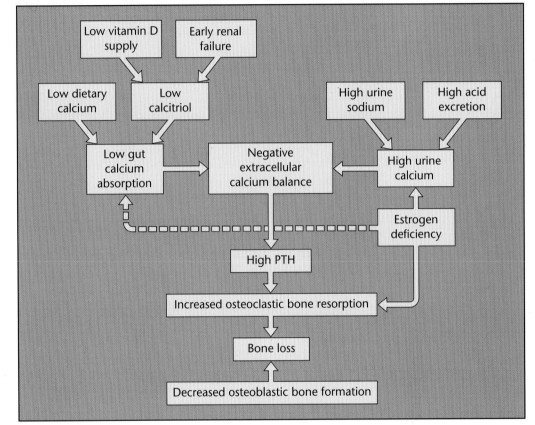

FIGURE 3-55.
Dietary factors contributing to age-related bone loss. Age-related bone loss is dependent on a negative extracellular calcium balance inducing a high parathyroid hormone. The negative extracellular balance is derived in approximately equal parts by a high urine calcium and relatively low gut calcium. The high urine calcium is driven by estrogen deficiency and excessive ingestion of salt and high-acid foods.

Dietary calcium deficiency is exacerbated by impaired gut calcium absorption resulting from relatively low circulating levels of calcitriol and 25-hydroxy vitamin D. These levels are low because of early renal failure, preventing the formation of calcitriol, and lack of vitamin D supply because of lack of exposure to sunlight. Estrogen deficiency also may play a role in the intrinsic defect in gut calcium absorption that occurs with aging.

The negative extracellular calcium balance induces a high parathyroid hormone level, which increases osteoclastic bone resorption. Because of the age-related osteoblastic defect, increased bone turnover is associated with bone loss. PTH—parathyroid hormone.

Antiresorptive Agents for Osteoporosis

Estrogens
Calcitonin
Selective estrogen-receptor modulators
Bisphosphonates

FIGURE 3-56.
Antiresorptive medications in current use fall into one of four categories: estrogens, calcitonin, selective estrogen-receptor modulators (SERMs), or bisphosphonates.

Potential Uses for Bisphosphonates

Osteoporosis
Hypercalcemia
Paget's disease
Fibrous dysplasia
Osteogenesis imperfecta
Multiple myeloma
Bone metastases
Myositis ossificans
Heterotopic ossification
Periodontal disease
Neuropathic arthropathy (Charcot's joint)

FIGURE 3-57.
Potential uses for biphosponates. The literature suggests that bisphosphonates may be beneficial in almost any condition characterized by increased bone remodeling.

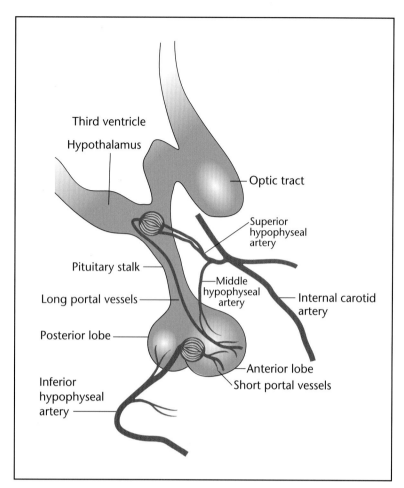

FIGURE 3-58.

Hypothalamic-pituitary communication. Because the anterior lobe is of ectodermal origin, it has no direct neuronal connections with the brain. Nevertheless, the hypothalamus is essential for pituitary function, exerting both trophic and regulatory effects over the major cell types in the pars distalis. Exertion of these effects is accomplished through massive vascular connections between the hypothalamus and the pars distalis. The superior hypophyseal arteries—a branch of the internal carotid arteries—give rise to a specialized capillary network, the portal capillary plexus, located in the base of the hypothalamus in a region called the median eminence (described in detail subsequently). These capillaries drain into the long portal veins that descend along the pituitary stalk to each of the capillary beds in the pars distalis. Thus, substances derived from the brain can be released into the portal capillary network and have direct access to the pars distalis. A small portion of the anterior pituitary may receive arterial blood from the middle hypophyseal artery (also called the trabecular or loral artery). Approximately 70% of the vascular supply derives from venous blood from the hypothalamus. The remaining 30% of the vascular supply to the anterior lobe derives from the posterior lobe through the short portal vessels. These vessels receive their blood supply from the inferior hypophyseal arteries, also a branch of the internal carotid arteries. (*Adapted from* Gay [90].)

ACROMEGALY

Etiology of Acromegaly

Excess growth hormone secretion
  Pituitary adenoma
    Somatotroph adenoma
    Mixed GH- and prolactin-cell adenoma
    Mammosomatotroph adenoma
  Pituitary carcinoma
Ectopic GH-releasing secretion
  Carcinoid tumor (59%)
  Pancreatic islet cell tumor (21%)
  Small cell carcinoma of lung (7%)
  Adrenal adenoma (3%)
Ectopic GH secretion

FIGURE 3-59.

Causes of acromegaly. Acromegaly is a rare disorder, with an estimated prevalence of 50 to 70 cases per 1 million persons. The disease occurs with equal frequency in men and women. Although acromegaly is most often diagnosed in patients in the fifth decade of life, the diagnosis is often delayed for 5 to 9 years because of subtle symptoms and physical changes that often go unnoticed in the early stages.

In 98% of cases, acromegaly is caused by a benign adenoma of the pituitary gland that is usually composed of somatotrophs that hypersecrete growth hormone (GH) alone. Pituitary adenomas that co-secrete both GH and prolactin occur in 30% to 40% of patients. Pituitary carcinoma causing GH excess and ectopic secretion of GH by breast, ovarian, or lung carcinoma are extremely rare. When a pituitary tumor is not seen on magnetic resonance imaging, ectopic secretion of GH-releasing factor should be considered.

Clinical Manifestations of Acromegaly

Effects of tumor mass
- Headaches
- Visual disturbances—visual field deficit, diplopia
- Hypopituitarism—decreased libido, erectile dysfunction, menstrual dysfunction

Effects of excess growth hormone secretion
- Thick and oily skin
- Coarsened facial features with frontal bossing and growth of mandible
- Deepened voice
- Enlargement of hands and feet
- Excessive sweating
- Galactorrhea
- Arthralgias
- Paresthesias, carpal tunnel syndrome
- Abnormal pulmonary function test results
- Obstructive sleep apnea
- Cardiovascular disease—hypertension, cardiomegaly, ventricular arrhythmias, congestive heart failure
- Muscular weakness
- Colonic polyps
- Increased incidence of malignancies
- Abnormal glucose metabolism
- Hypertriglyceridemia

FIGURE 3-60.

Clinical manifestations of acromegaly. These manifestations may be due to the effects of a pituitary mass lesion or to effects of excess GH secretion.

Transsphenoidal Surgery

Efficacy
Cures 50% to 60% of all tumors
Higher cure rate (up to 88%) in microadenomas
Complications (2562 cases), %
Mortality: 1.05
Major morbidity: 3.4
Vascular injury: 0.3
New visual loss: 0.4
Cranial nerve palsies: 0.1
Infection: 0.35
CSF rhinorrhea: 1.9
Diabetes insipidus (usually transient): 1.4
Symptomatic SIADH: 1.4

FIGURE 3-61.

Efficacy and safety of surgical treatment of acromegaly. The rate of surgical remission depends on the tumor size, invasiveness, and the preoperative GH level. The remission rate may be higher in patients with microadenomas (as high as 88% in one series) but is generally much lower in patients with macroadenomas (as low as 30%), which constitute most GH-secreting pituitary tumors [91–95]. The data on complications are from a series of 2562 cases of both GH-secreting and non–GH-secreting pituitary adenomas [96]. One potential complication, not listed here, hypopituitarism, has been found to develop postoperatively in no greater than 3% of patients with microadenomas [96].

Medical Therapy of Acromegaly

Therapeutic Class	Mode of Administration	Dose Range
Somatostatin analogue		
Octreotide	Subcutaneous	50–500 μg TID
Slow-release lanreotide	Intramuscular	30 mg q 10–14 days
Octreotide LAR	Intramuscular	10–40 mg q 28 days
Dopamine agonist		
Bromocriptine	Oral	2.5–10 mg three times daily
Pergolide	Oral	0.025–0.1 mg daily
Cabergoline	Oral	0.3–7.0 mg once weekly
Growth hormone receptor antagonist	Subcutaneous	Under investigation

FIGURE 3-62.

Names, modes of administration, and dose ranges of the three classes of medications used to treat acromegaly–somatostatin analogues, dopamine agonists, and growth hormone receptor antagonists. The latter class is still in the early stages of investigation.

Causes of Hypopituitarism

Genetic hormone deficiencies
  Growth hormone: GH-1 gene, GHRH receptor gene, Pit-1 gene, Prop-1 gene
  LH, FSH: Kallmann syndrome, LH-b gene, FSH-b gene
  TSH: Pit-1 gene, Prop-1 gene, TSH-b gene
  Prolactin: Pit-1 gene, Prop-1 gene
  Vasopressin: vasopressin/neurophysin II gene
Pituitary tumors
  Null cell adenoma
  Somatotroph, lactotroph, corticotroph, gonadotroph, thyrotroph adenoma
  Rathke's cleft tumor
Hypothalamic tumors
  Craniopharyngioma
  Hamartoma
  Neural and parasellar tumors: glioma, meningioma, pinealoma, chordoma
Vascular causes
  Pituitary apoplexy
  Pituitary infarct (Sheehan syndrome)
Cranial irradiation
Postoperative state (pituitary surgery)
Head trauma
Granulomatous disease
  Sarcoid, histiocytosis X, eosinophilic granuloma
Infectious disease
  Tuberculosis, syphilis, mycosis, meningitis, basilar abscess
Metastatic disease
Autoimmune
  Lymphocytic hypophysitis
Empty sella (rarely severe hypopituitarism)
Idiopathic
  Idiopathic growth hormone deficiency (presumed GHRH deficiency)
Functional hypothalamic origin
  Stress-related hypogonadism (amenorrhea in depressed patients, athletes)
  Stress-related GH deficiency (psychosocial dwarfism)
  Disease-related TSH deficiency (euthyroid sick)

FIGURE 3-63.

Causes of hypopituitarism. Some causes result in selective hormone deficiency, whereas others result in panhypopituitarism. In diseases that are destructive to pituitary tissue, growth hormone (GH) and gonadotropins usually are the earliest hormones to become deficient. Prolactin may be mildly elevated in otherwise hypopituitary patients because of stalk compression, which interferes with inhibitory control of prolactin from the hypothalamus. FSH—follicle-stimulating hormone; GHRH—growth hormone releasing hormone; LH—luteinizing hormone; TSH—thyrotropin.

Diagnostic Tests for Hypopituitarism

Thyroid axis
    Serum thyroxine
    Serum tri-iodothyronine
    Serum TSH
    TRH test
Adrenal axis
    Serum cortisol
    Serum ACTH
    Insulin tolerance test
    ACTH stimulation test
Gonadal axis
    Serum testosterone or estradiol
    Serum FSH
    Serum LH
    (GnRH stimulation test)
Growth hormone
    Serum growth hormone
    Serum IGF-I
    Insulin tolerance test
    Other provocative tests (*eg*, L-dopa, arginine, clonidine, GHRH, glucagon)
Prolactin
    Serum prolactin
    TRH test
Vasopressin
    Dehydration test
    Hypertonic saline infusion
    Plasma vasopressin
Pituitary imaging
    MRI or CT scan

FIGURE 3-64.

Diagnostic tests for hypopituitarism. Under normal circumstances, there is a negative feedback loop between cortisol and the hypothalamo-pituitary unit, resulting in appropriate levels of adrenocorticotropic hormone (ACTH) and cortisol. Metyrapone blocks the last step in cortisol biosynthesis (11-hydroxylation), with a decrease in cortisol production and accumulation of its precursor, 11-deoxycortisol. The latter is biologically inert and fails to exert negative feedback on the hypothalamo-pituitary unit. As a result, ACTH secretion is increased and the adrenal gland activated to produce more steroids. Because of the block in cortisol synthesis, the normal negative feedback on ACTH secretion is disrupted, and large amounts of 11-deoxycortisol are produced. Thus, the healthy subject reacts to metyrapone with a large overproduction of 11-deoxycortisol, which is the measured endpoint of the test. Patients with hypopituitarism cannot increase their ACTH secretion, and little adrenal activation occurs. Therefore, 11-deoxycortisol production remains abnormally low. Plasma ACTH can also be used as an endpoint, although that is not a standardized test.

The table lists a sampling of static and dynamic tests available to assess pituitary function and anatomy. Tests must be interpreted in light of the patient's prevailing physiopathologic condition. Testing in most instances proceeds in two or three stages, from baseline static tests to dynamic hormone stimulation tests to imaging procedures. ACTH—adrenocorticotropic hormone; CT—computed tomography; FSH—follicle-stimulating hormone; GHRH—growth hormone releasing hormone; GnRH—gonadotropin-releasing hormone; IGF-I—insulin-like growth factor I; LH—luteinizing hormone; MRI—magnetic resonance imaging; TRH—thyrotropin-releasing hormone; TSH—thyrotropin.

Clinical Features of Growth Hormone Deficiency in Adult Hypopituitarism

Background
  Need for GH treatment as a child
  Known pituitary pathology, with or without previous treatment
  Full conventional pituitary hormone replacement
Symptoms
  Abnormal body composition
    Reduced lean body mass
    Increased abdominal adiposity
  Reduced strength and exercise capacity
  Impaired psychological well-being
    Reduced vitality and energy
    Depressed mood
    Emotional lability
    Impaired self control
    Anxiety
    Increased social isolation
Signs
  Overweight with predominantly central (abdominal) adiposity
  Thin, dry skin; cool peripheries; poor venous access
  Reduced muscle strength
  Reduction in exercise performance
  Depressed affect, labile emotions
Investigations
  Stimulated GH level below 3 µg/L
  Low or low-normal serum IGF-I
  Elevated serum lipids, particularly LDL cholesterol
  Reduced lean body mass and increased fat mass
  Reduced bone mineral density

FIGURE 3-65.
Clinical features of GH deficiency in adult hypopituitarism. Since patients were on replacement therapy for thyroid, adrenal, and gonadal deficiency, the features listed are attributed to GH deficiency. Identical findings are present in patients with isolated GH deficiency. (*Adapted from* Carroll *et al.* [97].)

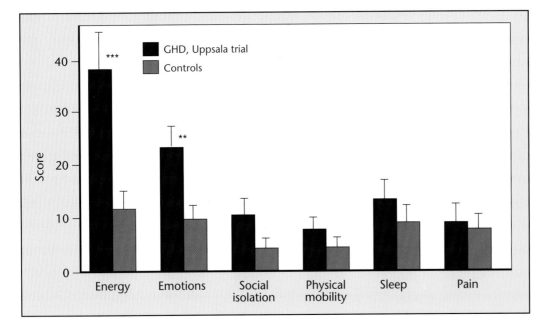

FIGURE 3-66.
Hypopituitarism and quality of life. Quality-of-life scores, as assessed by the Nottingham Health Profile, in 36 adults with panhypopituitarism compared to age- and sex-matched controls. Higher scores denote lower quality of life. Parameters assessed by the Nottingham Health Profile include energy, pain, emotional reaction, sleep, social isolation, and physical mobility. Similar conclusions are reached using other instruments of psychological assessment, such as the Hopkins Symptoms Checklist and the Psychological General Well-being Index. GHD—growth hormone deficiency. (*Adapted from* Burman *et al.* [98].)

Causes of Pathologic Hyperprolactinemia

Prolactinomas
Medications
Hypothalamic disorders
Nonfunctioning pituitary adenomas
Primary hypothyroidism
Pregnancy
Breast stimulation
Chest wall trauma
Renal failure
Idiopathic

FIGURE 3-67.

Causes of hyperprolactinemia. Although prolactinomas are the most common cause, any process that disrupts the hypothalamus or pituitary stalk or alters the synthesis or action of dopamine leads to hyperprolactinemia. Prolactin levels increase slightly during the mid-phase of the menstrual cycle and increase 10-fold during pregnancy. A careful history and physical examination, measurement of thyroid function, and a pregnancy test will exclude many causes of hyperprolactinemia. Idiopathic hyperprolactinemia refers to elevated prolactin levels without radiographic evidence of a pituitary tumor.

Medications Causing Hyperprolactinemia

Phenothiazines
Tricyclic antidepressants
Metoclopramide
Histamine receptor blockers
Estrogen
Reserpine
Calcium-channel blockers
Carbidopa

FIGURE 3-68.

Medications causing hyperprolactinemia. By altering dopaminergic inhibition, a variety of drugs cause prolactin hypersecretion. Antipsychotic agents act as dopamine receptor antagonists, carbidopa interferes with dopamine synthesis, and reserpine depletes central catecholamine levels. After discontinuation of drug therapy, prolactin levels return to normal in 3 to 4 days.

A. Clinical Presentation of Hyperprolactinemia in Women

Condition	Women Presenting With Condition, %
Amenorrhea and galactorrhea	81.0
Amenorrhea alone	12.0
Oligomenorrhea and galactorrhea	1.4
Regular menses and galactorrhea	1.4
Visual field defect	1.4
Other	2.8

B. Clinical Presentation of Hyperprolactinemia in Men

Condition	Men Presenting With Condition, %
Loss of libido/potency	47.0
Headache	13.0
Visual failure	13.0
Gynecomastia	6.0
Galactorrhea	2.0
Other	19.0

FIGURE 3-69.

Clinical presentation of hyperprolactinemia in women (A) and men (B). Women with prolactinomas usually present with amenorrhea, galactorrhea, and infertility. However, galactorrhea may occur alone, and some women with elevated prolactin levels have regular menses. Prolactinomas in women are often diagnosed after treatment with oral contraceptives, but case-control studies have shown no relationship between oral contraceptive use and the development of prolactin tumors [99].

Although men with hyperprolactinemia develop hypogonadism, they usually seek medical attention because of headaches or visual impairment. Up to one third of men with hyperprolactinemia have galactorrhea. Elevated prolactin levels may also affect sperm synthesis and metabolism. (Part A *adapted from* Schlechte *et al.* [100]; part B *adapted from* Walsh *et al.* [101].)

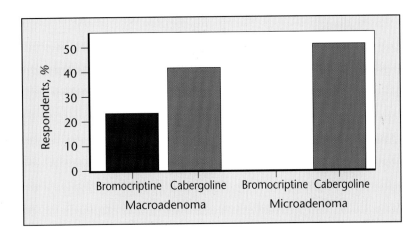

FIGURE 3-70.

The effect of bromocriptine and cabergoline on tumor size. Twenty-seven patients who were unresponsive to bromocriptine were treated with cabergoline. After 3 months of cabergoline therapy, tumors shrank significantly (25% to 50% of pretreatment tumor volume) in 42% of the macroadenomas and in 50% of the microadenomas. (*Adapted from* Colao *et al.* [102].)

THYROTROPIN-PRODUCING TUMORS

Clinical Characteristics of TSHomas*

Symptoms and Signs	No. Patients (%)
Sex	
Male	115
Female	140
Goiter	166/177 (94)
Abnormal visual fields	53/126 (42)
Ophthalmopathy	8/128 (6)
Acromegaly	42 (16)
Amenorrhea/galactorrhea	30 (12)

*N = 255.

FIGURE 3-71.

Clinical features of 255 patients with TSHomas. Unlike hyperthyroidism due to autoimmune thyroid disease, which occurs predominantly in women, TSHomas often are diagnosed in men. Goiters usually are diffuse, and macroadenomas may impair vision. Eye changes have been reported in several patients as a result of coexisting Graves' disease, and orbital involvement by tumor has been seen in several others. Cosecretion of growth hormone or prolactin can occur. (*Adapted from* Beck-Peccoz *et al.* [103].)

Baseline Laboratory Values in Patients with Thyrotropin-Secreting Pituitary Tumors*

Test	No. Patients (%)
T4/T3 elevated	All
TSH detectable	All
α-SU/TSH > 1.0	71/88 (81)
Growth hormone elevated	44
Prolactin elevated	30
LH/FSH elevated	4
ACTH elevated	0
Thyroid antibody positive	8/106 (8)
TSH-receptor antibody positive	3/73 (4)

*N = 255.

FIGURE 3-72.

Laboratory results in 255 patients with TSHomas. Serum thyroid hormones always are increased; TSH usually is elevated, but may be within the normal range, an inappropriate response when the thyroxine (T4) level is high. The molar ratio of the alpha subunit (a-SU) to TSH usually is greater than 1.0, suggesting unbalanced overproduction of a-SU. In patients with thyroid hormone resistance, this ratio is less than 1.0, making the test quite helpful in distinguishing between these two conditions. A simple way to calculate this ratio is to divide the a-SU value (normally expressed as ng/mL) by the TSH value (expressed as mIU/L), and multiply by 10. Autoimmune thyroid disease is present in the same percentages that would be expected in the healthy population. ACTH–adrenocorticotropic hormone; FSH–follicle-stimulating hormone; LH–luteinizing hormone; T3–triiodothyronine. (*Data from* Beck-Peccoz *et al.* [103].)

Congenital and Acquired Hypogonadotropic Disorders

Congenital disorders
  Idiopathic hypogonadotropic hypogonadism
  Fertile eunuch syndrome
  Prader-Willi syndrome
  Laurence-Moon-Biedl syndrome
  Basal encephalocele
  Multiple lentigines syndrome
  Cerebellar ataxia and hypogonadotropic hypogonadism
  Rud syndrome
  Miscellaneous disorders
Acquired disorders
  Functional disorders
    Anorexia nervosa and amenorrhea associated with weight loss
    Amenorrhea of athletes, joggers, and ballet dancers
    Correlations of feeding pattern and fertility in !KUNG San tribes
  Drug-related hypothalamic dysfunction: marijuana, postoral contraceptive amenorrhea
    Hypothalamic dysfunction with stress or systemic illness
    Hypothalamic dysfunction in polycystic ovarian disease
    Hyperprolactinemia and hypogonadotropism
    Hemochromatosis
  Organic disorders
    Neoplastic
    Inflammatory and infiltrative

FIGURE 3-73.

Clinical manifestations of hypogonadotropic hypogonadism. In early fetal life, testosterone is required for the development of the vasa efferentia, epididymis, vas deferens, and seminal vesicles from the Wolffian ducts. Because testosterone production by the fetal testis is being driven by human chorionic gonadotropin at this stage of development, patients with idiopathic hypogonadotropic hypogonadism have normal development of Wolffian structures. Testosterone is also responsible for the development of prostate and the male urethra from the urogenital sinus and for the fusion of the labioscrotal swellings and the urethral folds in the midline to form the scrotum and penis. Genital tubercle under the influence of dihydroxytestosterone forms the glans penis. Androgen deficiency or insensitivity in fetal life can therefore cause varying degrees of failure of the male sexual differentiation and ambiguity of external genitalia, hypospadia, or microphallus.

During pubertal development, increasing testosterone levels lead to development of secondary sex characteristics in the male, deepening of the voice, and epiphyseal fusion. Therefore, androgen deficiency before puberty presents with delay or failure of secondary sex characteristics, continued growth of the long bones (resulting in eunuchoidal proportions), and persistence of a high-pitched voice. Androgen deficiency occurring after pubertal development is associated with regression of secondary sex characteristics, decreased sexual desire and activity, loss of muscle mass, accumulation of aft mass, and osteoporosis.

Disorders associated with hypogonadotropic hypogonadism can be classified into congenital and acquired groups. Acquired disorders are much more common than congenital disorders.

A. Who Should Be Screened for Androgen Deficiency?

Men presenting with any of the following clinical profiles are at risk for androgen deficiency and should be evaluated:

Delayed pubertal development

Sexual dysfunction and loss of libido

Loss of secondary sex characteristics

Infertility

Breast enlargement

Minimal trauma fracture or osteoporosis before 40 years of age

Chronic diseases associated with sarcopenia, such as end-stage renal disease, HIV infection, chronic obstructive lung disease, and cancer cachexia

History of cancer chemotherapy or whole-body, cranial, or inguinal irradiation

History of use of such medications as glucocorticoids, ketoconazole, megestrol acetate, cimetidine, and cyclosporine

---

FIGURE 3-74.

Screening for androgen deficiency and diagnostic work-up. **A,** Because the clinical manifestations of androgen deficiency in men are often subtle, a high index of suspicion is the key to diagnosis. **B,** Diagnostic work-up of androgen-deficiency begins with general health evaluation. It is crucial to exclude systemic diseases, such as uncontrolled diabetes, cancer, HIV infection, kidney or liver disease, abuse of recreational drugs (such as cocaine, opiates, and marijuana), and current use of medications that alter testosterone production or metabolism (such as glucocorticoids, cyclosporine, ketoconazole, or megestrol acetate).

Total testosterone levels should then be measured, preferably in an early-morning specimen. If total testosterone levels are less than 200 ng/dL, this value should be verified by repeating the measurement and measuring serum LH and follicle-stimulating hormone FSH levels. Low testosterone levels along with high LH and FSH levels suggest primary testicular dysfunction; a karyotype can verify the diagnosis of Klinefelter syndrome, a common cause of primary testicular dysfunction. Low testosterone levels but normal LH and FSH levels suggest a defect at the hypothalamic-pituitary site. Measurement of prolactin levels and magnetic resonance imaging (MRI) can help exclude hyperprolactinemia and space-occupying lesions in such patients. By process of exclusion, one is left with the diagnosis of idiopathic hypogonadotropic hypogonadism.

In men with total testosterone levels between 200 and 350 ng/dL, repeating the total testosterone measurement and measuring the free testosterone level can be helpful. There is no consensus on which method for measurement of free testosterone levels is optimum, but authors agree that tracer analogue methods are not reliable. Because there is good correlation of clinical features of androgen deficiency with free testosterone levels measured by equilibrium dialysis or ammonium sulfate precipitation method, either of these methods can be used.

General health evaluation: rule out systemic disease, such as uncontrolled diabetes, cancer, HIV infection, kidney, liver or lung disease; abuse of recreational drugs, especially marijuana and cocaine; eating disorders; and excessive exercise

Total testosterone levels

< 200 ng/dL; Repeat testosterone measurement and measure LH and FSH

200–350 ng/dL: Repeat testosterone measurement, measure free testosterone*; If low, measure LH and FSH

> 350 ng/dL: No further work-up necessary

Low testosterone, high LH and FSH: Primary testicular dysfunction. Obtain a karyotype

Low testosterone; LH and FSH not evaluated: Hypothalamic-pituitary problem, Measure prolactin, get MRI scan

B

Pathophysiology of the Clinical Manifestations of Patients with Large Null-cell Adenomas

Signs and symptoms of mechanical effects of the expanding adenoma

Headaches caused by

Stretching of the dura

Increased intrasellar pressure

Visual abnormalities

Visual field deficit: superior extension

Decreased visual acuity: superiors extension

Ocular dysmolility: cavernous sinus invasion

CSF leak occasionally seen caused by inferior extension of the adenoma

Signs and symptoms of impaired pituitary hormone secretion; hypopituitarism

---

FIGURE 3-75.

Pathophysiology of the clinical manifestations of patients with large null-cell adenomas. There is no characteristic phenotypic presentation of patients with null-cell adenomas or of other intrasellar mass lesions. Instead, they present predominantly with signs and symptoms caused by the mechanical effects of the adenomas: headaches, visual symptoms, and hypopituitarism. The most common clinical manifestation of hypopituitarism in this setting is hypogonadism, presenting as diminished libido in men and amenorrhea in premenopausal women. Signs and symptoms of hypothyroidism or adrenal insufficiency also are seen [104].

About 60% of these patients have mild hyperprolactinemia, which could, at least theoretically, contribute to the development of hypogonadism in this setting. However, the degree of hyperprolactinemia is mild and is not sufficient to influence gonadal function. Furthermore, lowering serum prolactin levels with dopamine agonists does not affect gonadal function.

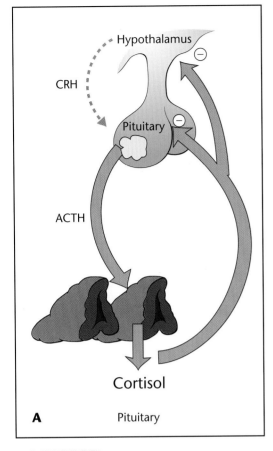

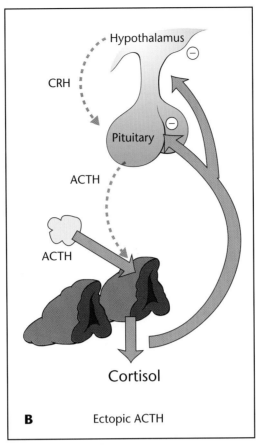

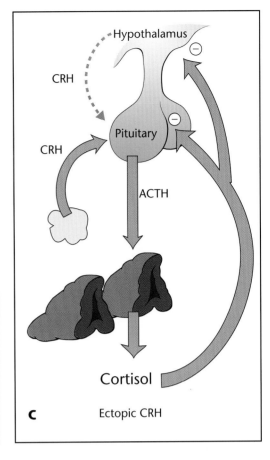

FIGURE 3-76.

Hypothalamic-pituitary-adrenal axis in adrenocorticotropic hormone (ACTH)–dependent Cushing's syndrome. In the normal hypothalamic-pituitary-adrenal axis, corticotropin-releasing hormone is synthesized in the hypothalamus in a pulsatile manner, then transverses the portal blood vessels surrounding the pituitary stalk to reach the anterior pituitary gland. There, corticotropin-releasing hormone triggers synthesis and secretion of adrenocorticotropic hormone, which is likewise released in a pulsatile pattern. Adrenocorticotropic hormone circulates through the body to reach the adrenal cortex, where it stimulates production and release of the glucocorticoid cortisol. Superimposed on the pulsatility is a diurnal rhythm, with cortisol levels highest in the early morning and lowest in the evening. Because of this diurnal variation and pulsatile release, measurements of random levels of cortisol are rarely useful because it is impossible to determine whether a peak, trough, or intermediate secretion point has been sampled.

The cortisol hypersecretion of endogenous Cushing's syndrome can result from a tumor of the pituitary gland (the originally described site [thus, this disease is called Cushing's disease], representing 65% to 75% of cases of Cushing's syndrome), the adrenal gland (approximately 15% of cases), or an ectopic site such as the lung (10% to 15% of cases). Pituitary and ectopic Cushing's syndrome is caused by excess secretion of ACTH, which, in turn, triggers excess adrenal cortisol production. These cases are therefore classified as ACTH-dependent Cushing's syndrome. The adrenal glands often become hypertrophied because of the excess ACTH stimulation. In pituitary Cushing's syndrome (**A**), both ACTH and cortisol production is increased. In ectopic ACTH production (**B**), pituitary levels of ACTH are suppressed by the high cortisol levels; however, ACTH is measurable because it is arising from the ectopic source. In the rare cases of ectopic corticotropin-releasing hormone (CRH) production (**C**), the tumor secretes CRH, triggering release of both pituitary ACTH and adrenal cortisol. Cases of ACTH-dependent Cushing's syndrome are not necessarily associated with elevated ACTH levels. These values are often in the normal to mildly elevated range, but this is inappropriate given the high levels of circulating cortisol.

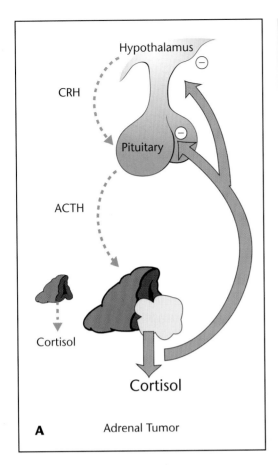

A   Adrenal Tumor

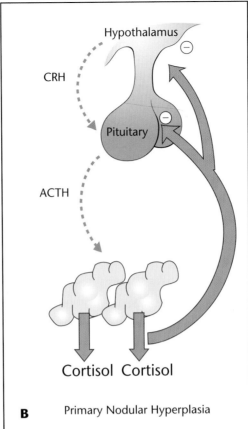

B   Primary Nodular Hyperplasia

FIGURE 3-77.

Hypothalamic-pituitary-adrenal axis in adrenocorticotropic hormone (ACTH)–independent Cushing's syndrome. Adrenal Cushing's syndrome results in autonomous production of cortisol, which suppresses ACTH production by the normal pituitary gland. Adrenal Cushing's syndrome is therefore called ACTH-independent Cushing's syndrome. This condition is usually due to a unilateral lesion that can be benign or malignant (A). Rarely, bilateral disease occurs (B). CRH—corticotropin-releasing hormone.

Clinical Features of Cushing's Disease

Features	Incidence, %
General	
Obesity	85
Hypertension	75
Headache	10
Skin	
Facial plethora	80
Hirsutism	75
Superficial fungal infections	50
Striae	50
Acne	35
Bruising	35
Hyperpigmentation	5
Neuropsychiatric	85
Gonadal dysfunction	
Menstrual disorders	75
Impotence/decreased libido	65
Musculoskeletal	
Osteopenia	80
Back pain	65
Weakness	50
Metabolic	
Glucose intolerance/diabetes	75/20
Kidney stones	15
Polyuria	10

FIGURE 3-78.

Clinical features of Cushing's syndrome. The first step in the evaluation of a patient with suspected Cushing's syndrome is to make the diagnosis, which begins with an evaluation of clinical features. The clinical picture can vary greatly among patients according to the duration and severity of cortisol excess and the relative contributions of glucocorticoid, mineralocorticoid, and adrenal androgen excess. Many of the features of Cushing's syndrome are nonspecific. However, findings that tend to predict that a patient has Cushing's syndrome rather than obesity and hypertension or hirsutism include the following: a centripetal distribution to the obesity (including supraclavicular and posterior cervical fat pads and abdominal obesity), osteoporosis, proximal myopathy (often associated with a thin appearance of the arms and legs relative to the truncal obesity), spontaneous ecchymoses, wide violaceous striae, and hypokalemia. (*Adapted from* Findling *et al.* [105].)

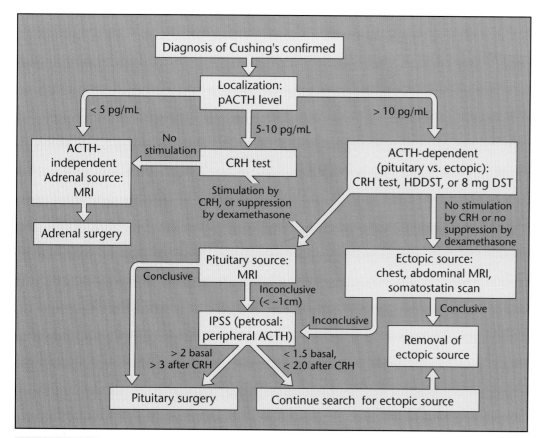

FIGURE 3-79.

Algorithm of localizing tests for Cushing's syndrome. In most cases, Cushing's syndrome is curable with removal of the tumor that has led to cortisol overproduction. This means that the localizing tests are critical because they determine which operation should be performed. The first step is to measure a plasma adrenocorticotropic hormone (ACTH) level. If ACTH is undetectable, the patient has ACTH-independent Cushing's syndrome (adrenal Cushing's syndrome); if the dexamethasone suppression test (DST) shows nonsuppression or the corticotropin-releasing hormone (CRH) test shows nonstimulation, the adrenal glands should be imaged to find the tumor. If the ACTH level is in the borderline suppressed range (approximately 5 to 10 pg/mL), patients should undergo a peripheral CRH test to determine whether they are ACTH independent (no stimulation) or ACTH dependent (stimulability by CRH). If the ACTH level is in the normal to elevated range, the patient has ACTH-dependent Cushing's syndrome and needs further testing to distinguish a pituitary from an ectopic source. If the CRH test shows stimulation or the high-dose DST shows suppression, a pituitary source is most likely and magnetic resonance imaging (MRI) of the head is performed. If there is no responsiveness to CRH or dexamethasone, an ectopic source is more likely and imaging of the chest (and, if necessary, other sites) is performed.

Some benign occult ectopic tumors exhibit suppressibility or stimulability identical to that seen in Cushing's syndrome, thereby creating a diagnostic problem. For patients whose hormone/dynamic testing suggests a pituitary source but who do not have a discrete lesion of approximately 1 cm on MRI of the head, bilateral inferior petrosal sinus sampling (IPSS) is recommended [106]. It is important to note that the absence of a lesion on pituitary scan does not rule out pituitary Cushing's syndrome because these lesions can be as small as 0.5 mm in size. Conversely, the presence of a small pituitary lesion does not establish the pituitary as the source because more than 10% of the normal population has pituitary incidentalomas. Pituitary lesions greater than 1 cm are not likely to be incidentalomas, and patients with such lesions do not need to undergo IPSS [107,108]. HDDST—high-dose dexamethasone suppression test. (*Adapted from* Meier and Biller [106].)

FIGURE 3-80.

Treatment of Cushing's syndrome. Surgical removal of the hormone-secreting tumor is the treatment of choice for Cushing's syndrome. Transsphenoidal adenomectomy, when performed by a surgeon with experience in pituitary surgery, has a cure rate of more than 80% and is associated with a recurrence rate of approximately 5% [109]. In addition, procedures performed by an experienced surgeon have low mortality and morbidity rates. Thoracotomy is the treatment of choice for a localized lung lesion associated with ectopic Cushing's syndrome, and other ectopic tumors are removed according to the appropriate approach to that site.

Adrenalectomy is the treatment of choice for patients with an adrenal tumor. Temporary adrenal insufficiency occurs after cure of Cushing's syndrome; this requires glucocorticoid administration for an average of 1 year. Patients with metastatic adrenal or ectopic tumors may not be operable and may require chemotherapy for the lesion and medical therapy to reduce adrenal cortisol production. The most common agents used for this purpose are ketoconazole, metyrapone, aminoglutethimide, and mitotane.

Treatment of Cushing's Syndrome

Pituitary
  Transsphenoidal adenomectomy
  If unsuccessful
    Radiation
      Stereotactic (proton, gamma, linac)
      Conventional
    Bilateral adrenalectomy
    Medical
Ectopic
  Thoracotomy (or other, depending on tumor location)
  Medical (for metastatic cancer)
Adrenal
  Unilateral adrenalectomy
  Bilateral adrenalectomy (for rare case of bilateral disease)
  Medical (for metastatic adrenal carcinoma)

DIABETES INSIPIDUS

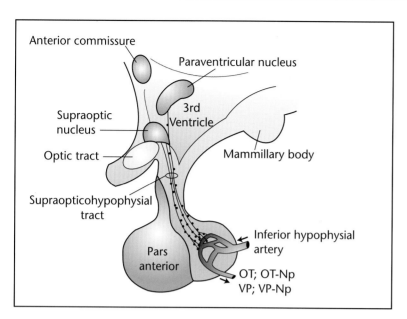

FIGURE 3-81.

Schematic of the neurohypophysis in the sagittal plane. Shown are the hypothalamic supraoptic and paraventricular nuclei, which are the sites of vasopressin synthesis, and the supraopticohypophysial tract coursing through the infundibular stalk. Vasopressinergic axons terminate in the posterior pituitary gland, the storage site for the synthesis and release of vasopressin into the peripheral circulation. NP-II—neurophysin II; OT—optic tract; VP—vasopressin. (*Adapted from* Reeves *et al.* [110].)

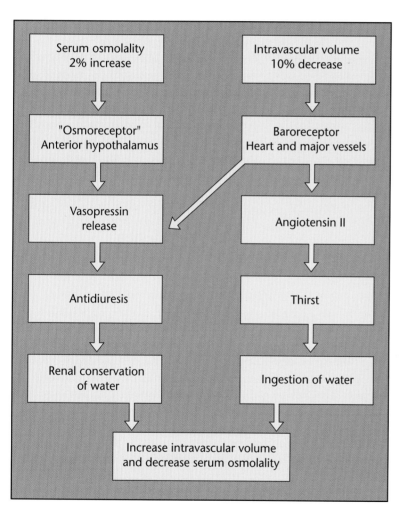

FIGURE 3-82.

Schematic of the physiologic regulation of vasopressin release by osmotic and volume stimuli. The major physiologic regulators of vasopressin secretion are plasma osmolality and intravascular volume. Osmoreceptors respond to changes in osmolality concentration, whereas baroreceptors respond to changes in intravascular volume. An increase in the serum osmolality concentration of as little as 2% causes shrinkage of the osmoreceptor cells (located in the anterior hypothalamus). This increase also causes stimulation of both thirst and vasopressin release from the posterior pituitary gland. Volume-dependent mechanisms operate independently of changes in osmolality concentration. Thirst and vasopressin release are stimulated when intravascular volume decreases by 10%. The acquisition and conservation of water both operate to restore intravascular volume and plasma osmolality levels to normal.

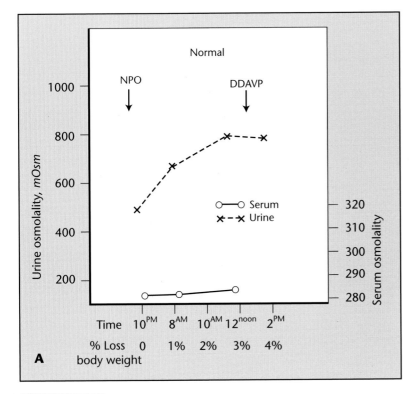

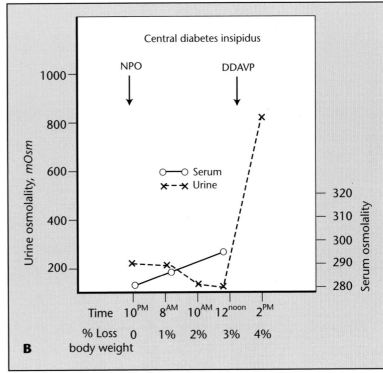

FIGURE 3-83

The water deprivation test. **A,** Results of this test in a normal person. **B,** Results in a patient with diabetes insipidus (DI). The diagnosis of diabetes insipidus in a patient with polyuria and polydipsia requires documentation of elevated levels of serum sodium and osmolality and low urine osmolality. In some instances the criteria are met without formal water deprivation. In these instances, hydration and a therapeutic trial of vasopressin or desmopressin are all that is required. First a blood sample is drawn to measure plasma vasopressin levels. In other instances, a water deprivation test is necessary. Because patients with complete vasopressin deficiency may become dehydrated quickly, the test is best done in a controlled setting where blood pressure and clinical status can be monitored. Maximal dehydration typically is achieved when the patient has lost 3% of total body weight. At that point, urine osmolality should be maximal owing to the combined stimuli of hyperosmolality and hypovolemia. Plasma vasopressin levels should then be measured. In patients with central diabetes insipidus, serum osmolality and

sodium levels usually are high, urine osmolality levels are low, urine output continues unabated, and plasma vasopressin concentrations are low or undetectable. With the administration of vasopressin or its analogue desmopressin, urine osmolality levels increase and urine volume decreases. Patients with nephrogenic diabetes insipidus respond similarly to those with central diabetes insipidus. The differentiating point is that those with nephrogenic diabetes insipidus have elevated circulating levels of plasma vasopressin at the point of maximal dehydration and do not respond to exogenously administered vasopressin or desmopressin. Patients with primary polydipsia will maintain normal serum osmolality concentrations, have maxmimal concentrations of urine osmolality, and will not further increase their urine osmolality levels in response to vasopressin or desmopressin. Note that the maximal concentration of urine osmolality may be submaximal owing to the washout of the medullary concentrating ability of the kidneys. DDAVP—1-desamino-8-D-arginine vasopressin; NPO—nothing by mouth.

Differential Diagnosis of Hyponatremia

Extracellular Fluid Volume	Urinary [Na⁺]*	Presumptive Diagnosis
↓	Low	Depletion (non-renal): GI, cutaneous, or blood ECF loss
	High	Depletion (renal): Diuretics, mineralocorticoid insufficiency (Addison's disease), salt-losing nephropathy
→	Low	Depletion (non-renal): Any cause + hypotonic fluid replacement
		Dilution (proximal): Hypothyroidism, early decreased effective arterial blood volume
		Dilution (distal): SIADH + fluid retention
	High	Dilution (distal): SIADH, glucocorticoid insufficiency
		Depletion (renal): Any cause + hypotonic fluid replacement (especially diuretic treatment)
↑	Low	Dilution (proximal): Decreased, effective arterial blood volume (CHF, cirrhosis, nephrosis)
	High	Dilution (proximal): Any cause + diuretics or improvement in underlying disease, renal failure

*Urine [Na⁺] values < 30 mEq/L are generally considered to be low and values > 30 mEq/d to be high, based on studies of responses to hyponatremic patients to infusions of isotonic saline.

FIGURE 3-84.

Differential diagnosis of hyponatremia. Because of the multiplicity of disorders causing hypo-osmolality and the fact that many involve more than one pathologic mechanism, a definitive diagnosis is not always possible at the time of initial presentation. Nonetheless, a relatively straightforward approach based on the commonly used parameters of extracellular fluid (ECF) volume status and urine sodium concentration generally allows adequate categorization of the underlying cause to allow appropriate decisions regarding initial therapy and further evaluation in most cases. The presence of clinically detectable hypovolemia always signifies total body solute depletion. A low urinary [Na⁺] indicates a non-renal cause of solute depletion. If the urinary [Na⁺] is high despite hypo-osmolality, renal causes of solute depletion are more likely responsible. Conversely, the presence of clinically detectable hypervolemia always signifies total body Na⁺ excess. In these patients, hypo-osmolality results from an even greater expansion of total body water caused by a marked reduction in the rate of water excretion, and, sometimes, an increased rate of water ingestion. The impairment in water excretion is secondary to a decreased effective arterial blood volume (EABV), which increases the reabsorption of glomerular filtrate not only in the proximal nephron but also in the distal and collecting tubules by stimulating AVP secretion [111]. These patients generally have a low urinary [Na⁺] because of secondary hyperaldosteronism, which also is a product of

decreased EABV. However, under certain conditions, urinary [Na⁺] may be elevated, usually secondary to concurrent diuretic therapy but also sometimes because of a solute diuresis (eg, glucosuria in diabetics) or after successful treatment of the underlying disease (eg, ionotropic therapy in patients with congestive heart failure). Many different hypo-osmolar disorders can potentially present clinically with euvolemia, in large part because it is difficult to detect modest changes in volume status using standard methods of clinical assessment. In such cases measurement of urinary [Na⁺] is an especially important first step. A high urinary [Na⁺] in euvolemic patients usually implies a distally mediated, dilution-induced hypo-osmolality such as SIADH. However, glucocorticoid deficiency can mimic SIADH so closely that these two disorders are often indistinguishable in terms of water balance. Hyponatremia from diuretic use also can present without clinically evident hypovolemia, and the urinary [Na+] often is elevated in such cases because of the renal tubular effects of the diuretics. A low urinary [Na⁺] suggests a depletion-induced hypo-osmolality from ECF losses with subsequent volume replacement by water or other hypotonic fluids. The solute generally is non-renal in origin. One important exception, however, is recent cessation of diuretic therapy, because urinary [Na⁺] can quickly decrease to low values within 12 to 24 hours after discontinuation of the drug.

Criteria for the Diagnosis of SIADH

Essential

Decreased effective osmolality of the extracellular fluid (POsm < 275 mOsm/kg H_2O)

Inappropriate urinary concentration (UOsm > 100 mOsm/kg H_2O with normal renal function) at some level of hypo-osmolality

Clinical euvolemia, as defined by the absence of signs of hypovolemia (orthostasis, tachycardia, decreased skin turgor, dry mucous membranes) or hypervolemia (subcutaneous edema, ascites)

Elevated urinary sodium excretion while on normal salt and water intake.

Absence of other potential causes of euvolemic hypo-osmolality: hypothyroidism, hypocortisolism (Addison's disease or pituitary ACTH insufficiency), renal failure and diuretic use

Supplemental

Abnormal water load test (inability to excrete at least 80% of a 20 mL/kg water load in 4 h and/or failure to dilute UOsm to < 100 mOsm/kg H_2O)

Plasma AVP level inappropriately elevated relative to plasma osmolality

No significant correction of plasma [Na$^+$] with volume expansion but improvement after fluid restriction

FIGURE 3-85.

Clinical criteria for the diagnosis of SIADH. SIADH is the most common cause of euvolemic hypo-osmolality. It also is the single most prevalent cause of hypo-osmolality of all causes encountered in clinical practice, with a prevalence ranging from 20% to 40% among all hypo-osmolar patients. The clinical criteria necessary to diagnose SIADH remain basically the same as those set forth by Bartter and Schwartz in 1967 [112]. This figure presents a modified summary of these criteria, along with several other clinical findings that support this diagnosis. Several points about each of these criteria deserve emphasis or qualification. 1) True hypo-osmolality must be present and hyponatremia secondary to pseudohyponatremia or hyperglycemia alone must be excluded. 2) Urinary concentration (osmolality) must be inappropriate for plasma hypo-osmolality. This does not mean that urine osmolality must be greater than plasma osmolality (a common misinterpretation of this criterion), but simply that the urine must be less than maximally dilute (ie, urine osmolality greater than 100 mOsm/kg H_2O). 3) Clinical euvolemia must be present to establish a diagnosis of SIADH, because both hypovolemia and hypervolemia strongly suggest different causes of hypo-osmolality. This does not mean that patients with SIADH cannot become hypovolemic or hypervolemic for other reasons, but in such cases it is impossible to diagnose the underlying inappropriate antidiuresis until the patient is rendered euvolemic and is found to have persistent hypo-osmolality. 4) The criterion of renal salt-wasting probably has caused the most confusion regarding diagnosis of SIADH. This criterion is included because of its usefulness in differentiating between hypo-osmolality caused by a decreased EABV (in which case renal Na$^+$ conservation occurs) and distal dilution-induced disorders, in which urinary Na$^+$ excretion is normal or increased secondary to ECF volume expansion. However, two qualifications limit the utility of urinary [Na$^+$] measurement in hypo-osmolar patients: urinary [Na$^+$] also is high when solute depletion is of renal origin, as with diuretic use or Addison's disease, and patients with SIADH can have low urinary Na$^+$ excretion if they subsequently become hypovolemic or solute depleted, conditions that sometimes follow severe salt and water restriction. Consequently, although high urinary Na$^+$ excretion is the rule in most patients with SIADH, its presence does not guarantee this diagnosis; conversely, its absence does not necessarily rule out the diagnosis. 5) SIADH remains a diagnosis of exclusion. Thus, the presence of other potential causes of euvolemic hypo-osmolality must always be excluded; this includes not only thyroid and adrenal dysfunction, but also diuretic use, because this can also sometimes present as euvolemic hypo-osmolality.

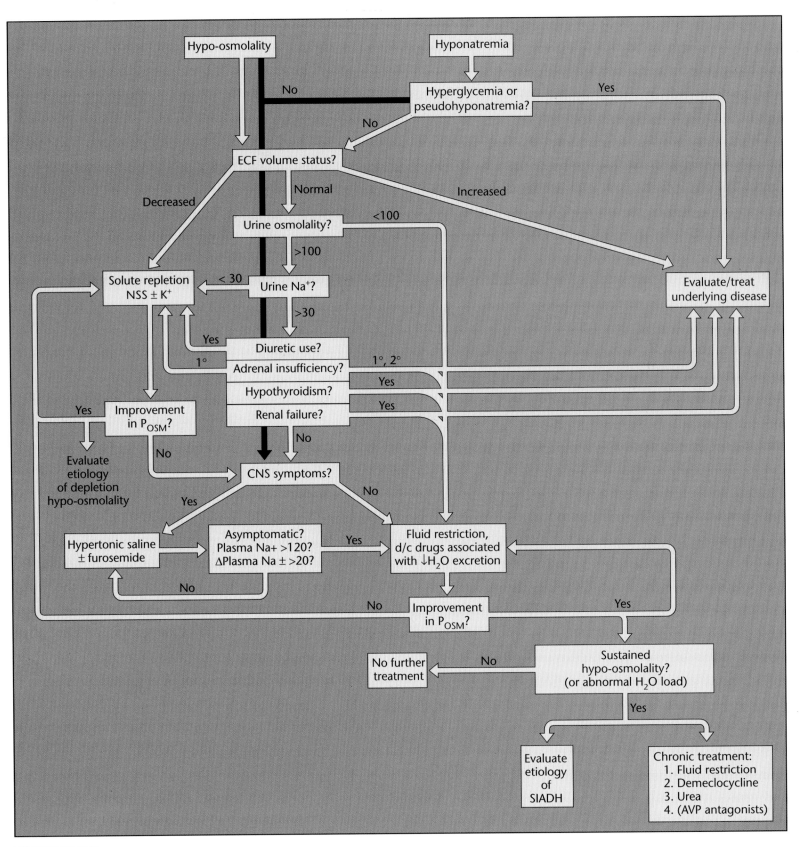

FIGURE 3-86.

Evaluation and treatment of hypo-osmolar patients. The dark arrow in the center emphasizes that the presence of central nervous system dysfunction resulting from hyponatremia should always be assessed immediately, so that appropriate therapy can be started as soon as possible in symptomatic patients while the outlined diagnostic evaluation is proceeding. ECF—extracellular fluid volume; NSS—normal (isotonic) saline; 1°—primary; 2°—secondary; Posm—plasma osmolality; d/c—discontinue; SIADH—syndrome of inappropriate antidiuretic hormone secretion. Numbers referring to osmolality are in mOsm/kg H₂O; numbers referring to Na⁺ concentration are in mEq/L. (*Adapted from* Verbalis [113]).

■ HUMAN NUTRITION AND OBESITY

Source and Action of Fibers

	Soluble Fibers	Insoluble Fibers
Food sources	Fruit such as apples and citrus	Wheat bran
	Oats	Whole grain breads and cereals
	Barley	Vegetables
	Legumes	
Action in the body	Delays gastrointestinal transit	Accelerates gastrointestinal transit
	Stimulates colonic fermentation	Increases fecal weight
	Delays glucose absorption	Slows starch hydrolysis
	Lowers blood cholesterol	Delays glucose absorption
Examples	Gums	Cellulose
	Pectins	Lignins
	Some hemicelluloses	Many hemicelluloses
	Mucilages	

FIGURE 3-87.
Fiber is an important nonnutrient constituent of food such as cereals, grains, fruits, and vegetables. Fiber can be classified as soluble or insoluble. (*Adapted from* Whitney and Rolfes [114].)

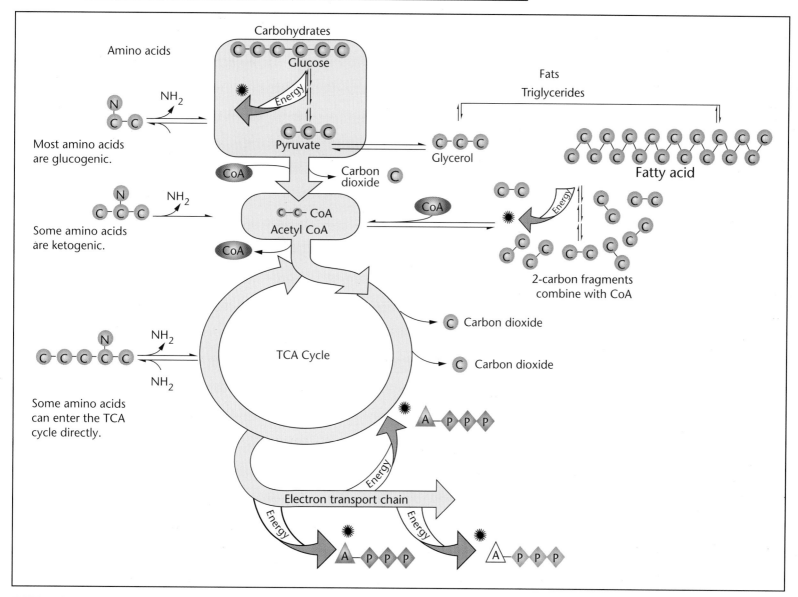

FIGURE 3-88.
Central pathways of energy metabolism. The digestion of carbohydrate yields glucose. Some of the glucose is stored as glycogen and some is taken into the brain and other cells to be broken down to provide energy. The digestion of fats yields glycerol and free fatty acids. Some fats are reassembled into triglycerides and stored as fat; others are broken down to provide energy. Protein digestion yields amino acids, some of which are used to build body protein. When a surplus of amino acids exists, or when there is inadequate carbohydrate or fat to meet energy needs, amino acids also can provide energy. Of the energy-containing nutrients, fat provides the most energy by weight. A—adenosine; C—carbon; CoA—coenzyme A; N—nitrogen; NH2—amino group; P—phosphate; TCA—tricarboxylic acid. (*Adapted from* Whitney and Rolfes [114].)

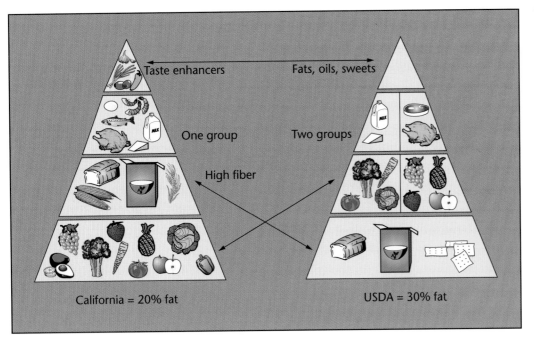

FIGURE 3-89.

Pyramid comparisons. Recommendations for dietary intake among populations often take the form of pyramids, with the base of the pyramid determining the basis of the diet. In the pyramid developed by the United States Department of Agriculture (USDA) in the late 1980s the base consists of cereals and grains, without an emphasis on the fiber content of those grains. The fruits and vegetables appear on the second level and are two separate groups. In a new pyramid developed in 1997 by the Center for Human Nutrition at the University of California at Los Angeles, a modified plant-based diet is recommended. The base consists of five to 11 servings of fruits and vegetables to provide unique phytonutrients for prevention of chronic diseases. The second level consists of six to nine servings of high-fiber cereals and grains to provide the benefits of fiber from this level as well as from fruits and vegetables. The protein level is made up of low-fat protein choices, including protein from plants (beans, rice, and soybeans) and animals (egg whites, chicken breast, turkey, low-fat fish, other seafood, and nonfat milk products). The top tier of the USDA pyramid has only dots representing fats and sweets with the mixed message "use sparingly." The top tier of the new California pyramid emphasizes taste enhancers including olives, avocados, garlic, onion, nuts, cheese, chili peppers, and monounsaturated or omega-3-rich oils. The overall fat recommendation of the USDA pyramid is 30% or less of calories from fat. The new pyramid reflects the decreased fat intake in the population by recommending 20% or less of calories from fat. This exercise illustrates how the science of nutrition can be used to influence dietary recommendations. (*Adapted from* Heber [115].)

VITAMINS AND MINERALS

Role of Vitamins in Health and Disease

Vitamin	Biochemical Function	Deficiency	Prevention/Treatment
Niacin	NAD, NADP component	Pellagra	Hypercholesterolemia
B_6	Transamination cofactor	Convulsions	Carpal tunnel syndrome
B_{12}	Transmethylation cofactor	Anemias	Cognitive dysfunction
Folic acid	Single carbon transport	Megaloblastic anemia	Hyperhomocysteinemia
C	Hydroxylation cofactor	Scurvy	Oxidative stress
D	Calcium transport	Rickets	Osteoporosis
E	Antioxidant	Hemolytic anemia	Relative anergy

FIGURE 3-90.

Role of vitamins in health and disease. Several dose-dependent biochemical functions have been identified for most vitamins, only some of which are related to their essentiality in preventing deficiency syndromes. The essentiality of niacin is based on its role in oxidation-reduction (redox) reactions (NAD, NADP), although this mechanism is unrelated to its hypocholesterolemic action at high doses. Pyridoxine is essential to the metabolic transformation of amino acids, which may be related to the epileptiform convulsions of deficiency and its analgesic pharmacology in tenosynovitis. Vitamin C at low intakes supports proline hydroxylation via iron reduction and prevents scurvy, whereas higher consumption provides enough redox capacity for ascorbate to function as an antioxidant. The antioxidant function of vitamin E maintains membrane integrity, but supplemental intake is associated with the inhibition of cyclooxygenase and stimulation of immune function.

Percentage of Individuals with Diets that Meet the RDA: Problem Minerals

Mineral	Population Meeting RDA, %	Groups at Highest Risk for Not Meeting RDA
Calcium	13.5–25.3	Females (12–70+)
Phosphorus	33.7	Females (12–19)
Magnesium	17.9–33.5	Males (12–29, 50+), females (12–70+)
Iron	22.1–27.7	Females (12–49)
Zinc	12.4–32.7	Children (1–5), males (40+), females (6+)

FIGURE 3-91.

Percentage of individuals with diets that meet the recommended dietary allowances (RDAs): problem minerals. Assessment of mineral intakes over a 2-day period reveals that no age/gender group meets 100% of the US RDA for all nutrients [116]. However, low mineral intake and risk of deficiency can be defined as intake of less than 66% of the RDA over time. Poor intake of calcium, phosphorus, magnesium, and zinc is associated with lower peak bone mineral density by 35 to 40 years of age and faster loss in postmenopausal women, resulting in an increased risk of osteoporosis; iron is necessary for collagen matrix production, providing a structural framework for bone. Poor iron intake is also associated with anemia and, in children, with cognitive impairment. Poor magnesium intake is also associated with atherosclerosis, diabetes, hypertension, migraine headaches, and stroke.

Changes in Serum Levels of Hormones in Obese Subjects after 12 Hours and after 7 Days of Fasting*

Parameter	12-Hour Fast	7-Day Fast
Triiodothyronine, *ng/dL*	130±15	59±5[†]
Free triiodothyronine, *pg/dL*	322±32	159±13[†]
Reverse triiodothyronine, *ng/dL*	35±3	57±5[†]
Thyroxine, *mg/dL*	9.1±0.7	9.3±0.8[†]
Free thyroxine, *ng/dL*	4.7±0.2	3.0±0.3[†]
Insulin, *mU/mL*	34±6	15±2[†]
Morning cortisol, *mg/dL*	19.1±2.1	26.4±3.4[†]
Urinary free cortisol, *mg/dL*	27.1±3.2	41.8±6.3[†]

*Data are expressed as the mean ± SEM for nine subjects.
[†]$P < 0.05$.

FIGURE 3-92.

Serum hormone level changes in obese subjects after 12 hours and after 7 days of fasting. In addition to insulin, other hormones that potentially affect the immune system, such as thyroid hormone and cortisol, change dramatically during starvation [117]. Such changes result in immunosuppression. (*Adapted from* Heber [117].)

DIAGNOSIS AND MANAGEMENT OF OBESITY

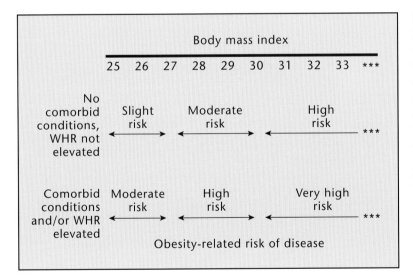

FIGURE 3-93.

Influence of comorbid conditions (hypertension, hyperlipidemia, diabetes mellitus, sleep apnea) or elevated waist-to-hip ratio (WHR) (or simply waist circumference) on how body mass index affects disease risk. The diagnosis of obesity must be considered in the context of comorbid diseases, and weight reduction should be used as a part of the therapy for these conditions. Body mass index can be defined by using widely available charts or calculated as the weight in pounds multiplied by the factor 705 and divided by the height in inches squared. (*Adapted from* National Institutes of Health [118].)

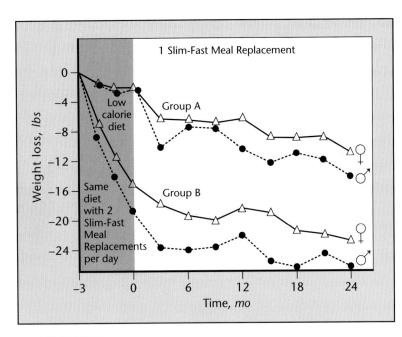

FIGURE 3-94.

Weight loss and weight maintenance with daily use of meal replacements (Slim-Fast Foods Co, West Palm Beach, FL). In this study, patients were told to restrict their favorite foods by counting calories between 1200 and 1500 calories per day or to use two meal replacements as part of an overall diet of 1200 to 1500 calories. The markedly increased weight loss in the meal replacement group over the first 12 weeks can be attributed to the enhanced dietary compliance mediated by the use of meal replacements. Both groups then ingested one meal replacement per day over 2 years, and both groups lost additional weight. (*Adapted from* Ditschuneit *et al.* [119].)

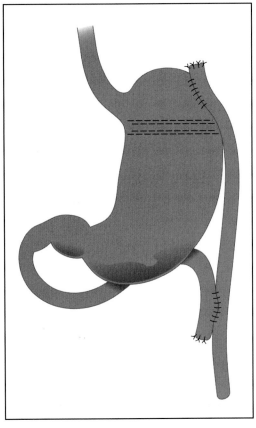

FIGURE 3-95.

Roux-en-Y gastric bypass. This surgery creates a small gastric pouch the size of a hard-boiled egg, where food that is well-chewed can enter the intestine. This results in a rapid-onset satiety response. The side effects of the operation include dumping syndrome and hypoglycemia. As with vertical banded gastroplasty, diet and lifestyle changes are needed. The side effects are more pronounced than those with vertical banded gastroplasty, but the results are also more predictable. Vitamin B12 must be administered bimonthly by injection because the area of the stomach that produces intrinsic factor is bypassed. This operation is preferred as the primary surgery for obesity at many of the academic medical centers that have comprehensive obesity programs. (*Adapted from* Shikora *et al.* [120].)

■ REFERENCES

1. Kaptein EM: Clinical application of free thyroxine determinations. *Clin Lab Med* 1993, 13:653–672.

2. Nelson JC, Wilcox RB: Analytical performance of free and total thyroxine assays. *Clin Chem* 1996, 42:146–154.

3. Persani L, Borgato S, Romoli R, *et al.*: Changes in the degree of sialylation of carbohydrate chains modify the biological properties of circulating thyrotropin isoforms in various physiological and pathological states. *J Clin Endocrinol Metab* 1998, 83:2486–2492.

4. Kaptein EM: Nonthyroidal illness. *Thyroid Int* 1998, 3:1–13.

5. Surks MI, Sievert R: Drugs and thyroid function. *N Engl J Med* 1995, 333:1688–1694.

6. Kaptein EM: Thyroid in vitro testing in non-thyroidal illness. *Exp Clin Endocrinol* 1994, 102:92–101.

7. Kaptein EM: Clinical relevance of thyroid hormone alterations in nonthyroidal illness. *Thyroid Int* 1997, 4:22–25.

8. Okabayashi T, Takeda K, Kawada M, *et al.*: Free thyroxine concentrations in serum measured by equilibrium dialysis in chronic renal failure. *Clin Chem* 1996, 42:1616–1620.

9. Surks MI, DeFesi CR: Normal serum free thyroid hormone concentrations in patients treated with phenytoin or carbamazepine. *J Am Med Assoc* 1996, 275:1495–1498.

10. Wilcox RB, Nelson JC: Heterogeneity in affinities of serum proteins for thyroxine among patients with non-thyroidal illness as indicated by the serum free thyroxine response to serum dilution. *Eur J Endocrinol* 1994, 131:9–13.

11. Burmeister LA: Reverse T3 does not reliably differentiate hypothyroid sick syndrome from euthyroid sick syndrome. *Thyroid* 1995, 5:435–441.

12. Samuels MH, Kramer R: Differential effects of short-term fasting on pulsatile thyrotropin, gonadotropin, and a-subunit secretion in healthy men: a clinical research center study. *J Clin Endocrinol Metab* 1996, 81:32–36.

13. Kosary CL, Ries LAG, Miller BA: SEER Cancer Statistic Review 1973–1992: tables and graphs. Bethesda, MD: National Cancer Institute; 1995. [NIH publication no. 96-2789.]

14. Landis SH, Murray T, Bolden S, *et al.*: Cancer statistics, 1998. *Cancer* 1998, 48:6–30.

15. Mazzaferri EL: Thyroid carcinoma: papillary and follicular. In *Endocrine Tumors*. Edited by Mazzaferri EL, Samaan N. Cambridge: Blackwell Scientific; 1993:278–333.

16. Larsen R, Ingban SH: In *Williams Textbook of Endocrinology*, edn. 8. Philadelphia, WB Saunders; 1992: 425.

17. Shapiro LE, Surks MI: Hypothyroidism. In *Principles and Practice of Endocrinology and Metabolism, edn 3*. Edited by Becker KL. Philadelphia: Lippincott, Williams and Wilkins, 2001.

18. Brent GA, Larsen PR. Treatment of hypothyroidism. In *Werner and Ingbar's The Thyroid*. Philadelphia: Lippincott-Raven; 1996:883–887.

19. Mariotti S, Franceschi C, Cossarizza A, *et al.*: The aging thyroid. *Endocr Rev* 1995, 16:686–710.

20. Jonas J-C, Sharma A, Hasenkamp W, *et al.*: Chronic hyperglycemia.triggers loss of pancreatic beta cell differentiation in an animal model of diabetes. *J Biol Chem* 1999, 274: 14112–14121.

21. Rhodes, CJ: Processing of the insulin molecule. In *Diabetes Mellitus*. Edited by LeRoith, D Taylor, SI and Olefsky, JM. Philadelphia: Lippincott-Raven; 1996:27–41.

22. Rhodes CJ Alarcon C: What b-cell defect could lead to hyperproinsulinemia in NIDDM: Some clues from recent advances made in understanding the proinsulin conversion mechanism. *Diabetes* 1994, 43:511–517.

23. Leahy JL, Cooper HE, Deal DA Weir GC: Chronic hyperglycemia is associated with impaired glucose influence on insulin secretion: a study in normal rats using chronic in vivo glucose infusions. *J Clin Invest* 1986, 77:908–915.

24. Brunzell JD, Robertson RP, Lerner RL, *et al.*: Relationships between fasting plasma glucose levels and insulin secretion during intravenous glucose tolerance tests. *J Clin Endocrinol Metab* 1976, 42:222–229.

25. Ward WK, Beard JC, Halter JB, *et al.*: Pathophysiology of insulin secretion in non-insulin-dependent diabetes mellitus. *Diabetes Care* 1984, 7:491–502.

26. Kitabachi AE, Wall BM:Diabetic ketoacidosis. *Med Clin North Am* 1995, 79:9–37.

27. Kitabchi AE, Umpierrez GE, Murphy MB, Barrett, *et al.*: Management of hyperglycemic crises in patients with diabetes mellitus. *Diabetes Care*. (In Press)

28. Bjellerup P, Kallner A, Kollind M: GLC determination of serum-ethylene glycol, interferences in ketotic patients. *J Toxicol Clin Toxicol* 1994, 32(1):85–87.

29. Morris LE, Kitabchi AE: Coma in the diabetic. *Diabetes mellitus: problems in management*. Edited by Schnatz JD Menlo Park, CA: Addison-Wesley Publishing. 1982, 234–251.

30. Chupin M, Charbonnel B, Chupin F: C-peptide levels in ketoacidosis and in hyperosmolar non-ketotic diabetic coma. *Acta Diabet* 1981, 18:123–128.

31. Schade DS, Eaton RP: Dose response to insulin in man: Differential effects on glucose and ketone body regulation. *J Clin Endocrinol Metab* 1977, 44:1038–1053.

32. Kitabchi AE, Fisher JN, Murphy MB, *et al.*: Diabetic ketoacidosis and the hyperglycemic hyperosmolar nonketotic state. In *Joslin's Diabetes Mellitus, 13th ed.* Kahn CR, Weir GC, eds. Lea & Febiger, Philadelphia, 1994, pp 738–770.

33. Kitabchi AE, Fisher JN: Insulin therapy of diabetic ketoacidosis: Physiologic versus pharmacologic doses of insulin and their routes of administration. In *Handbook of Diabetes Mellitus, vol 5*. Edited by Brownlee M. New York: Garland ATPM Press, 1981, 95–149.

34. Kulkarni RN, Bruning JC, Winnay JN, *et al.*: Tissue-specific knockout of the insulin receptor in pancreatic b cells creates an insulin secretory defect similar to that in Type 2 diabetes. *Cell* 1999, 96:329–339.

35. Tobe K, Sabe H, Yamamoto T, *et al.*: CSK enhances insulin-stimulated dephosphorylation of focal adhesion proteins. *Mol Cell Biol* 1996, 16:4765–4772.

36. Stumvoli M, Nurjhan N, Perriello G, *et al.*: Metabolic effects of metformin in non-insulin-dependent diabetes mellitus. *N Engl J Med* 1995, 333:550–554.

37. Inzucchi SE, Maggs DG, Spollett GR, *et al.*: Efficacy and metabolic effects of metformin and troglitazone in type II diabetes mellitus. *N Engl J Med* 1998, 338:867–872.

38. Jackson RS, Creemers JWM, Ohagi S, *et al.*: Obesity and impaired prohormone processing associated with mutations in the human prohormone convertase I gene. *Nat Genet* 1997, 16:303–306.

39. Ristow M, Muller-Wieland D, Pfeiffer A, *et al.*: Obesity associated with a mutation in a genetic regulator of adipocyte differentiation. *N Engl J Med* 1998, 339:953–959.

40. Stout RW: Hyperinsulinemia and atherosclerosis. *Diabetes* 1996, 45:S45–S46.

41. UK Prospective Diabetes Study (UKPDS) Group. Intensive blood-glucose control with sulphonylureas or insulin compared with conventional treatment and risk of complications in patients with type 2 diabetes (UKPDS 33). *Lancet* 1998, 352:837–853.

42. Turner RC: The U.K. Prospective Diabetes Study. A review. *Diabetes Care* 1998, 21:C35–C38.

43. Harris MI: Summary. In *Diabetes in America*. NIH Publication No. 95-1468. Edited by Harris MI, Cowie CC, Stern MP, *et al*. Washington, DC: US Government Printing Office; 1995:1–14.

44. Fagan TC, Deedwania PC: The cardiovascular dysmetabolic syndrome. *Am J Med* 1998, 105(1A):77S–82S.

45. Garber AJ: Vascular disease and lipids in diabetes. *Med Clin North Am* 1998, 82:931–948.

46. Harati Y: Diabetes and the nervous system. *Endocrinol Metab Clin North Am* 1996, 25:325–359.

47. Boulton AJM, Malik RA: Diabetic neuropathy. *Med Clin North Am* 1998, 82:909–929.

48. Levin ME: Foot lesions in patients with diabetes mellitus. *Endocrinol Metab Clin North Am* 1996, 25:447–462.

49. American Diabetes Association: Position Statement: Foot care in diabetes. *Diabetes Care* 1998, 21(suppl):S54–S55.

50. Krowelski AS, Warram JH, Valsania P, *et al.*: Evolving natural history of coronary artery disease in diabetes mellitus. *Am J Med* 1991, 90 (suppl 2A):56S–61S.

51. Kuusisito J, Mykannen L, Pyorala K, *et al.*: NIDDM and its metabolic control predict coronary artery disease in elderly subjects. *Diabetes* 1994, 43:960–967.

52. Warram JH, Krowleski AS: Use of the albumin/creatinine ratio in patient care and clinical studies. In *The Kidney and Hypertension in Diabetes Mellitus*. Edited by Mogensen CE. London: Kluwer Academic Publishers, 1998: 85–96.

53. Brownlee M: Advanced products of nonenzymatic glycosylation and the pathogenesis of diabetic complications. In *Diabetes Mellitus. Theory and Practice*. Edited by Rifkin H, Porte D. New York: Elsevier, 1990:279.

54. Diabetes Control and Complications Trial Research Group: Effect of intensive diabetes treatment on nerve conduction in the Diabetes Control and Complications Trial. *Ann Neurol* 1995 38(6):869–80.

55. Vinik AI, Newlon PG, Lauterio TJ, *et al.*: Nerve survival and regeneration in diabetes. *Diabetes Rev* 1995, 3:139–157. by Riflin H, Porte D. New York, Amsterdam, London: Elsevier, 1990:279.

56. Said G, Goulon-Gorcau C, Lacroix C, Moulonguet A: Nerve biopsy findings in different patterns of proximal diabetic neuropathy. *Ann Neurol* 1994, 35:559–569.

57. Krendel DA, Costigan DA, Hopkins LC: Successful treatment of neuropathies in patients with diabetes mellitus. *Arch Neurol* 1995, 52:1053–1061.

58. Vinik AL, Milicevic Z, Colen LB, *et al.*: Histopathological and electrophysiologic heterogeneity in patients with proximal diabetic neuropathy (PDN) [abstract]. Diabetes 1996, 769:209A.

59. Malik RA, Tesfaye S. Thompson SD, *et al.*: Transperineurial capillary abnormalities in the sural nerve of patients with diabetic neuropathy. *Microvasc Res* 1994, 48:236–245.

60. Dyck P, Hansen S, Karnes J: Capillary number and percentage closed in human diabetic sural nerve. *Proc Natl Acad Sci USA* 1985, 82:2513–2517.

61. Low P, Lagerlund T, McManis : Nerve blood flow and oxygen delivery in normal. diabetic. and ischemic neuropathy. *Int Rev Neurobiol* 1989, 33(1):355–438.

62. Yasuda H, Dyck P: Abnormalities of endoneurial microvessels and sural nerve pathology in diabetic neuropathy. *Neurology* 1987, 37:20–28.

63. Malik RA, Veves A, Masson EA, *et al.*: Endoneurial capillary abnormalities in human diabetic neuropathy. *J Neurol Neurosurg Psychiatry* 1992, 55:557–561.

64. Tuck RR, Schinelzer JD, Low PA: Endoneurial blood flow and oxygen tension in the sciatic nerves of rats ,with experimental diabetic neuropathy. *Brain* 1984, 107:935–950.

65. Newrick PG, Wilson AJ, Jakubowski J, *et al.*: Sural nerve oxygen tension in diabetes. *Brit Med J* 1986, 293:1053–1054.

66. Zachodne DW, Ho LT: Normal blood flow but lower oxygen tension in diabetes of' young rats: microenvironment and the influence of sympathectomy. *Can J Physiol Pharmacol* 1992, 70:651–659.

67. Hotta N, Koh N, Sakakibara F, *et al.*: Effect of proplionyl-L-carnitine on motor nerve conduction, autonomic cardiac function, and nerve blood flow in rats with streptozotòcin-induced diabetes: comparison with an aldose reductase inhibitor. *Diabetes* 1992, 41:587–591.

68. Service FJ: Hypoglycemias. In *Cecil's Textbook of Medicine, Update 4*. Edited by Smith LH Jr. Philadelphia: WB Saunders; 1989.

69. Service FJ: Clinical presentations and laboratory evaluation of hypoglycemic disorders in adults. In *Hypoglycemic Disorder: Pathogenesis, Diagnosis and Treatment*. Edited by Service FJ. Boston: GK Hall; 1983:73–95.

70. Cryer PE: Glucose counter-regulation: the physiological mechanisms that prevent or correct hypoglycemia. In *Hypoglycaemia and Diabetes: Clinical and Physiological Aspects*.Edited by Frier BM, Fisher BM. London: Edward Arnold; 1993:34–55.

71. Cooper C, Melton LJ III: Epidemiology of osteoporosis. *Trends Endocrinol Metab* 1992, 3:224–229

72. Riggs BL, Khosla S, Melton LJ: A unitary model for involutional osteoporosis: estrogen deficiency causes both type I and type II osteoporosis in postmenopausal women and contributes to bone loss in aging men. *J Bone Miner Res* 1998, 13:763–773.

73. Wasnish RD: Epidemiology of Osteoporosis. In *Primer on the Metabolic Bone Diseases and Disorders of Mineral Metabolism, edn 3*. Edited by Favus MJ. Philadelphia: Lippincott-Raven, 1996:249–251.

74. Kanis JA, McCloskey EV: Evaluation of the risk of hip fracture. *Bone* 1996, 18:127S–132S.

75. Melton LF, Atkinson EJ, O'Fallon M, *et al.*: Long-term fracture prediction by bone mineral assessed at different skeletal sites. *J Bone Min Res* 1993, 8:1227–1233.

76. Hutchinson TA, Polansky SM, Feinstein AR: Post-menopausal oestrogens protect against fractures of the hip and distal radius. *Lancet* 1979, 2:705–709.

77. Kreiger N, Kelsey JL, Holford TR, *et al.*: An epidemiologic study of hip fracture in postmenopausal women. *Am J Epidemiol* 1982, 116:141–148.

78. Paganini-Hill A, Ross RK, Gerkins VR, *et al.*: Menopausal estrogen therapy and hip fractures. *Ann Int Med* 1981, 95:28–31.

79. Weiss NS, Ure CL, Ballard JH, et al.: Decreased risk of fractures of the hip and lower forearm with postmenopausal use of estrogen. *N Engl J Med* 1980, 303:1195–1198.

80. Katznelson L, Finkelstein JS, Schoenfeld DA, *et al.*: Increase in bone density and lean body mass during testosterone administration in men with acquired hypogonadism. *J Clin Endocrinol Metab* 1996, 81:4358–4365.

81. Cryer PE, Kissane JM: Vertebral compression fractures with accelerated bone turnover in a patient with Cushing's disease (clinicopathologic conference). *Am J Med* 1980, 68:932–940.

82. Greenberger PA, Hendrix RW, Patterson R: Bone studies in patients on prolonged systemic corticosteroid therapy for asthma. *Clin Allergy* 1982, 12:363–368.

83. Sambrook PN, Birmingham J, Kempler S: Corticosteroid effects on proximal femur bone loss. *J Bone Miner Res* 1990, 5:1211–1216.

84. Gennari C, Civitelli R: Glucocorticoid-induced osteoporosis. *Clin Rheum Dis* 1986, 12:637–654.

85. LoCascio V, Bonucci E, Imbimbo B: Bone loss in response to long-term glucocorticoid therapy. *Bone Miner* 1990, 8:39–51.

86. Thompson JM, Modin GW, Arnaud CD, *et al.*: Not all postmenopausal women on chronic steroid and estrogen treatment are osteoporotic: predictors of bone mineral density. *Calcif Tissue Int* 1997, 61:377–381.

87. Reed IR, Heap SW: Determinants of vertebral mineral density in patients receiving long-term glucocorticoid therapy. *Arch Intern Med* 1990, 150:2545–2548.

88. Varanos S, Ansell BM, Reeve J: Vertebral collapse in juvenile chronic arthritis: its relationship with glucocorticoid therapy. *Calcif Tissue Int* 1987, 41:75–78.

89. Als OS, Gotfredsen A, Christiansen C: The effect of glucocorticoids on bone mass in rheumatoid arthritis patients: influence of menopausal state. *Arthritis Rheum* 1985, 28:369–375.

90. Gay VL: The hypothalamus: physiology and clinical use of releasing factors. *Fertil Steril* 1972, 23:50–63.

91. Ross DA, Wilson CB: Results of transsphenoidal microsurgery for growth hormone-secreting pituitary adenoma in a series of 214 patients. *J Neurosurg* 1988, 68:854–867.

92. Losa M, Oeckler R, Schopohl J, *et al.*: Evaluation of selective transsphenoidal adenomectomy by endocrinological testing and somatomedin-C measurement in acromegaly. *J Neurosurg* 1989, 70:561–567.

93. Fahlbusch R, Honegger J, Buchfelder M: Surgical management of acromegaly. *Endocrinol Metab Clin North Am* 1992, 21:669–692.

94. Davis DH, Laws ER, Ilstrup DM, *et al.*: Results of surgical treatment for growth hormone-secreting pituitary adenomas. *J Neurosurg* 1993, 79:70–75.

95. Freda PU, Wardlaw SL, Post KD: Long-term endocrinological follow-up evaluation in115 patients who underwent transsphenoidal surgery for acromegaly. *J Neurosurg* 1998, 89:353–358.

96. Laws ER, Thapar K: Pituitary Surgery. *Endocrinol Metab Clin North Am* 1999, 28:119–131.

97. Carroll PV, Christ ER, and the members of the Growth Hormone Research Society scientific committee: Growth hormone deficiency in adulthood and the effects of growth hormone replacement: a review. *J Clin Endocrinol Metab* 1998, 83:382–395.

98. Burman P, Broman JE, Hetta J, *et al.*: Quality of life in adults with growth hormone (GH) deficiency: Response to treatment with recombinant human GH in a placebo-controlled 21-month trial. *J Clin Endocrinol Metab* 1995, 80:3585–3590.

99. Pituitary Adenoma Study Group. Pituitary adenomas and oral contraceptives: a multicenter case control study. *Fertil Steril* 1983, 39:753–760.

100. Schlechte JA, Sherman B, Halmi N, *et al.*: Prolactin-secreting pituitary tumors in amenorrheic women: a comprehensive study. *Endocr Rev* 1980, 1:295–308.

101. Walsh JP, Pullan PT: Hyperprolactinaemia in males: a heterogeneous disorder. *Austral N Z J Med* 1997, 7:385–390.

102. Colao A, DiSarno A, Sarnacchiaro F, *et al.*: Prolactinomas resistant to standard dopamine agonists respond to chronic cabergoline treatment. *J Clin Endocrinol Metab* 1997, 82:876–883.

103. Beck-Peccoz P, Brucker-Davis F, Persani L, *et al.*: Thyrotropin-secreting pituitary tumors. *Endocr Rev* 1996, 17:610–638.

104. Arafah BM, Kailani S, Nekl KE, *et al.*: Immediate recovery of pituitary function after transsphenoidal resection of pituitary macroadenomas. *J Clin Endocrinol Metab* 1994, 79:348–354.

105. Findling JW, Aron DC, Tyrrell JB: Cushing disease. In *The Pituitary Gland*. Edited by Imura H. New York: Raven Press; 1985:441.

106. Meier C, Biller BMK: Clinical and biochemical evaluation of Cushing's syndrome. In *Endocrinology and Metabolism Clinics of North America. Diagnostic Evaluation Update*. Edited by Young WF, Klee GG. Philadelphia: W.B. Saunders; 1997:741–762.

107. Hall WA, Luciano MNG, Doppman JL, *et al.*: Pituitary magnetic resonance imaging in normal human volunteers: occult adenomas in the general population. *Ann Intern Med* 1994, 120:817–820.

108. Molitch ME, Russell EJ: The pituitary "incidentaloma." *Ann Intern Med* 1990, 112:925–931.

109. Mampalam TJ, Tyrrell JB, Wilson CB: Transsphenoidal microsurgery for Cushing's disease. A report of 216 cases. *Ann Intern Med* 1988, 109:487–493.

110. Reeves WB, Bichet DG, Andreoli TE: Posterior pituitary and water metabolism In *William's Textbook of Endocrinology, edn 9*. Edited by Wilson JD, Foster DW, Kronenberg, HM, Larsen PR. Philadelphia; WB Saunders: 1998:341–387.

111. Schrier RW: Body fluid volume regulation in health and disease: a unifying hypothesis. *Ann Int Med* 1990, 113:155–159.

112. Bartter FC, Schwartz WB: The syndrome of inappropriate secretion of antidiuretic hormone. *Am J Med* 1967, 42:790–806.

113. Verbalis JG: Inappropriate antidiuresis and other hypo-osmolar states. In *Principles and Practice of Endocrinology and Metabolism, edn 2*. Edited by Becker KL. Philadelphia: JB Lippincott; 1995:265–276.

114. Whitney EN, Rolfes SR: *Understanding Nutrition, edn 7*. Minneapolis-St. Paul: West Publishing Company, 1996:261.

115. Heber D: *The Resolution Diet*. Garden City Park, NY: The Avery Publishing Group; 1999.

116. U.S. Department of Agriculture, Agricultural Research Service: 1997 Data tables: results from USDA's 1994-96 Continuing Survey of Good Intakes by Individuals and 1994-96 Diet and Health Knowledge Survey. ARS Food Surveys Research Group. Available online under "Releases" at: http://www.barc.usda.gov/bhnrc/foodsurvey/home.htm.

117. Heber D: *Endocrinology, vol 3, part XI, edn 3*. Edited by DeGroot, Cahill, Martini *et al*. Philadelphia: WB Saunders; 1995:2663–2678.

118. Clinical Guidelines on the Identification, Evaluation, and Treatment of Overweight and Obesity in Adults. Bethesda, MD: National Institutes of Health; National Heart, Lung, and Blood Institute; 1998:VIII.

119. Ditschuneit HH, Flechtner-Mors M, Johnson TD, *et al.*: Metabolic and weight-loss effects of a long-term dietary intervention in obese patients. *Am J Clin Nutr* 1999, 69:198–204.

120. Shikora SA, Benotti PN, Forse RA: Surgical treatment of obesity. In *Obesity: Pathophysiology, Psychology and Treatment*. Edited by Blackburn and Kanders. New York: Chapman & Hall; 1994:264–282.

Dermatology

JEFFREY P. CALLEN

The dermatology chapter of this Atlas presents common and complex dermatoses and growths in a format that aids the practitioner with diagnosis. The algorithmic approach of first separating dermatologic disease into rashes or growths, then separating further is illustrated in Figures 4-1 and 4-2 [1]. It is preferable for the clinician to develop a differential diagnosis rather than attempt to match the patient's condition with a photograph depicted in this chapter. Appropriate diagnosis is most likely to result in a better chance that selected therapy will be appropriate. In addition, correct diagnosis allows one to predict prognosis more accurately [2].

■ PRINCIPLES OF DIAGNOSIS

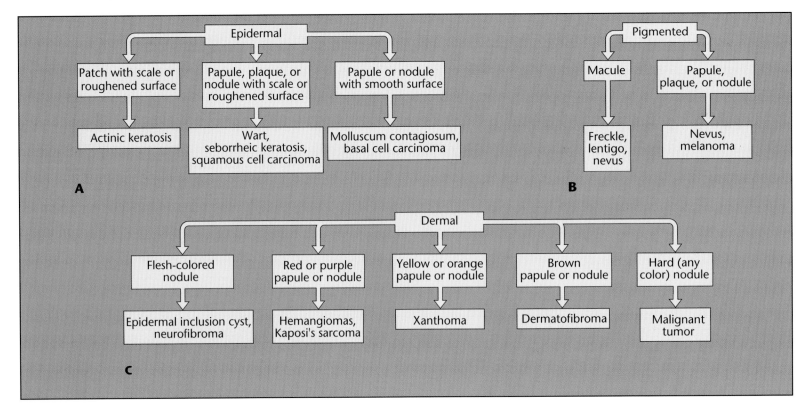

FIGURE 4-1.
Algorithm of epidermal (*panel A*), pigmented (*panel B*), and dermal   growths (*panel C*). (*Courtesy of* Donald P. Lookingbill.)

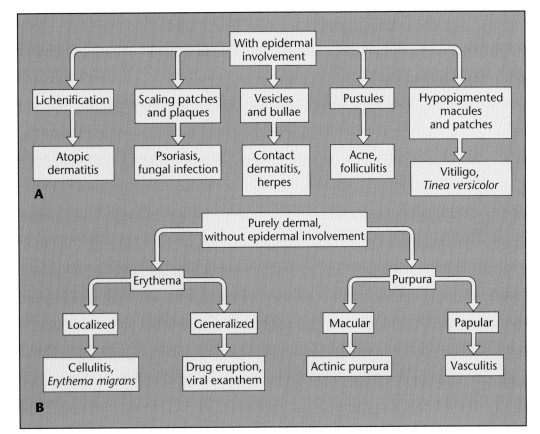

FIGURE 4-2.
Algorithm of rashes with epidermal development (*panel A*) and with purely dermal development (*panel B*). (*Courtesy of* Donald P. Lookingbill.)

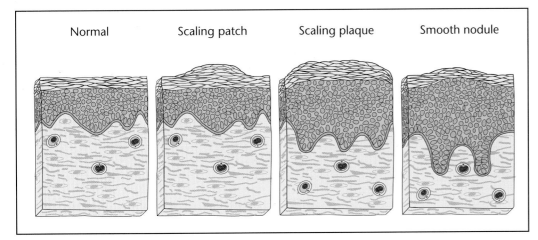

FIGURE 4-3.
Epidermal growths. These growths arise from thickening of the stratum corneum, the epidermis, or both. (*Courtesy of* Donald P. Lookingbill.)

Normal   Scaling patch   Scaling plaque   Smooth nodule

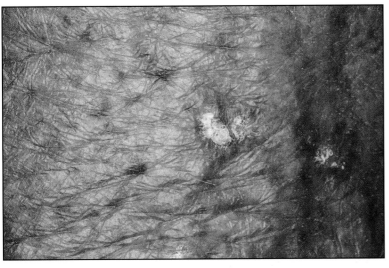

FIGURE 4-4.
Actinic keratoses. Epidermal growths appearing on exposed surfaces as a scaly papule or plaque.

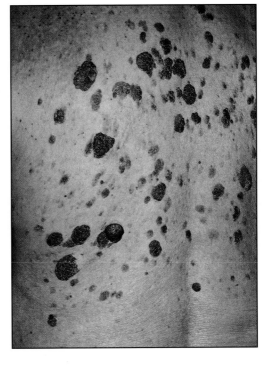

FIGURE 4-5.
Multiple seborrheic keratoses. Epidermal growths appearing as plaques, nodules, or both with a sharp margination and a verrucous surface. They appear to be "stuck on" the surface.

FIGURE 4-6.
Basal cell carcinoma, the most common form of cancer. Epidermal growth appearing as a smooth, pearly nodule.

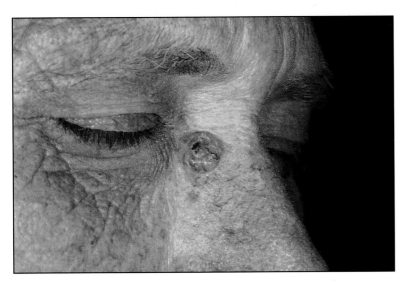

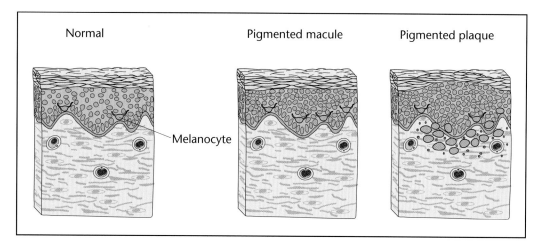

FIGURE 4-7.
Pigmented growths. These growths are due to increased pigment with or without an increase in pigment-producing cells. (*Courtesy of* Donald P. Lookingbill.)

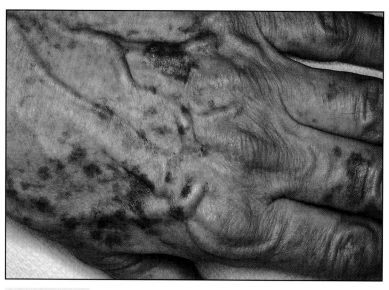

FIGURE 4-8.
Multiple lentigines. Pigmented growths appearing as macules on exposed surfaces.

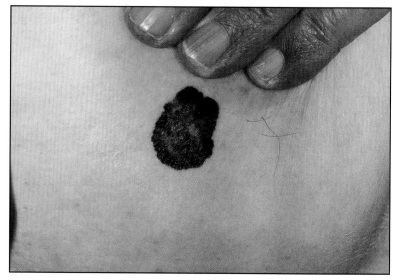

FIGURE 4-9.
Melanoma. Superficial spreading pigmented growth appearing as a plaque

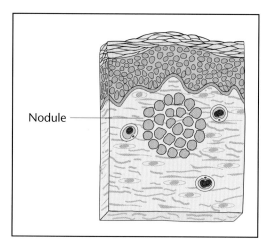

FIGURE 4-10.
Dermal growths. These nodules result from proliferation of cells in the dermis. (*Courtesy of* Donald P. Lookingbill.)

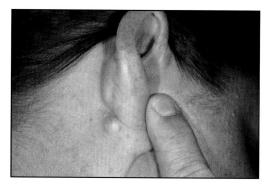

FIGURE 4-11.
Epidermal cyst. Dermal growth appearing as a flesh-colored nodule resulting from an epidermal-liined, keratin-containing cyst in the dermis.

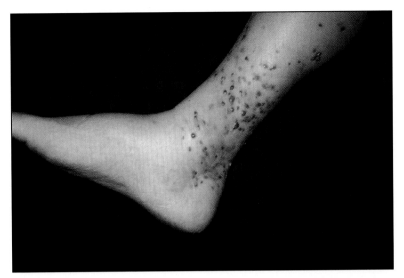

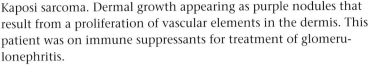

FIGURE 4-12.
Kaposi sarcoma. Dermal growth appearing as purple nodules that result from a proliferation of vascular elements in the dermis. This patient was on immune suppressants for treatment of glomerulonephritis.

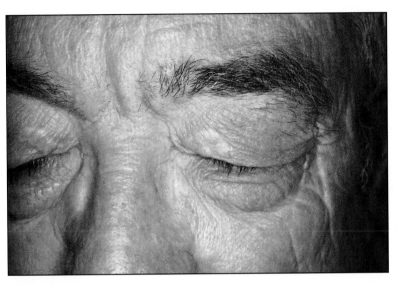

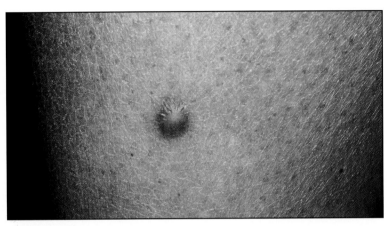

FIGURE 4-14.
Dermatofibroma. Dermal growth due to increased number of fibroblasts in the dermis.

FIGURE 4-13.
Xanthelasma. Dermal growth appearing as a yellow plaque derived from a collection of lipid-laden cells in the dermis.

FIGURE 4-15.
Metastatic squamous cell carcinoma. Dermal growth forming firm nodules from malignant cells that have aggregated in the dermis.

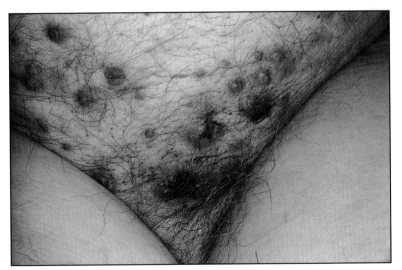

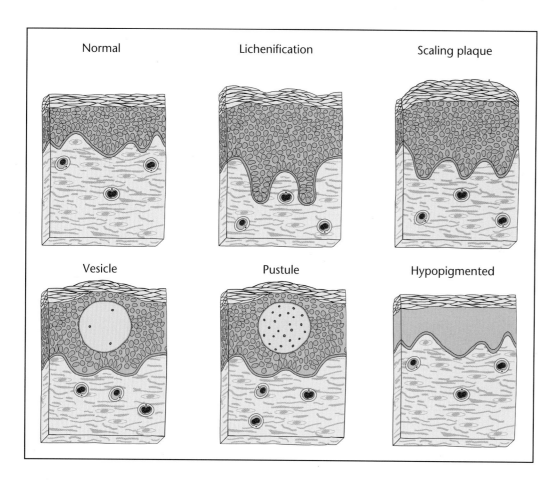

Normal   Lichenification   Scaling plaque

Vesicle   Pustule   Hypopigmented

FIGURE 4-16.
Rashes with epidermal involvement. These rashes are characterized by epidermal thickening (lichenification), scaling, disruption (vesicles and pustules), or hypopigmentation. (*Courtesy of* Donald P. Lookingbill.)

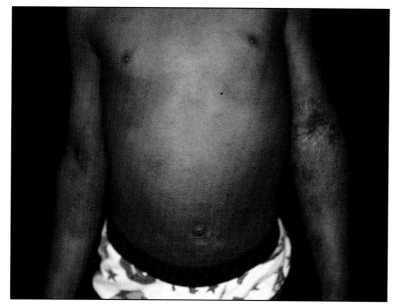

FIGURE 4-17.
Atopic dermatitis. Note the hyperpigmented, lichenified patches in the folds.

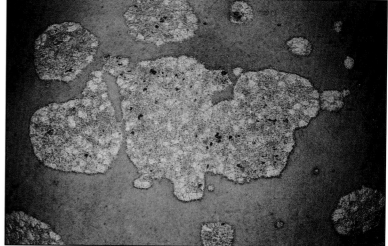

FIGURE 4-18.
Psoriasis vulgaris. Sharply marginated scaling plaques.

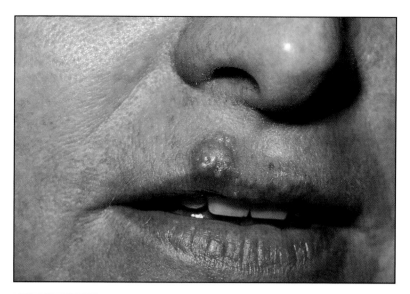

FIGURE 4-19.
Recurrent herpes simplex. Vesiculopustular eruption on the lip.

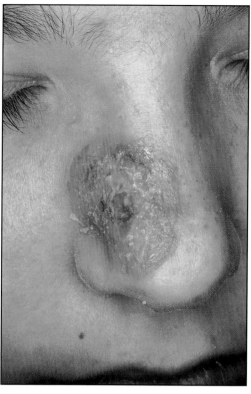

FIGURE 4-20.
Impetigo. Crusted erythematous patch on patient's nose.

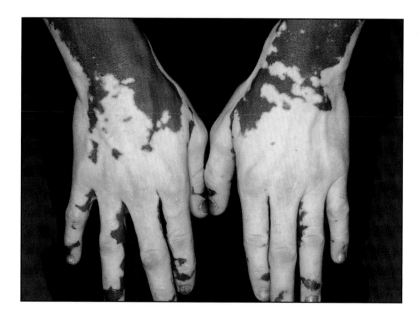

FIGURE 4-21.
Vitiligo. Hypopigmented patches.

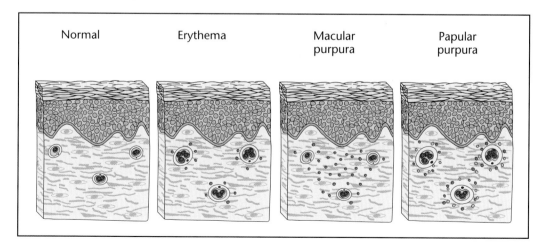

| Normal | Erythema | Macular purpura | Papular purpura |

FIGURE 4-22.
Purely dermal rashes. These rashes have no epidermal involvement. They are characterized by dermal vascular changes resulting in erythema (*ie,* blanchable redness) or purpura (*ie,* purple that is not blanchable). Noninflammatory purpura is macular; inflammatory purpura is papular (*ie,* palpable). (*Courtesy of* Donald P. Lookingbill.)

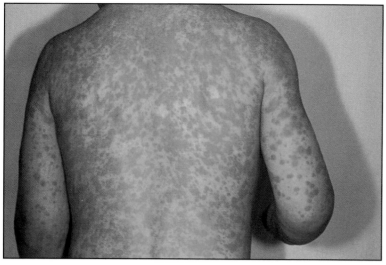

FIGURE 4-23.

Morbilliform drug eruption. Purely dermal rash characterized by confluent erythematous macules and papules.

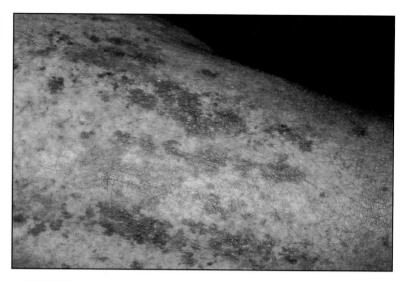

FIGURE 4-24.

Steroid-induced purpura. Purely dermal rash from noninflammatory extravasation of blood from fragile blood vessels.

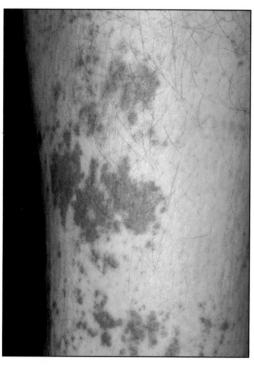

FIGURE 4-25.

Small vessel vasculitis. Purely dermal rash due to inflammatory necrosis of dermal blood vessels, resulting in palpable purpura.

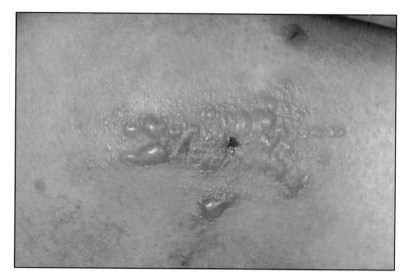

FIGURE 4-26.

Vesicles in a linear configuration. Streaks of vesicles and bullae due to allergic contact dermatitis from poison ivy (rhus dermatitis).

FIGURE 4-27.

Koebner phenomenon. Several disorders have the ability to appear on injured skin. This patient sustained a sunburn that resulted in an activation of psoriasis.

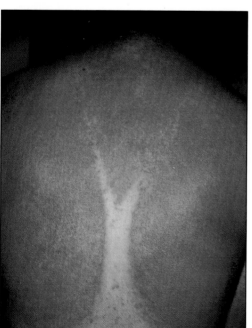

■ COMMON BACTERIAL INFECTIONS OF THE SKIN

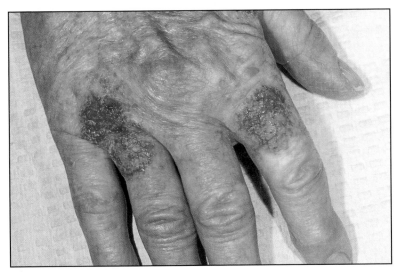

FIGURE 4-28.
Impetigo. Crusted erythematous patches on the dorsal hand.

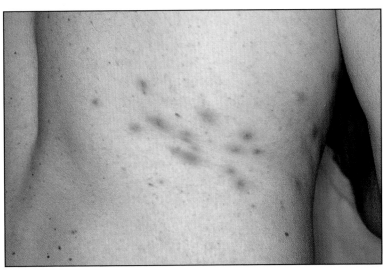

FIGURE 4-29.
Hot tub folliculitis. Erythematous pustules on the back. Self-limiting process due to *Pseudomonas aeruiginosa* infection.

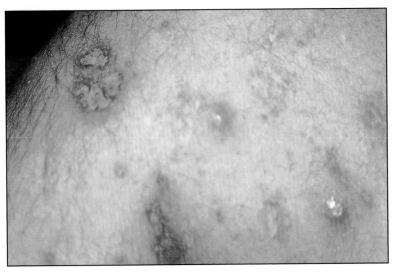

FIGURE 4-30.
Chronic folliculitis due to *Staphylococcus aureus* infection. (*Courtesy of* Neil Fenske, MD.)

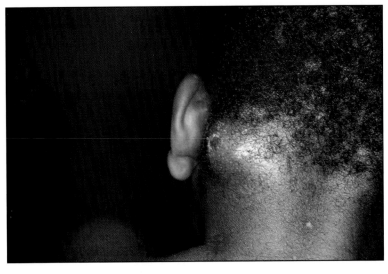

FIGURE 4-31.
Furuncle. Acute, tender nodule on the posterior neck of a boy with atopic dermatitis.

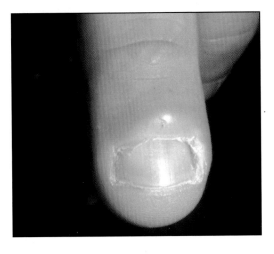

FIGURE 4-32.
Acute staphylococcal paronychia (note the acute swollen, inflamed erythematous paronychial folds). (*Courtesy of* Steven M. Hacker and Franklin P. Flowers.)

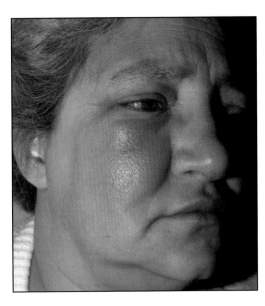

FIGURE 4-33.
Erysipelas. Note the erythematous and edematous skin with a sharply demarcated margin. (*Courtesy of* Steven M. Hacker and Franklin P. Flowers.)

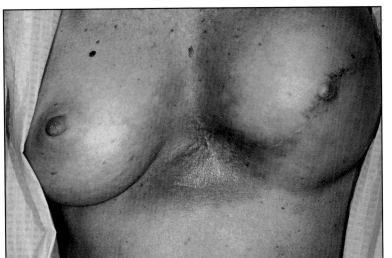

FIGURE 4-34.
Cellulitis. This woman had breast surgery that disrupted the lymphatics and resulted in a chronically infected erythematous patch on her mid-chest.

■ COMMON VIRAL INFECTIONS OF THE SKIN

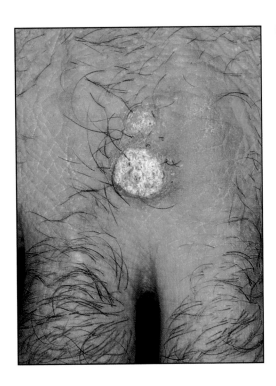

FIGURE 4-35.
Verruca vulgaris. Verrucous nodule on the dorsal hand.

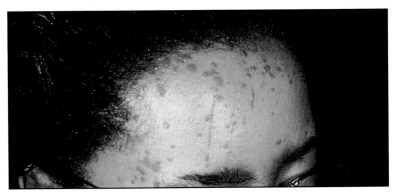

FIGURE 4-36.
Verruca plana. Flat warts on the forehead.

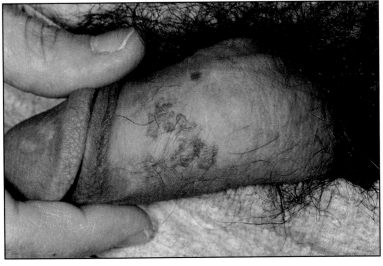

FIGURE 4-37.
Condyloma acuminata. Hyperpigmented verrucous lesions on the shaft of the penis.

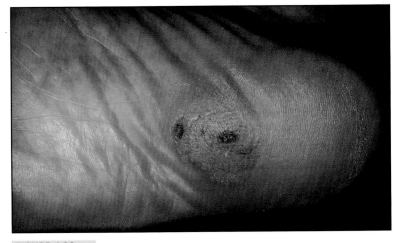

FIGURE 4-38.
Plantar wart. Verrucous plaque on the plantar surface of the foot.

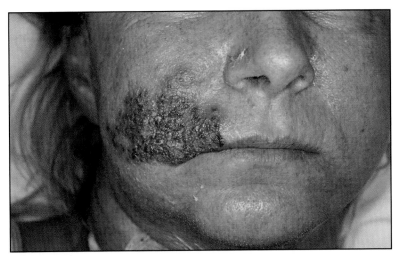

FIGURE 4-39.
Herpes simplex virus. Crusted, vesicular eruption of the cheek following a pnuemonitis.

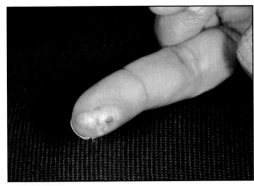

FIGURE 4-40.
Herpetic whitlow. Herpes simplex involving the finger. This appears to be more common in respiratory technicians or dentists.

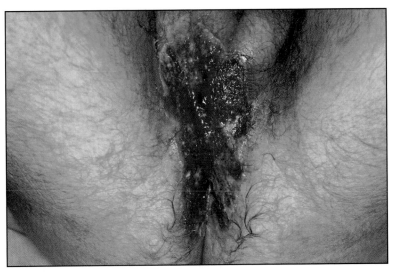

FIGURE 4-41.
Herpes simplex virus. Atypical appearance is associated with immunosuppression. In this case the patient is infected with HIV.

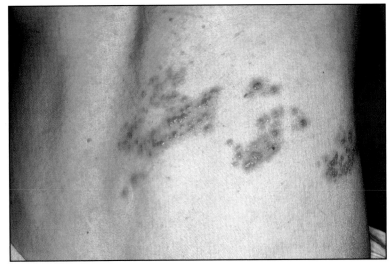

FIGURE 4-42.
Herpes zoster. Reoccurrence of the varicella virus. Vesicles usually appear in a dermatomal distribution.

FIGURE 4-43.
Molluscum contagiosum. Multiple umbilicated translucent papules are present on the forehead. This patient is infected with HIV.

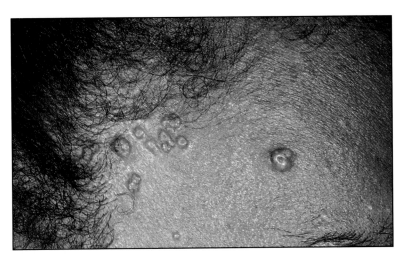

■ COMMON FUNGAL INFECTIONS OF THE SKIN

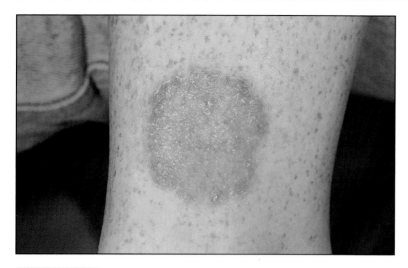

FIGURE 4-44.
Tinea corporis. Annular scaly patch.

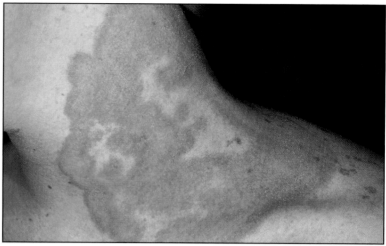

FIGURE 4-45.
Tinea corporis. This patient had applied a clotrimazole-betamethasone combination cream. Her dermatophyte was not suppressed by the antifungal and grew to form concentric and overlapping rings—"ringworm."

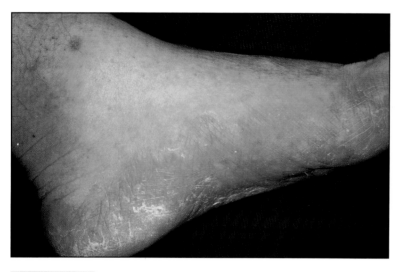

FIGURE 4-46.
Tinea pedis. Moccasin-type infection of the plantar surface, also known as "athlete's foot."

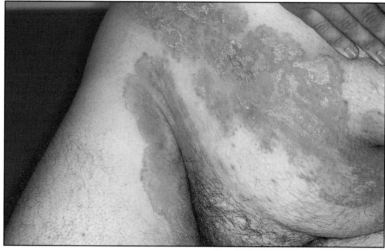

FIGURE 4-47.
Tinea cruris. Annular, scaly patches in the folds.

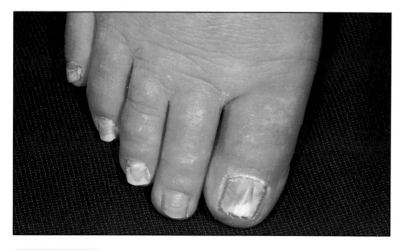

FIGURE 4-48.
Onychomycosis. Note thickening of the nail due to subungual hyperkeratosis with accompanying onycholysis. This patient had five episodes of cellulitis for which the onychomycosis was believed to be the source.

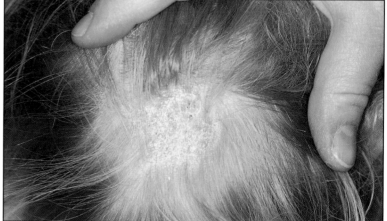

FIGURE 4-49.
Tinea capitis. Patch of alopecia.

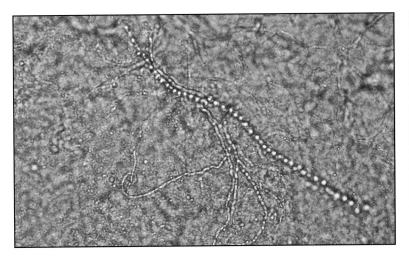

FIGURE 4-50.
Positive potassium hydroxide preparation. Note branching hyphae typical of dermatophyte infection. The exact organism must be determined by culture. (*Courtesy of* Boni E. Elewski.)

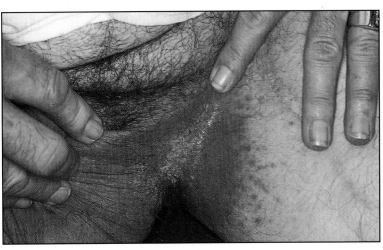

FIGURE 4-51.
Candida intertrigo. Note the satellite pustules outside of the boundary of this inguinal rash.

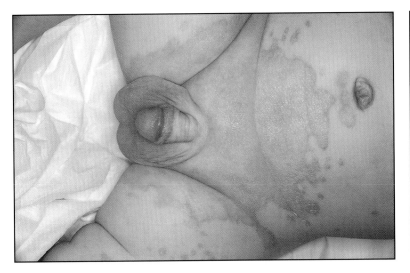

FIGURE 4-52.
Diaper dermatitis. *Candida* intertrigo in a baby.

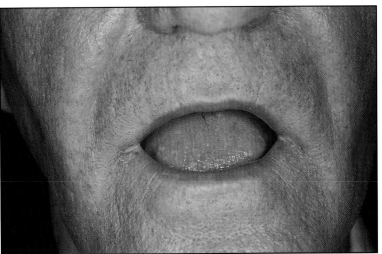

FIGURE 4-53.
Angular cheilitis. Erythematous patches at the corners of the mouth, also known as "perleche."

■ MALIGNANT EPIDERMAL TUMORS

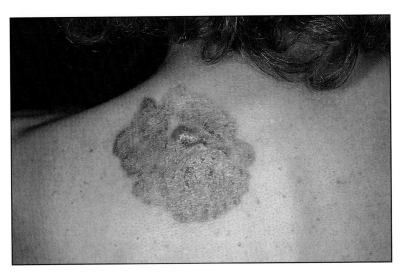

FIGURE 4-54.
Superficial basal cell carcinoma on the upper back. Red, scaly plaque is typical of superficial basal cell carcinoma.

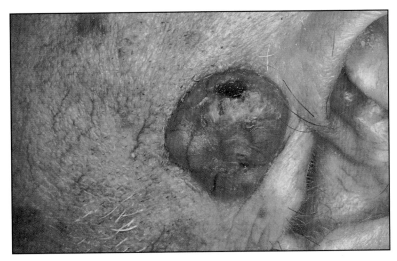

FIGURE 4-55.
Nodular basal cell carcinoma. Note the translucent (pearly) nodule with telangiectasia.

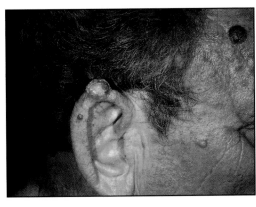

FIGURE 4-56.
Squamous cell carcinoma. Note the nodular lesion on the rim of the ear. This patient had a solid organ transplant. In this instance, the tumors are much more prone to aggressive behavior.

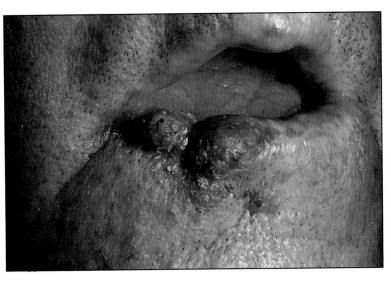

FIGURE 4-57.
Squamous cell carcinoma. Note the verrucous lesion of the lip. This location is one associated with aggressive tumor behavior.

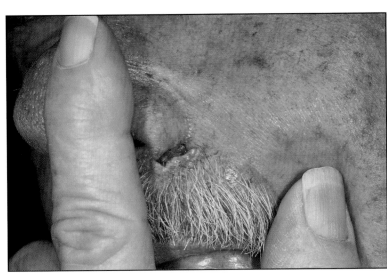

FIGURE 4-58.
Basal cell carcinoma. Note the subtle lesion in the nasolabial fold. This location is associated with deeper invasion, and treatment with micrographic surgery is indicated.

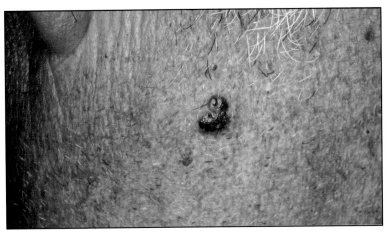

FIGURE 4-59.
Pigmented basal cell carcinoma, darkly pigmented lesion. The presence of a translucent quality to the surface is a helpful clinical clue in distinguishing this lesion from melanoma.

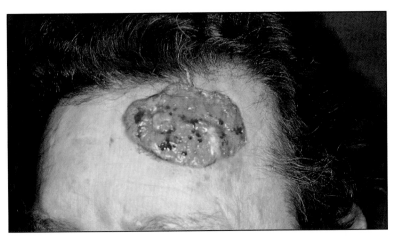

FIGURE 4-60.
Basal cell carcinoma. The patient ignored this large primary lesion for several years.

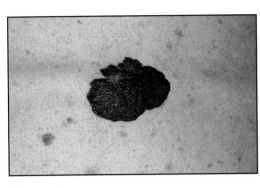

FIGURE 4-61.
Superficial spreading melanoma. Note the large, darkly pigmented, irregular lesion.

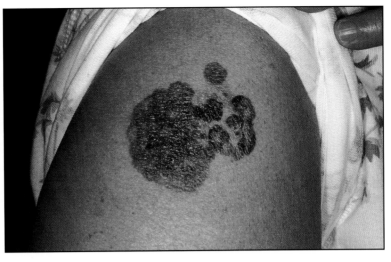

FIGURE 4-62.
Superficial spreading melanoma. Note the large, irregularly pigmented lesion on the shoulder.

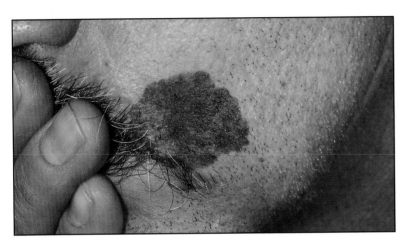

FIGURE 4-63.
Lentigo maligna melanoma. Note the irregularly pigmented lesion on the face.

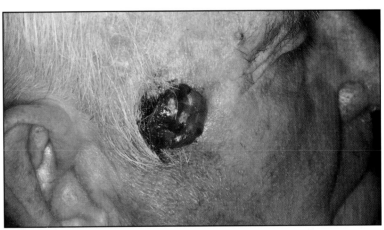

FIGURE 4-64.
Nodular melanoma. A large pigmented lesion on the face.

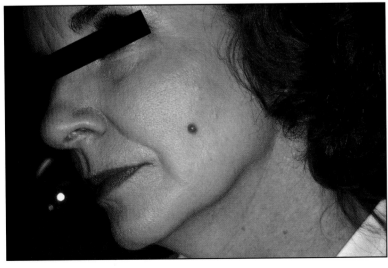

FIGURE 4-65.
Metastatic melanoma. This erythematous lesion appeared on the cheek about 1 year after the removal of a melanoma from this patient's foot.

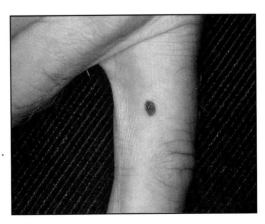

FIGURE 4-66.
Junctional nevus. A small, uniformly pigmented macule.

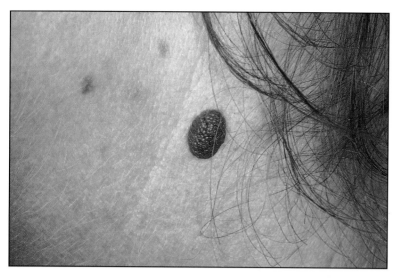

FIGURE 4-67.
Compound nevus. A sharply marginated papule or nodule with pigment.

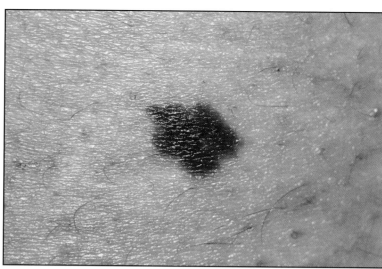

FIGURE 4-68.
Dysplastic or atypical mole. These lesions have some, but not all, of the features that suggest melanoma.

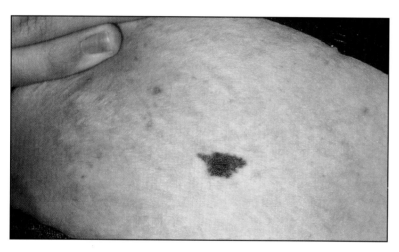

FIGURE 4-69.
Dysplastic or atypical mole on the forearm. These lesions have some, but not all, of the features that suggest melanoma.

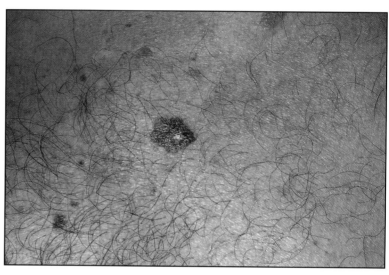

FIGURE 4-70.
Dysplastic or atypical mole. These lesions have some, but not all, of the features that suggest melanoma.

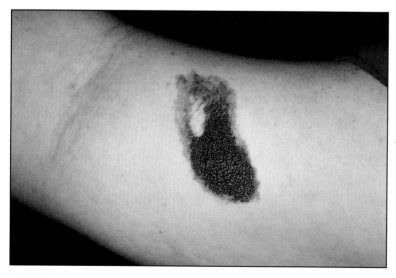

FIGURE 4-71.
Congenital nevocellular nevus. Large pigmented patch.

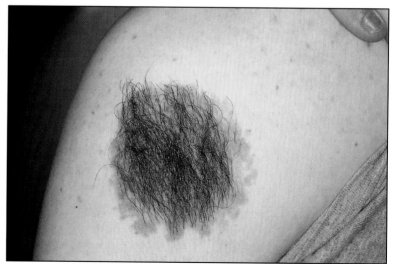

FIGURE 4-72
Congenital nevocellular nevus. Large, hairy, pigmented patch.

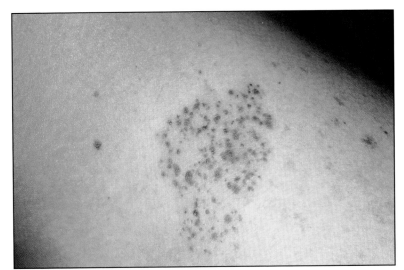

■ COMMON CUTANEOUS TUMORS

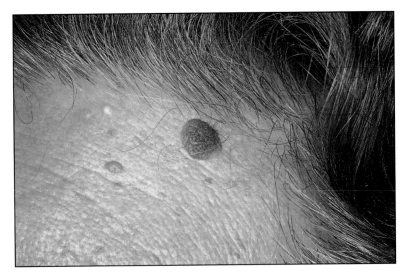

FIGURE 4-74.
Seborrheic keratosis. Note the sharply marginated, verrucous, tan lesion on the neck.

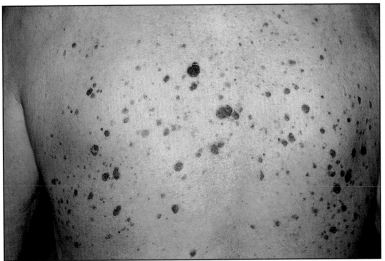

FIGURE 4-75.
Multiple seborrheic keratoses.

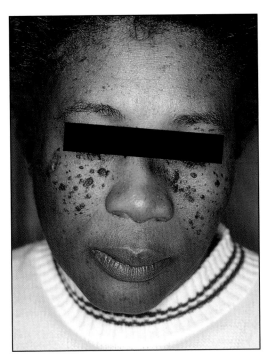

FIGURE 4-76.
Dermatosis papulosa nigra. Multiple verrucous papules on the cheeks. Persons of color are more prone to these lesions.

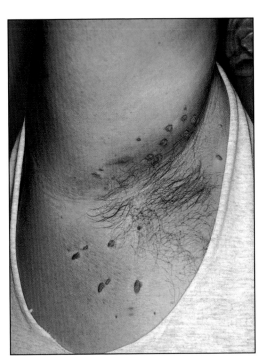

FIGURE 4-77.
Skin tags. Multiple flesh-colored pedunculated lesions. The axilla, neck, and groin are common sites.

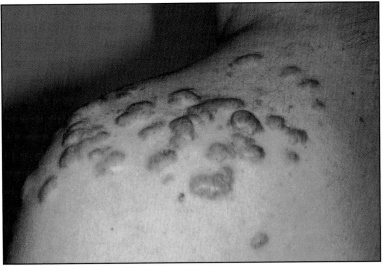

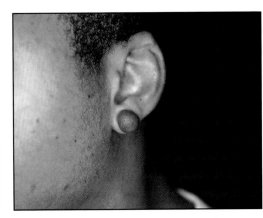

FIGURE 4-79.
Keloid. This lesion occurred following ear piercing.

FIGURE 4-78.
Keloids. Multiple lesions on the back of this young man followed relatively minor acne.

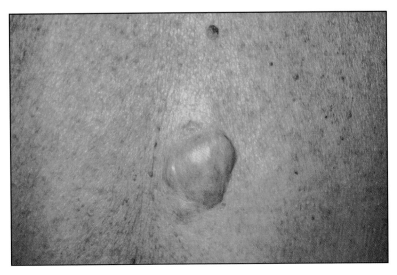

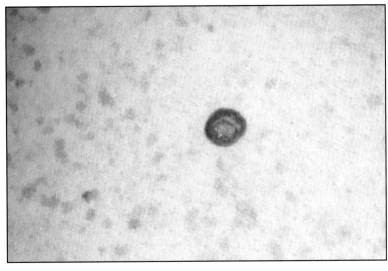

FIGURE 4-80.
Neurofibroma. Note the soft, fleshy tumor.

FIGURE 4-81.
Cherry angioma. These lesions are common, increase with age, often appear on the trunk, and are rarely symptomatic.

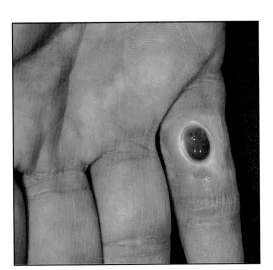

FIGURE 4-82.
Pyogenic granuloma. These lesions often follow minor trauma and commonly bleed. Destruction is the usual method of treatment.

■ PSORIASIS

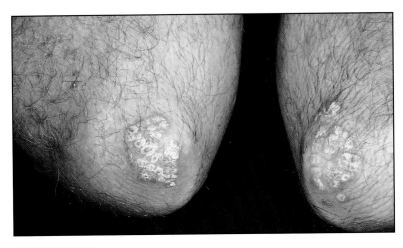

FIGURE 4-83.
Psoriasis vulgaris. Typical scaling plaques on the elbows are shown.

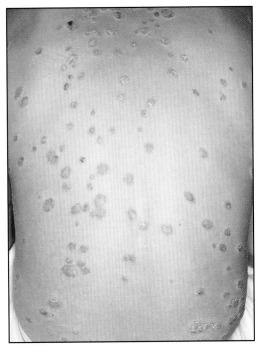

FIGURE 4-84.
Guttate psoriasis. Note the small, scaling plaques on the back. This variant of psoriasis often follows a strep-tococcal infection and is more common in children and adolescents.

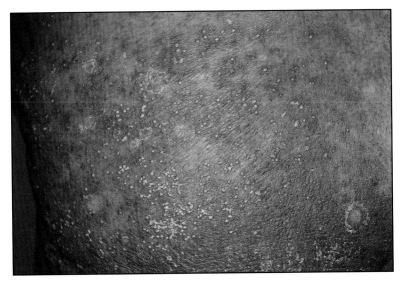

FIGURE 4-85.
Generalized pustular psoriasis. Erythroderma with superficial pustules.

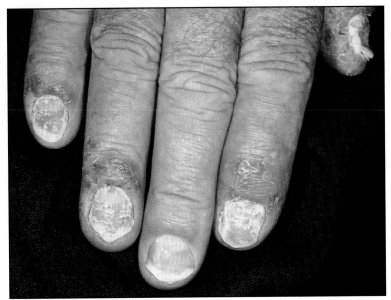

FIGURE 4-86.
Nail involvement of psoriasis. Pitting and subungual hyperkeratosis are seen in this patient.

ECZEMAS

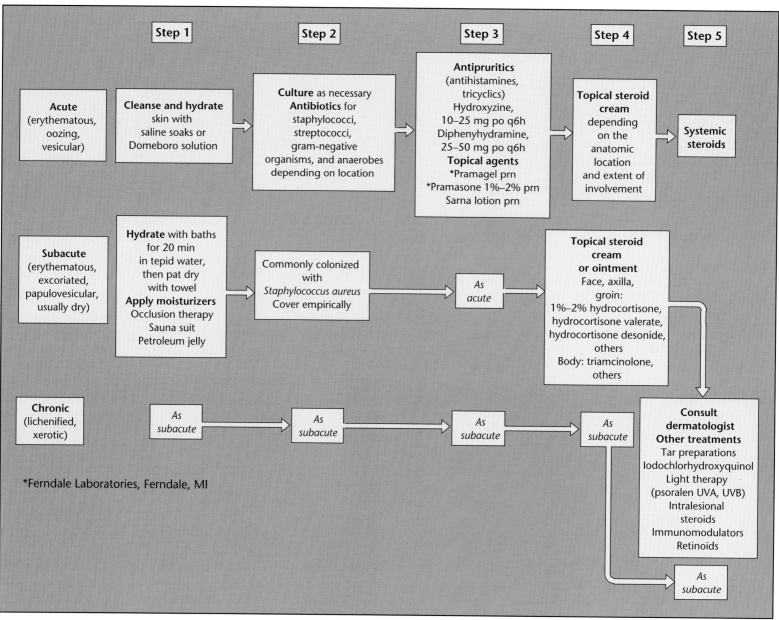

FIGURE 4-87.

General principles of eczema treatment according to reaction stage. po—orally; prn—as needed; q6h—every 6 hours. UVA—ultraviolet A; UVB—ultraviolet B. (*Courtesy of* Terence Hopkins and Richard AF Clark.)

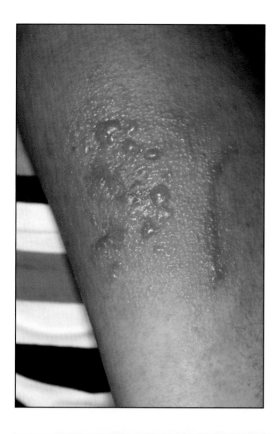

FIGURE 4-88.
Acute contact dermatitis due to poison ivy contact. (*Courtesy of* George Nahass.)

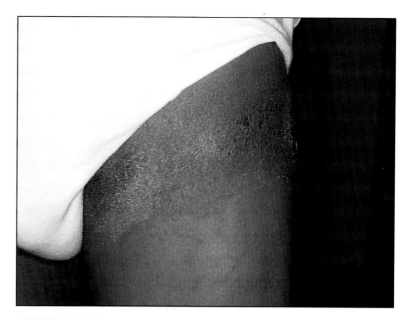

FIGURE 4-89.
Chronic contact dermatitis due to latex in the lining of the underwear.

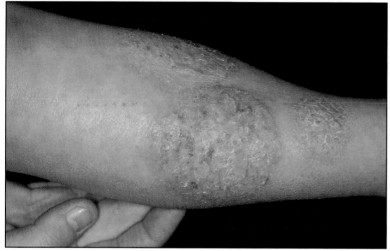

FIGURE 4-90.
Atopic dermatitis. Note the nummular patches on the leg of this child with atopic dermatitis.

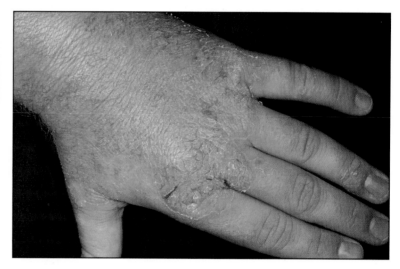

FIGURE 4-91.
Chronic hand dermatitis. Erythematous, scaly eruption of the dorsal hand.

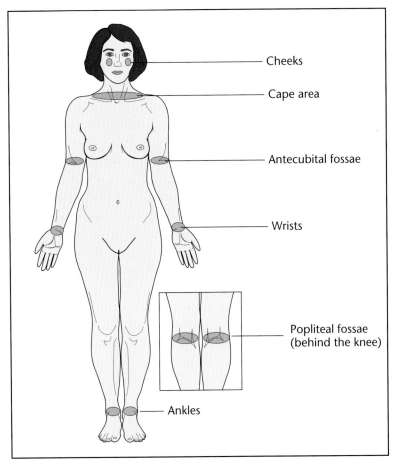

Cheeks

Cape area

Antecubital fossae

Wrists

Popliteal fossae
(behind the knee)

Ankles

FIGURE 4-92.
Characteristic distribution of eczema in older children and adults
with atopic dermatitis. (*Courtesy of* Terence Hopkins and Richard AF
Clark.)

FIGURE 4-93.
Seborrheic dermatitis has a predilection for
the seborrheic areas of the body. (*Courtesy of*
Terence Hopkins and Richard AF Clark.)

FIGURE 4-94.
Acute hand dermatitis, also known as
pompholyx.

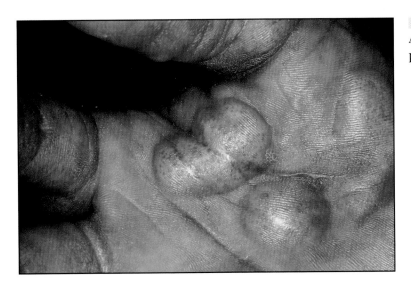

ACNE VULGARIS AND ROSACEA

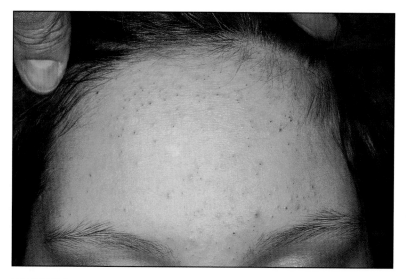

FIGURE 4-95.
Acne vulgaris. Comedonal lesions are prominent on this patient's forehead.

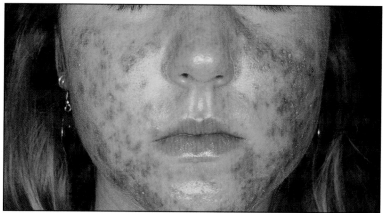

FIGURE 4-96.
Acne vulgaris; papulopustular lesions.

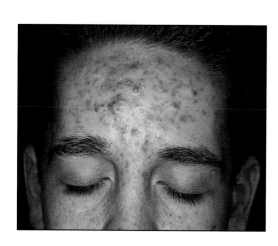

FIGURE 4-98.
Acne vulgaris. This patient has polycystic ovaries.

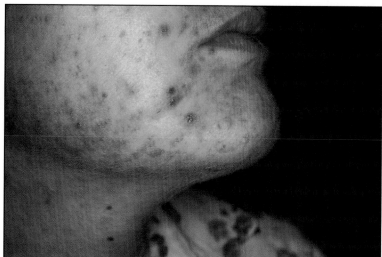

FIGURE 4-97.
Acne vulgaris; cystic lesions.

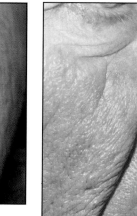

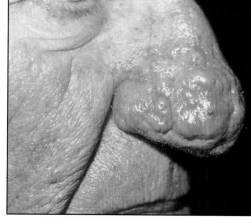

FIGURE 4-99.
Rosacea. Note erythematous papules and pustules. Comedones are absent.

FIGURE 4-100.
Rhinophyma. A consequence of chronically active rosacea that is more common in men.

■ PRURITUS

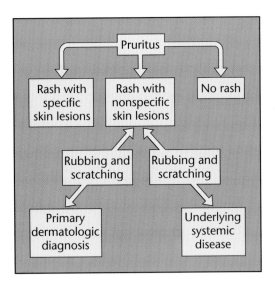

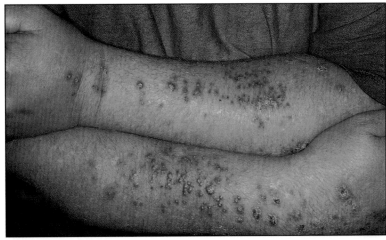

FIGURE 4-101.
Clinical algorithm for evaluation of pruritus. (*Courtesy of* Seth G. Kates and Jeffrey D. Bernhard.)

FIGURE 4-102.
Neurotic excoriations. This patient constantly picks at her skin and developed excoriated nodular lesions.

FIGURE 4-103.
Kyrle's disease. This patient is on chronic hemodialysis and has lesions that are pruritic. Biopsy revealed a perforation of the epidermis.

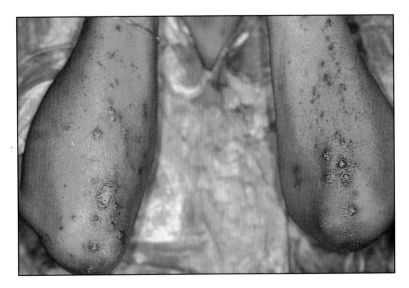

■ LEG ULCERS

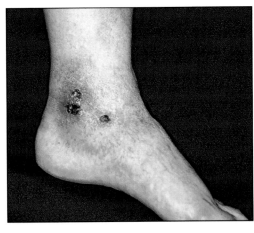

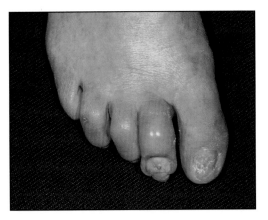

FIGURE 4-105.
Arterial ulcer. Vascular insufficiency led to development of an ulcer of the toe in this patient.

FIGURE 4-104.
Venous ulcer. Stasis dermatitis with ulceration over the medial maleolus.

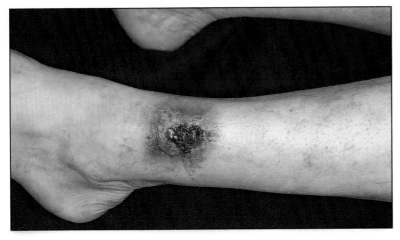

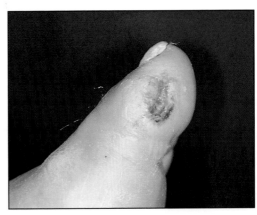

FIGURE 4-107.
Neurotrophic ulcer. This is a patient with diabetes mellitus and neuropathy. The ulcer developed due to minor trauma that was not appreciated by the patient.

FIGURE 4-106.
Ulcer in a patient with antiphospholipid antibody syndrome. This patient has high levels of anticardiolipin antibody.

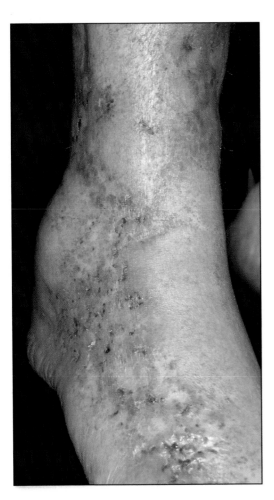

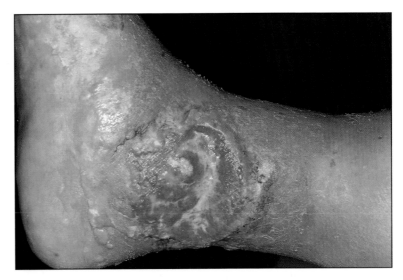

FIGURE 4-108.
Livedoid vasculopathy This patient has small ulcerations and purpura due to clogging of the small cutaneous vessels. Smoking exacerbates this process.

FIGURE 4-109.
Pyoderma gangrenosum. This is an inflammatory ulcer of unknown cause. About half of the patients will have inflammatory bowel disease, arthritis, or hematologic abnormalities.

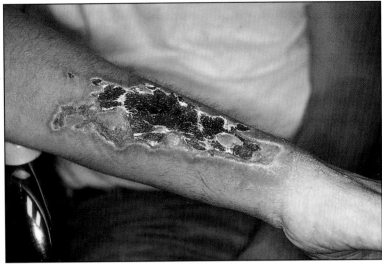

FIGURE 4-110.
Factitial ulceration. This patient used lye to cause an ulceration.

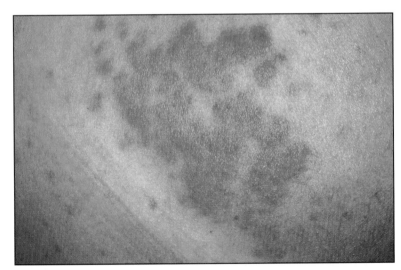

FIGURE 4-111.
Ulcerated necrobiosis lipoidica. This lesion is more common in patients with diabetes and can ulcerate.

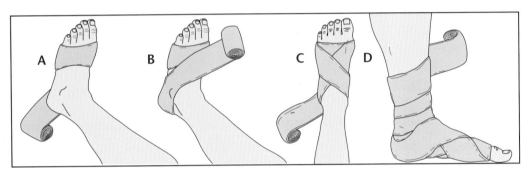

FIGURE 4-112.
Unna boot application. (*Courtesy of* Jeffrey B. Pardes and Vincent Falanga.)

■ PHOTOSENSITIVITY

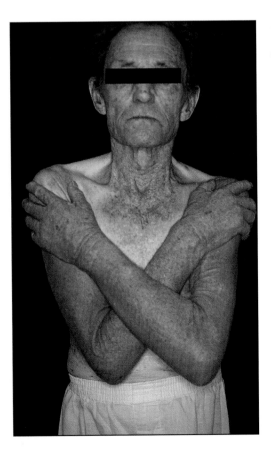

FIGURE 4-113.
Photosensitivity. This patient was on hydrochlorothiazide and developed a rash in a photodistribution.

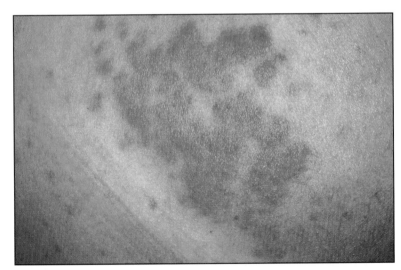

FIGURE 4-114.
Polymorphous light eruption. These lesions appear early in the spring or with excess light exposure. Diseases such as lupus erythematosus should be excluded.

■ COLLAGEN VASCULAR DISORDERS

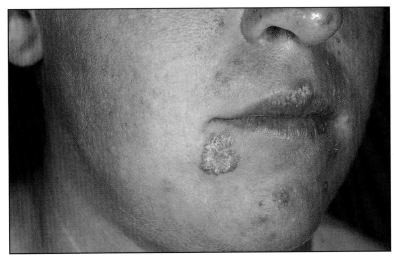

FIGURE 4-115.
Chronic cutaneous lupus erythematosus. Discoid lesions with erythema and adherent scale. These lesions are commonly observed on exposed surfaces and in the scalp.

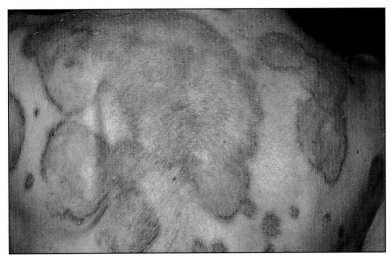

FIGURE 4-116.
Subacute cutaneous lupus erythematosus. Annular erythematous lesions.

FIGURE 4-117.
Subacute cutaneous lupus erythematosus, papulosquamous variant. At times, this condition may be difficult to distinguish from psoriasis or lichen planus.

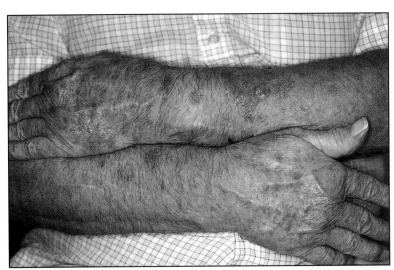

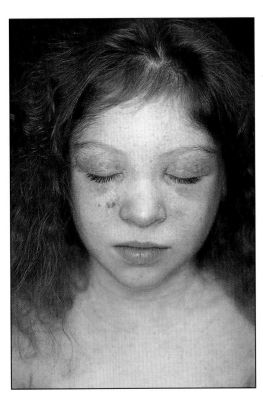

FIGURE 4-119.
Dermatomyositis. This young girl developed inflammatory myopathy in conjunction with a very typical heliotrope eruption around the eyelids and typical lesions elsewhere on her body.

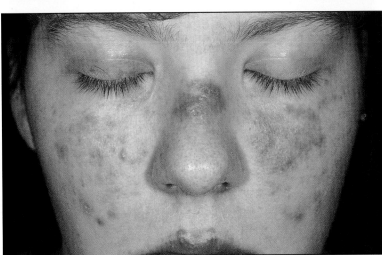

FIGURE 4-118.
Systemic lupus erythematosus. Malar rash is present in this patient.

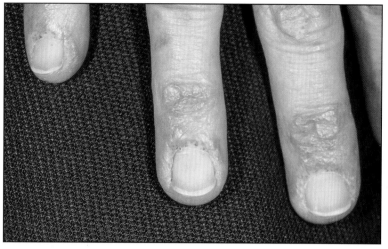

FIGURE 4-120.

Dermatomyositis, Gottron's papules. Erythematous to violaceous papules and plaques over the bony prominences. Also of note in this patient are the accompanying cuticular overgrowth and small hemorrhagic areas of the nail folds.

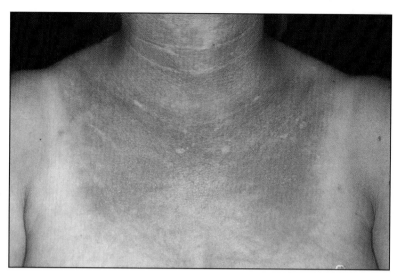

FIGURE 4-121.

Dermatomyositis. Poikilodermatous changes in a photodistribution.

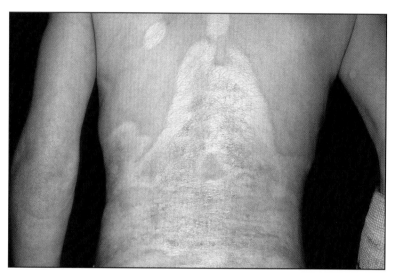

FIGURE 4-122.
Generalized morphea.

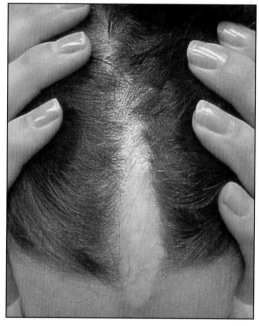

FIGURE 4-123.
En coup de sabre. Localized linear scleroderma.

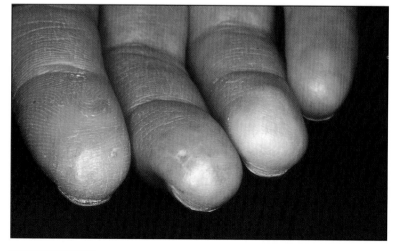

FIGURE 4-124.
Raynaud's phenomenon. Note the small pits of the fingertips from chronic, recurrent ischemia.

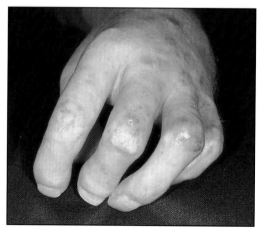

FIGURE 4-125.
CREST (calcinosis, Raynaud's phenomenon, esophageal dysmotility, sclerodactyly, and telangiectasia) syndrome. This patient has systemic sclerosis manifested by CREST.

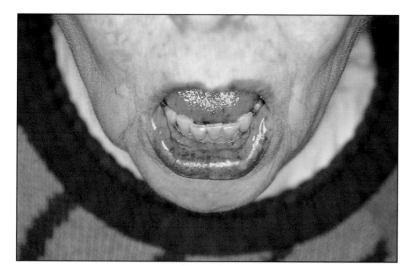

FIGURE 4-126.
CREST (calcinosis, Raynaud's phenomenon, esophageal dysmotility, sclerodactyly, and telangiectasia) syndrome. Note the prominent, matlike, telangiectasia on the lips and tongue. These lesions are similar to those seen in patients with hereditary hemorrhagic telangiectasia.

■ URTICARIA AND OTHER REACTIVE DERMATOSES

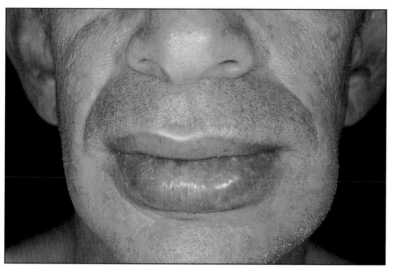

FIGURE 4-127.
Angioedema This patient developed acute swelling due to ticlodipine.

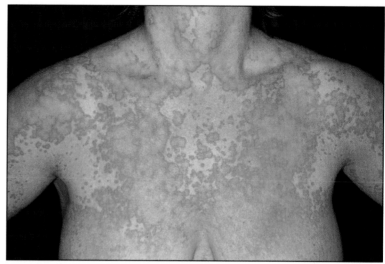

FIGURE 4-128.
Urticaria.

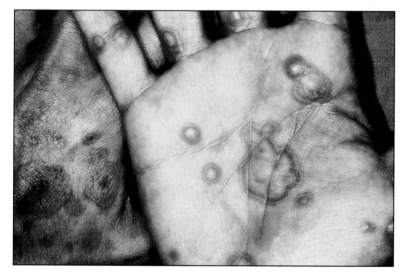

FIGURE 4-129.
Erythema multiforme. Targetoid lesions with central blistering are seen on the palm of the hand.

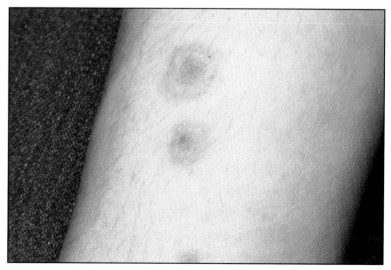

FIGURE 4-130.
Erythema multiforme. Targetoid lesions in this patient developed recurrently as a reaction to recurrent herpes simplex.

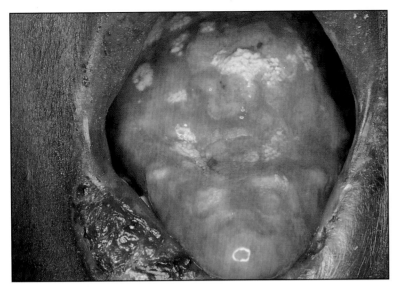

FIGURE 4-131.
Recurrent erythema multiforme secondary to infection with herpes simplex virus

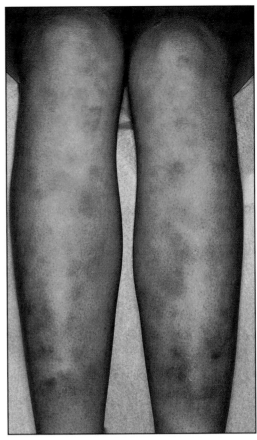

FIGURE 4-132.
Erythema nodosum. Tender, red nodules on the anterior legs.

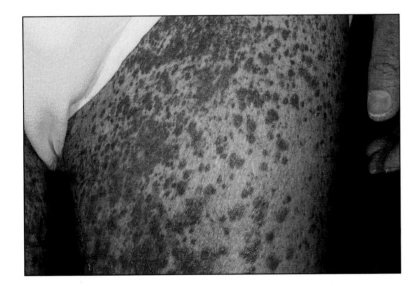

FIGURE 4-133.
Small-vessel vasculitis. Palpable purpura.

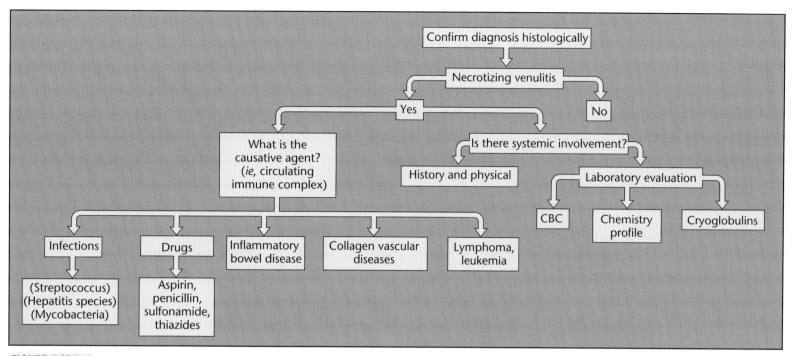

FIGURE 4-134.

Patient evaluation procedure for necrotizing vasculitis. CBC—complete blood count. (*Courtesy of* Jamie A. Alpert and Joseph L. Jorizzo.)

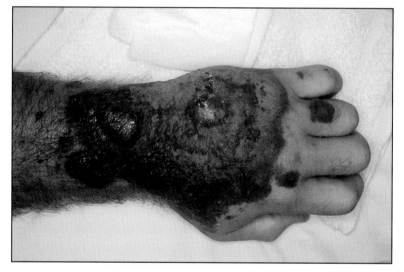

FIGURE 4-135.

Sweet's syndrome. This patient has acute myelogenous leukemia and developed tender plaques on the dorsal surfaces of the hands. Hemorrhage is present due to accompanying thrombocytopenia.

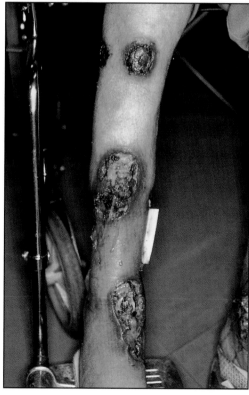

FIGURE 4-136.

Pyoderma gangrenosum. Multiple ulcers are present.

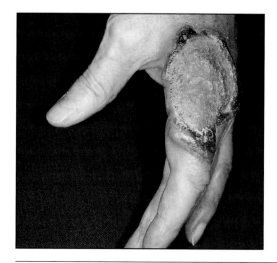

FIGURE 4-137.

Atypical pyoderma gangrenosum. This patient had polycythemia vera.

■ DRUG ERUPTIONS

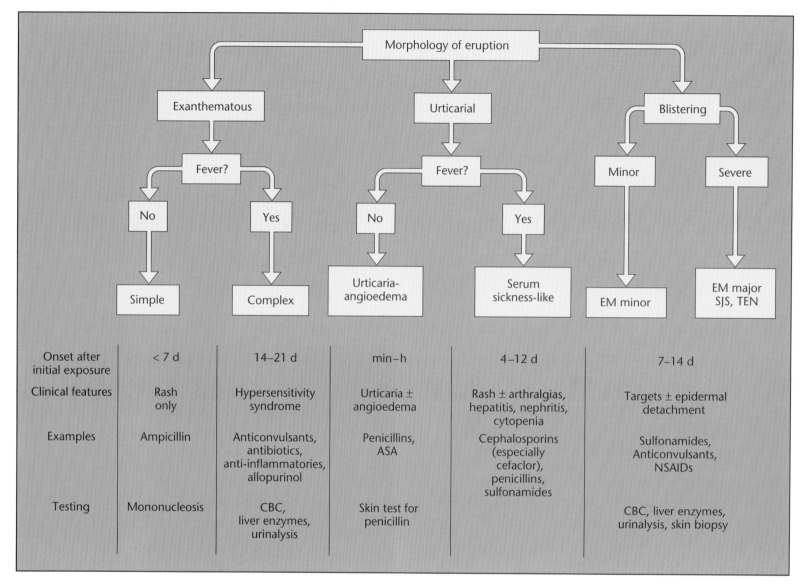

	Exanthematous		Urticarial		Blistering	
	Simple	Complex	Urticaria-angioedema	Serum sickness-like	EM minor	EM major SJS, TEN
Onset after initial exposure	< 7 d	14–21 d	min–h	4–12 d	7–14 d	
Clinical features	Rash only	Hypersensitivity syndrome	Urticaria ± angioedema	Rash ± arthralgias, hepatitis, nephritis, cytopenia	Targets ± epidermal detachment	
Examples	Ampicillin	Anticonvulsants, antibiotics, anti-inflammatories, allopurinol	Penicillins, ASA	Cephalosporins (especially cefaclor), penicillins, sulfonamides	Sulfonamides, Anticonvulsants, NSAIDs	
Testing	Mononucleosis	CBC, liver enzymes, urinalysis	Skin test for penicillin		CBC, liver enzymes, urinalysis, skin biopsy	

FIGURE 4-138.
Algorithm to aid the clinical diagnosis of drug rashes. ASA—acetyl-salicyclic acid; CBC—complete blood count; EM—erythema multi-forme; NSAIDs—nonsteroidal anti-inflammatory drugs; SJS Stevens-Johnson syndrome; TEN—toxic epidermal necrolysis. (*Courtesy of Paul I. Oh and Neil H. Shear.*)

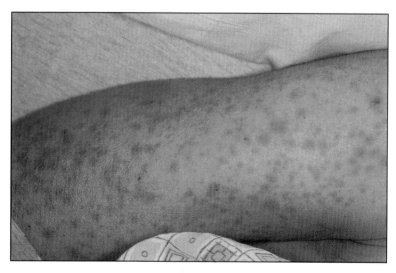

FIGURE 4-139.
Morbilliform drug eruption due to trimethoprim-sulfamethoxazole administration.

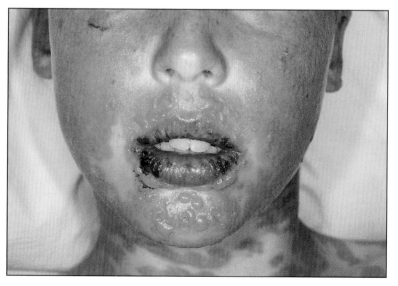

FIGURE 4-140.
Stevens-Johnson syndrome. Adolescent with erythema multiforme-like lesions and widespread blisters on the face and neck.

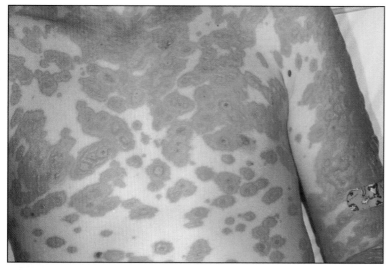

FIGURE 4-141.
Stevens-Johnson syndrome. Same patient as in Fig. 4-140. Adolescent with erythema multiforme-like lesions and widespread blisters on the chest and upper arm.

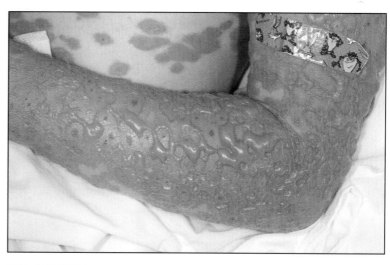

FIGURE 4-142.
Stevens-Johnson syndrome. Same patient as Fig. 4-140. Adolescent with erythema multiforme-like lesions and widespread blisters on the lower arm.

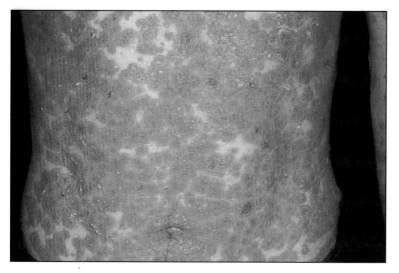

FIGURE 4-143.
Toxic epidermal necrolysis. This patient began with erythema multiforme-like lesions but developed an almost 100% slough of his epidermis.

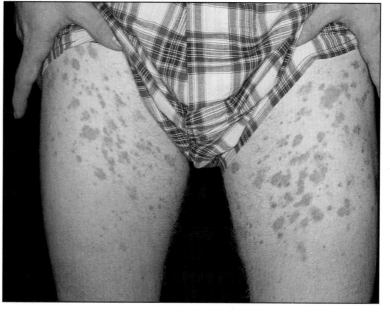

FIGURE 4-144.
Drug eruption due to gold. This young man developed a pityriasis rosea-like eruption from ingestion of a gold-containing liquor.

■ LIFE-THREATENING DERMATOSES

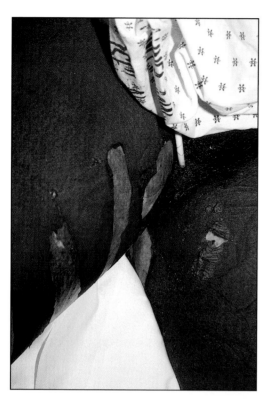

FIGURE 4-145.
Toxic epidermal necrolysis. Allopurinol was the cause of this patient's problem.

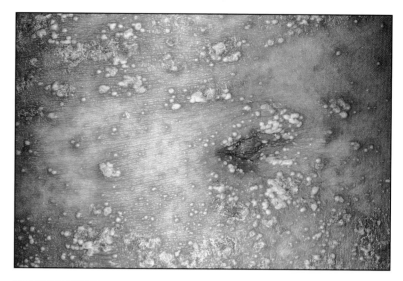

FIGURE 4-146.
Generalized pustular psoriasis.

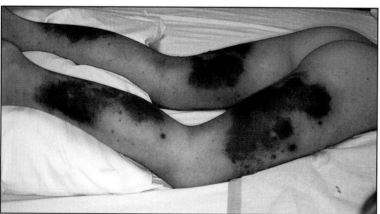

FIGURE 4-147.
Purpura fulminans. This process followed varicella.

■ CUTANEOUS MANIFESTATIONS OF INTERNAL MALIGNANCY

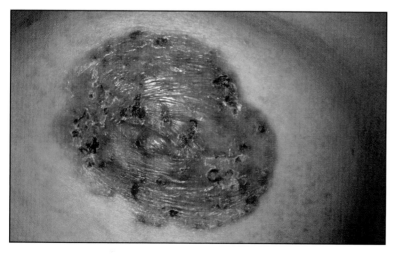

FIGURE 4-148.
Paget's disease of the breast. This reflects an underlying ductal adenocarcinoma.

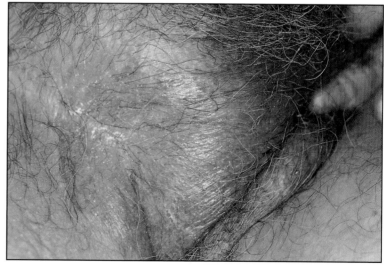

FIGURE 4-149.
Extramammary Paget's disease. An erythematous patch on the scrotal skin is often, but not always, reflective of an underlying malignancy.

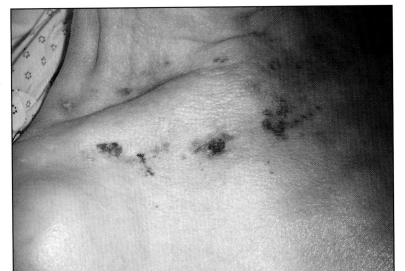

FIGURE 4-150.
Primary systemic amyloidosis. Such patients almost always have myeloma.

■ IMMUNOBULLOUS DISEASES

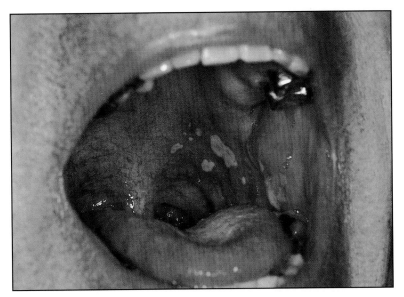

FIGURE 4-151.
Pemphigus vulgaris. This blistering disease often begins with erosions and ulceration of the oral mucousa.

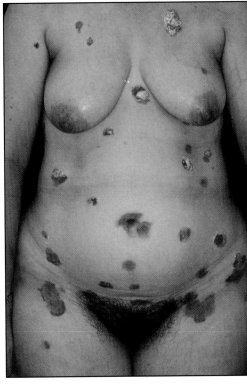

FIGURE 4-152.
Pemphigus vulgaris. Multiple crusted erosions.

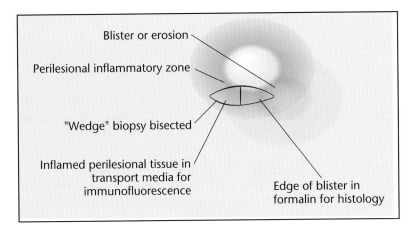

Blister or erosion

Perilesional inflammatory zone

"Wedge" biopsy bisected

Inflamed perilesional tissue in transport media for immunofluorescence

Edge of blister in formalin for histology

FIGURE 4-153.
A biopsy technique that is appropriate for the vast majority of immunobullous disorders. The physician should identify a blister or erosion and perform a "wedge" biopsy, as indicated. The proximal half of the biopsied specimen that includes the edge of the blister or erosion should be submitted in formalin for histologic examination. The portion of the specimen that is distal to the lesion but still encompasses some clinically inflamed skin in the perilesional area should be placed in immunofluorescent transport media and can subsequently be tested by direct immunofluorescence. Alternatively, if the physician is uncomfortable performing a wedge biopsy, two individual 3-mm punch biopsies can be performed on the edge of the lesion and the perilesional skin. This technique gives an optimum chance for completing the diagnostic criteria in the majority of bullous diseases. (*Courtesy of* Grant J. Anhalt.)

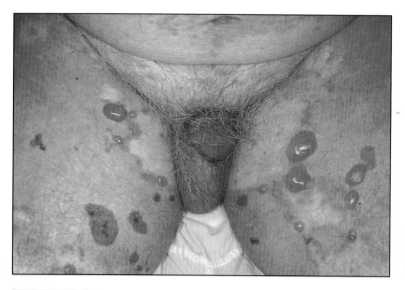

FIGURE 4-154.

Bullous pemphigoid. Tense blisters on an urticarial base. This condition occurs more frequently in elderly patients.

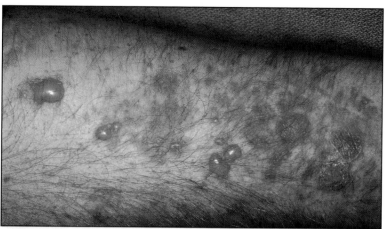

FIGURE 4-155.

Dermatitis herpetiformis (DH). Grouped vesicles and bullae are present. Patients with DH often have a gluten-sensitive enteropathy.

■ CUTANEOUS MANIFESTATIONS OF SYSTEMIC DISEASE

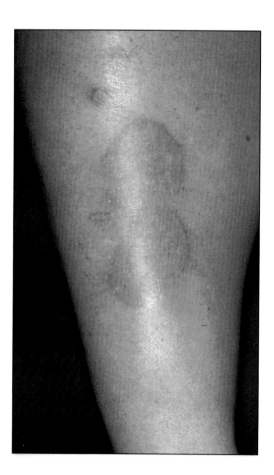

FIGURE 4-156.
Necrobiosis lipoidica. Most, but not all, patients have diabetes mellitus.

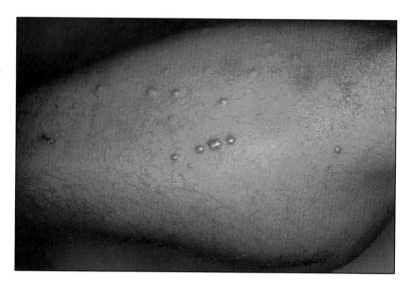

FIGURE 4-157.

Eruptive xanthomas. This patient's diabetes mellitus was discovered when his hyperlipidemia was diagnosed following the development of these lesions.

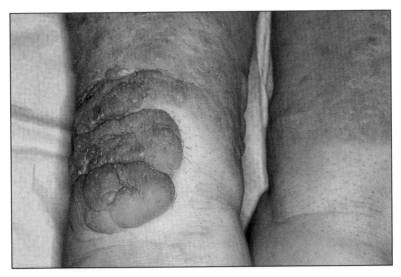

FIGURE 4-158.
Pretibial myxedema. This infiltrative process is linked to Grave's disease.

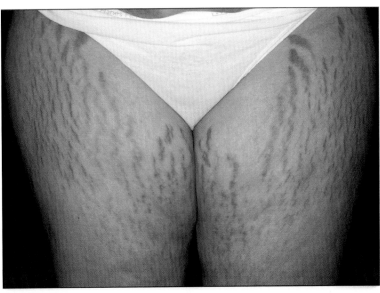

FIGURE 4-159.
Cushing's disease. This patient had excessive weight gain, paranoid ideations, hypertension, and these striae. Her diagnosis was suggested upon dermatologic referral.

FIGURE 4-160.
Acanthosis nigricans. Velvety, hyperpigmented skin on the intertriginous surfaces. Obese patients are often insulin resistant and may have polycystic ovaries.

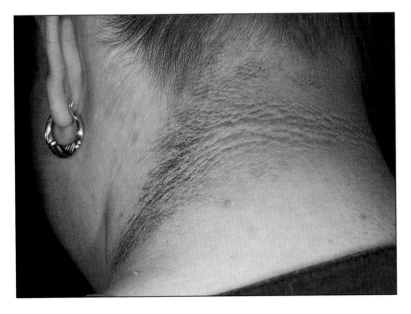

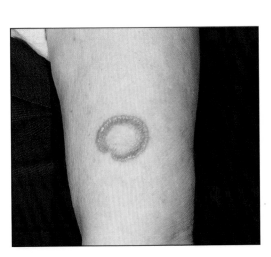

FIGURE 4-161.
Sarcoidosis. Annular infiltrated lesion.

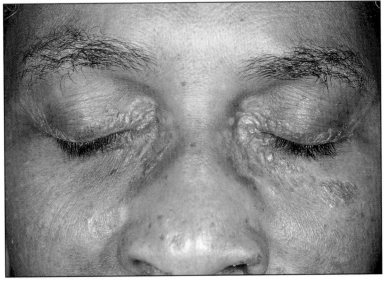

FIGURE 4-162.
Sarcoidosis. Violaceous papules and plaques on the eyelids and nose.

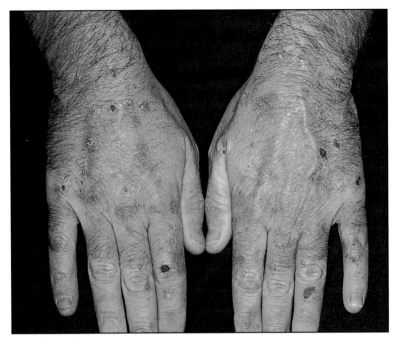

FIGURE 4-163.
Porphyria cutanea tarda. This patient has co-existing hepatitis C.

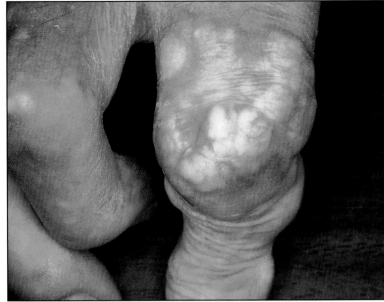

FIGURE 4-164.
Tophaceous gout. Yellow, firm, papules on the fingers.

■ ACKNOWLEDGMENT

This chapter utilizes some of the photographs from *Current Practice of Medicine*,
Volume 1. I am again grateful to the contributors to that work.

■ REFERENCES

1. Lookingbill DP, Marks JGM: *Principles of Dermatology*, edn 3. Philadelphia: WB Saunders; 2000.

2. Callen JP, Greer KE, Paller AS, Swinyer LJ: *Color Atlas of Dermatology*, edn 2. Philadelphia: WB Saunders; 2000.

Rheumatology

GENE G. HUNDER

The specialty of rheumatology includes a diverse group of diseases that involves joints and surrounding structures, muscles, and connective tissues. Arthritic diseases are among the most common medical problems in the world, and in the United States arthritis is the number one cause of disability. Many of these illnesses also involve other organs, adding to their diagnostic and therapeutic complexity. Most conditions tend to be chronic and often lead to disability and sometimes early death. Over 100 arthritic diseases have been described.

Rheumatoid arthritis is the most common inflammatory arthritis and affects approximately one percent of the world's population. It is a chronic polyarticular disease that frequently leads to joint destruction. Multiple genetic factors are involved in its development, the best known of which is the B lymphocyte alloantigen HLA-DR4, which is present in about 70% of patients. In more severe cases, extra-articular manifestations develop with the formation of rheumatoid nodules, sicca syndrome, Felty's syndrome (leukopenia and splenomegaly), pleurisy, pulmonary fibrosis, pericarditis, and vasculitis.

Osteoarthritis is characterized by structural deterioration of articular cartilage. As this process develops, osteophytes form at the joint margins. Ligamentous structures may also degenerate, adding to joint malfunction and joint instability. A mild inflammatory component also exists early in the disease. Osteoarthritis is present in varying degrees in all older persons.

The common forms of crystal-induced arthritis are gout and pseudogout or calcium pyrophosphate dehydrate deposition disease. Hydroxyapatite crystals also are involved in degenerative joint disease in some patients. Patients with gout who are untreated often develop tophaceous deposits, which gradually result in permanent joint damage. Deposits may also be extra-articular. Elevated blood urate develops from either excessive production or reduced renal excretion. Pseudogout tends to occur in selected joints such as the ankles, knees, and wrists, but may be more widespread. Radiographs may show chondrocalcinosis in numerous joints.

Lupus erythematosus has a highly variable course with involvement of a single or several organs. It affects women much more commonly than men. Excessive B-cell activity results in numerous autoantibodies that appear to contribute to the formation of immune complexes and the tissue inflammation. In scleroderma, thickening of the skin causes restriction of normal movements. The pathogenesis of scleroderma is poorly understood. It is not uncommon for patients with connective tissue disorders to have overlapping features and not fit a well-defined category.

Vasculitides are also a diverse group of syndromes characterized by necrotizing inflammatory lesions scattered throughout the vascular tree. Different forms of vasculitis are distinguished from each other by demographics of the patient population affected, predominant location of the blood vessels affected, histopathologic appearance of vascular lesions, and pathogenic factors.

Spondyloarthropathies are characterized by the presence of involvement of the spinal joints and surrounding structures as well as other joints. The alloantigen HLA-B27 forms a link among these various conditions.

Osteoporosis involves the skeleton in a systemic fashion and is characterized by low bone mass and deterioration of the micro-architecture of bone tissue. This leads to enhanced bone fragility and an increased rate of fractures. In osteomalacia, there is an excessive unmineralized osteoid tissue that also leads to weakness of bone structure. Paget's disease is a common process involving approximately 3% of the adult population. In many persons it is mild, but it may become extensive. Infectious arthritis is an uncommon but devastating process often leading to destruction of the joint tissues. It frequently occurs in one or two at a time but may become more systemic. Almost any organism may affect the joints.

■ RHEUMATOID ARTHRITIS, JUVENILE RHEUMATOID ARTHRITIS, AND RELATED CONDITIONS

The Differential Diagnosis of Polyarthritis

Spondyloarthropathies
Ankylosing spondylitis
Reiter's syndrome
Inflammatory bowel disease
Behçet's syndrome
Enteric infections, especially *Yersinia, Salmonella, Shigella, Campylobacter jejuni*
Whipple's disease
Psoriatic arthritis

Infectious
Bacterial endocarditis
HIV infection
Bacterial sepsis
Viral syndromes, especially hepatitis B, parvovirus, rubella, Epstein-Barr, others
Acute rheumatic fever
Lyme disease
Gonococcal arthritis

Metabolic and Endocrine Disorders
Gout
Pseudogout (calcium pyrophosphate dihydrate deposition disease)
Hemochromatosis
Hemoglobinopathies
Hyper- and hypothyroidism
Hyperlipoproteinemia
Hypertrophic osteoarthropathy

Connective Tissue Syndromes
Systemic lupus erythematosus
Dermatomyositis/polymyositis
Mixed connective tissue disease
Scleroderma

Other
Still's disease
Relapsing polychondritis
Familial Mediterranean fever
Intermittent hydrarthrosis
Hypereosinophilic syndrome
Malignancy
Osteoarthritis
Sarcoidosis
Multicentric reticulohistiocytosis
Vasculitis
Polymyalgia rheumatica and giant cell arteritis
Heritable polyarthropathies

FIGURE 5-1.

Differential diagnosis of polyarthritis. The differential diagnosis of polyarthritis, arthritis of six or more joints, is extensive. A careful history, persistence of symmetric joint swelling, and the typical laboratory and radiographic features aid in establishing an accurate diagnosis of rheumatoid arthritis. HIV—human immunodeficiency virus. (*Courtesy of* Eric L. Matteson and Thomas G. Mason.)

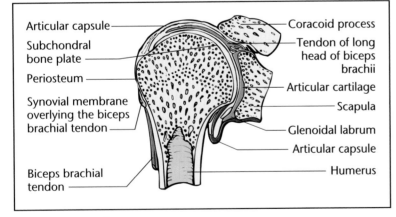

FIGURE 5-2.

Diagram of a diarthrodial joint: the glenohumeral articulation. Diarthrodial joints have articular surfaces of cartilage that are surrounded by a fibrous capsule. The articular capsule is adjoined to tendons, periosteum, ligaments, and fascia. The synovium covers the internal aspect of the capsule and the intercapsular periosteum, but not the articular surface itself. (*Courtesy of* Eric L. Matteson and Thomas G. Mason.)

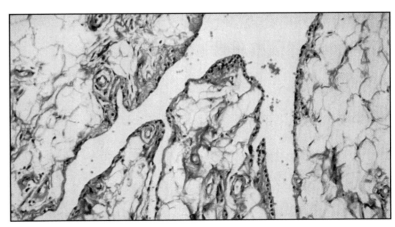

FIGURE 5-3.

Histology of normal articular synovium. The normal synovial membrane is composed of a flat layer, usually one or two cells thick, overlying the subsynovial stroma. Unlike other membranes, the cells of the synovial lining do not contain true epithelial tissue or basement membranes. Synovial blood vessels course throughout the stroma. There are two major types of synoviocytes: type A is macrophage-like, and type B is fibroblast-like (hematoxylin and eosin, medium power) [1]. (*Courtesy of* Thomas A. Gaffey.)

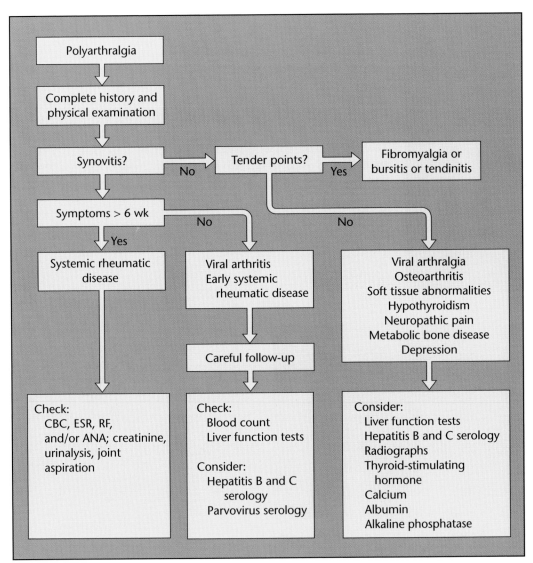

FIGURE 5-4.
Initial evaluation of the patient with poly-arthritis. A careful history and physical examination are essential. Disease features and time course help to guide the initial workup and management. Polyarthritis per-sisting for more than 6 weeks is consistent with rheumatoid arthritis; viral syndromes with polyarthritis are usually self-limited. Arthralgias may be accompanied by muscle pain. In the absence of true joint swelling, proximal weakness and elevated creatine phosphokinase levels suggest myositis. Patients over 50 years of age with arthralgias and myalgias may have polymyalgia rheumatica. Initial laboratory tests include a complete blood count (CBC), erythrocyte sedimentation rate (WEST), and rheumatoid factor (RF) among others. A joint aspiration may be helpful to demonstrate inflamma-tion and rule out infection and crystalline diseases in the appropriate clinical setting. ANA—antinuclear antibodies; ESR—erythro-cyte sedimentation rate. (*Adapted from* Ad Hoc Committee on Clinical Guidelines [2].)

Epidemiology of Rheumatoid Arthritis

Gender	Female–male ratio is 3:1
Incidence	Annually 25–30 new cases/100,000 population
Prevalence	Occurs in 1% of the adult population of North America and Europe
	The prevalence in males over 65 years of age is about 1.9%, and for females about 5.0%
Genetics	Greatest risks in persons who are HLA-DR4 and HLA-DR1 positive
Pattern at age of onset	Usually polyarticular, affecting the wrist, metacarpophalangeal, and proximal interphalangeal joints. At onset 20% of patients have monoarticular disease, whereas 80% have multiple (two or more) joints involved.
Peak age of onset	Between about 20–50 years of age

FIGURE 5-5.
Epidemiology of rheumatoid arthritis. Rheumatoid arthritis affects approximately 1% to 2% of the adult population worldwide. The incidence of rheumatoid arthritis is approximately 30 cases per 100,000 person years for women between the ages of 18 and 64. Genetic factors play a role; monozygotic twins have an 11-fold increase in risk compared with dizygotic twins, although pene-trance is low (34% in monozygotic, 3% in dizygotic twins) [3]. There are probably several genetic loci predisposing to the develop-ment of rheumatoid arthritis, including the class II major histocom-patibility complex alleles DR4. These alleles likely regulate the immune response to a putative environmental agent important in the etiology of the disease. (*Courtesy of* Eric L. Matteson and Thomas G. Mason.)

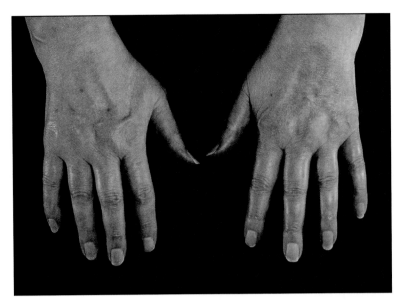

FIGURE 5-6.
Symmetric synovitis in early rheumatoid arthritis. Symmetric involvement of the hands is a hallmark of rheumatoid arthritis. In early disease, there may be swelling of the wrists, metacarpophalangeal joints, or the proximal interphalangeal joints. There is no deformity. The proximal interphalangeal swelling may appear to be fusiform, as is evident in several digits in this patient. There is bilateral involvement of the metacarpophalangeals and the wrists of this 54-year-old woman, who had had synovitis for about 10 weeks at the time this photograph was taken. (*Courtesy of* Eric L. Matteson and Thomas G. Mason.)

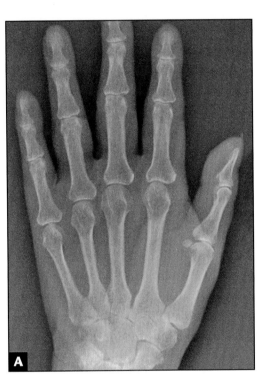
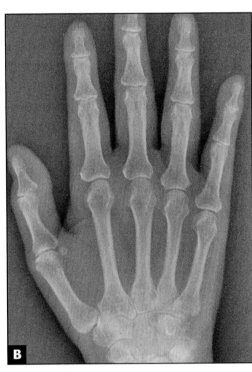

FIGURE 5-7.
Radiographic features of aggressive, early rheumatoid arthritis. Evidence of soft tissue swelling of the metacarpophalangeal and proximal interphalangeal joints can be seen on the hand radiograph of this 61-year-old woman with rheumatoid arthritis for 1 year. In the early, pre-erosive stage, juxta-articular osteoporosis appears, caused by the inflammation of the surrounding synovium. There is symmetric joint space narrowing of several metacarpophalangeal and proximal interphalangeal joints of both hands and subtle erosions of the right third and both fourth metacarpophalangeal joints. The carpus is involved as well, and the carpal margins are becoming indistinct, reflecting continued active synovitis. Soft tissue swelling from synovitis is present at the wrists and many of the digits. (*Courtesy of* Eric L. Matteson and Thomas G. Mason.)

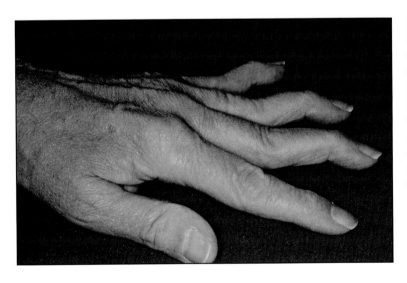

FIGURE 5-8.
Swan neck deformity. The swan neck deformity is caused by joint swelling and associated tenosynovitis with subsequent contracture of the intrinsic (lumbrical and interosseous) hand muscles. There is flexion at the metacarpophalangeal, hyperextension at the proximal interphalangeal, and flexion at the distal interphalangeal joint evident in fingers, especially the third, fourth, and fifth, but to a lesser extent also in the index finger. In early disease the deformity can be passively corrected; later, functional impairment may result from inability to flex at the proximal interphalangeal joint so that the patient is unable to make a fist. (*Courtesy of* Eric L. Matteson and Thomas G. Mason.)

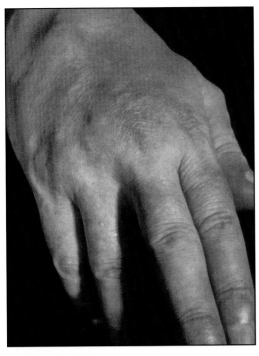

FIGURE 5-9.
Rupture of finger extensors in rheumatoid arthritis. Rupture of the extensors of the fourth and fifth digits is caused by active synovitis and invasive synovial proliferation. Wrist instability with prominence of the eroded ulnar styloid process can also shear the ulnar tendons. (*Courtesy of* Eric L. Matteson and Thomas G. Mason.)

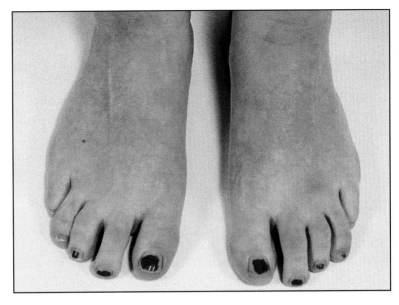

FIGURE 5-10.
Symmetric synovitis of the feet in early rheumatoid arthritis. Swelling of the right second and third toes and the second toe of the left foot in a 26-year-old patient with rheumatoid arthritis of 6 months' duration. There is also swelling of the first to third metatarsophalangeal joints of the right foot and the first to fourth metatarsophalangeals of the left foot. This swelling may be apparent on visual inspection, but digital palpation by the examiner confirms the synovitis. The skin proximal to the affected metatarsophalangeals often appears swollen, as it is in this patient. (*Courtesy of* Eric L. Matteson and Thomas G. Mason.)

FIGURE 5-11.
Wrist synovitis—magnetic resonance imaging (MRI). MRI permits detailed study of soft tissue and bones and can demonstrate the extent of proliferative and erosive disease at an earlier stage and in more detail than conventional radiographic techniques. The T1-weighted image shows multiple erosions in the carpus and distal ulna as well as defined areas of decreased signal. Synovial proliferation is present, especially at the distal carpal row and proximal metacarpophalangeal joint. (*Courtesy of* Richard P. Polisson, MD.)

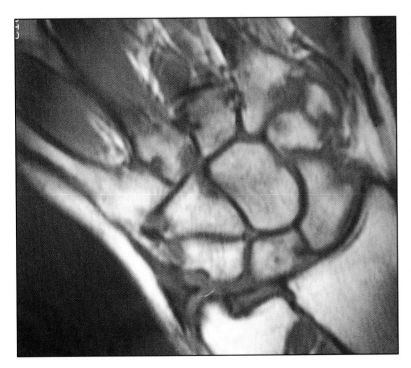

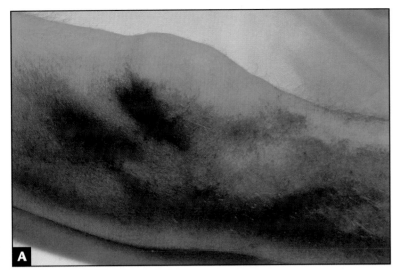

A

B

FIGURE 5-12.

Demonstration of the "bulge sign." **A,** Although massive swelling is obvious, the presence of lesser knee swelling can be demonstrated using the "bulge sign." **B,** To elicit this sign, the examiner compresses the intra-articular fluid from the medial aspect of the knee and then strokes the lateral aspect, forcing the fluid to appear at the medial aspect, or vise versa. (*Courtesy of* Eric L. Matteson and Thomas G. Mason.)

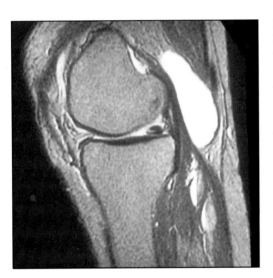

FIGURE 5-13.

Baker's cyst—magnetic resonance image (MRI). MRI demonstrates a Baker's cyst in a patient with well-controlled, early rheumatoid arthritis and previous knee trauma. There is an extensive horizontal tear involving the body and posterior horn of the medial meniscus associated with degeneration of the meniscus and some loss of articular cartilage. There is a minimal amount of fluid in the knee joint. A 4 × 2 cm Baker's cyst is seen posteromedially. A few smaller cysts are seen inferiorly. Fluid levels are likely related to debris. (*Courtesy of* Michael E. Torchia.)

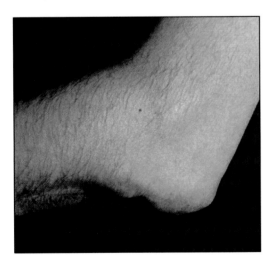

FIGURE 5-14.

Bursitis and nodulosis. Subcutaneous rheumatoid nodules commonly form over pressure points such as the olecranon (arm rest), feet (shoe wear and plantar surfaces), and fingers (gripping), and scapula, occiput, ischium, and sacrum from sitting and lying. The nodules are firm, and may be mobile or, when adherent to the periosteum, fixed. As in this patient with nodules and olecranon bursitis, the nodules may be within subcutaneous tissue overlying the bursae. Only about 20% of patients with rheumatoid arthritis develop rheumatoid nodules, and most patients with rheumatoid nodules are positive for rheumatoid factor. Although nodules usually regress with improvement of disease activity, in some patients methotrexate treatment promotes nodule formation. (*Courtesy of* Eric L. Matteson and Thomas G. Mason.)

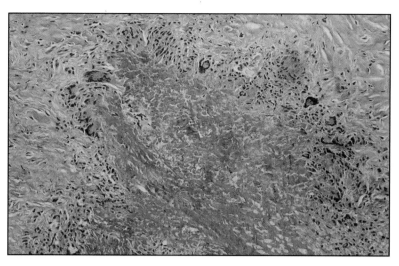

FIGURE 5-15.

Granulomatous transformation of a rheumatoid nodule is evident. There is prominent central fibrinoid necrosis, surrounding palisading histiocytes, and an outer layer of chronic fibrosing connective tissue with inflammatory cells including plasma cells, lymphocytes and fibroblasts (hematoxylin and eosin, low power). (*Courtesy of* Thomas A. Gaffey.)

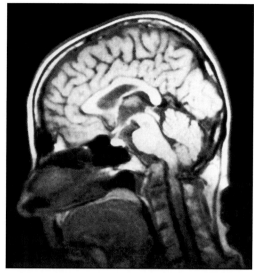

FIGURE 5-16.

Magnetic resonance image of basilar invagination. The T1-weighted sagittal view demonstrates impingement of the brain stem with protrusion of the eroded odontoid process into the foramen magnum. (*Courtesy of* Miguel E. Cabenela.)

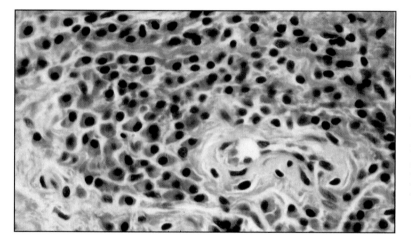

FIGURE 5-17.

Synovitis in rheumatoid arthritis. Synovial biopsy is rarely performed as a diagnostic procedure to confirm the diagnosis of rheumatoid arthritis. The histopathologic changes are characteristic but not specific for rheumatoid arthritis. Features of the inflamed synovium include synovial hyperplasia, angiogenesis, subsynovial fibrosis, perivascular infiltrates, and the presence of plasma cells. Macrophages, mast cells, histiocytes, and multinucleated giant cells may also be seen. These features are present throughout the disease course. As in this photomicrograph, there are marked perivascular lymphoplasmacytic infiltrates, a hallmark of active disease (hematoxylin and eosin, high power). (*Courtesy of* Thomas A. Gaffey.)

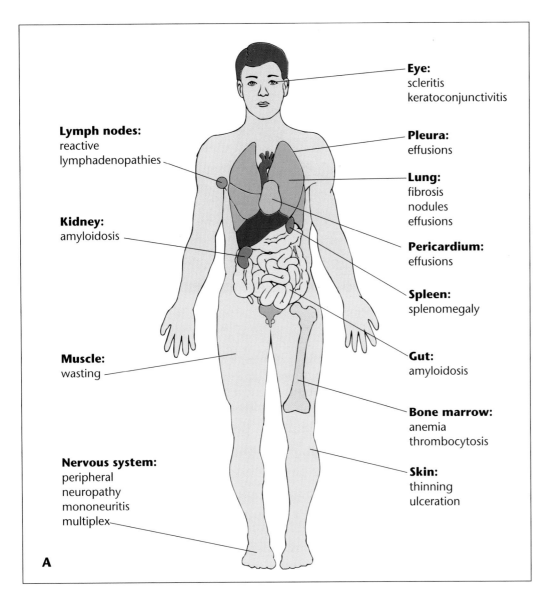

Eye:
scleritis
keratoconjunctivitis

Lymph nodes:
reactive
lymphadenopathies

Pleura:
effusions

Lung:
fibrosis
nodules
effusions

Kidney:
amyloidosis

Pericardium:
effusions

Spleen:
splenomegaly

Muscle:
wasting

Gut:
amyloidosis

Bone marrow:
anemia
thrombocytosis

Nervous system:
peripheral
neuropathy
mononeuritis
multiplex

Skin:
thinning
ulceration

A

FIGURE 5-18.
Systemic rheumatoid arthritis. **A**, Extra-articular disease manifestations affect about 42% of patients with rheumatoid arthritis and can include multiple organ systems. [5]. **B**, Constitutional symptoms and signs. Constitutional symptoms and signs can vary with disease activity. Most patients with active arthritis experience more than one hour of morning stiffness.

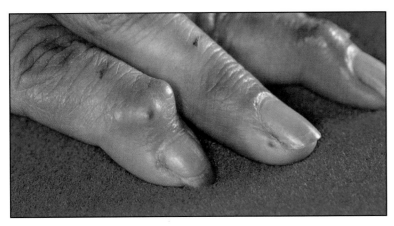

FIGURE 5-19.
Rheumatoid vasculopathy. Rheumatoid vasculopathy is a rather unusual manifestation of small vessel arteritis. This condition manifests as small, well-localized infarctions that may occur over rheumatoid nodules (nodules on the third and fifth distal interphalangeal joints of this patient), or present as nail fold infarctions (ulnar aspect of the fourth and fifth digits). When they occur in isolation or with leg ulcers only, without evidence of other systemic inflammation, gangrene, or a sensorimotor neuropathy, they usually do not require specific treatment, especially increased immunosuppression or higher doses of corticosteroids. (*Courtesy of Eric L. Matteson and Thomas G. Mason.*)

Classification of Synovial Effusions

Fluid	Appearance	Leukocyte Count/mm³
Normal	Clear, colorless	< 200, with < 25% PMNs
Noninflammatory	Clear, yellow	200–2000 with < 25% PMNs
Inflammatory	Cloudy, yellow	2000–100,000 with > 50% PMNs
Septic	Purulent	> 80,000 with > 75% PMNs

FIGURE 5-20.

Classification of synovial effusions. Normal and noninflammatory synovial fluid (such as may be seen in osteoarthritis) is viscous with low cellularity. In inflammation, the fluid becomes turbid, and viscosity decreases. In patients taking glucocorticosteroids, antimetabolites, and immunosuppressive agents, the cell count is an unreliable indicator of the possibility of infection, because cell counts in these patients may not be dramatically increased and are indistinguishable from patients with active synovitis but uninfected joints. PMN—polymorphonuclear neutrophil leukocytes. (*Adapted from* Schumacher and Reginato [5].)

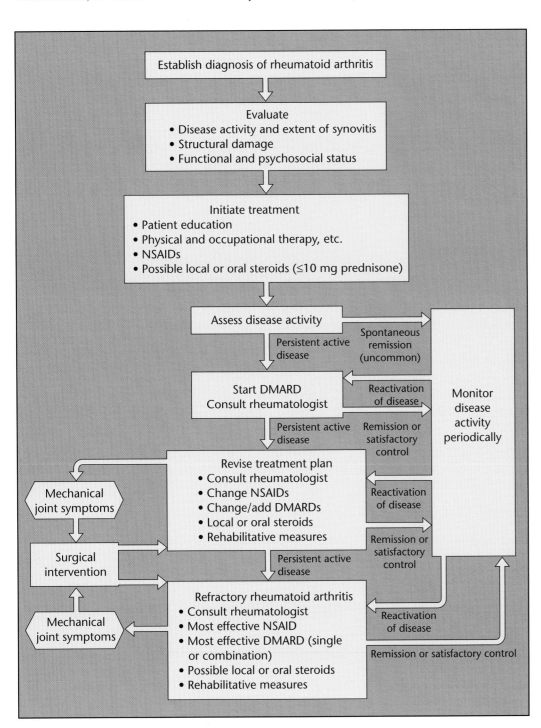

FIGURE 5-21.

Management of rheumatoid arthritis. This algorithm outlines the management of rheumatoid arthritis. After the diagnosis has been established, early therapeutic intervention is important to control disease, preserve function, and improve disease outcome. Initial interventions to control symptoms include the use of nonsteroidal anti-inflammatory drugs (NSAIDs) and sometimes glucocorticosteroids. For patients in whom the diagnosis is established, slower-acting second-line drugs should be initiated early in the disease course. The disease process is dynamic, and frequent reevaluation is necessary to good disease management. Consultation with a rheumatologist helps to guide diagnostic and therapeutic decision making. DMARDs—disease modifying antirheumatic drugs. (*Adapted from* Ad Hoc Subcommittee on Clinical Guidelines [6].)

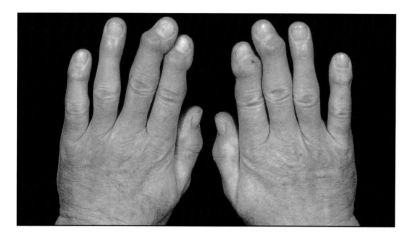

FIGURE 5-22.
Osteoarthritis classified. Osteoarthritis, the most prevalent form of arthritis in the United States, is characterized by progressive loss of the articular cartilage that comprises the normal weight-bearing surface of the joint and remodeling of the bone beneath and adjacent to that cartilage. The swelling and angular deformities of the distal interphalangeal joints of the second and third fingers seen here are caused by osteoarthritis in these joints. (*Courtesy of* Stephen L. Myers.)

Clinical Subsets of Primary Osteoarthritis

Generalized osteoarthritis: affects hands, hips, knees, first CMC and MTP joints, cervical or lumbar spine.

Primary generalized or nodal osteoarthritis: involves DIP and IP joints, females:males 10:1

Erosive osteoarthritis: red, swollen DIP or IP joints; often first CMC, hip, and knee symptoms

FIGURE 5-23.
Primary osteoarthritis. Several clinical subsets of patients with primary or idiopathic osteoarthritis have been described, although many patients cannot readily be classified into one of these categories on the basis of existing radiographic criteria. To date, useful genetic or immunologic markers that distinguish these subsets of patients have not been identified. Most clinicians will recall patients with *generalized osteoarthritis* that involves three or more joints, who have, for example, symptoms in their spine, knees, hips, in the first carpometacarpophalangeal joint (CMC) at the base of the thumb, the distal fingers, and the great toe. The wrists, elbows, and shoulder are typically spared. A second group of patients with generalized osteoarthritis includes women who develop painful swelling of several distal interphalangeal (DIP) or proximal interphalangeal (IP) joints within a year or two of menopause and have a strong family history of osteoarthritis. They have been described as having *nodal osteoarthritis*. Another subset of patients have *erosive osteoarthritis* characterized by the erythema and tenderness that develops in multiple DIP and IP joints and by the development of "erosive" changes and osteophytes at these sites. MTP—metatarsophalangeal. (*Courtesy of* Stephen L. Myers.)

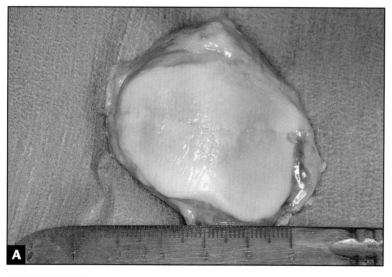

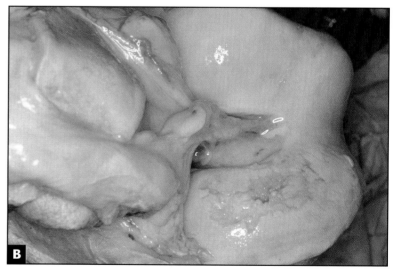

FIGURE 5-24.
Fibrillated cartilage. **A,** This osteoarthritic patella shows thinned, fibrillated cartilage that has a "crab-meat" appearance. Patients with patellofemoral osteoarthritis often benefit from exercise programs that include isometric strengthening of the quadriceps muscle.

B, The suprapatellar bursa of this osteoarthritic knee was opened, and the patella was dislocated to expose a large area of eroded cartilage on the medial femoral condyle. Thinning and erosion of the patellar cartilage are also visible.

(*Continued*)

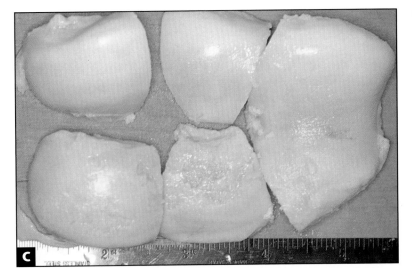

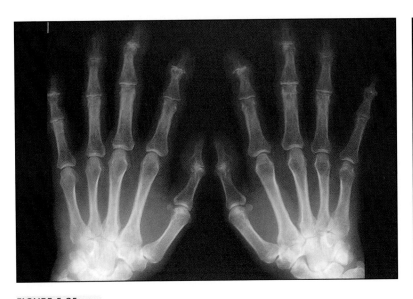

FIGURE 5-24. (*CONTINUED*)

C, An osteoarthritic femoral condyle was sawed into sections to display the distribution of roughened, pitted, and fibrillated articular surfaces. The most severe changes in this knee were located on the central and "habitually loaded" area of the medial condyle. In patients with end-stage osteoarthritis who undergo knee arthroplasty, this area often contains no cartilage, and the subchondral bone is exposed. (*Courtesy of* Stephen L. Myers.)

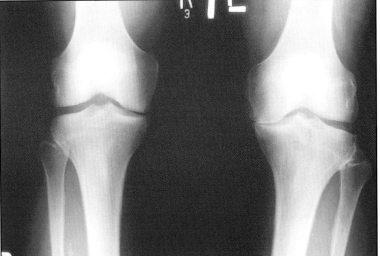

FIGURE 5-25.
Heberden's and Bouchard's nodes. The radiographic changes that accompany the development of Heberden's and Bouchard's nodes in the distal interphalangeal (DIP) and proximal interphalangeal joints (PIP), respectively, include soft tissue swelling, angular deformities of the distal digits, osteophytes, loss of joint space, and subchondral cysts. (*Courtesy of* Stephen L. Myers.)

FIGURE 5-26.
Tibiofemoral joint space, standing view in this radiograph obtained with the patient standing. The tibiofemoral joint space in the medial compartment of the left knee is abnormally narrow, compared with that in the right knee. Marginal osteophytes are visible. Radiographs that have been obtained with the patient supine cannot be relied on to indicate the severity of joint space narrowing, and thus of cartilage loss, in the osteoarthritic knee.

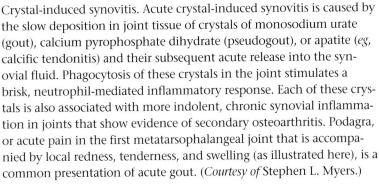

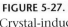

FIGURE 5-27.
Crystal-induced synovitis. Acute crystal-induced synovitis is caused by the slow deposition in joint tissue of crystals of monosodium urate (gout), calcium pyrophosphate dihydrate (pseudogout), or apatite (*eg*, calcific tendonitis) and their subsequent acute release into the synovial fluid. Phagocytosis of these crystals in the joint stimulates a brisk, neutrophil-mediated inflammatory response. Each of these crystals is also associated with more indolent, chronic synovial inflammation in joints that show evidence of secondary osteoarthritis. Podagra, or acute pain in the first metatarsophalangeal joint that is accompanied by local redness, tenderness, and swelling (as illustrated here), is a common presentation of acute gout. (*Courtesy of* Stephen L. Myers.)

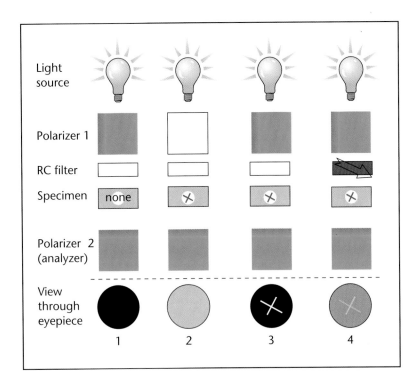

FIGURE 5-28.

Polarizing microscopy. The unique elements of a polarizing microscope equipped for the identification of birefringement (*ie*, light-bending) crystals, including monosodium urate and calcium pyrophosphate dihydrate (CPPD), are two optical polarizers and a first-order red compensator (RC) filter. In this diagram, 1) no light reaches the eyepiece when the polarizers are correctly adjusted for crystal viewing, and neither the RC filter nor a specimen of crystal is in the optical path; 2) if one polarizer is removed (or rotated 90°), crystals are nearly transparent and can be difficult to identify; 3) urate and CPPD crystals are easily seen when a correct, perpendicular alignment of the polarizers has been obtained; 4) the addition of the RC filter to the optical path changes the background from black to magenta, enabling urate and CPPD crystals to be distinguished by their color and orientation, as well as by their shape. Urate crystals are always *negatively* birefringement, and when the long axis of this crystal parallels the optical axis of the RC filter (*black arrow*), it appears yellow. If the urate crystal is rotated clockwise or counterclockwise, its color fades and then changes to blue as its long axis falls perpendicular to the axis of the RC. In contrast, crystals of CPPD are *positively* birefringement and appear blue when their long axis is aligned with the axis of the RC filter. Because they have opposite birefringence, if two parallel crystals of CPPD and urate are viewed with the RC filter in place, one crystal appears blue and the other yellow. (*Courtesy of* Stephen L. Myers.)

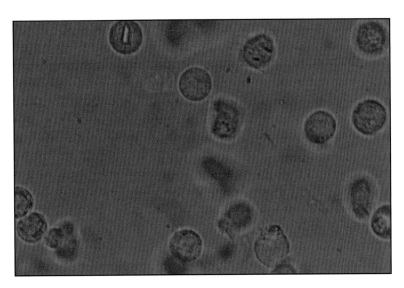

FIGURE 5-29.

Synovial fluid leukocytes. Synovial fluid aspirated from a painful knee during an acute attack of arthritis was photographed with a polarizing microscope (10×) equipped with a first-order red compensator filter. Numerous synovial fluid leukocytes are visible, and several contain blunt or rhomboid-shaped crystals of calcium pyrophosphate monohydrate (CPPD). These crystals are positively birefringent, and when their long axis is aligned with the optical axis of the red compensator they appear blue. When they lie perpendicular to this axis, CPPD appears yellow. (*Courtesy of* Stephen L. Myers.)

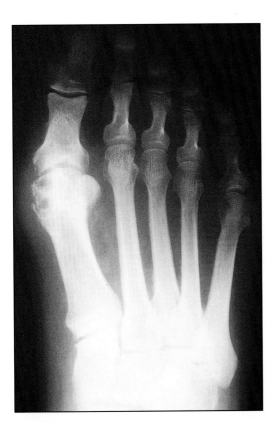

FIGURE 5-30.

Erosions. The erosion of the medial aspect of the first metatarsal head in this patient with a 1-year history of gout appears cystic and has an "overhanging edge" of cortical bone that helps distinguish it from the erosions seen in other inflammatory arthropathies, as well as from osteoarthritis. Aspiration of this site is likely to yield urate crystals even in the absence of podagra. (*Courtesy of* Stephen L. Myers.)

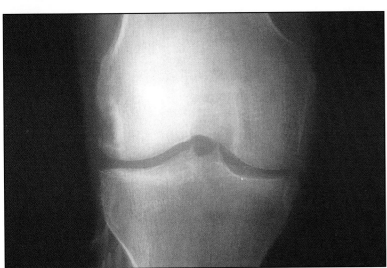

FIGURE 5-31.

Chondrocalcinosis. This knee radiograph shows chondrocalcinosis, a faint white line parallel to the contours of the femoral condyle midway between the femur and tibial plateau, in a patient with pseudogout. The lateral tibial femoral compartment is slightly narrowed on this standing view, indicating concomitant osteoarthritis. Because deposits of nonbirefringent calcium-containing crystals (*ie*, basic calcium phosphate or apatite) also produce chondrocalcinosis, it is necessary to find calcium pyrophosphate dihydrate crystals in the synovial fluid to diagnose pseudogout [6]. (*Courtesy of* Stephen L. Myers.)

SYSTEMIC LUPUS ERYTHEMATOSUS, ANTIPHOSPHOLIPID SYNDROME, SCLERODERMA, AND INFLAMMATORY MYOPATHIES

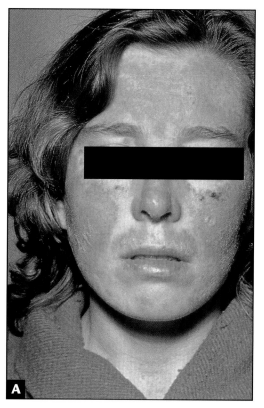

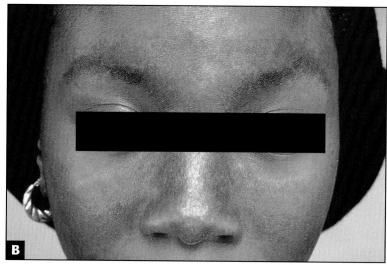

FIGURE 5-32.

Systemic lupus erythematosus. **A,** Butterfly rash. Classic lupus rash on the cheeks, nose, and forehead. The distribution varies, and the classic rash is now seen in a minority of patients as milder cases of lupus are diagnosed. **B,** Rash and hyperpigmentation in active lupus. In addition to the classic butterfly rash on the nose and cheeks, note the marked involvement of the eyebrows and skin above the eyebrows. In pigmented skin, hyper- or hypopigmentation can occur. (*Courtesy of* Graham R.V. Hughes and Munther A. Khamashta.)

Principal Pathologic Features

General
Fibrinoid necrosis
Hematoxylin bodies
Deposition of immune complexes along basement membranes

Skin
Discoid lupus—follicular plugging and scarring
Systemic lupus—immune complexes in dermal/epidermal junction

Kidneys
Immune complex deposition
Focal or diffuse glomerulonephritis
Fibrinoid necrosis of arterioles or arteries

Cerebral
Microinfarcts
Choroid plexus immune complexes

Heart
Pericarditis
Myocarditis
Libman-Sacks endocarditis

Blood Vessels
Arteriolitis and capillaritis
Microthrombi

Spleen
"Onion-skin" thickening

Joints
Fibrinoid deposition

Lungs and Pleura
Fibrinoid adhesions
Effusions
Interstitial pneumonitis
Recurrent atelectasis

FIGURE 5-33.

Principal pathologic features of systemic lupus erythematosus. The most striking histologic feature is the so-called fibrinoid necrosis, which affects particularly the small arteries, arterioles, and capillaries (as distinct from polyarteritis nodosa, which affects predominantly medium-sized vessels such as the coronary and mesenteric arteries) [8]. (*Courtesy of* Graham R.V. Hughes and Munther A. Khamashta.)

Modified World Health Organization Classification of Renal Pathology of Lupus Nephritis

I. Normal glomeruli
II. Mesangial glomerulonephritis
III. Focal proliferative glomerulonephritis
IV. Diffuse proliferative glomerulonephritis
    A. Hypercellularity only (without segmental necrotizing lesions)
    B. With active necrotizing lesions
    C. With active and sclerosing lesions
    D. With sclerosing lesions
V. Membranous nephropathy
VI. Sclerosing nephropathy

FIGURE 5-34.

Modified World Health Organization (WHO) classification of renal pathology of lupus nephritis. Renal biopsy is initially important in differentiating patients with potentially reversible or steroid-responsive lesions (mesangial or focal proliferative) from those with diffuse proliferative disease requiring more aggressive immunosuppression and those minimally or unresponsive to therapy (membranous nephropathy). Follow-up biopsy is sometimes helpful in guiding changes in or withdrawal of treatment. Management of terminal chronic renal failure does not differ from that of other causes and systemic lupus erythematosus is not usually a contraindication to transplantation. (*Courtesy of* Graham R.V. Hughes and Munther A. Khamashta.)

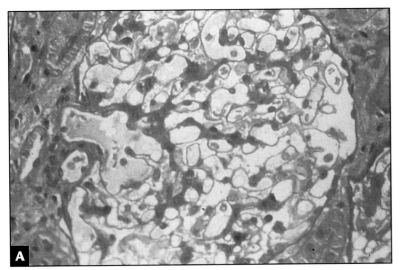

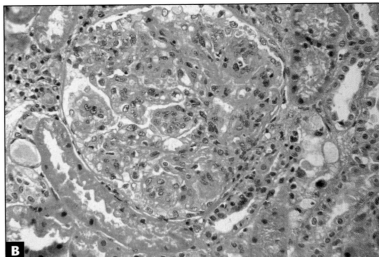

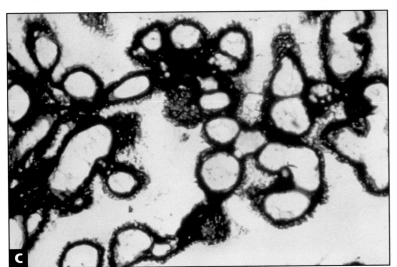

FIGURE 5-35.

Light microscopy of the major World Health Organization (WHO) classes of lupus nephritis. **A**, Mesangial lupus nephritis, WHO class II (hematoxylin and eosin). **B**, Diffuse proliferative lupus nephritis, WHO class IV (hematoxylin and eosin). **C**, Membranous lupus nephritis, WHO class V (silver methenamine).

Drug-induced and Idiopathic Lupus: Autoantibody–Disease Associations

	Idiopathic Lupus, %	Drug-induced Lupus, %
ANA	> 95	100
LE cells	75	90
Anti-histone	60	> 95
Anti-dsDNA	60	< 5
Anti-Sm	25	< 5
Anti-RNP	35	< 5
Anti-Ro	30	< 5
Anti-La	15	< 5

FIGURE 5-36.

Drug-induced and idiopathic lupus: autoantibody–disease associations. Antinuclear antibody (ANA) tests are almost invariably positive in patients with drug-induced lupus and lupus cells are plentiful. However, anti-ds-DNA antibodies are usually absent or in low titer. Anti-histone antibodies are positive in most patients with drug-induced lupus. (*Courtesy of* Graham R.V. Hughes and Munther A. Khamashta.)

Drug Therapy in Systemic Lupus Erythematosus

Drug	Indications
Nonsteroidal anti-inflammatories*	Synovitis and mild systemic illness
Antimalarials*	Synovitis and cutaneous disease
Corticosteroids	Moderate to severe systemic disease, including nephritis, vasculitis, neuropathy, and other vital organ involvement
Immunosuppressives*	Severe disease, including nephritis
Plasma exchange (use still not proven)	Severe vasculitis and nephritis; used in combination with corticosteroids and immunosuppressives

* Useful steroid-sparing agents.

FIGURE 5-37.

Therapeutic approach for systemic lupus erythematosus. Patients must be evaluated fully to determine the extent of organ involvement, so that treatment can be tailored to individual needs. (*Courtesy of* Graham R.V. Hughes and Munther A. Khamashta.)

FIGURE 5-38.

Definition—Hughes' syndrome. In 1983, a distinct syndrome was described associated with both venous and (importantly) arterial thrombosis. The syndrome is marked by the presence of circulating antiphospholipid antibodies. A major feature of this syndrome in women is recurrent pregnancy loss; treatment in these patients is centered on anticoagulation rather than immunosuppression or anti-inflammatory therapy [9,10].

Antiphospholipid Syndrome: Clinical Features

Feature	Patients, %
Venous thrombosis	48
Arterial thrombosis	38
Thrombocytopenia	32
Recurrent pregnancy loss	55

Clinical Associations in Antiphospholipid Syndrome

Major Features

Venous thrombosis: Deep venous thrombosis, Budd-Chiari syndrome, and pulmonary thromboembolism

Arterial thrombosis: Strokes, transient ischemic attacks, multi-infarct dementia, myocardial infarctions

Recurrent pregnancy loss

Thrombocytopenia

Associated Clinical Features

Leg ulcers, livedo reticularis, thrombophlebitis, and Sneddon's syndrome

Migraine headaches

Heart valve lesions

Transverse myelitis, chorea, and epilepsy

Hemolytic anemia, Coombs positivity, and Evans syndrome

Pulmonary hypertension

Others (Less Common)

Splinter hemorrhages

Labile hypertension and accelerated atherosclerosis

Ischemic necrosis of bone

Addison's disease

Guillain-Barré syndrome and pseudo-multiple sclerosis

Renal artery and vein thrombosis and renal microangiopathy

Retinal artery and vein thrombosis

Amaurosis fugax

Digital gangrene

FIGURE 5-39.

Clinical associations in antiphospholipid syndrome. (*Courtesy of* Graham R.V. Hughes and Munther A. Khamashta.)

Treatment of the Different Antiphospholipid-Associated Clinical Manifestations

Clinical Situation	Suggested Treatment
Asymptomatic individuals	Observation ± low-dose aspirin
Recurrent deep venous thrombosis ± pulmonary embolism	Life-long oral anticoagulants (INR ≥ 3)
Large vessel arterial occlusion (*ie*, stroke)	Life-long oral anticoagulants (INR ≥ 3) ± low-dose aspirin
Transient ischemic attack	Low-dose aspirin
Recurrent transient ischemic attacks	Life-long oral anticoagulants (INR ≥ 3) ± low-dose aspirin
Catastrophic antiphospholipid syndrome	Oral anticoagulants (INR ≥ 3) + plasmapheresis ± corticosteroids or immunosuppressives
History of first trimester pregnancy loss	Low-dose aspirin
History of second or third trimester fetal loss	Low-dose aspirin ± subcutaneous heparin
Severe thrombocytopenia (< 20,000)	Corticosteroids

FIGURE 5-40.
Therapeutic approach to the different clinical manifestations of antiphospholid syndrome. INR—International normalized ratio.

Classification of Scleroderma

Systemic scleroderma
  Diffuse cutaneous scleroderma
  Limited cutaneous scleroderma
  CREST syndrome
Localized scleroderma
  Morphea
  Linear scleroderma
Overlap syndromes
Scleroderma-like syndromes

FIGURE 5-41.
Classification of scleroderma. CREST—calcinosis, Raynaud's esophageal dysmotility, sclerodactyly, telangiectasia. (*Courtesy of* Graham R.V. Hughes and Munther A. Khamashta.)

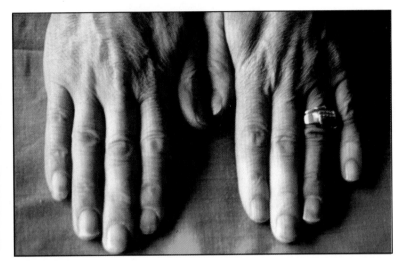

FIGURE 5-42.
Raynaud's phenomenon. Mild to moderate Raynaud's phenomenon occurs in over 75% of patients with scleroderma and may precede other disease manifestations. It should arouse suspicion in women over the age of 35 years, especially when there is considerable edema. The Raynaud's may be confined to a single digit or, as shown in this case, to two or three digits. (*Courtesy of* Graham R.V. Hughes and Munther A. Khamashta.)

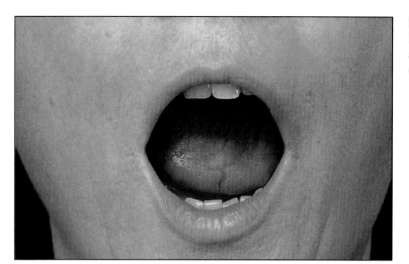

FIGURE 5-43.
Facial changes in scleroderma. Tightness of the skin is apparent around the mouth in a patient with scleroderma. (*Courtesy of* Graham R.V. Hughes and Munther A. Khamashta.)

Classification of the Idiopathic Inflammatory Myopathies

Major Forms
Dermatomyositis
  Adult form
  Juvenile form
Polymyositis
Inclusion body myositis

Other Forms
Polymyositis associated with other connective tissue diseases
Sarcoid myopathy
Myositis in graft-versus-host disease
Eosinophilic polymyositis
Focal myositis
Proliferative myositis
Myositis ossificans

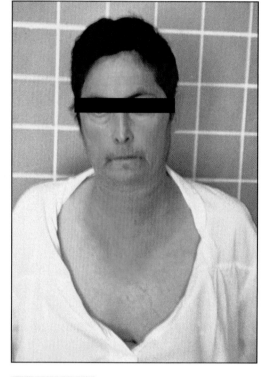

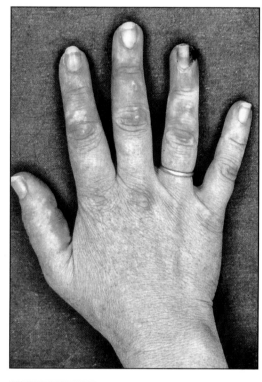

FIGURE 5-44.
Classification of the idiopathic inflammatory myopathies [11]. (*Courtesy of* Graham R.V. Hughes and Munther A. Khamashta.)

FIGURE 5-45.
This woman has acute onset dermatomyositis. Note the classic rash over light-exposed areas on the neck, upper chest, and cheeks. (*Courtesy of* Graham R.V. Hughes and Munther A. Khamashta.)

FIGURE 5-46.
Gottron's papules. Typical appearance of dermatomyositis with thickened patches on the dorsal surface of the knuckles. (*Courtesy of* Graham R.V. Hughes and Munther A. Khamashta.)

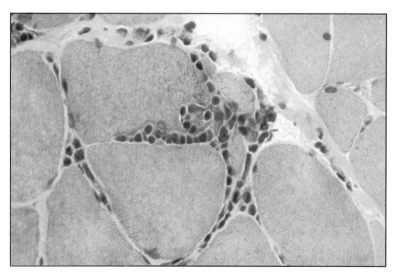

FIGURE 5-47.
Idiopathic inflammatory myopathies. Muscle biopsy (photomicrograph). Care must be taken in the selection of the location, processing, and interpretation of the muscle biopsy. A muscle selected for biopsy should be moderately weak, without marked atrophy, and free of recent trauma, such as intramuscular injection or electromyographic testing. Selection of a biopsy site is also aided by choosing the corresponding muscle on the opposite side of the body of one showing electromyographic changes or use of magnetic resonance imaging. In this photomicrograph, marked variability in the size of the muscle cells and mononuclear inflammatory infiltrate in the endomysial space is seen in a patient with polymyositis. Note the typical "partial cellular invasion" phenomenon, characterized by the presence of inflammatory cells beneath the basal membrane of otherwise normal appearing muscle cells (trichrome stain, ×350). (*Courtesy of* Jose-Maria Grau.)

VASCULITIDES

Practical Classification of Vasculitides

Primary Vasculitides

Affecting large-, medium-, and small-sized blood vessels
  Takayasu arteritis
  Giant cell (temporal) arteritis
  Isolated angitis of the central nervous system
Affecting predominantly medium- and small-sized blood vessels
  Polyarteritis nodosa
  Churg-Strauss syndrome
  Wegener's granulomatosis
Affecting predominantly small-sized blood vessels
  Microscopic polyangiitis
  Henoch-Schönlein purpura
  Cutaneous leukocytoclastic angitis
Miscellaneous conditions
  Buerger's disease
  Cogan's syndrome
  Kawasaki disease

Secondary Vasculitides

Infection-related vasculitis
Vasculitis secondary to connective tissue disease
Drug hypersensitivity-related vasculitis
Vasculitis secondary to mixed essential cryoglobulinemia
Malignancy-related vasculitis
Hypocomplementemic urticarial vasculitis
Post-organ transplant vasculitis
Pseudovasculitic syndromes (myxoma, endocarditis, Sneddon's syndrome)

FIGURE 5-48.

Lie's classification of vasculitides [12]. This classification is based on clinical and pathologic criteria. We advocate the use of similar clinical and pathologic findings to classify the vasculitides, for example, lung and renal involvement to help separate polyarteritis nodosa and microscopic polyangiitis, the use of laboratory tests (antineutrophil cytoplasmic antibodies, hepatitis B virus or hepatitis C virus infection), and angiographic data [11], and realizing that individual patients may have findings that overlap the clinical diagnostic categories [13,14]. (*Courtesy of* Loic Guillevin.)

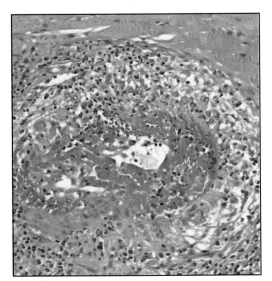

FIGURE 5-49.

Muscle biopsy showing vasculitis involving a medium-sized muscular artery. Fibrinoid necrosis, endothelial modifications, and adventitial leukocyte infiltrate are seen (×100). (*Courtesy of* Loic Guillevin.)

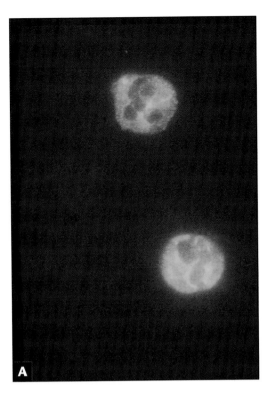

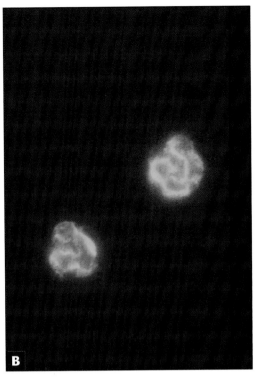

FIGURE 5-50.

Antineutrophil cytoplasmic antibodies (ANCA). ANCA are implicated in several systemic vasculitides. They are found in approximately 80% of systemic Wegener's (WG) granulomatosis, 50% of localized WG, 50% to 60% of microscopic polyangiitis (MPA) and Churg-Strauss syndrome (CSS) [13]. ANCA are present in less than 10% of classic polyarteritis nodosa. At present, ANCA should be considered as reflecting small-sized vessel involvement. In WG, a cytoplasmic (c) fluorescent staining pattern (**A**) is observed and antibodies directed against proteinase 3 (PR3) are responsible. These antibodies are also detected by enzyme-linked immunosorbent assay (ELISA). Anti-PR3 antibodies are highly specific to WG. Conversely, in MPA, CSS, and in rare cases of WG, the fluorescence pattern is perinuclear (p) (**B**). Antibodies producing this pattern are directed against myeloperoxidase (MPO). These antibodies can also be detected by ELISA. p-ANCA are less specific for vasculitis than c-ANCA and can be found in other diseases (inflammatory colitis, infections). (*Courtesy of* Loic Guillevin.)

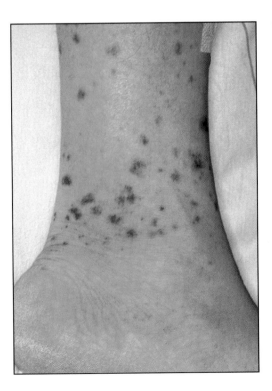

FIGURE 5-51.
Purpura. Palpable purpura is frequent in vasculitis affecting vessels of the skin. It is frequent in microscopic polyangiitis and reflects small-sized vessel involvement. Infiltration of the purpuric area and local necrosis are the most characteristic features of vascular purpura. (*Courtesy of* Loic Guillevin.)

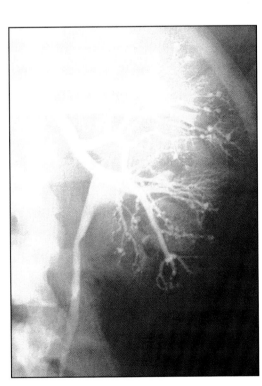

FIGURE 5-52.
Renal angiogram. Multiple kidney aneurysms are seen in a patient with polyarteritis nodusa. Hematuria was present secondary to areas of ischemia and infarction of renal tissue. (*Courtesy of* Loic Guillevin.)

Differential Diagnosis of Polyarteritis Nodosa and Microscopic Polyangiitis

Criteria	PAN	MPA
Histology		
Type of vasculitis	Necrotizing with mixed cells, rarely granulomatous	Necrotizing with mixed cells, not granulomatous
Type of vessels involved	Medium- and small-sized muscle arteries, sometimes arterioles	Small vessels (*ie,* capillaries, venules or arterioles)
		Small- and medium-sized arteries may be also affected
Distribution and localization		
Kidney		
Renal vasculitis with renovascular hypertension, renal infarcts, and microaneurysms	Yes	No
Rapidly progressive glomerulonephritis	No	Very common
Lung		
Pulmonary hemorrhage	No	Yes
Peripheral neuropathy	50%–80%	10%–20%
Relapses	Rare	Frequent
Laboratory data		
pANCA	Rare (< 10%)	Yes (50%–80%)
HBV infection present	Yes (uncommon)	No
Abnormal angiography (microaneurysms, stenoses)	Yes (variable)	No

FIGURE 5-53.

Differences between polyarteritis nodosa (PAN) and microscopic polyangiitis (MPA). MPA is now recognized as an entity distinct from PAN (or classic PAN). Glomerulonephritis and lung hemorrhage are the two manifestations that distinguish MPA from PAN because they are never observed in PAN. According to the Chapel Hill criteria [15], MPA would not be limited to pulmonary-renal syndrome and every type of vasculitis respecting the Chapel Hill criteria could be considered MPA. pANCA—perinuclear antineutrophil cytoplasmic antibodies; HBV—hepatitis B virus. (*Adapted from* Lhote and Guillerin [16]).

Frequency of Clinical Manifestations of Wegener's Granulomatosis

	Walton	Cordier	Hoffman	Anderson
Year	1958	1990	1992	19.92
Reference	[17]	[18]	[19]	[20]
Patients, *n*	56	77	158	265
Age, *y* (range)	45 (12–75)	46.5 (17–80)	41 (9–78)	50 (10–83)
Sex ratio (M/F)	1.5	1	1	1.2
Fever, weight loss, %		83	50	
Lung manifestations, %	100	100	85	73
Ear, nose, throat symptoms, %	89	75	92	87
Kidney involvement, %	90	74	77	60
Arthritis, %	34	34	67	20
Skin manifestations, %	46	29	46	25
Neurologic manifestations, %	29	30	15	
Ocular manifestations, %	41	29	52	14

FIGURE 5-54.

Main clinical symptoms of systemic Wegener's granulomatosis in four series of patients [17–20]. (*Courtesy of* Loic Guillevin.)

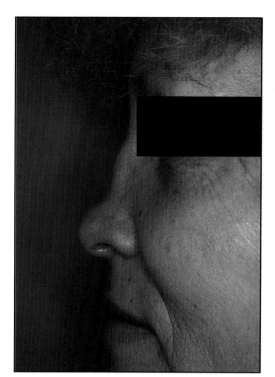

FIGURE 5-55.

Saddle nose. Cartilage neurosis and collapse occur in systemic or localized Wegener's granulomatosis. This symptom often causes a disfiguring sequel to the disease.

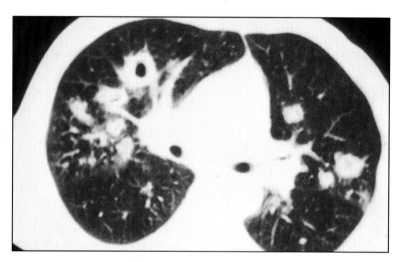

FIGURE 5-56.

Nodules. Pulmonary involvement in Wegener's granulomatosis. Computed tomography scan of the lungs shows several nodules, some with thick-walled cavities. Some nodules were not visible on a standard radiograph. Computed tomography scanning with thin slices is the major radiologic investigation for diagnosis and follow-up of Wegener's granulomatosis. (*Courtesy of* Loic Guillevin.)

Criteria for Classification of Takayasu Arteritis

Criterion	Definition
1. Age at disease onset ≤ 40 y	Development of symptoms or findings related to Takayasu arteritis at age of ≤ 40 y
2. Claudication of extremities	Development and worsening of fatigue and discomfort in muscles of one or more extremities while in use, especially the upper extremities
3. Decreased brachial artery pulse	Decreased pulsation of one or both brachial arteries
4. Blood pressure difference > 10 mm Hg	Difference of >10 mm Hg in systolic blood pressure between arms
5. Bruit over subclavian arteries or aorta	Bruit audible on auscultation over one or both subclavian arteries or abdominal aorta
6. Arteriogram abnormality	Arteriographic narrowing or occlusion of the entire aorta, its primary branches, or large arteries in the proximal upper or lower extremities, not due to atherosclerosis, fibromuscular dysplasia, or similar causes; changes usually focal or segmental

FIGURE 5-57.

American College of Rheumatology 1990 classification criteria for Takayasu arteritis [21]. Takayasu arteritis is a primary inflammatory vasculitis that affects large vessels, mainly the aorta and its major branches [21,22]. This rare disease, also called "pulseless disease," is usually observed in young women. It is difficult to diagnose because many nonspecific symptoms are present, including fever, myalgias, arthralgias, weight loss, and anemia. Vasculitis comprises granulomatous changes in the media and adventitia. The disease progresses slowly to intimal hyperplasia, medial degeneration, and fibrosis. For the purpose of classification, a patient shall be said to have Takayasu arteritis when at least three of the six criteria are present. The presence of any three or more criteria yields a sensitivity of 90.0% and a specificity of 97.8%. (*Courtesy of* Loic Guillevin.)

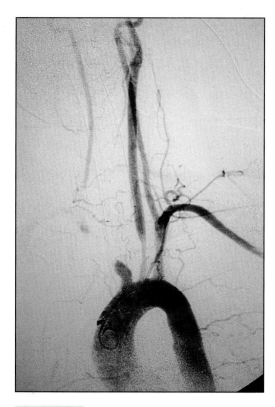

FIGURE 5-58.
Angiography. This angiogram of the aortic arch shows the long stenosis of the left carotid artery and the obstruction of the brachiocephalic arterial trunk. The right vertebral artery is seen after a few centimeters of total obstruction of the subclavian artery. The right carotid artery appears to have been obstructed and is not seen on this angiogram.

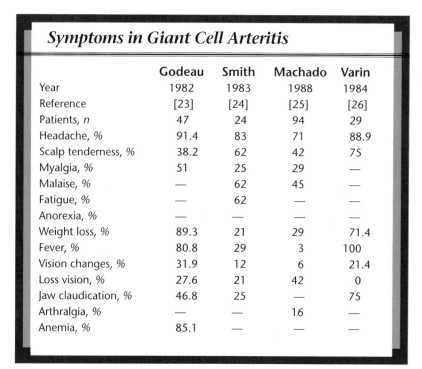

Symptoms in Giant Cell Arteritis

	Godeau	Smith	Machado	Varin
Year	1982	1983	1988	1984
Reference	[23]	[24]	[25]	[26]
Patients, n	47	24	94	29
Headache, %	91.4	83	71	88.9
Scalp tenderness, %	38.2	62	42	75
Myalgia, %	51	25	29	—
Malaise, %	—	62	45	—
Fatigue, %	—	62	—	—
Anorexia, %	—	—	—	—
Weight loss, %	89.3	21	29	71.4
Fever, %	80.8	29	3	100
Vision changes, %	31.9	12	6	21.4
Loss vision, %	27.6	21	42	0
Jaw claudication, %	46.8	25	—	75
Arthralgia, %	—	—	16	—
Anemia, %	85.1	—	—	—

FIGURE 5-59.
Main clinical manifestations of giant cell arteritis in four series of patients [23–26]. NS—not significant.

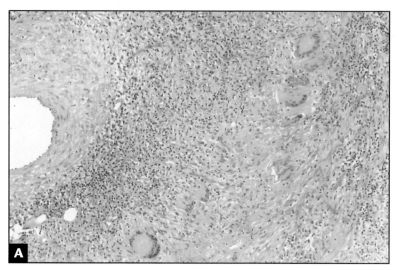

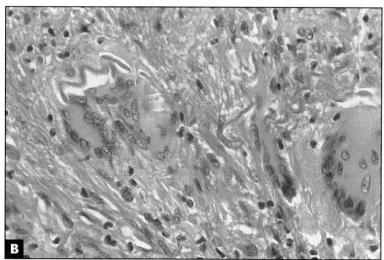

FIGURE 5-60.
Temporal artery biopsy. **A,** This biopsy shows extensive infiltration of the media with lymphocytes and macrophages (granulomatous inflammation). Several multinucleated giant cells are seen.

B, Higher magnification of the same specimen shows fragmentation of the internal elastic lamina next to multinucleated giant cells.

Main Characteristics of Cryoglobulinemia

Type	Immunoglobin Characteristics	Associated Disease	Immunoglobulin Type	Etiology
I	Monoclonal only	Multiple myeloma	Mainly IgG	Unknown
		Waldenström's macroglobulinemia	IgM	HCV? (47)
II	Monoclonal Ig and polyclonal Ig	Essential cryoglobulinemia	IgG and IgM	HCV (>80%^)
III	Polyclonal Ig	Essential cryoglobulinemia	Polyclonal, all types	Other virus unknown

FIGURE 5-61.

Classification and etiologies of cryoglobulinemia. Cryoglobulinemia is characterized by the presence of abnormal proteins that precipitate when plasma is cooled at temperatures below 37°C. Cryoglobulinemias are classified into three groups [27]. The main clinical manifestations consist of a systemic vasculitis, arthralgia, myalgias, vascular purpura, Raynaud's phenomenon, glomerulonephritis, peripheral neuropathy, and cardiac involvement [28–30]. The disease is thought to develop secondary to vascular deposition of immune complexes and may be triggered by viral antigens. Hematologic malignancies are always present in type I cryoglobulinemia. Type III, formerly called essential cryoglobulinemia, is, in most cases, caused by hepatitis C virus (HCV) infection. Type II is an intermediate situation in which benign or malignant neoplastic disease can be found. In type II HCV-related cryoglobulinemia, IgM k are found in most patients [27].

Predictive Mortality Value of the Five Factor Score

FFS	Death, %	Survival, %	Relative Risk (RR)	Patients, n
0	12	88	0.63	217
1	26.25	73.75	1.38	80
≥ 2	45.95	54.05	2.4	37
Total	64	273		337

FIGURE 5-62.

Prognostic factors and treatment of systemic vasculitides. Vasculitis treatments should be chosen according to classification, etiology, pathogenetic mechanisms, severity, and predictable outcome. In virus-associated vasculitides, treatment is based on the combination of antiviral agents and symptomatic or immunomodulating therapies [31]. Hepatitis B virus–related polyarteritis nodosa and hepatitis C virus–related cryoglobulinemia [29] respond to interferon-α and plasma exchanges. Responses are excellent in hepatitis B virus polyarteritis nodosa [31] but usually partial in hepatitis C virus cryoglobulinemia, and relapses occur in the majority of cases. Microscopic polyangiitis, classic polyarteritis nodosa, Wegener's granulomatosis, and other vasculitides respond to steroids and cytotoxic agents, mainly cyclophosphamide [32]. Optimal treatment duration and ways of administration can vary from one disease to another. Plasma exchanges are not recommended as the first-line treatment. Intravenous immunoglobulins and other immunomodulating treatments are indicated in some limited cases, and better definition of their indications requires further prospective studies.

This table shows the prognostic factors of polyarteritis nodosa, microscopic polyangiitis, and Churg-Strauss syndrome. A prognostic five factor score (FFS) [33] was established and comprises the following items: levels of creatininemia greater than 1.58 mg/dL and proteinuria greater than 1 g/d, presence of severe gastrointestinal tract involvement, cardiomyopathy, and central nervous system involvement. The presence of each factor was accorded one point. Three classes of scores were defined to predict mortality after 5 years: 0. when no factor was noted; 1, when one factor was present; and 2, when two or more factors were present. The FFS can be correlated with outcome. $P < 0.01$ for scores 0 versus 1 or 1 versus 2 [33]. (*Courtesy of Loic Guillevin.*)

SPONDYLOARTHROPATHIES

The Concept of Spondyloarthropathy

Disease Subgroups
Ankylosing spondylitis
Reactive arthritis (Reiter's syndrome)
Enteropathic arthritis
Psoriatic arthritis
Undifferentiated spondyloarthropathy
Juvenile spondyloarthropathy

All These Share Rheumatologic Features
Sacroiliac and spinal (axial) involvement
Enthesitis at long attachments of ligaments and tendons
    causing: Achilles tendonitis and plantar fasciitis,
    syndesmophyte formation ("bamboo spine"), sacroiliitis
    (due to a combination of enthesitis and synovitis), and
    periosteal reaction ("whiskering") at gluteal tuberosity and
    other parts of pelvis and other sites
Peripheral, often asymmetric, inflammatory arthritis and
    dactylitis ("sausage" digits)

Share Extra-articular Features
Propensity to ocular inflammation (acute anterior uveitis
    conjunctivitis)
Mucocutaneous lesions, variable for the subgroups
Rare aortic incompetence or heart block
Lack of association with rheumatoid factor and rheumatoid
    nodules

Share Genetic Predisposition
Strong association with HLA-B27 gene
Familial clustering

FIGURE 5-63.

The concept of spondyloarthropathy. The clinical spectrum of the rheumatologic diseases included under the term *spondylo-arthropathies* consists of ankylosing spondylitis, reactive arthritis or Reiter's syndrome, spondyloarthritis associated with psoriasis and chronic inflammatory bowel diseases, and a form of juvenile chronic arthritis (pauciarticular, late-onset type) [34–37]. All forms of the spondyloarthropathies are associated with the histocompatibility antigen HLA-B27, although the strength of this association varies markedly not only among the various disease forms but also among the various ethnic and racial groups worldwide [38,39]. These diseases tend to occur more often among young men who are in their late teens and early twenties and may start with features such as enthesitis (inflammatory lesions of the entheses, *ie*, sites of ligamentous of tendinous attachments to bone) or dactylitis oligoarthritis, and in some cases may progress to sacroiliitis and spondylitis, with or without extra-articular features such as acute anterior uveitis or mucocutaneous lesions [35,36]. The clinical features typical of the spondyloarthropathies may occur in different combinations so that the existing classification criteria may be inappropriate for a subset of such patients. For example, there are now well-defined HLA-B27–associated clinical syndromes such as seronegative oligoarthritis or polyarthritis (mostly affecting joints of the lower extremities), dactylitis, and enthesitis (plantar fascitis or calcaneal periostitis, Achilles tendonitis, and tenderness of tibial tubercles) [40]. The overall prevalence of this form of undifferentiated spondyloarthropathy may be higher than that of reactive arthritis in some parts of the world [32,40–42]. *Courtesy of Muhammad Asim Khan.*)

Clinical Features of Ankylosing Spondylitis

Skeletal
Axial arthritis, such as sacroiliitis and spondylitis
Arthritis of "girdle joints" (hips and shoulders)
Peripheral arthritis uncommon
Others: enthesopathy, osteoporosis, vertebral fractures,
    spondylodiscitis, pseudoarthrosis

Extraskeletal
Acute anterior uveitis
Cardiovascular involvement
Pulmonary involvement
Cauda equina syndrome
Enteric mucosal lesions
Amyloidosis

FIGURE 5-64.

Clinical features of ankylosing spondylitis. Ankylosing spondylitis is a chronic systemic inflammatory disorder of undetermined etiology, usually beginning in early adulthood, primarily affecting the axial skeleton (sacroiliitis being its hallmark), but can also exhibit some extra-articular features. Acute anterior uveitis is the most common extra-articular feature, occurring in 25% to 30% of patients. The prevalence of the disease generally varies with the prevalence of HLA-B27 gene in the population. Studies in Eurocaucasoid populations suggest that the disease prevalence in the adult population is close to 0.2% [34,35,37]. It is three times more common in males, and the clinical and radiographic features seem to evolve more slowly in females.

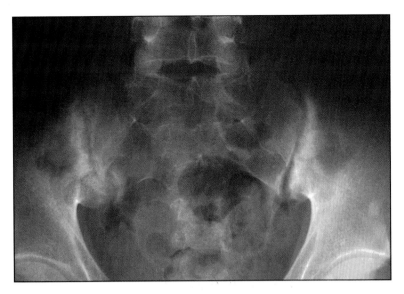

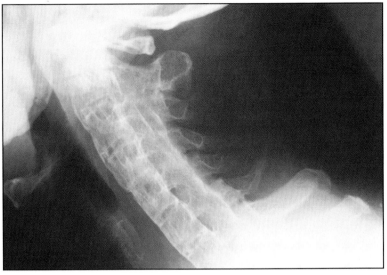

FIGURE 5-65.

Bilateral sacroiliitis. Anteroposterior radiographic view of the pelvis showing bilateral sacroiliitis in ankylosing spondylitis. There are erosions and blurring of the subchondral bone plate and reactive bone sclerosis that are more prominent on the iliac side of the joint. (*Courtesy of* Muhammad Asim Khan.)

FIGURE 5-66.

"Bamboo spine." This lateral view of the cervical spine shows a rigid and forward stooping cervical spine of a patient with severe ankylosing spondylitis for more than 35 years. The spine is completely ankylosed ("bamboo spine" due to syndesmophytes and fused facet [apophyseal] joints). Spinal osteoporosis is also present. Such patients are prone to spinal fracture. In fact, this patient had sustained lower cervical spine fracture that day and it could not be visualized on this radiograph. However, it was easily detected on a magnetic resonance imaging scan. (*Courtesy of* Muhammad Asim Khan.)

Salient Principles of Management of Ankylosing Spondylitis

No cure, but most patients can be well managed with NSAIDs

A concerned (primary) physician providing continuity of care; consultation as needed by a rheumatologist, ophthalmologist, orthopedist, etc.

Education of the patient about the disease to help increase compliance

Importance of daily exercises to preserve good posture and minimize limitation of chest expansion; swimming is the best exercise; appropriate sports and recreations; sleeping on firm mattress; avoiding pillows under the head, if possible; avoidance of smoking and prevention of spinal trauma

Supportive measures and counseling with regard to social, sexual, and vocational aspects; importance of patient support groups

Family counseling; thorough family history; physical examination of the relatives may disclose remarkable disease aggregation and many undiagnosed or misdiagnosed affected relatives in some families

Surgical measures: arthroplasty, correction of deformity, etc.

Early diagnosis is important, as is the early recognition and treatment of extraskeletal manifestations, such as acute anterior uveitis (iritis), and of the associated diseases or complications

---

FIGURE 5-67.

Management of ankylosing spondylitis. Most patients with ankylosing spondylitis can be well managed, even though there is currently no known method to cure or prevent the disease and there is no special diet or any specific food that has a role in its initiation or exacerbation. Aspirin seldom provides an adequate therapeutic response, but other nonsteroidal anti-inflammatory drugs (NSAIDs) are more helpful and should be used in full therapeutic anti-inflammatory doses during active phase of the disease. The patients should be informed about this because otherwise they may use the drugs occasionally and for their analgesic effect only. The responses by patients differ, as do the side effects, and it is worthwhile to search out the best alternative NSAID that works for each individual.

When the disease is not being adequately controlled by NSAIDs, or for those intolerant to such drugs, sulfasalazine may be effective in those with peripheral arthritis, but it has no appreciable influence on purely axial disease and on peripheral enthesitis [43]. Because of its efficacy in inflammatory bowel disease and psoriasis, sulfasalazine may be especially useful for ankylosing spondylitis associated with

those diseases. A few patients with severe ankylosing spondylitis with peripheral joint involvement unresponsive to NSAIDs and sulfasalazine have sometimes responded to oral methotrexate therapy [44,45]. D-Penicillamine is not effective, and antimalarial drugs and gold have not been well studied in ankylosing spondylitis. Oral corticosteroids have no therapeutic value in the long-term management of the musculoskeletal aspects of this disease because of their serious side effects, and they do not halt disease progression.

Recalcitrant enthesitis and persistent synovitis may respond to a local corticosteroid injection, and therapeutic contribution of injection into the sacroiliac joints is being evaluated [46]. There seems to be a consensus that spinal radiotherapy has no role in the modern management of patients with ankylosing spondylitis because of the high risk of leukemia and aplastic anemia. There are occasional uncontrolled reports of efficacy of low-dose external beam radiotherapy of persistent peripheral enthesitis and synovitis resistant to standard treatments.

(Continued)

FIGURE 5-67. (*CONTINUED*)

Splints, braces, and corsets are generally not helpful and are not advised. Pregnancy does not usually affect the disease symptoms, and fertility, course of pregnancy, and childbirth have been reported to be normal [47].

The patient should walk erect, keeping the spine as straight as possible and sleep on a firm mattress using as thin a pillow as possible. Physical activity that places prolonged strain on the back muscles, such as prolonged stooping or bending, should be avoided. Regular exercises are of fundamental importance in preventing or minimizing deformity. Spinal extension exercises and deep-breathing exercises should be done routinely once or twice daily, and smoking should be avoided. Formal physical therapy is of value especially in teaching the patient the proper posture, appropriate exercises, and recreational sports, and the need for maintaining the exercise program. Group exercise sessions that include hydrotherapy in warm water are helpful. Regular swimming is considered to be one of the best exercises for these patients. Some patients have difficulty driving their car because

of the impaired neck mobility, and they may find special wide-view mirrors to be helpful. Patient support groups enlist enthusiastic patient cooperation and provide information about the disease and advice about life and health insurance, jobs, working environment, wide-view mirrors, and other useful items.

Acute anterior uveitis requires prompt and vigorous treatment with dilation of the pupil and use of corticosteroid eyedrops. Systemic steroids or immunosuppressives may be needed for rare patients with severe refractory uveitis. The patient should be informed about the possibility of recurrences of acute iritis. Total hip arthroplasty gives very good results and prevents partial or total disability from severe hip disease. Vertebral wedge osteotomy may be needed for correction of severe kyphosis in some patients, although it carries a relatively high risk of paraplegia. Cardiac complications may require aortic valve replacement or pacemaker implantation. Apical pulmonary fibrosis and cavitation are not easy to manage; surgical resection may rarely be required. (*Adapted from* Khan *et al* [48].)

■ OSTEOPOROSIS

FIGURE 5-68.

Clinical features of osteoporosis. Patients with osteoporosis may have no warning signs until the first fracture occurs. Gradual height loss and dorsal kyphosis may result from microfractures or complete fractures of vertebral bodies. Acute back pain is caused by stretching of the periosteum, whereas chronic back pain derives from paraspinal muscles and other local soft tissues. Progressive thoracic kyphosis with encroachment of the ribs onto the pelvic brim may decrease the space available for abdominal contents and lead to gastrointestinal symptoms such as nausea and early satiety.

Clinical Features of Osteoporosis

May be asymptomatic

Height loss

Dorsal kyphosis

Back pain

Restrictive lung disease

Protuberant abdomen with early satiety

■ DISEASES OF BONE AND CONNECTIVE TISSUE

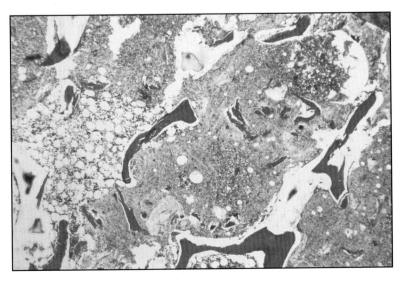

FIGURE 5-69.

Histopathology of osteoporosis. This hematoxylin and eosin-stained slide displays decreased bone mass from thinning of the trabeculae and loss of microarchitectural connectivity, the two cardinal features of osteoporosis. Both of these qualities lead to increased fragility of bone and a subsequent increase in fracture risk. There is also an increased number of fat cells seen among the marrow elements, a common finding as trabecular bone volume decreases with age. (*Courtesy of* Michael J. Maricic and Marcia Ko.)

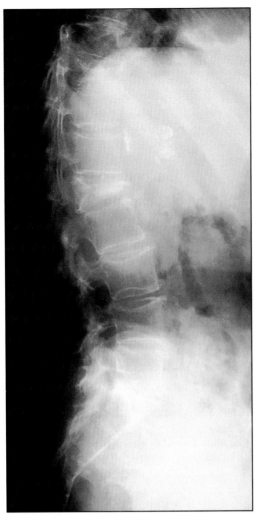

FIGURE 5-70.

Crush fracture, lumbar vertebra. Diffuse osteopenia and a crush fracture of L1 are present. Central end-plate deformities of L3 and L4 are also present. (*Courtesy of* Michael J. Maricic and Marcia Ko.)

Comparison of Available Bone Density Techniques

Site	DXA	QCT	pDXA	RA
Precision, %	1–2	2–4	1–2	1–2
Accuracy, %	3–5	5–15	2–5	5
Radiation dose, *uSv*	1–2	50	< 1	5

Note: Annual background radiation equals approximately 2000 uSv.

FIGURE 5-71.

Comparison of bone density tests. Dual energy x-ray absorptiometry (DXA) is currently considered the gold standard for measuring bone density because of its high precision and accuracy, low radiation, and ability to measure central sites such as the hip and spine [49]. Quantitative computed tomography (QCT) scans are able to discriminate trabecular bone better than the other techniques, which may be helpful in certain research applications. The radiation dose, however, is much higher than with other techniques. Peripheral techniques such as peripheral DXA (pDXA) and radiographic absorptiometry (RA) are highly precise and accurate. Their major limitation is their inability to measure central sites such as the hip and spine.

Bone mineral density as assessed by DXA has been able to predict the relative risk for future fracture of the hip and other bones. Large epidemiologic studies [50] have shown that for each 1 standard deviation (SD; approximately 10%) below a mean peak normal bone mass (T score on Hologic densitometer or young adult Z score on the Lunar), the risk of future spinal fracture is increased approximately twofold. The predictive value for low hip density is slightly higher at about 2.6-fold for each 1 SD decrease. When combined with a history of prevalent fracture after menopause (which by itself increases future fracture risk) there is a synergistic increase in future fracture risk. The major value of obtaining bone mineral density in patients is to determine whether the patient has osteopenia significant enough to result in a nontraumatic fracture, to assess the relative risk of future fracture, and to follow response to treatment. (*Courtesy of* Michael J. Maricic and Marcia Ko.)

WHO Criteria for Osteoporosis

Diagnosis	T Score
Normal	≥-1.0 SD
Osteopenia	-1.0 to -2.5 SD
Osteoporosis	≤ -2.5 SD
Severe osteoporosis	≤ -2.5 SD (with fragility fractures)

FIGURE 5-72.

Criteria for the diagnosis of osteoporosis. In 1993, a World Health Organization (WHO) consensus conference established criteria for the densitometric diagnosis of osteoporosis in postmenopausal women. A T score (comparison to peak normal mean bone density) above or better than -1 standard deviation (SD) is considered normal. A T score of worse than or below -2.5 SD represents osteoporosis. The intermediate category (between -1.0 and -2.5 SD) is labeled osteopenia, or low bone mass. (*Courtesy of* Michael J. Maricic and Marcia Ko.)

Indications for Bone Density Measurement

In estrogen-deficient women, to make decisions about therapy

In patients with vertebral abnormalities or radiographic osteopenia, to establish a diagnosis of osteoporosis

In patients receiving long-term glucocorticoid therapy, to diagnose low bone mass to adjust therapy

In patients with primary asymptomatic hyperparathyroidism, to diagnose low bone mass to identify those at risk of severe skeletal disease who may be candidates for surgical intervention

To monitor response to treatment

FIGURE 5-73.

Indications for bone density measurement. In general, bone density measurement should be performed only when it will influence therapeutic decisions. The results of bone density measurement have been shown to influence patient acceptance of hormone replacement therapy, and this would be the most common indication for its use. Dual energy x-ray absorptiometry (DXA) may also be extremely useful in the patient beginning long-term glucocorticoid use to categorize the patient's present risk of fracture and to aid in the tapering of glucocorticoids or the use of prophylactic agents. When using DXA to monitor response to treatment, because of the precision error of the test, only decreases of more than 5% should be considered significant for the purpose of changing treatment. (*Courtesy of* Michael J. Maricic and Marcia Ko.)

Nonpharmacologic Management of Osteoporosis

Patient education

Avoid smoking, excessive alcohol intake

Fall prevention intervention

Physical therapy

  Weight-bearing exercise

  Exercise to strengthen paraspinal muscles

  Balance and lower extremity strengthening

FIGURE 5-74.

Nonpharmacologic management of osteoporosis. Management of osteoporosis begins with patient education. Risk factor reduction such as avoidance of nicotine and alcohol are mandatory. Fall prevention includes avoiding drugs that may cause sedation or hypotension, checking the patient for proper vision and hearing, and avoiding obstacles in the home that may cause falls. Physical therapy should be given to all patients, even those who have not yet sustained a fracture. (*Courtesy of* Michael J. Maricic and Marcia Ko.)

Pharmacologic Therapies for Osteoporosis

Calcium

Vitamin D

Hormone replacement therapy

Calcitonin nasal spray

Bisphosphonates

SERMS

FIGURE 5-75.

Pharmacologic therapies for osteoporosis. Medical treatment for osteoporosis should always begin with vitamin D (400 to 800 IU/d) and calcium (1000 mg/d) for premenopausal women and women on hormone replacement therapy (HRT), and 1500 mg/d for estrogen-deficient women and older men. HRT is currently the standard for prevention and treatment because of its global health benefits. Calcitonin nasal spray (200 IU/d) and alendronate (5 mg/d for prevention or 10 mg/d for treatment) are useful alternatives in women who cannot or will not take HR. Other bisphosphonates have been approved more recently. Selective estrogen replacement modulators (SERMS) may play a significant role in osteoporosis in the near future. (*Courtesy of* Michael J. Maricic and Marcia Ko.)

Bacterial Arthritis: Which Organism to Suspect?

Organism	Age, y			
	< 2	2–15	16–50	> 50
Staphylococcus	40%	50%	15%	75%
Streptococcus	25%	35%	5%	10%
Haemophilus	30%	2%	—	—
Gonococcus	—	5%	75%	—
Gram-negative	3%	5%	5%	10%

FIGURE 5-76.

Bacterial arthritis. The demographics of the patient, especially age, can help to predict the organism causing septic arthritis. Nongonococcal infectious arthritis is usually monoarticular, most often affecting the large joints. Pain, often followed by swelling, is relatively abrupt in onset. Local signs of inflammation are usually present, although constitutional complaints can overshadow local features. Any delay in diagnosis and effective treatment can increase the likelihood and severity of joint damage, especially if the infection is with a virulent organism. First and foremost in the evaluation of such patients is analysis of the synovial fluid: culture, Gram stain (positive in 50%–75% of cases), cell count (10,000–30,000 cells/mm^3 early in the septic process; 50,000–100,000 cell/mm^3 later, usually with neutrophil predominance), glucose and protein determinations, and examination for intracellular crystals. The only contraindication to this rule is surrounding or overlying soft tissue infection; it is usually unwise to penetrate an area of cellulitis to tap a joint. Because cellulitis and bursitis do not penetrate an intact joint capsule, differentiating between these and septic arthritis is crucial (*see* Fig. 5-78). Blood cultures may be positive in up to 50% of patients with septic arthritis. Radiographs are normal in the earliest stages of septic arthritis, although they may be useful to rule out trauma and act as a baseline. Bone scans are positive in 4 to 7 days, but they are not specific and so are not especially useful except for sacroiliac joint infections, where the diagnosis may be obscure. (*Courtesy of* Leonard Sigal.)

Differential Diagnosis of Septic Arthritis

Periarthritis (periarticular inflammatory disease), *eg*, cellulitis, bursitis

Osteomyelitis

Trauma; disruption of internal structures, *eg*, meniscal or ligamentous tear; fracture

Crystal-induced inflammation, *eg*, monosodium urate (gout), calcium pyrophosphate dihydrate ("pseudogout")

Intra-articular hemorrhage: hemophilia or other bleeding disorders, hemorrhage may follow inapparent trauma

Viral—often polyarticular; often with a rash

Tuberculosis—chronic, monarthritis, insidious onset, minimal inflammatory changes (*see* section on mycobacteria)

Presentation of chronic rheumatologic disease, *eg*, Reiter's syndrome, rheumatoid arthritis

FIGURE 5-77.

Differential diagnosis of septic arthritis. When evaluating a patient with a painful and inflamed joint, when septic arthritis is a consideration, the processes listed would be included within the differential diagnosis. Spinal septic arthritis (septic diskitis) should be suspected in patients with chronic unrelenting back pain, fever, and marked local spine tenderness. Children with septic diskitis may present with no local pain, but refuse to walk. The thoracolumbar region is most commonly affected. The infection usually crosses the disk space on imaging studies, a finding that differentiates septic diskitis from malignancy. (*Courtesy of* Leonard Sigal.)

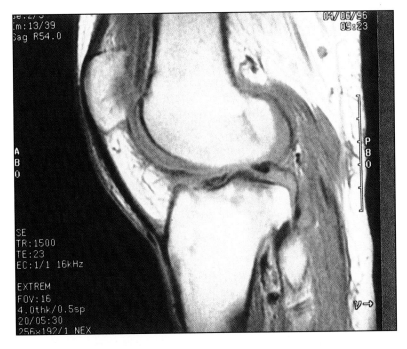

FIGURE 5-78.

Changes of septic arthritis on magnetic resonance imaging (MRI). The MRI of the right knee was performed on a 1.5 Tesla magnet. Synovial proliferation with internal debris is seen. Osseous structures demonstrate edema on both sides of the joint (most notable in the posterior aspect of the lateral tibial condyle), compatible with septic arthritis. Focal loculation of fluid seen between the tibial spines appears to be eroding bone and may represent focal erosion related to the septic arthritis. Similar changes also increased signal intensity within the posterior horn of the medial meniscus (shown here), extending to the inferior articular surface, and represents a complex tear. (*Courtesy of* Robert Epstein, MD.)

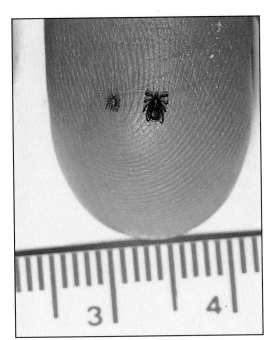

FIGURE 5-79.

Ixodes scapularis ticks. Nymph and adult specimens are shown on a normal finger, with a background scale drawn in centimeters for comparison. The etiologic agent of Lyme disease, *Borrelia burgdorferi*, was isolated from Ixodid ticks captured on Long Island and then grown from patient samples. Lyme disease is spread by the bite of infected Ixodid ticks: I. scapularis in the northeastern, southeastern, and midwestern United States (in the northeast previously called *Ixodid dammini*, but now thought to be identical with *I. scapularis*); *Ixodid pacificus* in California and Oregon; *Ixodid ricinus* in Europe; and *Ixodid persulcatus* in Asia. Ixodid ticks have a four-stage life cycle. The egg mass is laid in the leaf clutter at the base of the forest. Larvae hatch from the mass and, in the northeastern and midwestern regions, feed in the summer and fall, typically from *Peromyscus leucopus*, the white-footed field mouse, although other animals will do as well. Fewer than 1% of eggs are infected with *B. burgdorferi*; the spirochete is obtained with the initial blood meal. White-footed field mice maintain a persistent, although apparently asymptomatic, spirochetemia throughout their lives. Once the larval tick feeds, it falls off and after molting, it emerges in the early spring as a nymph. The nymph typically waits on a leaf of grass or low-lying shrub until something warm and exhaling carbon dioxide happens along; it will then grasp its potential host. The most common host of the nymph is a mouse, but other mammals, including dogs, cows, horses, humans, and birds, can also provide the blood meal. Once fed, the nymphs molt. Adults appear in the fall and winter, typically taking their blood meal from white-tailed deer (*Odocolieus virginianus*) or other large mammals.

The percentage of nymphs infected with the spirochete is only half that of adult ticks. Nonetheless, 90% or more of cases of Lyme disease are spread by nymphs because adults are less abundant, larger (found and removed more quickly and easily), and active at a time when fewer people are outside. The tick takes 24 hours or longer to attach. During that time *B. burgdorferi* lies dormant on the inner aspect of the tick's midgut. As the blood meal reaches the midgut, spirochetes proliferate and escape the gut, ultimately reaching the tick's salivary glands, where the excess water of the blood meal is passed back into the host along with the spirochete. (*Courtesy of* Leonard Sigal.)

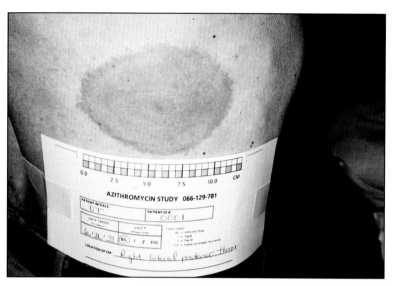

FIGURE 5-80.

Single erythema migrans. The hallmark of early localized Lyme disease, and the only pathognomonic finding, is erythema migrans. The rash occurs at the site of the tick bite (recalled by only about 30% of patients) a mean of 7 to 10 days (range, 1–30 days) after the

bite; most erythema migrans rashes are noted in the spring, summer, and early fall, as expected from the time nymphs are looking for their blood meal. Erythema migrans consists of an erythema expanding to a large circular or annular lesion, starting as a papule or macule, often with central clearing. It is typically found in the inguina, axilla, midriff, or behind the knee, the most common sites for tick bites. The rash is usually asymptomatic, but it may burn or itch and may be associated with a virus-like illness. The lesion may persist for 4 weeks before fading spontaneously.

The differential diagnosis of erythema migrans should include cellulitis, fixed drug eruption, tinea, plant dermatitis, granuloma annulare, and urticaria.

A transient erythema may develop at the site of a tick bite, within hours of the bite. Probably due to a reaction to components of the tick's saliva, this resolves within a day or two and should not be confused with erythema migrans. The bite of a spider (*eg,* brown recluse spider) is found on exposed skin and causes painful and rapidly expanding lesions that may undergo central necrosis.

An example of single erythema migrans is shown on the back with the appearance of a "bull's eye." The lesion occurred at the site of a tick bite and slowly spread over the course of a few days. (*Courtesy of* Leonard Sigal.)

Criteria for Positive Western Blot (Immunoblot) Analysis in the Serologic Confirmation of Infection With *Borrelia Burgdorferi* (*Lyme Disease*)		
Duration of Disease	**Isotype Tested**	**Bands to be Considered**
First few weeks of infection	IgM	Two of the following: ospC (23), 39, 41*
After first weeks of infection	IgG	Five of the following: 18, 21, 28, 30, 39, 41, 45, 58, 66, 93

* Alternate criteria for IgM reactivity, proposed by a Centers for Disease Control and Prevention conference.

FIGURE 5-81.

Criteria for positive Western blot (immunoblot) analysis in the serologic confirmation of infection with *Borrelia burgdorferi* (Lyme disease). The alternate criteria for IgM reactivity were proposed by the Centers for Disease Control and Prevention. IgM criteria should not be used in the confirmation of purported infection of more than a few weeks' duration. (*Criteria derived from* Dressler *et al.* [51].)

■ ARTHRITIS AND SYSTEMIC DISEASE

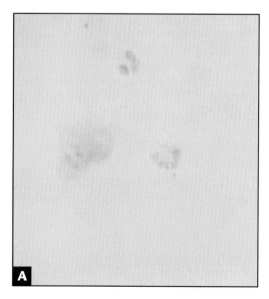

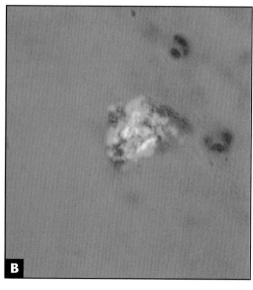

A   **B**

FIGURE 5-82.

Synovial fluid analysis in amyloid arthropathy. Synovial fluid analysis may often yield diagnostic findings in patients with amyloid arthropathy. The slide shows synovial fluid from a shoulder of a 64-year-old patient with primary amyloidosis. The sample of synovial fluid was prepared in a cytocentrifuge and stained with Congo red. **A,** Synovial fluid elements were examined with light microscopy. **B,** Polarized light microscopy reveals apple-green birefringence, which is diagnostic of amyloid [52].

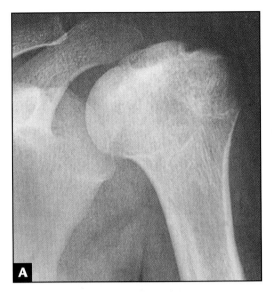

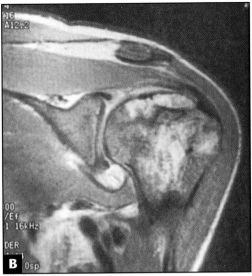

FIGURE 5-83.
Avascular necrosis of the shoulder in sickle cell disease. **A,** Radiograph and **B,** magnetic resonance imaging scan of left shoulder. The most common arthropathy in patients with sickle cell anemia is related to avascular necrosis of subchondral bone. Hip and shoulder involvement are most common [53]. (*Courtesy of* Thomas H. Berquist.)

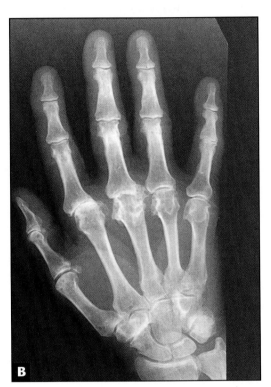

FIGURE 5-84.
Arthropathy associated with hemochromatosis. In hemochromatosis, degenerative changes at metacarpophalangeal joints are common. Beak-type osteophytes in this location are distinctive. Chondrocalcinosis of the wrist is also present. (*Courtesy of* William W. Ginsburg.)

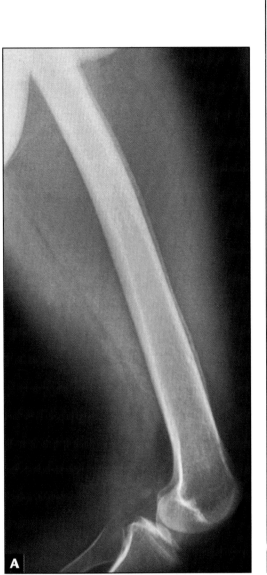

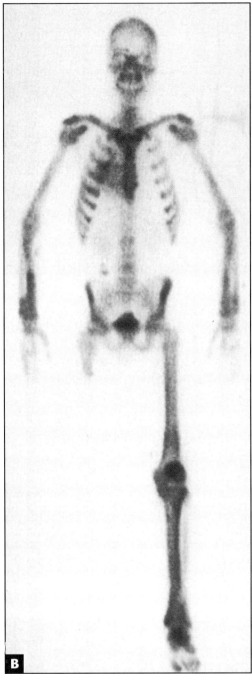

FIGURE 5-85.

Hypertrophic osteoarthropathy secondary to pulmonary metastatic osteogenic sarcoma. The 20-year-old patient presented with cough and chest pain 7 years after right above-the-knee amputation for osteogenic sarcoma of the distal femur. **A,** Plain radiograph of left femur revealed extensive, smooth, lamellated periosteal new bone formation, consistent with hypertrophic osteoarthropathy. **B,** The bone scan on the left shows mild, irregular increased uptake involving the left femur and tibia as well as the distal humeri and radii. The right lung uptake reflects the metastatic involvement. A chest radiograph revealed a large mass in the right midlung (not shown). (*Courtesy of* Thomas H. Berquist.)

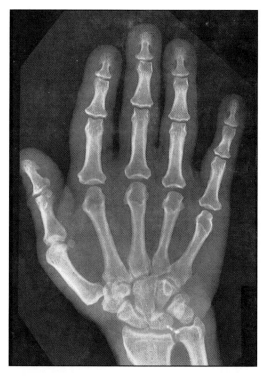

FIGURE 5-86.
Acromegaly. Hand radiograph. Joint space widening is present owing to stimulation of cartilage growth by excess growth hormone. An increase in soft tissue density and spadelike deformity of the distal tufts is also seen. (Courtesy of Thomas H. Berquist)

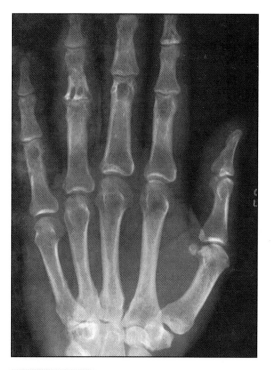

FIGURE 5-87.
Osseous lesions in chronic sarcoidosis. Hand radiograph. Chronic sarcoid arthritis is characterized by a persistent or remitting polyarthritis, often with dactylitis. Cutaneous lesions are often present. Synovial biopsy reveals characteristic granulomas. Although generally nonerosive, the association with osseous lesions may lead to destructive, often cystic, bony changes [54]. (Courtesy of Thomas H. Berquist.)

■ REFERENCES

1. Firestein GS: Etiology and pathogenesis of rheumatoid arthritis. In *Textbook of Rheumatology*, edn 5. Edited by Kelley WN, Harris ED, Rudy S, Sledge CB. Philadelphia: WB Saunders; 1997:851–897.

2. Ad Hoc Committee on Clinical Guidelines: Guidelines for the initial evaluation of the adult patient with acute musculoskeletal symptoms. *Arthritis Rheum* 1996, 39:1–8.

3. Mitchell DM: Rheumatoid arthritis. In *Rheumatoid Arthritis: Epidemiology, Etiology, Diagnosis and Treatment.* Edited by Utsinger PO, Zvaifler NJ, Ehrlich GE. Philadelphia: JB Lippincott; 1985:133–150

4. Turesson C, O'Fallon WM, Matteson EL, *et al.*: Occurrence of extraarticular disease manifestations is associated with excess mortality in a population-based cohort of patients with rheumatoid arthritis [submitted].

5. Schumacher HR Jr, Reginato AJ: *Atlas of Synovial Fluid Analysis and Crystal Identification.* Philadelphia: Lea & Febiger; 1991.

6. Ad Hoc Subcommittee on Clinical Guidelines for the management of rheumatoid arthritis. *Arthritis Rheum* 1996, 39:713–722.

7. Haverson PB: Calcium crystal-associated diseases. *Curr Opin Rheumatol* 1996, 8:259–265.

8. Hugher GRV: Systemic lupus erythematosus. In *Connective Tissue Diseases*, edn 4. Edited by Hughers GRV. Oxford: Blackwell Scientific Publications; 1994:4–74.

9. Khamashta MA, Mackworth-Young C: Antiphospholipid (Hughes) syndrome—a treatable cause of recurrent pregnancy loss. *Br Med J* 1997, 314:244.

10. Hunt BJ, Khamashta MA: Managemnet of the Hughes syndrome. *Clin Exp Rheumatol* 1996, 14:115-117.

11. Grau JM, Casademont J, Urbano-Marquez A: Polymyositis-dermatomyositis. In *Autoimmune Connective Tissue Disease.* Edited by Kamashta MA, Font J, Hughes GRV. Barcelona: Doyma; 1993:73–84.

12. LeRoy EC, Black C, Fleischmajer R, *et al.*: Scleroderma (systemic sclerosis): classification, subsets and pathogenesis. *J Rheumatol* 1988, 15:202–205.

13. Lie J: Nomenclature and classification of vasculitis: Plus ca change, plus c'est la mème chose. *Arthritis Rheum* 1994, 37:181–186.

14. Guillevin L, Lhote F, Amouroux J, Gheradi R, *et al.*: Antineutrophil cytoplasmic antibodies, abnormal angiograms and pathological findings in polyarteritis nodosa and Churg-Strauss syndrome: indications for the classification of vasculitides of the polyarteritis nodosa group. *Br J Rheumatol* 1996, 35:958–964.

15. Jennette JC, Falk RJ, Andrassy K, *et al.*: Nomenclature of systemic vasculitides. Proposal of an international consensus conference. *Arthritis Rheum* 1994, 37:187–192.

16. Lhote F, Guillevin L: Polyarteritis nodosa, microscopic polyangiitis, and Churg-Strauss syndrome. Clinical aspects and treatment. *Rheum Dis Clin North Am* 1995, 21:911–947.

17. Walton E: Giant-cell granuloma of respiratory tract (Wegener's granulomatosis). *Br Med J* 1958, 2:265.

18. Cordier JF, Valeyre D, Guillevin L, *et al.*: Pulmonary Wegener's granulomatosis. A clinical and imaging study of 77 cases. *Chest* 1990, 97:906–912.

19. Hoffman GS, Kerr GS, Leavitt RY, *et al.*: Wegener granulomatosis: an analysis of 158 patients. *Ann Intern Med* 1992, 116:488–498.

20. Anderson G, Coles ET, Crane M, *et al.*: Wegener's granuloma. A series of 265 British cases seen between 1975 and 1985. A report by a sub-committee of the British Thoracic Society Research Committee. *Q J Med* 1992, 83:427–438.

21. Arend W, Michel B, Block D, *et al.*: The American College of Rheumatology 1990 criteria for the classification of Takayasu arteritis. *Arthritis Rheum* 1990, 33:1129–1234.

22. Hata A, Noda M, Moriwaki R, Numano F: Angiographic findings of Takayasu's arteritis: new classification. *Int J Cardio* 1996, 54:S155–S163.

23. Godeau P, Aubert I, Guillevin L, *et al.*: Aspect clinique, évolution et prognostic de las maladie de Horton. *Ann Med Interne (Paris)* 1982, 133:393–400.

24. Smith CA, Fidler WI, Pinals RS: The epidemiology of giant ell arteritis. Report of a 10-year study in Shelby County, Tennessee. *Arthritis Rheum* 1983, 26:1214.

25. Machado EB, Michet CT, Ballard DJ, *et al.*: Trends in incidence and clinical presentation of temporal arteritis in Olmstead County, Minnesota, 1950–85. *Arthritis Rheum* 1988, 31:745–749.

26. Varin J, Guillot de Suduiratut C, Muffat-Joly M, *et al.*: Aspects clinques et épidémiologiques do la maladie de Horton selon le mileu de recrutement, ophtalmologique ou de Médecine Interne. *Ann Mé Interne (Paris)* 1994, 145:398–404.

27. Brouet JC, Clauvel JP, Danon F, *et al.*: Biologic and clinical significance of cryoglobulins. A report of 86 cases. *Am J Med* 1974, 57(5):775–788.

28. Gorevic PD, Kassab HJ, Levo Y, *et al.*: Mixed cryoglobulinemia: clinical aspects and long-term follow-up of 40 patients. *Am J Med* 1980, 69(2):287–308.

29. Ferri C, Marzo E, Longombardo G, *et al.*: Interferon-alpha in mixed cryoglobulinemia patients—A randomized, crossover-controlled trial. *Blood* 1993, 81:1132–1136.

30. Cohen P, Nguyen QT, Deny P, *et al.*: Treatment of mixed cryoglobulinemia with recombinant interferon alpha and adjuvant therapies. A prospective study on 20 patients. *Ann Med Interne (Paris)* 1996;147(2):81–86.

31. Guillebin L, Lhote F, Cohen P, *et al.*: Polyarteritis nodosa related to hepatits B virus. A prospective study with long-term observation of 41 patients. *Medicine (Baltimore)* 1995, 74:238–253.

32. Gross WL: New developments in the treatment of systemic vasculitis. *Curr Opin Rheumatol* 1994, 6:11–19.

33. Guillevin L, Lhote F, Gayraud M, *et al.*: Prognostic factors is polyarteritis nodosa and Churg-Strauss syndrome. A prospective study in 342 patients. *Medicine (Baltimore)* 1996, 75:17–28.

34. Khan MA, ed: Ankylosing spondylitis and related spondyloarthropathies. *Spine: State of the Art Reviews* Philadelphia: Hanley & Belfus; 1990:

35. Khan MA, ed: Spondyloarthropathies. *Rheum Dis Clin North Am* 1992, 18:1–276.

36. Richens J, McGill PE: The spondyloarthropathies. *Baillieres Clin Rheumatol* 1995, 9:95–109.

37. van der Linder S: Ankylosing spondylitis. In *Textbook of Rheumatolgoy*, edn 5. Edited by Kelly WN, Harris ED, Ruddy S, Sledge CB. Philadelphia: WB Saunders; 1996:969–982.

38. Zeidler H, Mau W, Khan MA: Undifferentiated spondyloarthropathies. *Rheum Dis Clin North Am* 1992, 18:187–202.

39. Khan MA: Ankylosing spondylitis: Clinical features. In *Rheumatology*, edn 2. Edited by Klippel JH, Dieppe PA. London: Mosby-Wolfe; 1994:3.25.1–3.25.10.

40. Khan MA: HLA-B27 and its subtypes in world populations. *Curr Opin Rheumatol* 1995, 7:263–269.

41. Carlos Lopez-Larrea, ed: *HLA-B27 in the Development of Spondyloarthropathies*. Austin, TX: Chapman & Hall (RG Landes Company); 1997.

42. Burgos-Vargos R, Vasquez-Mellado J: The early clinical recognition of juvenile-onset ankylosing spondylitis and its differentiation from juvenile rheumatoid arthritis. *Arthritis Rheum* 1995, 22:899–903.

43. Khan MA: Medical and surgical treatment of spondyloarthropathies. *Curr Opin Rheumatol* 1990, 2:592–599.

44. Toivanen A, Khan MA: Therapeutic dilemma in ankylosing spondylitis and related spondylarthropathies. *Rheum Rev* 1994, 3:21–27.

45. Lehtinen A, Lerisalo-Repo M, Taavisainen M: Persistence of enthesopathic changes in patients with spondylarthropathy during a six month follow-up. *Clin Exp Rheumatol* 1995, 13:733–736.

46. Lehtinen A, Lerisalo-Repo M, Taavisainen M: Persistence of enthesopathic changes in patients with spondylarthropathy during a six month follow-up. *Clin Exp Rheumatol* 1995, 13:733–736.

47. Gran JT, Husby G: Ankylosing spondylitis in women. *Semin Arthritis Rheum* 1990, 19:303–312.

48. Khan MA, Skosey JR: Ankylosing spondylitis and related spondyl-arthropathies. In *Immunological Diseases*, edn 4. Edited by Samter M, Talmage DW, Frank MM, *et al.*: Boston: Little, Brown; 1988:1509–1538.

49. Miller PD, Bonnick SL, Rosen CJ, *et al.*: Clinical utility of bone mass measurement in adults: consensus of an international panel. *Sem Arthritis Rheum* 1996, 25:361–372.

50. Ross PF, Davis JW, Epstein RS, Wasnich RD: Pre-existing fractures and bone mass predict vertebral fracture incidence in women. *Ann Intern Med* 1991, 114:919–923.

51. Dressler F, Whalen JA, Reinhardt BN, Steere AC: Western blotting in the serodiagnosis of Lyme disease. *J Infect Dis* 1993, 167:392–400.

52. Lakhanpal S, Li CY, Getz MA, *et al.*: Synovial fluid analysis for diagnosis of amyloid arthropathy. *Arthritis Rheum* 1987, 30:419–423.

53. David HG, Bridgman SA, Davies SC, *et al.*: The shoulder in the sickle-cell disease. *J Bone Joint Surg Br* 1993, 75:538–545.

54. Totemchokchyakarn K, Ball GV: Sarcoid arthropathy. *Bull Rheum Dis* 1997, 46(3):3–5.

Allergy and Immunology

PHILLIP L. LIEBERMAN

Allergic diseases, especially those of the skin, lend themselves quite readily to pictorial representation. This chapter takes advantage of this fact and presents figures in several areas: rhinitis, sinusitis, allergic diseases of the eye, allergic diseases of the skin, insect stings and bites, and vasculitis.

Most of the figures are illustrative of the physical signs accompanying allergic disease of these organs. They are intended to point out to the viewer instructive differential diagnostic features and facilitate the diagnosis and therefore the management of the disorders represented.

The section on rhinitis emphasizes the importance of an adequate nasal examination. This cannot be accomplished without the use of a nasal speculum, and is best accomplished with a speculum plus a very strong source of light such as a head mirror.

The diagnosis and management of sinusitis have been revolutionized with the development of computed tomography (CT) scanning and functional endoscopic surgery. Therefore, the images of sinus disease contained in this chapter include a comparison of a CT scan with a routine radiograph. In addition, the effects of functional endoscopic surgery are depicted.

The physical examination of the eye and the differential diagnosis of eye disease involving the conjunctiva are often neglected in the training of primary care physicians. The figures and text collected for this chapter are intended to enhance the skills of the primary care physician related to the diagnosis and differential diagnosis of conditions affecting the conjunctiva.

Perhaps allergic skin disease most readily lends itself to pictorial review. Therefore, included in this chapter are examples of urticarias, contact dermatitis, and mastocytosis.

There are very few resources in medicine that discuss and illustrate insect bites and stings. This chapter contains vivid illustrations of the insects responsible for human disease with their bites and stings. It also contains representative figures showing the cutaneous results of such bites and stings.

Differential Diagnosis Between Allergic and Nonallergic Rhinitis

Manifestation	Allergic Rhinitis	Chronic Nonallergic Rhinitis
Age of onset	Usually before age 20 years	Usually after age 30 years
Seasonality	Usually with seasonal variation; spring, fall	Usually perennial but not infrequently worse during weather changes such as those occurring during fall and early spring
Exacerbating factors	Allergen exposure	Irritant exposure, weather conditions
Nature of symptoms		
Pruritus	Common	Rare
Congestion	Common	Common
Sneezing	Prominent	Usually not prominent but can be dominant in some cases
Postnasal drainage	Not prominent	Prominent
Other related manifestations (eg, allergic conjunctivitis, atopic dermatitis)	Often present	Absent
Family history	Usually present	Usually absent
Physical appearance	Variable; classically described as pale, boggy, swollen; may appear normal	Variable, erythematous
Ancillary studies	Allergy skin test results always positive	Allergy skin test results negative
Nasal eosinophilia	Usually present	Present 15% to 20% of the time (nonallergic rhinitis with eosinophilia)
Peripheral eosinophilia	Often present, especially during allergy season	Absent

FIGURE 6-1.

Differential diagnosis between allergic and nonallergic rhinitis. Although it is commonly thought that all rhinitis is "allergic," this is not true. In fact, in an adult population, perhaps 50% of people with chronic symptoms of rhinitis have no allergy whatsoever. Therefore, it is important to make a distinction between allergic and chronic nonallergic rhinitis. The treatment of these two disorders differs.

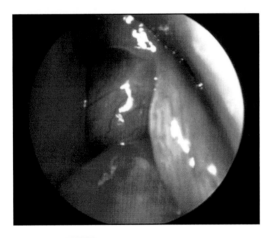

FIGURE 6-2.

Nasal polyps. Nasal polyps occur in patients with chronic rhinitis and in children with cystic fibrosis. They can usually be distinguished from normal nasal turbinates by their color. They have a gunmetal-gray or bluish-gray tint. They are also distinguished from turbinates because they are mobile when touched with a cotton-tipped applicator and manipulation does not cause pain (turbinates are immobile and manipulation produces pain). This figure shows a typical nasal polyp behind the turbinate [1].

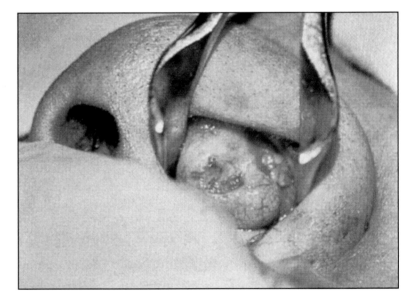

FIGURE 6-3.

Surgical removal of nasal polyp. Surgical removal is often necessary for the therapy of nasal polyps. Polyps can also be shrunk medically (using medical polypectomy) with corticosteroids. (*From* Lieberman *et al.* [2]; with permission.)

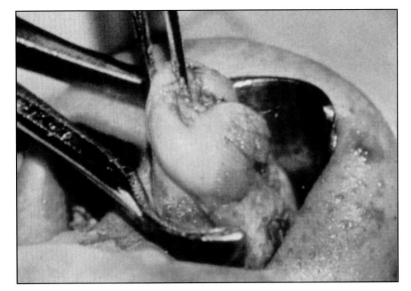

FIGURE 6-4.

Surgical removal of nasal polyp in an aspirin-sensitive asthmatic. This is the same procedure seen in Figure 6-3 in a more advanced stage of removal. (*From* Lieberman *et al.* [3]; with permission.)

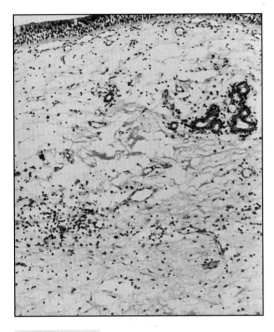

FIGURE 6-5.

Histology of nasal polyps. Photomicrograph of a nasal polyp revealing edema fluid, pseudostratified epithelium, and an inflammatory cell infiltrate. Polyps are repositories of inflammatory mediators, such as leukotrienes and histamine. In patients with allergic nasal disease, exposure to allergen causes release of these mediators and therefore exacerbates symptoms. Most patients with polyps have marked eosinophilia of their nasal secretions. Any patient with nasal polyps should be warned about the possibility of nonsteroidal anti-inflammatory drug (NSAID) sensitivity, since such patients are at increased risk of developing wheezing and rhinitis after ingestion of NSAIDs. (*Courtesy of* Raymond G. Slavin.)

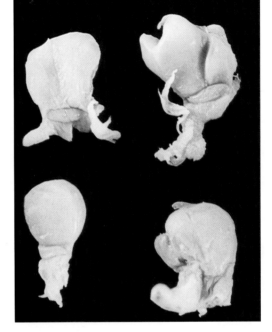

FIGURE 6-6.

Nasal polyps after removal. All four of these were removed from the same patient. (*Courtesy of* Raymond G. Slavin.)

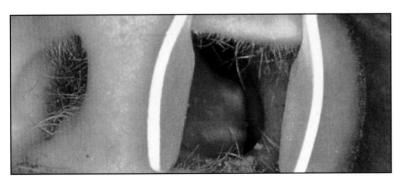

FIGURE 6-7.

Severe nasal septal deviation. In this instance, the septum is deviated to the left and obstructs approximately 80% to 90% of the nasal airways. (*From* Bull [4]; with permission.)

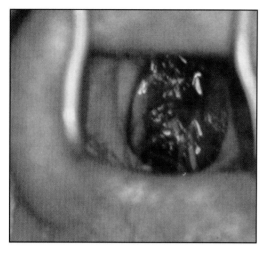

FIGURE 6-8.
Nasal tumor. Pigmentation of any polypoid structure or a polyp that bleeds should arouse suspicion of a nasal carcinoma or a malignant granuloma. These are usually unilateral, as opposed to polyps, which are usually bilateral. Both are associated with sinusitis. In nasal polyps, the sinusitis usually involves several sinuses; in nasal tumors, there is usually unilateral involvement of the maxillary or ethmoid sinus on the same side as the tumor. Although bleeding is a hallmark of nasal tumors, polyps are not usually associated with bleeding. (*From* Bull [4]; with permission.)

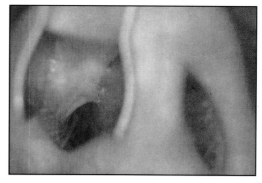

FIGURE 6-9.
Synechia formed between the turbinates and the septum following nasal trauma. Such synechia can occur as complications of septoplasties. They are usually easily visible on anterior nasal examination. (*From* Bull [4]; with permission.)

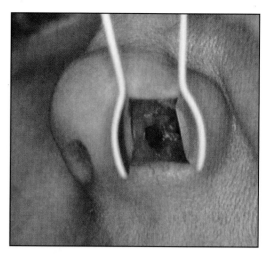

FIGURE 6-10.
Nasal septal perforation. Septal perforations produce alterations in nasal air flow, and thus patients often perceive nasal obstruction [1]. Many perforations fail to produce any symptoms whatsoever. However, patients often notice nasal bleeding occurring at the edges of the perforation. Perforations can be due to the use of nasal sprays or cocaine. (*From* Bull [4]; with permission.)

■ SINUSITIS

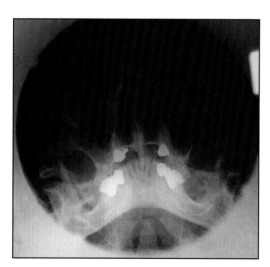

FIGURE 6-11.
Sinus radiograph showing haziness of the left maxillary antrum and bilateral muco-periosteal thickening of both maxillary antra. (*Courtesy of* Raymond G. Slavin.)

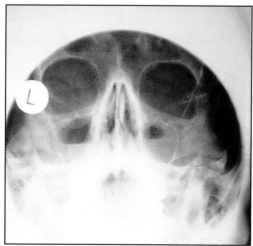

FIGURE 6-12.
Sinus radiograph demonstrating bilateral air fluid levels in both maxillary antra. (*Courtesy of* Raymond G. Slavin.)

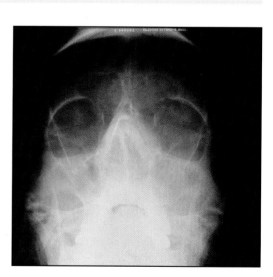

FIGURE 6-13.
Radiograph showing bilateral maxillary opacification with thickening of the mucosa. The thickening of the mucosa seen in this instance indicates a chronic hyperplastic process and is distinguished from the acute air fluid levels seen in Figure 6-11. (*Courtesy of* Raymond G. Slavin.)

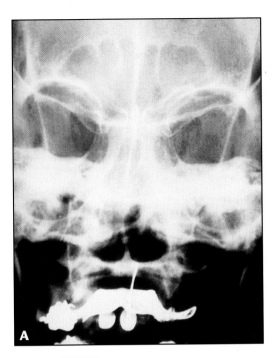
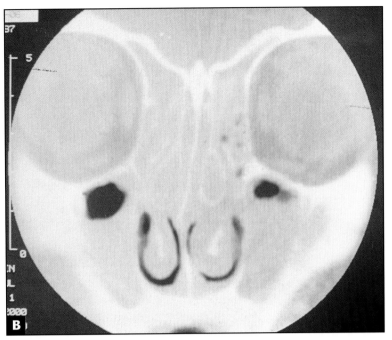

FIGURE 6-14.

Diagnosis of sinusitis. Comparison of a sinus radiograph (**A**) with a computed tomography (CT) scan (**B**) for diagnosis of sinusitis. Even though the ethmoid sinuses appear normal on the radiograph, they appear opacified on the CT scan. CT scans are far superior to radiographs for diagnosing sinusitis.

CT scanning has revolutionized the diagnosis of sinusitis. This is especially true for the diagnosis of ethmoid and sphenoid sinusitis. However, maxillary sinusitis can also be present on CT scan and absent on sinus radiograph. CT scans have altered our conception of the pathogenesis and frequency of sinusitis. For example, it was once thought that since pathology of the maxillary sinuses could be seen more easily on radiographs, they were the most common sinuses to be affected by sinusitis. However, with the advent of CT scans, it was learned that ethmoid involvement rivals that of the maxillary sinuses and may be the most common sinus involved, especially in children. (*Courtesy of* Raymond G. Slavin.)

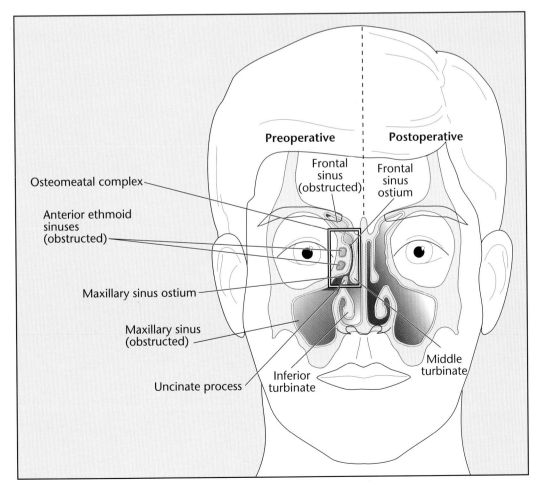

FIGURE 6-15.

The osteomeatal complex. The maxillary, ethmoid, and frontal sinusitis are seen on the *left*. Functional endoscopic surgery (*right*) removes the uncinate process, enlarging the maxillary ostium; exonerates the anterior ethmoids; and enlarges the frontal ostium. (*Adapted from* Lockey [5].)

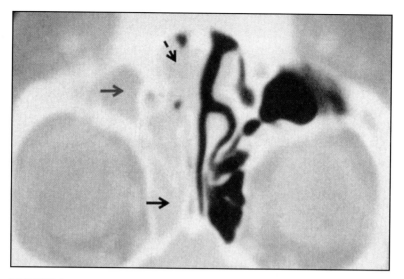

FIGURE 6-16.

The ostiomeatal complex in a patient with nasal polyposis and opacification of the left frontal and ethmoid sinuses (*solid black arrow*), left maxillary sinus (*red arrow*), and nasal passage (*dashed black arrow*). (*From* Lockey [5]; with permission.)

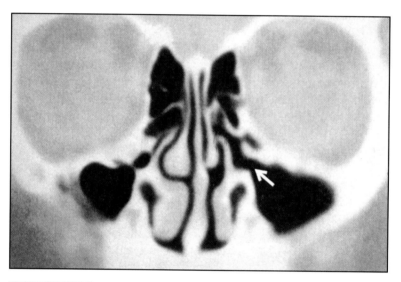

FIGURE 6-17.

The same patient seen in Figure 6-16 10 days after therapy with glucocorticosteroids. The *white arrow* indicates an open maxillary sinus ostium and ostiomeatal complex. (*From* Lockey [5]; with permission.)

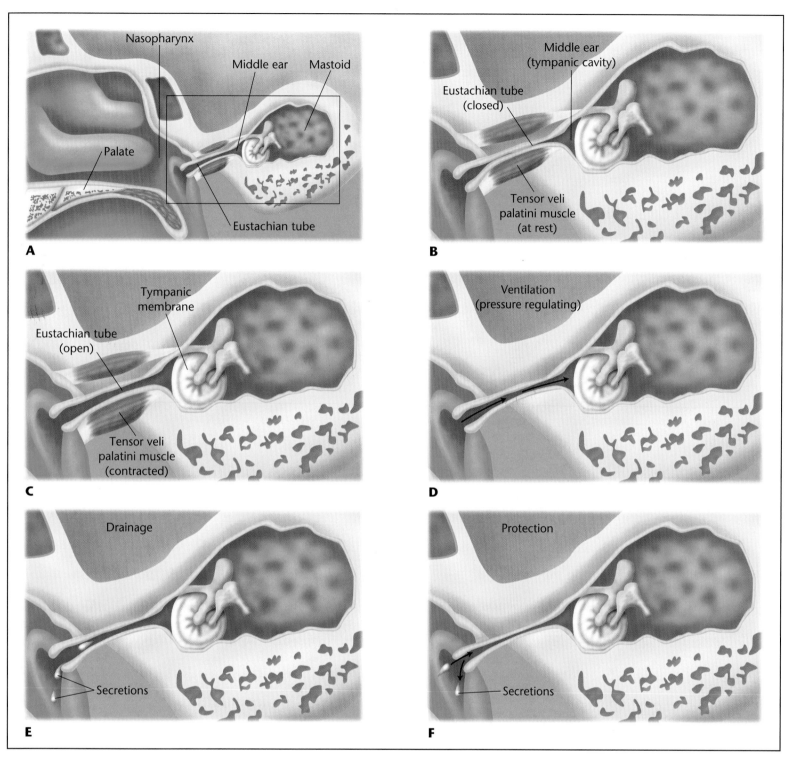

FIGURE 6-18.

Role of eustachian tube dysfunction in the development of otitis media. The eustachian tube connects the middle ear and the nasopharynx, and its function is partially controlled by the tensor veli palatini muscle. When the muscle is at rest, the tube is almost always closed. When the muscle contracts during swallowing, yawning, or crying, the tube opens. Functions of the eustachian tube include ventilation of the middle ear to regulate pressure, drainage, and clearance of middle ear secretions and protection of the middle ear from nasopharyngeal secretions. The use of animal models has documented that experimental obstruction of the eustachian tube results in middle ear underpressures and middle ear effusion by transudation, which are hallmark features of otitis media [6].

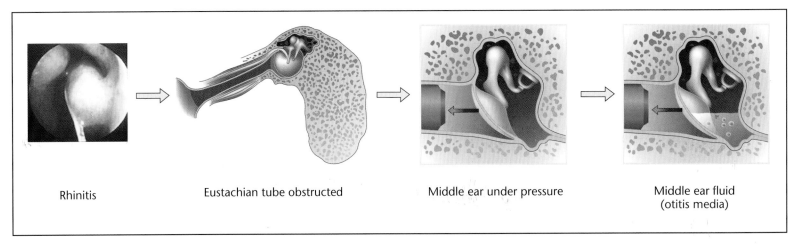

Rhinitis | Eustachian tube obstructed | Middle ear under pressure | Middle ear fluid (otitis media)

FIGURE 6-19.

Role of allergic rhinitis in the development of otitis media. Several lines of evidence support the hypothesis that allergic rhinitis contributes to the development of otitis media. Allergic rhinitis has been shown to be present in approximately 50% of patients in whom otitis media with effusion was diagnosed, and otitis media with effusion has been shown to be present in approximately 20% of patients in whom allergic rhinitis was diagnosed [6]. Elevations of IgE and inflammatory mediators released during IgE-mediated degranulation reactions, including prostaglandin D_2, tryptase, histamine, eosinophil products, and cytokines, have been detected in middle ear effusions of children with otitis media. Experimental histamine and allergen inhalation by allergic subjects has been shown to result in both early (within 30 minutes) and late (2 to 12 hours post challenge)

eustachian tube dysfunction. The results of this laboratory model were confirmed in a natural history model, in which untreated grass-allergic subjects followed during grass pollen season also developed eustachian tube dysfunction. A similar study showed the development of middle ear underpressures during pollen season [6]. Despite the confirmed phenomenon of allergen-induced eustachian tube dysfunction and middle ear underpressures, conclusive evidence of allergen-induced middle ear fluid has not been forthcoming in either human or animal models. However, it is conceivable that an interaction between allergy and viral upper respiratory infections may play a role in predisposing to otitis media in patients with allergic rhinitis. This possibility is strengthened by the regular, extensive overlap between respiratory viral and allergen seasons.

Respiratory virus

Increased eustachian tube obstruction
Abnormal immune/ inflammatory response

FIGURE 6-20.

Role of viruses in the development of otitis media. The most well-supported immediate cause of otitis media is a preceding or concurrent viral upper respiratory infection. Indeed, otitis media is one of the most frequent complications of viral upper respiratory infections, with epidemiologic studies documenting that more than 50% of new episodes of otitis media are diagnosed immediately after or concurrent with a viral upper respiratory infection [7–10]. A causal relationship between the two disorders was documented in experimental studies. Using an adult experimental model of infection, otitis media has been observed as a complication of rhinovirus and influenza virus in approximately 3% and 20% of subjects, respectively [11]. In those studies, there was a sequential development of nasal inflammation, impaired eustachian tube function, abnormal middle ear pressures, and the development of otitis media. In clinical studies, a significantly lesser incidence of acute otitis media was reported for infants and children immunized with an influenza virus vaccine compared with nonimmunized controls during a seasonal influenza epidemic [12].

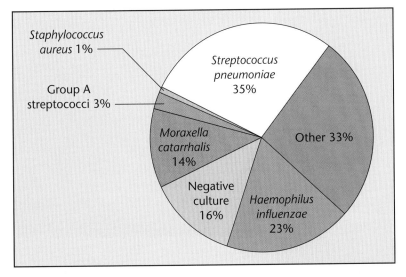

FIGURE 6-21.

Distribution of bacterial pathogens in otitis media. Bacteria are frequently isolated from middle ear fluids of children with otitis media, and less frequently from children with chronic otitis media [13]. The bacteriology of acute otitis media in adults is very similar to that in children. A number of bacteria cultured from middle ear aspirates have developed mechanisms of resistance against commonly employed antimicrobial agents [14]. Certain strains of *Haemophilus influenzae* and *Moraxella catarrhalis* produce the enzyme capable of degrading the β-lactam ring of penicillin-like antibiotics. Penicillin-resistant *Streptococcus pneumoniae* is also recognized as an increasingly significant and geographically variable problem. (*Adapted from* McBride [15].)

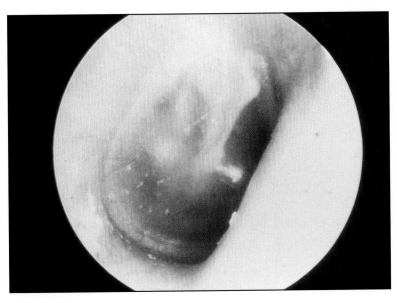

FIGURE 6-22.

Normal tympanic membrane. The tympanic membrane is thin, translucent, neutrally positioned, and mobile. The ossicles, particularly the malleus, are easily visualized. (*From* McBride [15]; with permission.)

FIGURE 6-23.

Acute otitis media with air fluid levels. Bubbles formed by the presence of both air and fluid and separated by grayish-yellow menisci are readily visible. The combination of this finding, along with fever and otalgia, is consistent with an acute infection. (*From* McBride [15]; with permission.)

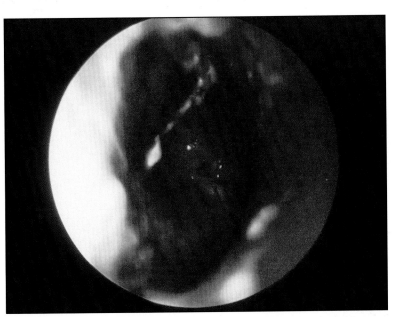

FIGURE 6-24.

Acute otitis media with perforation. Increased middle ear pressure associated with acute otitis media may result in perforation of the tympanic membrane. The tympanic membrane is erythmatous and thickened. Acute otorrhea through a perforation of the tympanic membrane is common. (*From* McBride [15]; with permission.)

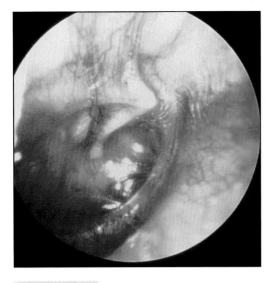

FIGURE 6-25.

Chronic otitis media with effusion. The tympanic membrane is retracted and thickened. A clear, yellow effusion is visible behind the tympanic membrane. Mobility is decreased. Patients with chronic otitis media with effusion are not acutely ill but often have decreased hearing. (*From* McBride [15]; with permission.)

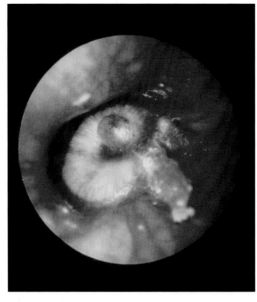

FIGURE 6-26.

Tympanosclerosis. Scarring and thickening of the tympanic membrane are common sequelae of recurrent acute or chronic otitis media. If large, tympanosclerosis may cause a mild conductive hearing loss. (*From* McBride [15]; with permission.)

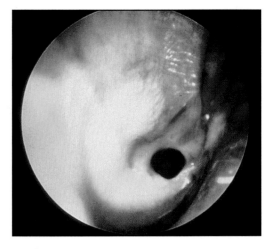

FIGURE 6-27.

Chronic perforation. Chronic perforation of the tympanic membrane is another sequela of recurrent acute or chronic otitis media; it may persist after tympanostomy tubes have been extruded. This tympanic membrane is also markedly thickened and scarred in a large arc. A large perforation may interfere with hearing. An opening in the tympanic membrane may allow water to enter the middle ear during bathing and swimming, which could cause infection with discharge from the ear. (*From* McBride [15]; with permission.)

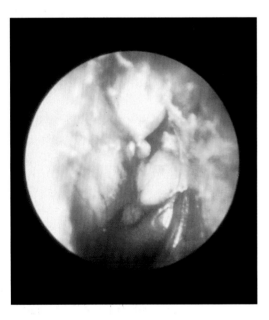

FIGURE 6-28.

Cholesteatoma. A cholesteatoma is the most common and one of the most serious mass lesions of the tympanic membrane [16]. It is an accumulation of desquamated epithelium or keratin that often appears as a white mass behind or involving the tympanic membrane; it may be congenital or acquired. The acquired type is commonly caused by recurrent acute or chronic otitis media, but can also be iatrogenic (after tympanostomy tube placement or other procedures). Cholesteatoma can enlarge and erode the bone, including the ossicles, causing hearing loss. They can also become infected, leading to a foul-smelling discharge from the ear. A cholesteatoma needs to be removed surgically. The recurrence rate is high, which necessitates long-term follow-up. (*From* McBride [15]; with permission.)

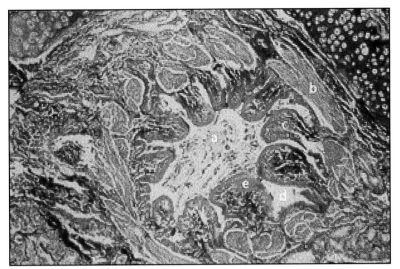

FIGURE 6-29.

Pathologic features of the asthmatic airway. This postmortem specimen depicts most of the characteristic features of an asthmatic airway caused by chronic inflammation. Hypertrophied and hyperplastic smooth muscle, mucosal edema, and increased mucus secretion contribute to the bronchoconstriction. Thickening of basement membrane and subepithelial fibrosis decreases the usual elasticity of the airway, leading to ineffective bronchodilation with treatment. These structural changes are collectively known as "airway remodeling." Biopsy studies have shown increased numbers of activated eosinophils, mast cells, and T lymphocytes in the airway mucosa and lumen. These changes may be present even when asthma is asymptomatic, and their extent appears to be correlated with the clinical severity of the disease [3]. a—mucus plug containing cells and debris; b—smooth muscle hypertrophy and hyperplasia; c—thickening of basement membrane and subepithelial fibrosis; d—damaged epithelium; e—hypertrophied mucous gland.

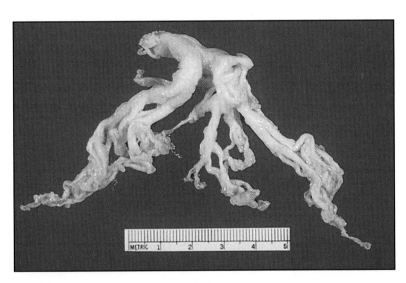

FIGURE 6-30.

Mucus plug. In chronic asthma, copious amounts of tenacious mucus are secreted by the hypertrophied submucosal glands. This mucus, along with plasma exudates, inflammatory and epithelial cells, and cellular debris, produces the mucus plug. It commonly blocks small airways, causing segmental collapse of the lung (atelectasis), but in severe exacerbation it may block the major bronchial tree, causing severe airflow obstruction and leading to death. Sometimes these plugs are seen as airway casts called *Cushmann's spirals*. (*From* Klatt [18]; with permission.)

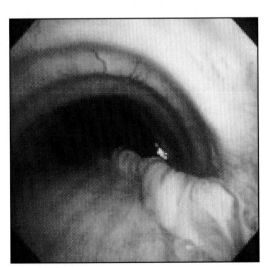

FIGURE 6-31.

Mucus plug. Bronchoscopic view showing lumen with mucus plug. (*From* McLennan [19]; with permission.)

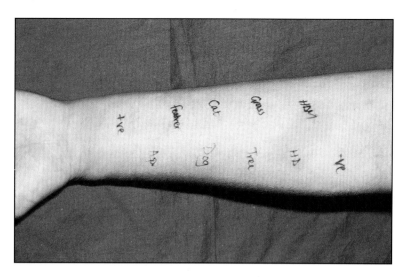

FIGURE 6-32.

Skin prick testing. Skin prick testing with allergens provides objective information about the atopic status, but the results must be interpreted in relation to the patient's history. In asthma, the skin prick test is done against common aeroallergens such as house dust mite, grass pollen, cat, dog, and any putative allergens that cause asthma symptoms on their exposure. A drop of allergen solution is placed in the flexor aspect of the forearm and a prick through the solution is made using a sterile lancet. Negative saline and histamine are used as negative and positive controls, respectively. A positive test is a wheal larger than 2 mm, or greater than the negative control. Skin tests should not be performed in the presence of severe eczema, and the subject should not take antihistamines during the test period.

■ ALLERGIC DISEASES OF THE EYE

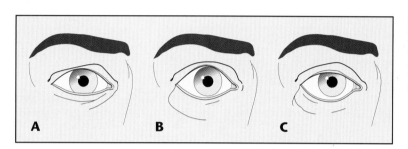

FIGURE 6-33.

Examination of the external eye. The position of the eyelid is important to note on external examination of the eye. **A**, The normal eye. **B**, The appearance of the eyelid in exophthalmus. **C**, The appearance of the eyelid in ptosis. (*Courtesy of* Leonard Bielory.)

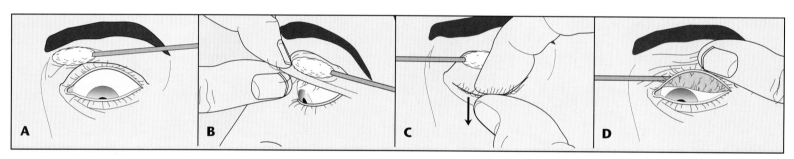

FIGURE 6-34.

The technique for the examination of the conjunctival surface of the upper eyelid. Proper examination requires inversion of the upper eyelid, which is done by **A**, placing a cotton-tipped swab above the eyelid; **B**, while the patient looks down, gently grasping the upper eyelash; **C**, pulling down the upper eyelid while placing pressure on the cotton swab; and **D**, lifting the eyelid up and over the surface of the cotton swab. (*Courtesy of* Leonard Bielory.)

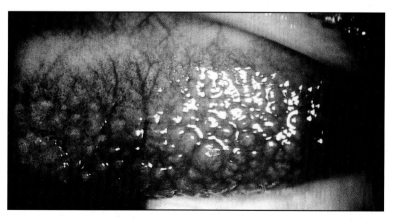

FIGURE 6-35.

Vernal conjunctivitis. These typical findings of vernal conjunctivitis can only be seen after eversion of the upper lid. Shown here is the typical "cobblestoning" produced by papillary hypertrophy. This cobblestone appearance is produced by an inflammatory exudate. Changes seen here in vernal conjunctivitis can also occur in the giant papillary conjunctivitis associated with the wearing of contact lenses. (*Courtesy of* Leonard Bielory.)

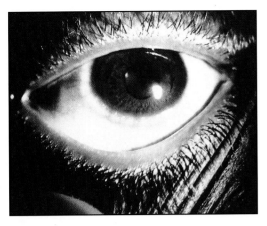

FIGURE 6-36.
Vernal conjunctivitis without the "cobblestoning" seen in Figure 6-35. Vernal conjunctivitis can also present as a limbal infiltrate of inflammatory cells, commonly in the upper limbus. The blood vessels are not prominent, and there is no mucus. Trantas dots (collections of eosinophils) can be present. They appear as small grayish-white epithelial collections of cellular debris. (*Courtesy of* Leonard Bielory.)

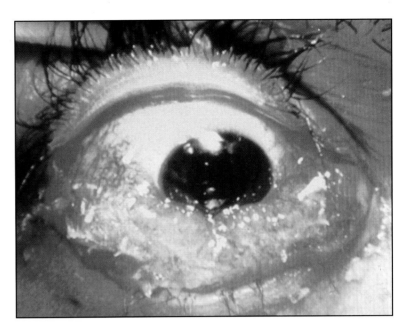

FIGURE 6-37.
Allergic conjunctivitis. Allergic conjunctivitis can occur in an acute and severe form when there is manual contamination of the conjunctiva by allergen. In this instance, a patient who was allergic to cats had been petting a cat and then touched his eye. There is marked edema of the lower conjunctival surface. This is often described by patients as "fried egg" in appearance, since the bulbar conjunctiva "bubbles up." This gives the appearance of the white of an egg as it is being fried. (*From* Lieberman *et al.* [20]; with permission.)

FIGURE 6-38.
Dermatoconjunctivitis. Eyelid dermatitis is one of the most common forms of contact dermatitis. In this instance, it is accompanied by conjunctivitis. When both conjunctivitis and dermatitis are present, the culprit is almost always eye drops. In this instance, the patient was using neomycin eyedrops for an infective conjunctivitis that healed, leaving a residual contact dermatoconjunctivitis [21]. (*From* Lieberman *et al.* [20]; with permission.)

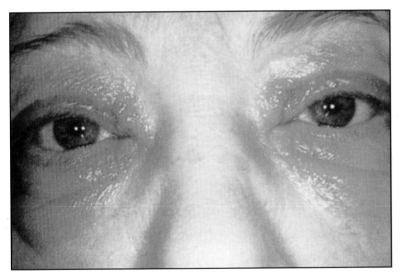

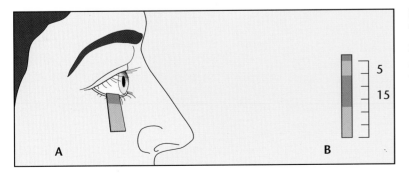

FIGURE 6-39.
Tear secretion measured by the Schirmer test. One of the conditions mimicking allergic conjunctivitis in adults, especially women over the age of 50, is conjunctivitis sicca. This produces a burning sensation, which is often described by the patient as itching. A simple test to detect the presence of decreased tearing is the Schirmer test. **A,** A piece of filter paper is placed in the inferior cul-de-sac of an unanesthetized eye at the junction of the lateral one third and the medial two thirds of the eyelid. **B,** Normal tear secretion wets more than 10 mm of filter paper at 5 minutes. Wetting of the test paper can be easily discerned by using paper (Eagle Vision, Memphis, Tennessee) that changes color on contact with tears. (*Courtesy of* Leonard Bielory.)

Differential Diagnosis of Conjunctival Inflammatory Disorders

	AC	VC	AKC	GPC	Signs Contact	Bacterial	Viral	Chlamydial	KCS	BC
Predominant cell type	Mast cell EOS	Lymph EOS	Lymph EOS	Lymph EOS	Lymph	PMN	PMN mono lymph	Mono lymph	Lymph mono	Mono lymph
Chemosis	+	±	±	±	—	±	±	±	—	±
Lymph node	—	—	—	—	—	+	++	±	—	—
Cobblestoning	—	++	++	++	—	—	±	+	—	—
Discharge	Clear mucoid	Stringy mucoid	Stringy mucoid	Clear white	±	++ Mucopurulent	Clear mucoid	++ Mucopurulent	± Mucoid	++ Mucopurulent
Eyelid involvement	—	+	+	—	++	—	—	—	—	++
Symptoms										
Pruritus	+	++	++	++	+	—	—	—	—	+
Gritty sensation	±	±	±	+	—	+	+	+	+++	++
Seasonal variation	+	+	±	±	—	±	±	±	—	—

+—present; —not present; ±—may or may not be present; AC—allergic conjunctivitis; AKC—atopic keratoconjunctivitis; BC—blepharoconjunctivitis; EOS—eosinophil; GPC—giant papillary conjunctivitis; KCS—keratoconjunctivitis sicca; lymph—lymphocyte; mono—monocyte; PMN—polymophonuclear cells; VC—vernal conjunctivitis.

FIGURE 6-40.

Differential diagnosis of conjunctival inflammatory disorders. (*Courtesy of* Leonard Bielory.)

■ ALLERGIC SKIN DISEASES

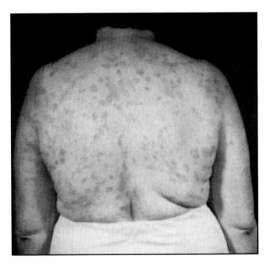

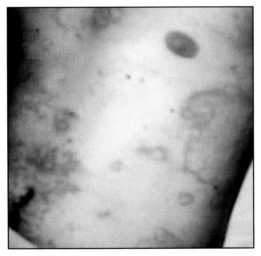

FIGURE 6-41.

Chronic idiopathic urticaria. Urticarial lesions are elevated, highly pruritic, and evanescent, each lesion usually persisting at the same site for no more than a few hours. (*From* Lieberman *et al.* [8]; with permission.)

FIGURE 6-42.

Large urticaria with serpiginous border caused by drug-induced serum sickness. The urticaria associated with serum sickness can be vasculitic in nature, as opposed to the more common idiopathic form. The latter may be less pruritic, and each lesion can persist at the same site for longer than 24 hours. (*Courtesy of* Roger W. Fox.)

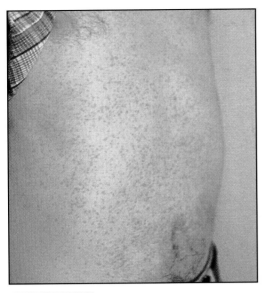

FIGURE 6-43.
Cholinergic urticaria. Cholinergic urticaria is a form of urticaria that occurs whenever there is sweating. It is actually the production of sweating that seems to precipitate the urticarial episode. Thus, any stimulus that causes sweating can produce cholinergic urticaria. It can therefore occur during exercise, during hot showers, with fever, or with emotional upset. The typical appearance of cholinergic urticaria is seen here. The lesions are initially punctate and morbilliform in nature. They are not as pruritic as are the lesions of acute or chronic idiopathic urticaria. With cessation of the stimulus producing the lesion, there is spontaneous resolution. However, if the stimulus continues (for example continuation of exercise), these punctate lesions will coalesce and can form giant urticaria [23]. (*From* Lieberman *et al.* [22]; with permission.)

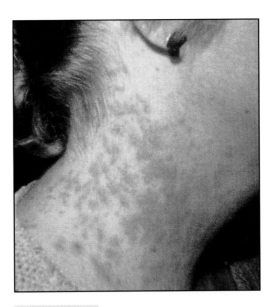

FIGURE 6-44.
Cholinergic urticaria. There is coalescence of punctate lesions with wheal and flare. The neck and trunk are the most common sites for cholinergic urticaria, and lesions usually appear first in these locations. (*Courtesy of* Roger W. Fox.)

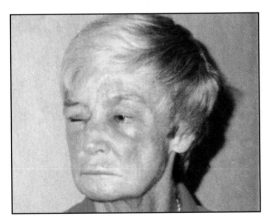

FIGURE 6-45.
Facial angioedema. Angioedema and urticaria often occur together in the same patient. However, either can occur alone. In this instance, angioedema was present without urticaria. The most common sites for the occurrence of angioedema are the eye, lip, tongue, pharynx, and digits. Angioedema occurring without urticaria, especially when there is a family history of angioedema or in the elderly, should prompt the consideration of C1 inhibitor deficiency syndrome. If urticaria is present, this disorder can be ruled out. (*Courtesy of* Roger W. Fox.)

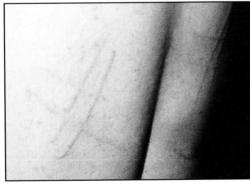

FIGURE 6-46.
Dermatographism after stroking the back. Dermatographism is the most common physical urticaria. It is present in almost all cases of chronic idiopathic urticaria. However, dermographic urticaria can occur alone. In this instance, the patient will not develop urticarial lesions unless he scratches. It is thought that the pruritus is initially produced by the leakage of small amounts of histamine from cutaneous mast cells. When the patient scratches, it induces a more significant release of histamines by traumatizing cutaneous mast cells and urticarial lesions that appear along the scratch marks. It is interesting to note that at least 50% of cases of dermatographic urticaria can be transferred by serum (transfer of IgE). (*Courtesy of* Roger W. Fox.)

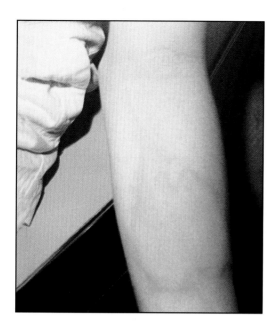

FIGURE 6-47.

Ice-cube test in a patient with cold urticaria. This test is performed by wrapping an ice cube in waxed paper or placing it in a plastic sandwich bag and then applying it to the skin surface. Characteristically the ice cube is left on the skin for approximately 5 minutes and then removed. In approximately 50% of patients with urticaria produced by cold exposure, an urticarial lesion will develop upon rewarming at the site of the ice cube placement. Cold urticaria is the second most common form of physical urticaria. Cold urticaria, like dermographic urticaria, is associated with mast-cell degranulation and subsequent histamine release from the areas exposed to the cold. Thus, patients with cold urticaria should avoid situations that might expose large skin surfaces to cold since massive amounts of histamine can be released and result in anaphylaxis. An example of such exposure would be jumping into a cold pool. (*Courtesy of* Roger W. Fox.)

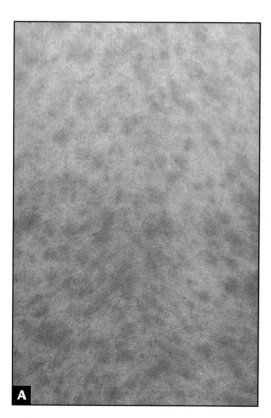

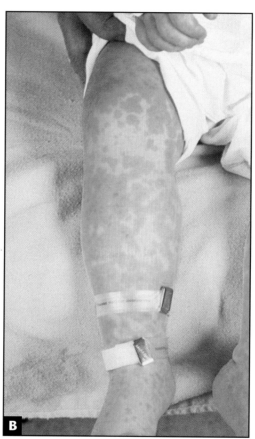

FIGURE 6-48.

Typical adverse drug reactions. The most common manifestation of an adverse drug reaction is a rash. **A,** Most drug-induced skin eruptions are morbilliform or maculopapular erythema [24]. These rashes are almost always generalized, more confluent in intertriginous areas, and usually spare the face, palms, and soles [25]. Pruritus is a frequent symptom but may be absent. This rash must be differentiated from similar, viral-induced eruptions.
It is virtually impossible to identify the causative agent based solely on the morphology of the lesions, and practically any drug can trigger such a reaction [25]. **B,** Typical amoxicillin rash, which occurs in 5% to 13% of patients [26]. Approximately 33% of patients with penicillin allergy (positive history and skin test) presented with this rash [27].

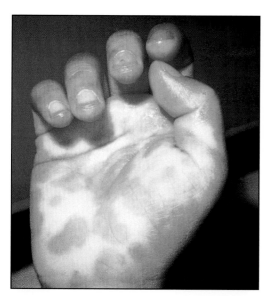

FIGURE 6-49.

Erythema multiforme, minor. This dermatosis consists of multiple, symmetric, persistent macules and papules in which some lesions are "iris" or "targetoid" in appearance. The areas commonly involved are extensor surfaces, palms, soles, and sites of trauma [28]. One mucosal surface may be involved with superficial erosions in approximately 25% of cases. Most cases are of either infectious (*eg*, herpes simplex virus) or idiopathic origin [28]. Drugs may be the cause in 10% to 20% of cases. The child depicted in this figure had extensive involvement of the trunk and extremities, including the palms and soles. In this case the skin reaction was considered to be associated with phenytoin seizure therapy.

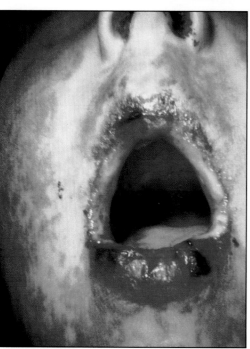

FIGURE 6-50.

Stevens-Johnson syndrome (erythema multiforme, major). In addition to the target lesions of erythema multiforme, the skin in Stevens-Johnson syndrome (SJS) is more extensively involved with widespread blistering pruritic macules of the face, trunk, and proximal extremities [26]. At least two mucosal surfaces are involved. The syndrome is usually associated with toxicity, fever, and visceral organ involvement [25,29]. This patient apparently reacted to a β-lactam antibiotic. Note the involvement of the face, mouth, nose, and (not shown) eyes.

Between 43% and 100% of cases of SJS are associated with drugs [25,28,29]. The usual drugs identified are antibiotics, including β-lactams, sulfonamides, and now others such as vancomycin plus anticonvulsant medications. Mortality has been reported to range from 1% to 5% [28,29].

Studies suggest that this syndrome resembles graft-versus-host disease and that it represents an immune reaction directed towards a cell-bound drug metabolite. Although therapeutic use of corticosteroids in this syndrome has been controversial, some experts are strongly committed to their use at the earliest stage of disease possible [25,29].

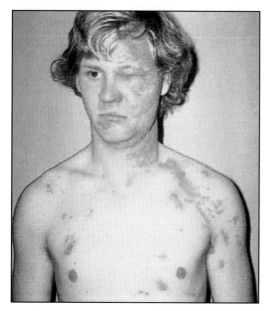

FIGURE 6-51.

Classical poison ivy dermatitis. Note the linear streaking on the thorax and shoulder. This linear streaking is characteristic of contact dermatitis, especially poison ivy dermatitis, and is produced by scratching. Also note the periorbital edema, which could be confused with angioedema if skin lesions were not prominent (*see* Fig. 6-45). (*From* Lieberman *et al.* [30]; with permission.)

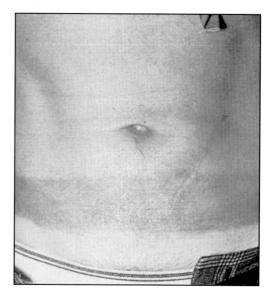

FIGURE 6-52.

Waistband dermatitis due to latex elastic. This is a classic example of how the allergen can be identified by the distribution of the lesion [31]. (*From* Lieberman *et al.* [30]; with permission.)

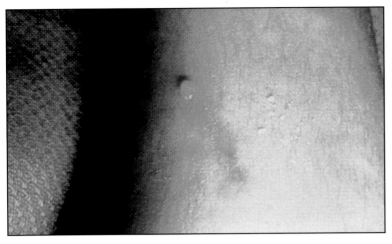

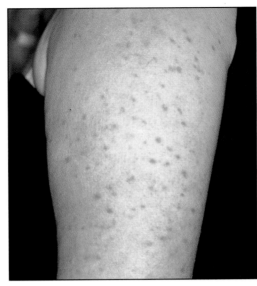

FIGURE 6-54.
Urticaria pigmentosa in an adult. Discrete lesions are randomly disrupted over the arm. (*Courtesy of* Dean D. Metcalfe.)

FIGURE 6-53.
Very early contact dermatitis showing a tense blister formation. This should be contrasted with Figure 6-38 (*From* Lieberman *et al.* [30]; with permission.)

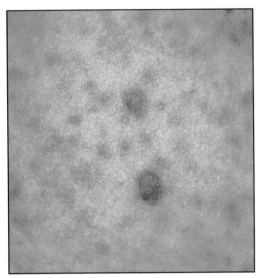

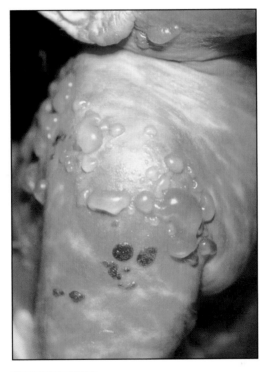

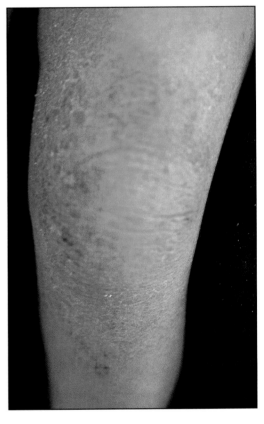

FIGURE 6-55.
Close-up view of an urticaria pigmentosa lesion. These lesions are pigmented brown and are elevated above the skin surface. Scratching such a lesion produces urtication and a wheal-and-flare reaction at the site of the lesion as mast cells are degranulated by the trauma. This is known as Darrier's sign. (*Courtesy of* Dean D. Metcalfe.)

FIGURE 6-56.
Bullous mastocytosis in a child. It is of note that the contents of mast cells can, when released suddenly, produce bullae in the skin. Note the resemblance of these blisters to those formed during the acute phase of poison ivy (*see* Fig. 6-53). (*Courtesy of* Dean D. Metcalfe.)

FIGURE 6-57.
Lichenification in chronic atopic dermatitis. Long-standing atopic dermatitis with poor skin hydration and ongoing inflammatory disease results in the hyperpigmented, thickened skin known as lichenification.

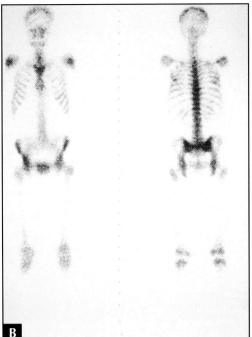
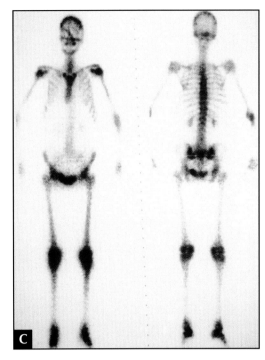

FIGURE 6-58.

Systemic manifestations of urticaria pigmentosa. These systemic manifestations can be seen especially in association with systemic mastocytosis. One of the most dramatic of these is osteoporosis. Shown here are the effects of invasion of the marrow with mast cells and the effect of histamine on bone catabolism. Results of technetium bone scans are usually normal (**A**) early in mastocytosis, but the bone scan will often become abnormal as the disease progresses. Bone scans usually progress from unifocal or multifocal abnormalities (**B**) to diffuse patterns of abnormality (**C**). *Panels B and C* were obtained from two patients with indolent systemic mastocytosis. (*Courtesy of* Dean D. Metcalfe.)

■ INSECT STINGS AND BITES

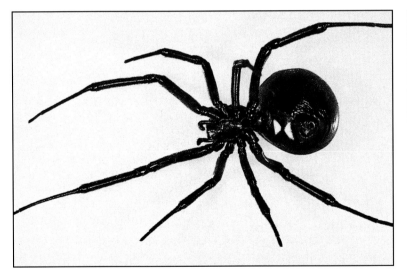

FIGURE 6-59.

Black widow spider (*Latrodectus mactans*). Black widow spiders cohabitate with humans and are often found near buildings. They can be recognized by the red hourglass configuration on the abdomen. These spiders can be found in abandoned houses, water meter boxes, and in areas under park benches or tables. The poison is primarily a neurotoxin and affects the nervous system. There is an antivenom available for black widow spider bites. However, in most instances the effects of the bite are self-limited and no antivenom is needed. (*From* Lockey *et al.* [32]; with permission.)

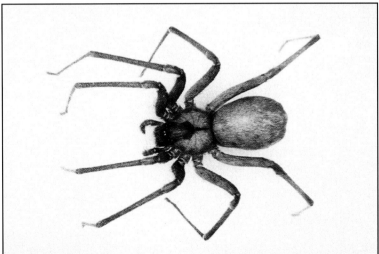

FIGURE 6-60.

Brown recluse spider (*Loxosceles reclusa*). It is also known as the fiddleback spider because of the dark fiddle structure seen on its back. Its venom is cytotoxic, causing local tissue necrosis that can produce a prolonged period of tissue damage with delayed wound healing. There is no specific treatment for the bite of the brown recluse. Surgical debridement is often necessary. (*From* Lockey *et al.* [33]; with permission.)

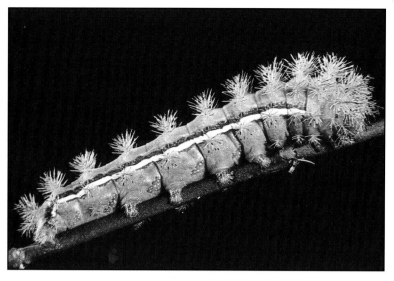

FIGURE 6-61.

Io caterpillar (*Automeris io*). The Io caterpillar is a beautiful caterpillar that is more than 2 inches long. It is pale green with yellow spines, and along each side are a red stripe and a yellow stripe. These stiff spines contain a poison that can produce a severe stinging injury. There is no specific treatment. (*From* Lockey *et al.* [32]; with permission.)

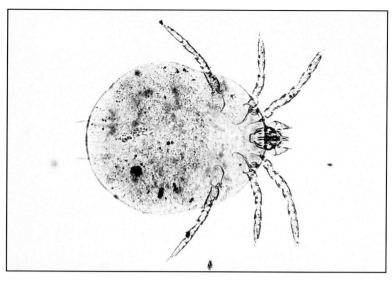

FIGURE 6-62.

Chigger or red bug (*Trombicula* sp.). Chiggers or red bugs prefer damp areas where there is thick vegetation. They ensconce themselves on plants and wait for a host to pass. Red bugs invade the body where clothing lies adjacent to skin (under a belt or shoe tops). They attach themselves to the skin with their mouth parts and inject salivary juices into the tissue. The mites feed on damaged tissue, causing intensely pruritic erythematous papules. The lesions are extremely aggravating but self-limited. There is no specific therapy. (*From* Lockey *et al.* [32]; with permission.)

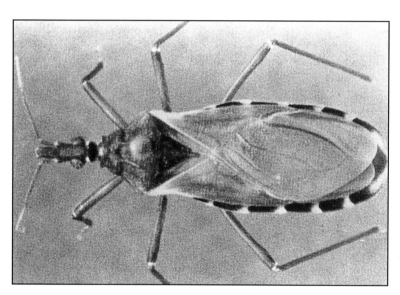

FIGURE 6-63.

Triatoma. *Triatoma* are known as kissing bugs, assassin bugs, or cone-nose bugs. They are of the order *Hemiptera*, genus *Triatoma*. They are found from Texas to California and occasionally have been noted in the southeastern United States. They typically bite at night while the victim is asleep. Such bites have been known to cause nocturnal anaphylaxis due to sensitization to saliva components. (*Courtesy of* Richard F. Lockey.)

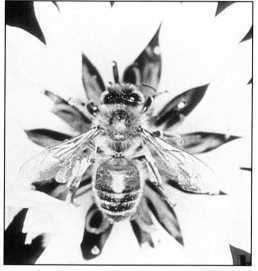

FIGURE 6-64.

Honey bee (*Apis mellifera*). Honey bees are the only *Hymenoptera* with a barbed stinger. Therefore, they "commit suicide" when they sting, since the barb holds the stinger within the skin and eviscerates the bee as it flies away, leaving the stinger attached to the venom sac. The venom sac, even after evisceration, undergoes contractile movement; thus, there is continued injection of venom even after departure of the bee. Care must be taken in removing the stinger and the venom sac. If the venom sac is grasped and squeezed, envenomation will be enhanced. Thus the stinger should be carefully scraped away with a fingernail or knife blade. (*Courtesy of* Miles, Pharmaceutical Division—Allergy Products, Spokane, WA.)

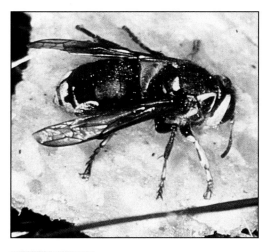

FIGURE 6-65.

Hornet. Hornets feed on organic debris left in the ground and create paper nests in the eaves of houses or in trees. Their venom is closely related to that of yellow jackets. (*Courtesy of* Miles, Pharmaceutical Division—Allergy Products, Spokane, WA.)

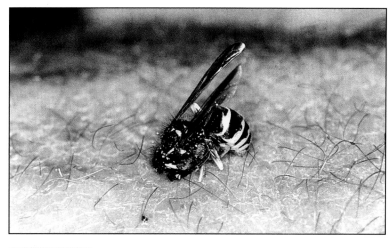

FIGURE 6-66.

An actual *Hymenoptera* envenomation. Note that the stinger is located posteriorly. Members of the *Hymenoptera* family are bees, yellow jackets, wasps, hornets, and fire ants. (*Courtesy of* Miles, Pharmaceutical Division—Allergy Products, Spokane, WA.)

FIGURE 6-67.

The stinger of a *Hymenoptera*. The stinger is attached to the venom sac. The sac itself is a thick-walled muscular reservoir that stores the venom produced in the acid glands. It is egg shaped and approximately 1 to 2 mm in diameter. For Vespid (yellow jacket, paper wasp, and hornet) venom production, thousands of nests must be collected. Venom-sac dissection is tedious and labor intensive. (*Courtesy of* Miles, Pharmaceutical Division—Allergy Products, Spokane, WA.)

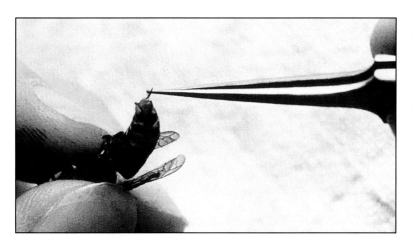

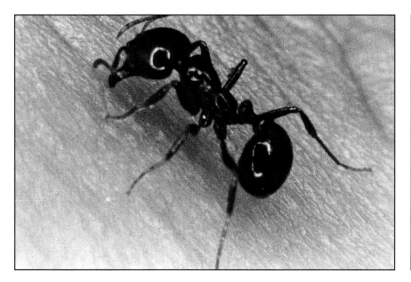

FIGURE 6-68.

Imported fire ant (*Solenopsis invecta*). The worker ant is from 0.125 to 0.25 inches long and can vary in color from reddish brown to dark brown. The ant attaches itself to the skin with the mandible and then produces multiple stings with its abdominal stinger. Each sting can form a sterile pustule. In addition, fire ant stings can cause anaphylaxis. (*Courtesy of* Richard F. Lockey.)

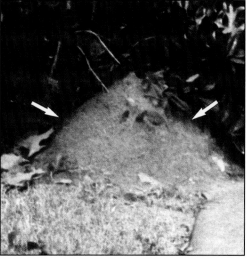

FIGURE 6-69.

Nest of the imported fire ant. These nests consist of large mounds that can be as high as 10 to 15 inches. They have a crust-like surface (*arrows*). Nests may be present in sandy soil with little or no mound structure. Imported fire ants aggressively defend their nests and attack, stinging repeatedly, when they are disturbed [33]. (*Courtesy of* R. deShazo.)

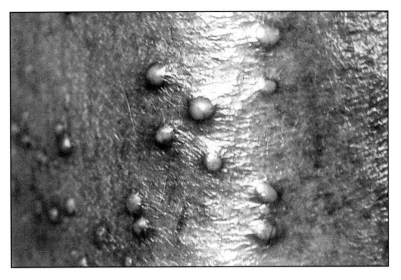

FIGURE 6-70.

Wheal-and-flare response to the sting of the imported fire ant. This response occurs immediately, and then within 24 hours, a sterile pustule forms at the site of each sting. These pustules usually resolve within 10 days. There is no specific therapy for these local reactions. (*From* Lockey [34]; with permission.)

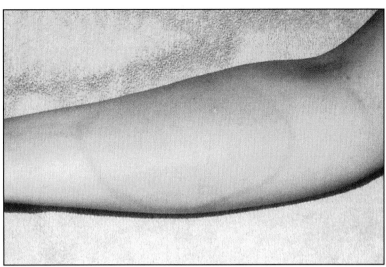

FIGURE 6-71.

Local reaction from the sting of the imported fire ant. Large local reactions often result from the sting of the imported fire ant. In this patient, shown 6 hours after three stings from a single fire ant, much of the forearm is covered with an erythematous and edematous lesion that is pruritic and painful. The reaction peaked at 48 hours. (*From* Lockey [34]; with permission.)

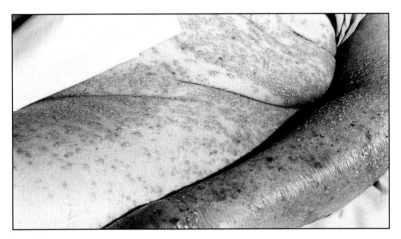

FIGURE 6-72.

Lesions from the sting of the imported fire ant. Fire ants invaded the home of this 84 year old woman with senile dementia who was confined to bed because of a history of multiple hip fractures. She was stung at least 10,000 times, as illustrated by the typical pustular eruptions. She developed neither toxic nor immunologic sequelae from the stings. Lesions such as these can become secondarily infected. Patients can also become sensitized and develop subsequent anaphylaxis on re-sting. Transient neurologic sequelae from imported fire ant stings have also been reported. (*From* Diaz *et al.* [35]; with permission.)

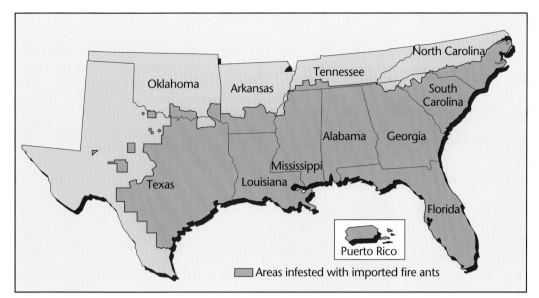

FIGURE 6-73.
Areas of the United States (and United States Caribbean possessions) infested with imported fire ants. The distribution of fire ants appears to be growing. They are marching northward and have been found as far north as Virginia. In addition, they are moving westward, and isolated colonies have been found in New Mexico and Arizona. A cold-tolerant hybrid adds to the possibility of greater spread. Their native habitat is South America. (*Adapted from* Lockey [34].)

■ VASCULITIS

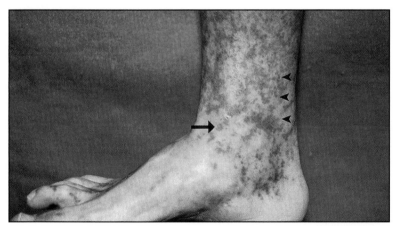

FIGURE 6-74.
Hypersensitivity vasculitis. The classical sign of hypersensitivity vasculitis is the palpable purpura (*arrow*). These usually appear over the lower extremities. They are the gross manifestation of a hypersensitivity vasculitis, leukocytoclastic vasculitis. Also shown are petechiae (*arrowheads*). (*Courtesy of* Dennis K. Ledford.)

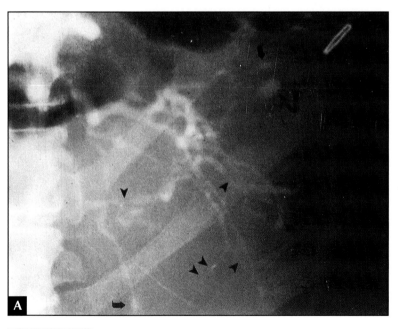

FIGURE 6-75.
Polyarteritis. Polyarteritis is a vasculitis of the small muscular arteries characterized by aneurysm formation [36]. These aneurysms can be clearly seen on arteriograms. **A,** An arteriogram of polyarteritis demonstrating irregular narrowing of the muscular arteries (*arrow heads*) with microaneurysm formation (*arrow*). **B,** A positive print (which reverses light and dark areas in the figure) of a renal arteriogram demonstrating multiple aneurysms typical of polyarteritis nodosa. (*Courtesy of* Dennis K. Ledford.)

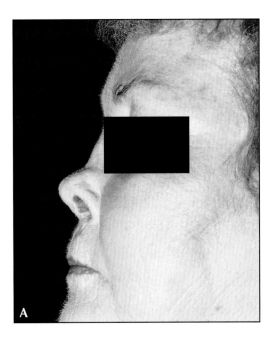

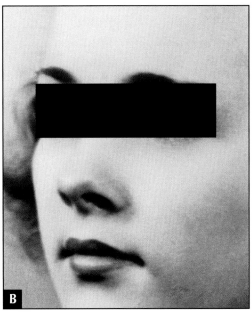

FIGURE 6-76.

Nasal septal collapse in Wegener's granulomatosis. Wegener's granulomatosis is characterized by the presence of destructive granuloma in the upper airways [36]. **A,** These can destroy nasal cartilage and produce the characteristic saddle-nose deformity. **B,** The same patient prior to the onset of the disease. (*Courtesy of* Dennis K. Ledford.)

■ REFERENCES

1. Lieberman PL: Rhinitis. In *Allergic Diseases, Diagnosis and Treatment.* Edited by Lieberman PL, Anderson J. Totowa, NJ: Humana Press; 1997:131–151.

2. Lieberman PL, Crawford LV, eds: Rhinitis. In *Management of the Allergic Patient: A Text for the Primary Care Physician.* New York: Appleton-Century-Crofts; 1982:155–168.

3. Lieberman PL, Crawford LV, eds: Management of asthma in the adult. In *Management of the Allergic Patient: A Text for the Primary Care Physician.* New York: Appleton-Century-Crofts; 1982:187–215.

4. Bull TR, ed: *A Colour Atlas of ENT Diagnosis* edn 2. London: Wolfe Medical Publishers; 1987:123–155.

5. Lockey RF: Management of chronic sinusitis. *Hosp Pract* 1996, vol:142.

6. Skoner DP, Casselbrant M: Diseases of the ear. In *Allergy, Asthma, and Immunology from Infancy to Adulthood* edn 3. Edited by Bierman CW, Pearlman DS, *et al.* Philadelphia: WB Saunders; 1996:411–427.

7. Heikkinen T, Thint M, Chonmaitree T: Prevalence of various respiratory viruses in the middle ear during acute otitis media. *N Engl J Med* 1999, 340:260–264.

8. Hirano T, Kurono Y, Ichimiya I, *et al.*: Effects of influenza A virus on lectin-blending patterns in murine nasopharyngeal mucosa and on bacterial colonization. *Otolaryngol Head Neck Surg* 1999, 121:616–621.

9. Pitkaranta A, Jero J, Arruda E, *et al.*: Polymerase chain reaction-based detection of rhinovirus, respiratory syncytial virus, and coronavirus in otitis media with effusion. *J Pediatr* 1998, 133:390–394.

10. Chonmaitree T, Hendrickson KJ: Detection of respiratory viruses in the middle ear fluids of children with acute otitis media by multiplex reverse transcription: polymerase chain reaction assay. *Pediatr Infect Dis J* 2000, 19:258–260.

11. Doyle WJ, Skoner DP, Alper CM, *et al.*: Effect of rimantadine treatment on clinical manifestations and otologic complications in adults experimentally infected with influenza A (H1N1) virus. *J Infect Dis* 1998, 177:1260–1265.

12. Belshe RB, Mendelman PM, Treanor J, *et al.*: The efficacy of live attenuated, cold-adapted, trivalent, intranasal influenza virus vaccine in children. *N Engl J Med* 1998, 338:1405–1412.

13. Commisso R, Romero-Orellano F, Montanaro PB, *et al.*: Acute otitis media: bacteriology and bacterial resistance in 205 pediatric patients. *Int J Pediatr Otorhinolaryngol* 2000, 56:23–31.

14. Nagai K, Davies TA, Dewasse BE, *et al.*: In vitro development of resistance to ceftriazone, cefprozil and azithromycin in Streptococcus pneumoniae. *J Antimicrob Chemother* 2000, 46:909–915.

15. McBride TP, Davis HW, Reilly JS: Otolaryngology. In *Atlas of Pediatric Physical Diagnosis* edn 3. Edited by Zitelli BJ, Davis HW. St. Louis: Mosby-Wolfe; 1997:683–728.

16. Cohen JT, Hochman II, DeRowe A, Fliss DM: Complications of acute otitis media and sinusitis. *Curr Infect Dis Rep* 2000, 2:130–140.

17. Vignola AM, Chanez P, Campbell AM, *et al.*: Airway inflammation in mild intermittent and in persistent asthma. *Am J Respir Crit Care Med* 1998, 157:403–409.

18. Klatt EC: WebPath: the Internet pathology laboratory for medical education. Available at: http://www-medlib.med.utah.edu/WebPath/LUNGHTML/LUNG051.html. Accessed June 11, 2001.

19. McLennan G: *Virtual Hospital Bronchoscopy Atlas: Left Bronchus Mucus Plugs.* Iowa City, Iowa: University of Iowa College of Medicine; 2001. vailable at: http://www.vh.org/Providers/TeachingFiles/Bronchoscopy/pages/LeftBronchus/MucusPlug.html. Accessed June 11, 2001.

20. Lieberman PL, Crawford LV, eds: Anaphylaxis and anaphylactic reactions. In *Management of the Allergic Patient: A Text for the Primary Care Physician.* New York: Appleton-Century-Crofts; 1982:300–309.

21. Guin J: Contact dermatitis and other contact reactions. In *Allergic Diseases, Diagnosis and Treatment.* Edited by Lieberman PL, Anderson J. Totowa, NJ: Humana Press; 1997:233–255.

22. Lieberman PL, Crawford LV, eds: Urticaria. In *Management of the Allergic Patient: A Text for the Primary Care Physician.* New York: Appleton-Century-Crofts; 1982:269–282.

23. Ledford DK: Urticaria and angioedema. In *Allergic Diseases, Diagnosis and Treatment.* Edited by Lieberman PL, Anderson J. Totowa, NJ: Humana Press; 1997:189–205.

24. Anderson JA: Allergic reactions to drugs and biological agents. *JAMA* 1992, 268:2845–2857.

25. Beltrami VS: Cutaneous manifestations of adverse drug reactions. *Immunology Allergy Clin North Am*1998, 18:867–895.

26. Bernstein IL, Gruchalla RS, Lee RE, *et al.*: Disease management in drug hypersensitivity: a practice parameter. *Ann Allergy Asthma Immunol* 1999, 83:665–700.

27. Solensky R, Earl HS, Gruchalla RS: Penicillin allergy: prevalence of vague history in skin test-positive patients. *Ann Allergy Asthma Immunol* 2000, 85:195–199.

28. Anderson JA:Antibiotic drug allergy in children. *Current Opinion in Pediatrics* 1994, 6:656–660.

29. Tripathi A, DittoAM, Grammer LC, *et al.*: Corticosteroid therapy in an additional 13 cases of Stevens-Johnson syndrome: a total series of 67 cases. *Allergy Asthma Proc* 2000, 21:101–105.

30. Lieberman PL, Crawford LV, eds: Contact dermatitis. In *Management of the Allergic Patient: A Text for the Primary Care Physician*. New York: Appleton-Century-Crofts; 1982:300–309.

31. Terr A: Cell-mediated hypersensitivity diseases. In *Medical Immunology* edn 9. Edited by Stites DP, Terr A, Parslow T. Stamford, CT; Appleton and Lange; 1997:425–432.

32. Lockey RF, Stewart GE II, Maxwell LS: *Florida's Poisonous Plants, Snakes, Insects* edn 3. Tampa, FL: Lewis S. Maxwell; 1992.

33. Gern J, Busse W: Diagnosis and treatment of insect sting allergy. In *Contemporary Diagnosis and Management of Allergic Diseases and Asthma* edn 2. Edited by Gern J, Busse W. Newtown, PA: Handbooks in Health Care Co; 1998.

34. Lockey RF: The imported fire ant: immunopathologic significance. *Hosp Pract* 1990, 25:109–124.

35. Diaz JD, Lockey RF, Stablein JJ, Mines HK: Multiple stings by imported fire ants (*Solenopsis Invicta*, Buren), without systemic effects. *South Med J* 1989, 82:775–777.

36. Cupps TR: Cardiac and vascular diseases. In *Medical Immunology* edn 9. Edited by Stites DP, Terr A, Parslow T. Stamford, CT: Appleton and Lange; 1997:513–527.

Infectious Diseases

GERALD L. MANDELL

The diagnosis and management of patients with infectious diseases is based in large part on visual clues. Skin and mucous membrane lesions, eye findings, imaging studies, Gram stains, culture plates, insect vectors, and preparations of blood, urine, pus, cerebrospinal fluid, and biopsy specimens are studied to establish the proper diagnosis and to choose the most effective therapy. The images included in this chapter encompass a wide variety of infectious diseases with emphasis on those conditions most likely to be encountered by the internist. Topics include AIDS, infections of the skin, soft tissues, bones and joints, central nervous system, eyes, ears, nose and throat, respiratory system, abdomen, urinary tract, sexual organs, heart, and blood vessels. The images selected for this chapter will aid the physician in dealing with patients with known and suspected infectious diseases.

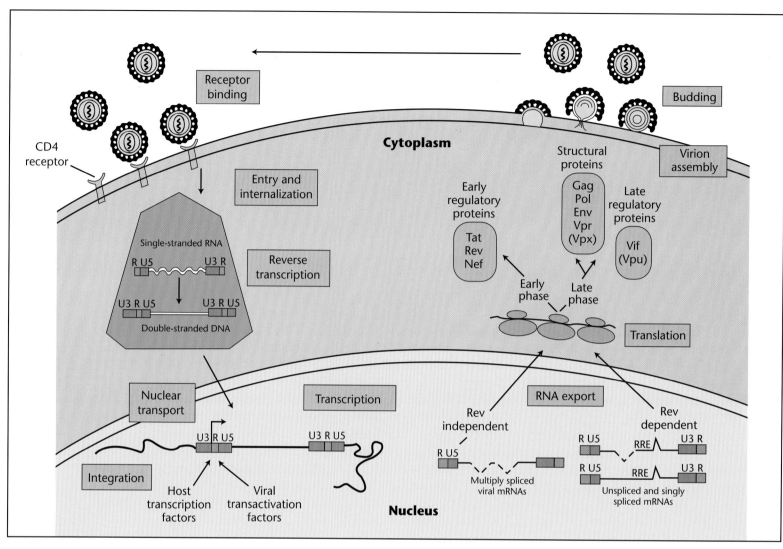

FIGURE 7-1.

Viral replication. Once HIV enters a cell, undergoes reverse transcription, and is integrated into the nucleus (integration), several host transcriptional and viral activational factors stimulate viral replication (transcription). Regulatory proteins, such as Tat, Rev, and Nef, are generally produced early and, in the case of Tat, stimulate the virus to replicate. Rev-dependent messenger RNA (mRNA) usually results in unspliced or singly spliced RNA products via the "chaperone" effect of Rev, which escorts the unspliced message from the nucleus to the cytoplasm. Once in the cytoplasm, the long messages are translated into structural proteins, such as Gag, Pol, and Env, usually as a later event in the replication cycle (translation, late regulatory proteins). The production of these proteins is augmented by the help of late regulatory proteins such as Vif. Once the proteins and genomic RNA have been produced, they aggregate near the cell surface, where an immature virion buds on the cell membrane. After release of the immature virion from the cell, the activity of the protease gene results in development of a mature virion [1]. RRE—Rev-responsive elements. (*Adapted from* Hahn [2].)

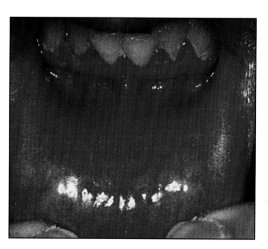

FIGURE 7-2.

Mucocutaneous inflammation in primary HIV-1 infection. Mucocutaneous inflammation and ulceration are distinctive features of primary HIV-1 infection. Inflammation of the buccal mucosa and gingiva is common, and ulceration has been reported at these sites as well as the palate and esophagus. The ulcers are generally round or oval and sharply demarcated, with surrounding mucosa that appears normal [3–5].

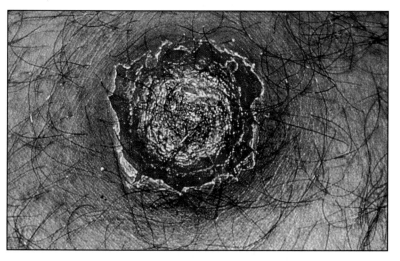

FIGURE 7-3.

Unusual skin manifestations. Cryptococcosis, cytomegalovirus disease, and non-Hodgkin's lymphoma (shown here) are common AIDS illnesses that generally present when immune deficiency is severe (CD4+ T-lymphocyte count < 100/μL). Although unusual, all three conditions can manifest as skin lesions. Non-Hodgkin's lymphoma was diagnosed following biopsy of a large (4–5 cm diameter), partly necrotic lesion involving the lower limb.

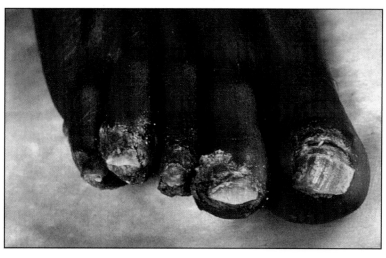

FIGURE 7-4.

Onychomycosis. Tinea infections of the nails usually cause marked thickening and discoloration with opacification of several nails in these patients. Although topical antifungal preparations are not useful, systemic antifungal agents such as Lamisil, fluconazole, and itraconazole are effective treatment for fungal infections of the nails. In general, those patients who are prone to such fungal infections tend to have rather extensive involvement of their skin and nails, which is resistant to the conventional forms of treatment.

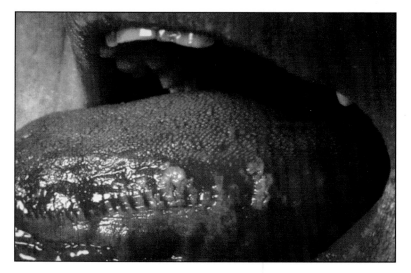

FIGURE 7-5.

Oral hairy leukoplakia. The appearance of symptomatic verrucous white excrescences on the lateral margins of the tongue (hairy leukoplakia) is frequently seen in HIV-positive persons, often prior to the development of symptomatic HIV disease. These lesions are believed to be due to the Epstein-Barr virus, which is found to be present under electron microscopic examination. Occasionally, such lesions occur on the other mucosal surfaces of the mouth. The lesions clinically mimic "thrush" but are not readily scraped off as with oral candidiasis.

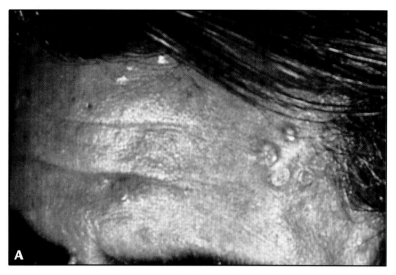

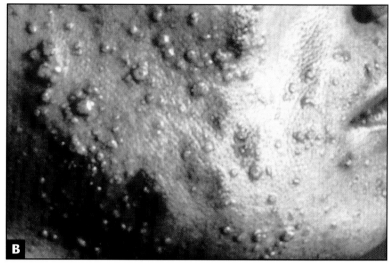

FIGURE 7-6.

Molluscum contagiosum. Widespread papular skin lesions of molluscum contagiosum, which is due to the human poxvirus, are frequently seen in HIV-infected hosts, especially those with low CD4+ lymphocyte counts. **A** and **B,** The asymptomatic, "waxy," skin-colored to pink papules of molluscum contagiosum (*panel A*), which can vary in size from 1 mm to > 1 cm, are often found widely scattered on the skin or in localized clusters, sometimes coalescing into "giant" molluscum lesions (*panel B*). In the center of each papule is a slightly depressed crusted "core," which when squeezed exudes a "cheesy" white matter. Local destructive surgical treatments including curettage and electrocauterization are usually effective, although immunocompromised patients tend to develop new lesions throughout the course of their illness. The skin lesions of disseminated systematic fungal infections such as cryptococcosis may mimic molluscum contagiosum in AIDS patients.

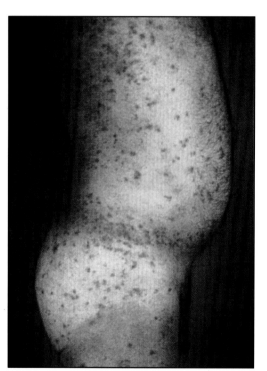

FIGURE 7-7.

Scabies. Ectoparasitic infection of the skin with scabies tend to be more severe and widespread in patients who are immunocompromised. Widespread excoriated, pruritic, tiny red papules develop that are usually more concentrated in the anogenital regions (especially the glans penis), wrist, axillae, waist, webs between the fingers, as well as the intertriginous folds. Microscopic examination of the scrapings or biopsy specimens from these papules reveal the presence of scabitic mites *Sarcoptes scabiei* and their eggs located within burrows in the epidermis. Repeated topical treatments with lindane (Kwell), crotamiton (Eurax), or permethrin (Elimite) will usually rid the host of infestation. The itchy red papules may persist for some time despite adequate treatment, due to a localized delayed hypersensitivity reaction to the residual proteins from the killed parasites within the skin. In such cases, both the physician and patient often assume that the infestation has not been adequately treated. Such posttreatment reactions are effectively treated with an antihistamine and the topical application of topical steroid creams until the symptoms subside.

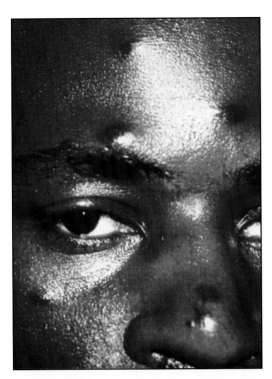

FIGURE 7-8.

Bacillary epithelioid angiomatosis (BEA). BEA is an unusual infection characterized by multiple, tender, red vascular lesions of the skin and subcutaneous tissues caused by *Bartonella henselae*, a species of *Rickettsia* closely related to the organisms that cause "cat scratch" disease. This agent is sensitive to a variety of systemic antibiotics including erythromycin and tetracycline. The vascular proliferative lesions of BEA are most frequently seen in the skin but also occur subcutaneously and can involve the internal organs in patients with AIDS. These skin lesions may clinically resemble those of Kaposi's sarcoma, although histologically, BEA is similar to pyogenic granuloma rather than Kaposi's sarcoma. The causative organisms of BEA are readily detectable in specially stained tissue sections. The skin lesions of BEA can also mimic the skin eruption associated with verruca peruana due to infection with another bacteria, *Bartonella* sp. Because BEA can be fatal, early diagnosis and initiation of appropriate antibiotic treatment can be life-saving.

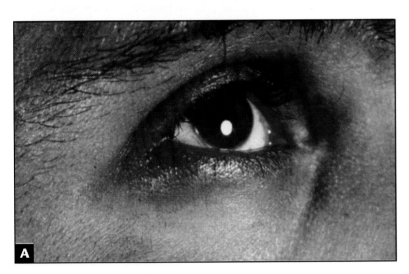

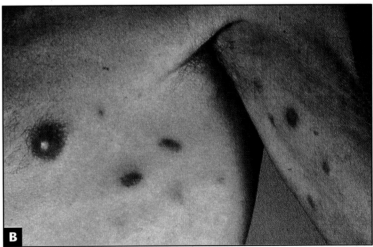

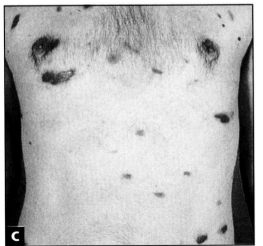

FIGURE 7-9.

AIDS-related Kaposi's sarcoma. An aggressive and disseminated form of Kaposi's sarcoma is the most frequently reported neoplastic disorder associated with AIDS. Remarkably, 95% of all of the AIDS-related "epidemic" form of Kaposi's sarcoma occurring in North America, Europe, and Australia has been seen among homosexual or bisexual men, suggesting that in this population, Kaposi's sarcoma may be due to a sexually transmissible agent other than HIV. The Kaposi's sarcoma tumors are seen most often on the skin and mucosa as asymptomatic, pink to deep purple or dark brown, round to oval-shaped patches, which eventually become thickened plaques and nodular tumors. They appear as single lesions or in clusters, at the same or distant sites. **A,** A faint early patch-stage lesion, which resembles a bruise, can even occur in the lower eyelid area. **B** and **C,** Remarkably, in AIDS patients, the lesions almost always have a symmetric distribution over the skin along the lines of skin cleavage.

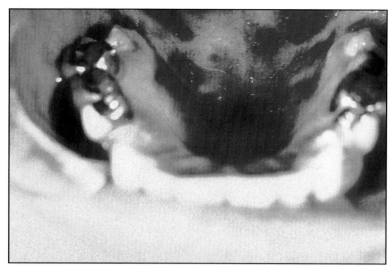

FIGURE 7-10.

Oral Kaposi's sarcoma lesions are usually flat asymptomatic patches or plaques on the hard or soft palate. Nodular tumor lesions on the oral mucosa, including the pharynx, tongue, or gingiva, can interfere with swallowing and speech. These lesions tend to ulcerate and bleed, become secondarily infected, and be very painful. Although usually asymptomatic, tumor lesions of the gastrointestinal tract may cause occasional bleeding.

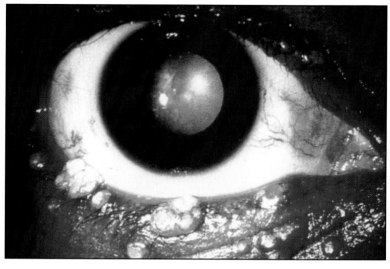

FIGURE 7-11.

Molluscum contagiosum of the eyelid margin. Progressive infection of the eyelids and face with this large DNA pox virus is associated in HIV-infected patients with advanced stages of AIDS [6]. Secondary keratoconjunctivitis can occur; epibulbar nodules are rare. Curettage, local excision, and cryotherapy can be attempted for eyelid margin lesions but recurrence is likely [7]. Recurrence may occur because of subclinical infection of epidermis up to 1.0 cm lateral to clinically visible lesions.

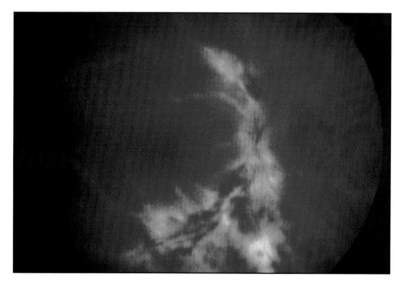

FIGURE 7-12.

Fulminant, edematous cytomegalovirus retinitis complicated by a mild vitreous reaction and diffuse periphlebitis or "frosted branch angiitis" [8]. Two months later, the retinitis was in remission on ganciclovir, 5 mg/kg daily. The retinal vessels appeared normal. The median time to complete response to medication was 31 ± 10 days [9]. Recurrent retinitis with progression into new areas of retina was noted after 150 days of therapy. The median time to progression after treatment is started is 60 days [10]. Despite an increase in ganciclovir dose, the retinitis continued to progress and a new lesion appeared next to the optic nerve head. In addition, retinal detachment became present in the temporal half of the retina due to hole formation in the area of active retinitis. Retinal detachment occurs in about 25% of patients with cytomegalovirus retinitis [11].

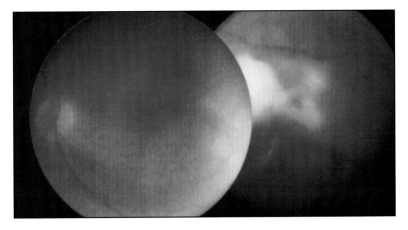

FIGURE 7-13.

Toxoplasmic chorioretinitis. This episode is the second reactivation of toxoplasmic chorioretinitis in this 32-year-old man. The first episode was complicated by retinal detachment, which was successfully repaired with 20/25 vision. The chorioretinitis remained under good control on sulfadiazine 500 mg twice daily and pyrimethamine 25 mg daily for 4 years. Reactivation occurred suddenly with decrease in vision to 4/200 due to vitreous cellular inflammation and subretinal fluid exudation in the macula. The figure is hazy due to vitreous opacification. Dark gray pigmentation corresponds to the old, healed lesion. The yellow exudate is the active lesion. The marked vitreous opacification, large amount of subretinal exudation, full-thickness involvement of retina, and response to increased doses of sulfadiazine and pyrimethamine distinguish this lesion from the more common cytomegalovirus retinitis. Clindamycin or atovaquone are possible alternate treatments in patients who cannot tolerate sulfa medications [12–14].

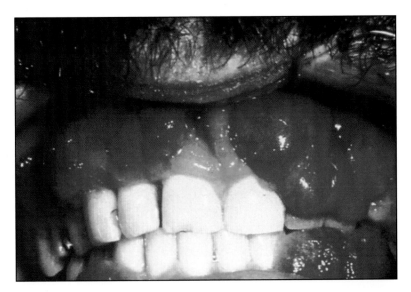

FIGURE 7-14.

Kaposi's sarcoma of the maxillary and mandibular gingiva. Multiple and extensive nodular purple lesions are apparent on the gingiva in this patient. The gingiva is the second commonest intraoral site, and these lesions often become infected with dental plaque microorganisms, causing severe pain. Careful debridement, scaling, and curettage result in reduction of inflammation, making surgical excision or radiotherapy more effective.

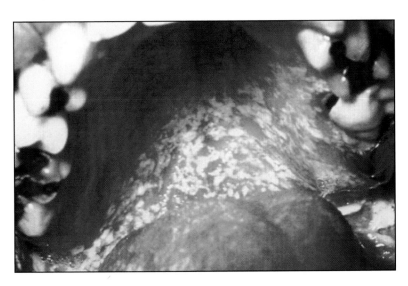

FIGURE 7-15.

Pseudomembranous candidiasis of the palate. A creamy-white plaque consisting of fungal hyphae, desquamated epithelial cells, and polymorphonuclear cells can be easily removed, leaving a red surface. These lesions can appear at any location in the mouth and oropharynx. There may be symptoms of burning or changes in taste [15].

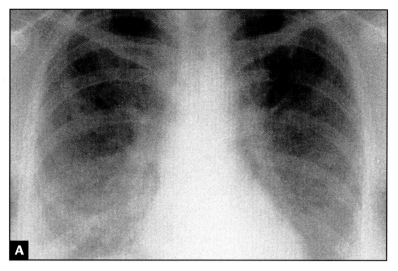

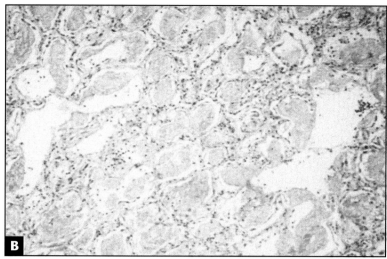

FIGURE 7-16.

Pneumocystis carinii pneumonia. **A,** Chest radiograph showing typical changes of *P. carinii* pneumonia. There are bilateral diffuse pulmonary infiltrates [16]. **B,** An open lung biopsy (hematoxylin-eosin stain) shows most alveoli are filled with foamy pink material, typical of *P. carinii* pneumonia. Profound ventilation-perfusion mismatching causes severe hypoxemia [17].

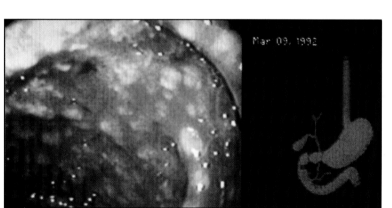

FIGURE 7-17.

Mycobacterium avium complex may infiltrate the small bowel of AIDS patients with low CD4 counts. In addition to systemic symptoms such as fever, it may result in severe malabsorption with weight loss and diarrhea. Such malabsorption also complicates therapy, as the oral drugs routinely used to treat *M. avium* complex would be poorly absorbed in this situation. When biopsy and culture-proven infiltration of the small bowel occurs, therapy may need to include intravenous modalities as well, such as amikacin and one of the intravenous quinolones [18,19]. (*Courtesy of* D. Pleskow.)

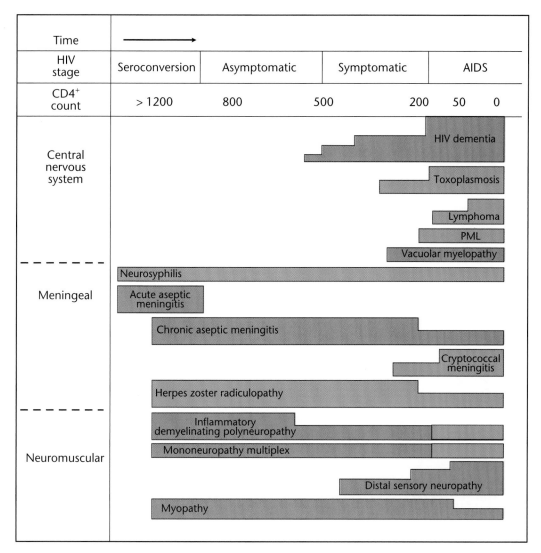

FIGURE 7-18.

Time line of primary (*pink*) and secondary (*green*) neurologic complications of HIV infection. As patients progress from seroconversion to progressive HIV disease, a constellation of central and peripheral neurologic complications may occur, in isolation or together. The CD4 cell count is the best predictor of the likelihood of a specific disorder and thus provides guidance for empiric and prophylactic therapy. (*Adapted from* Johnson *et al.* [20].)

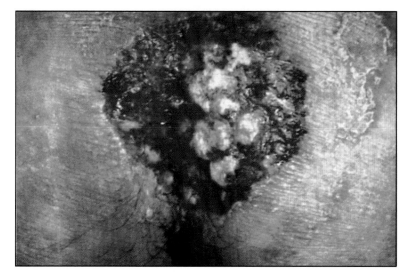

FIGURE 7-19.

Chronic mucocutaneous herpes simplex infection. Recurrent mucocutaneous herpes simplex virus (HSV) infections are common in the general population. In the immune competent host, these recurrences are self-limited, but in patients with severe immune suppression, such as those with advanced HIV disease, recurrences may be progressive. These herpetic lesions are nonhealing and expand relentlessly over time if not treated with effective antiviral therapy. The drug of choice for these infections is acyclovir. In some patients with advanced immune suppression who have received repeated courses of acyclovir, an acyclovir-resistant mutant population of virus may emerge. The exact incidence of this complication in patients with AIDS is unknown, but it appears to be relatively uncommon, given the common occurrence of HSV infections in patients with AIDS and their frequent treatment with acyclovir. The patient in this figure had chronic mucocutaneous herpes simplex type 2 infection of the sacrum, which was unresponsive to oral and intravenous acyclovir. The lesion healed completely with intravenous foscarnet therapy, which is active against acyclovir-resistant strains of HSV.

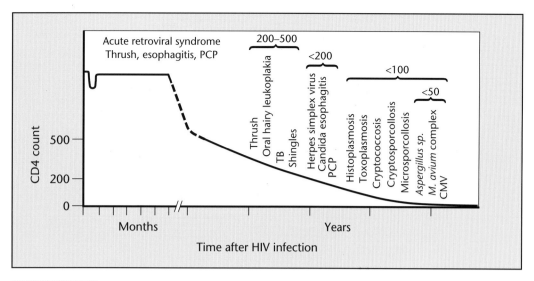

FIGURE 7-20.

Opportunistic infections in HIV disease. The appearance of opportunistic infections in the course of HIV disease is primarily a function of declining CD4+ cell counts. The spectrum of opportunistic infections, however, is also dependent on the prevalence of a given infection in a given area, with an increased prevalence of some diseases being seen in hyperendemic areas, such as histoplasmosis in the Ohio and Mississippi River valleys, coccidioidomycosis in the southwest, and tuberculosis in New York City. Because of improved survival and increased use of primary prophylaxis, many opportunistic infections seem to be appearing at lower CD4+ counts now than they did in the mid-1980s. Because the immunosuppression of AIDS is chronic and progressive, lifelong suppressive therapy is generally required once a patient has had a serious opportunistic infection. CMV—cytomegalovirus; PCP—*Pneumocystis carinii* pneumonia; TB—tuberculosis.

■ SKIN, SOFT TISSUE, BONE, AND JOINT INFECTIONS

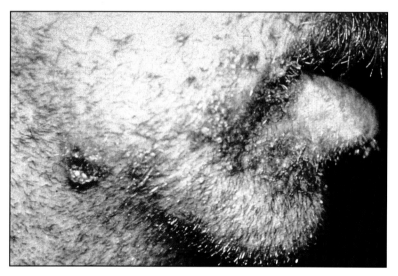

FIGURE 7-21.

Impetigo. Thick, adherent, golden ("honey-colored") crusts surmounting an erythematous base are present around the mouth and on the jaw. These findings are characteristic of non-bullous impetigo, which typically occurs on the face or extremities. More common in children than adults, impetigo often follows minor trauma, such as abrasions and insect bites, and is more prevalent in tropical climates, crowded living conditions, and circumstances of poor hygiene. Cultures of impetigo most frequently yield *Staphylococcus aureus* alone, less commonly a mixture of *S. aureus* and *Streptococcus pyogenes* (group A streptococci), and, least often, streptococci alone. Treatment is topical mupirocin or an oral antistaphylococcal antibiotic.

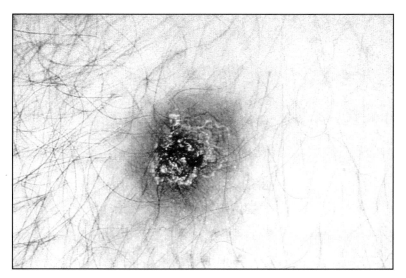

FIGURE 7-22.

Ecthyma. Erythematous ulcerations with adherent crusts, most commonly on the lower extremities, characterize ecthyma. It begins as vesicles or bullae, which rupture to form scabs. Unlike impetigo, the infection penetrates to the dermis to produce ulcerations below the crust and heals with scarring. As in nonbullous impetigo, ecthyma often follows skin trauma in patients with poor hygiene, and the cause may be *Staphylococcus aureus*, *Streptococcus pyogenes*, or both. Treatment is topical mupirocin or an oral antistaphylococcal antibiotic.

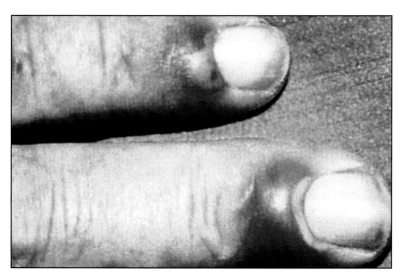

FIGURE 7-23.

Paronychia. Erythema, swelling, and accumulated pus are present proximal to the nail plates on these fingers. *Staphylococcus aureus* is the isolate in about 60% of finger paronychia. Predisposing factors include trauma, finger sucking, and protracted or repeated exposure to water. Streptococci and mouth anaerobes are frequent isolates in those not due to *S. aureus*. Gentle separation of the cuticle from the underlying nail plate with a scalpel blade provides drainage of the pus. Topical or systemic antimicrobials are rarely necessary.

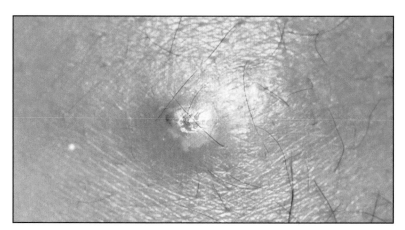

FIGURE 7-24.

Furuncle. A furuncle (boil) is a deeper infection of the hair follicle than folliculitis and consists of an inflammatory nodule with a pustular center through which a hair emerges. By contrast, a carbuncle involves several adjacent hair follicles, creating an inflammatory mass with pus discharging from several follicular orifices. Furuncles commonly occur on the face, neck, upper extremities, and buttocks. Treatment is incision and drainage, with oral antistaphylococcal antibiotics reserved for those with numerous lesions, substantial surrounding cellulitis, or fever. Some patients develop recurrent episodes of furunculosis. Occasionally, a white cell disorder such as Job's syndrome may be responsible, but most victims are otherwise healthy and have colonization of the anterior nares with *Staphylococcus aureus*, as does about 30% of the general population. Why some nasal carriers develop skin infections and others do not is unknown, but trauma to the skin is often an important factor.

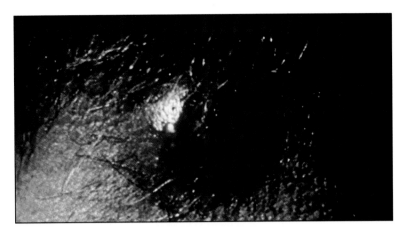

FIGURE 7-25.

Carbuncle. A large violaceous nodule has formed on the back of the neck with a pustule near its left border. A carbuncle is a staphylococcal infection involving several adjacent hair follicles. It typically occurs on the posterior neck, especially in diabetics, and begins as a nodule that enlarges to form an inflammatory mass with pus discharging from several follicular openings. Other common sites are the shoulders, hips, and thighs. Treatment consists of incision and drainage. Systemic antibiotics are unnecessary unless substantial surrounding cellulitis or fever is present.

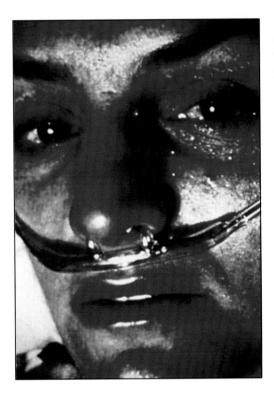

FIGURE 7-26.

Staphylococcal toxic shock syndrome. The bulbar conjunctivae are reddened in this young woman with menstrual-related toxic shock syndrome. Hyperemia of the mucous membranes, including the vagina, pharynx, and conjunctivae is common in this disorder. Sometimes, subconjunctival hemorrhages occur, and erosions can develop in the oral cavity and vagina.

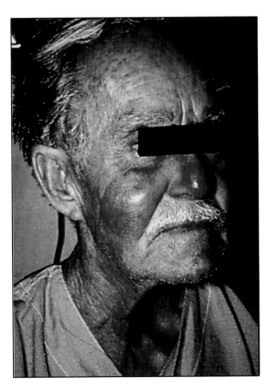

FIGURE 7-27.

Erysipelas. In the characteristic appearance of erysipelas, a brilliant red or salmon red, painful confluent erythema in a "butterfly" distribution involves the nasal eminence, cheeks, and nose with abrupt borders along the nasolabial fold. The erythema increases over a course of 3–6 days and usually resolves in 7–10 days. Erysipelas has been associated with high fevers, bacteremia, and possible death, even in modern times. The fluctuation in severity may reflect cyclical changes in the virulence of group A-β hemolytic streptococci.

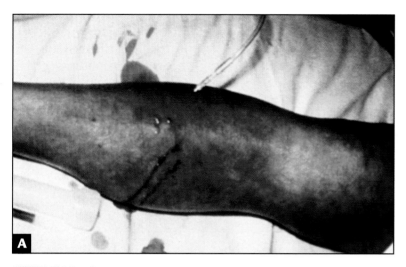

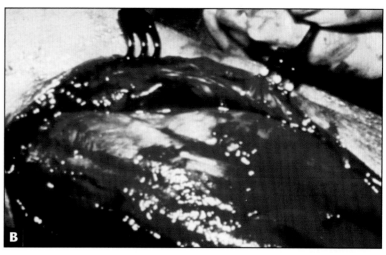

FIGURE 7-28.

Necrotizing fasciitis and myositis. The patient had sudden onset of excruciating pain and signs of systemic toxicity. **A,** Note the swelling of the leg and two small purple or violaceous bullae on the anterior shin, whereas the adjacent skin appears healthy. The pressures in the anterior and lateral compartments were measured by placing a needle in the deep tissue (hence the blood at the sampling site). Pressures were elevated and surgical exploration was performed. **B,** The fascia overlying the deep musculature was friable and brownish to dishwater-gray in appearance, establishing a diagnosis of necrotizing fasciitis. Deeper exploration of muscle compartments is warranted in such cases.

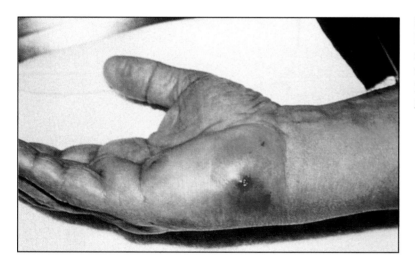

FIGURE 7-29.

Dog bite wound to the hand. Two days after injury, the hand shows swelling of the hypothenar eminence with surrounding cellulitis and underlying abscess formation. This patient's wound grew seven isolates: α-streptococci, EF-4, *Pasteurella multocida, Moraxella* sp., *Fusobacterium nucleatum, Prevotella oralis,* and *Peptostreptococcus* sp.

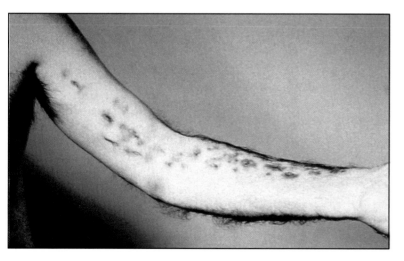

FIGURE 7-30.

Sporotrichosis. Lymphocutaneous sporotrichosis, the most common clinical syndrome caused by *Sporothrix schenckii*, usually begins with a solitary lesion followed by red nodules ascending along superficial lymphatics. The disease, which is acquired most commonly from the soil, but occasionally from animals, especially cats, has no systemic symptoms. Diagnosis is by culture; the organism is rarely seen in biopsy material. Saturated solution of potassium iodide administered orally or itraconazole is considered effective therapy.

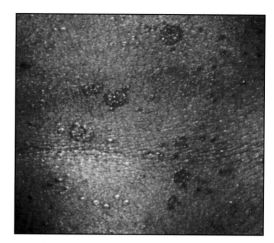

FIGURE 7-31.
Swimmer's itch. A pruritic, erythematous, papular rash is acquired by exposure to water contaminated by avian schistosomal species. It usually occurs in swimmers or fishermen. A rash occurs 5–14 days after water exposure and is caused by an allergic response to disintegration of cercariae in the skin. The rash is self-limited.

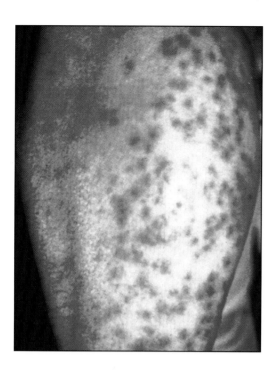

FIGURE 7-32.
Hyperpigmented tinea versicolor (Latin *versicolor*, of many colors). Round, hyperpigmented, barely palpable plaques and some perifollicular patches are evident on the upper abdomen.

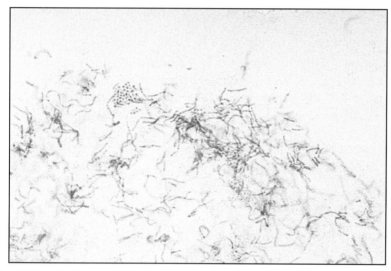

FIGURE 7-33.
KOH wet mount of tinea versicolor. Adding a small amount of Parker's blue-black ink to the KOH stains *Pityrosporon* organisms blue and facilitates their identification from skin scrapings.

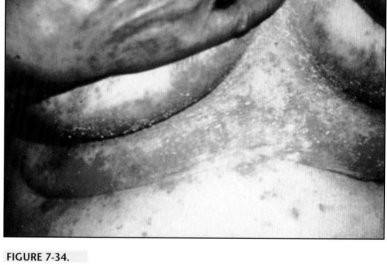

FIGURE 7-34.
Intertriginous candidiasis. The typical appearance of candidiasis is with bright red erythema and satellite papules and pustules, occurring in the axillae, groin, or other skin folds, as beneath pendulous breasts in this woman. The vigorous neutrophilic response is thought to be due to release of complement-derived chemotactic factors by fungal polysaccharides.

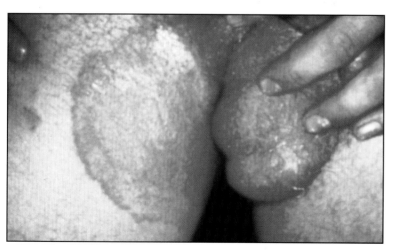

FIGURE 7-35.
Chronic tinea cruris. Asymmetrical distribution on the medial thighs, lack of scrotal skin involvement, and the papular erythematous border are characteristic of chronic tinea cruris. The best area to sample for a wet mount is the scaling just central to the papular erythematous border. Extension of tinea cruris to the buttock area occurred in this patient. Little inflammation accompanies this chronic stable infection.

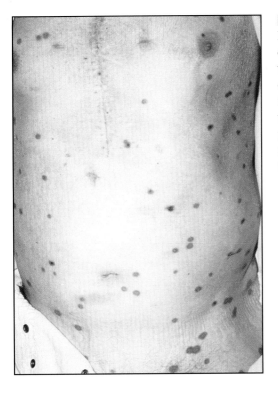

FIGURE 7-36.
Disseminated candidiasis. A patient whose neutrophil count was recovering developed a rash with tiny central pustules, indicating an early neutrophilic response.

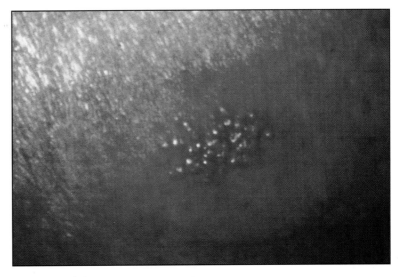

FIGURE 7-37.
Herpes simplex virus (HSV). *Herpesvirus hominis* is the causative agent in herpes simplex infections and is characterized by two major serologic types. Type I HSV (HSV-1) usually causes infections on the head, neck, and upper torso. Type 2 HSV (HSV-2) usually causes recurrent genital herpes infections and is primarily responsible for neonatal herpes. Both types of HSV cause primary and recurrent infections. This figure illustrates a classic example of recurrent HSV-1 infection. Note the grouped vesicles and pustules on an erythematous base. (*Courtesy of* M. Welch.)

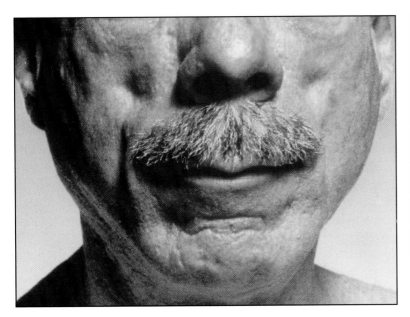

FIGURE 7-38.
Fat redistribution and metabolic change. Prominent loss of fat in face with deep indentations in cheeks. Potential contributing factors include age, use and duration of use of highly active antiretroviral therapy, in general; use and duration of use of specific antiretrovirals such as protease inhibitors and stavudine, duration of HIV infection, and HIV RNA levels.

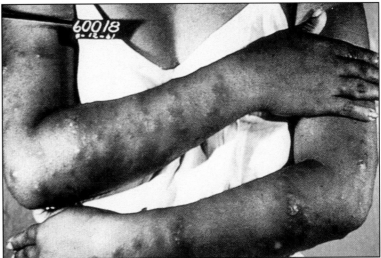

FIGURE 7-39.
A patient with several cutaneous and subcutaneous inflammatory erythema nodosum leprosum (ENL) lesions. As in this patient, at times these lesions may pustulate and ulcerate. ENL appears to be caused by circulating immune complexes. It is associated with elevated levels of tumor necrosis factor (TNF) and a local increase in cell-mediated immunity, as manifested by increased numbers of T-helper cells, interleukin-2, interferon-γ, and a loss of suppressor T-cell activity. Corticosteroids or thalidomide is effective therapeutically, with thalidomide acting by inhibiting TNF synthesis [21].

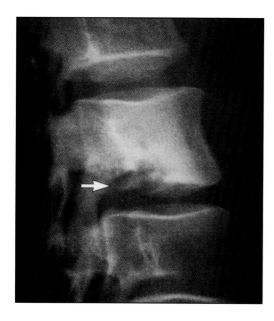

FIGURE 7-40.

Tuberculosis of the spine. A radiograph shows osteolytic destruction in the body of L3 (*arrow*) extending into the disk and posteriorly into the isthmus of the inferior articular process. The adjacent disk space is narrowed. This patient experienced low back pain and low-grade fevers for the previous 2 months. Pain was aggravated by bending, straining, and lifting heavy objects. The patient was PPD positive, and a chest film did not show evidence of tuberculosis. The needle biopsy from the L3 area was nondiagnostic by microscopic examination but subsequently grew *Mycobacterium tuberculosis* on culture. Approximately 50% of skeletal tuberculosis involves the spine, with the thoracolumbar spine being the most common site. Active or even inactive pulmonary tuberculosis is not present in most cases; almost all patients are PPD positive. Mycobacteria reach the vertebral body by the hematogenous route. Infection initially involves the subchondral bone of the vertebral body, but may spread to other vertebrae beneath the anterior and/or posterior longitudinal ligaments or into the adjacent disk leading to disk space narrowing. Collapse of vertebrae and destruction of the disk may result in the development of kyphosis or a gibbous deformity and can cause cord compression and paraplegia. Infection can spread to the paraspinal tissue, forming a psoas abscess, which may extend into the groin and thigh. Paraspinal abscesses can also invade internal organs, such as the esophagus, bronchus, lung, and even aorta. Other sites of axial involvement include the sacroiliac joints and ribs.

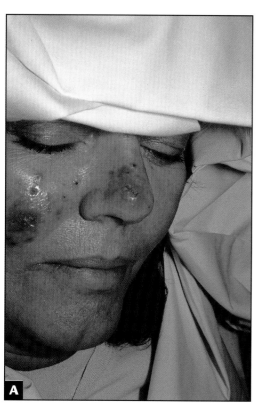

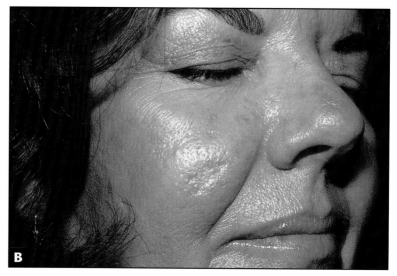

FIGURE 7-41.

Lesions of the nose and malar region in a patient with blastomycosis. The patient is shown prior to therapy (**A**) and following completion of 6 months' therapy with itraconazole (**B**). Note that the lesions are ulcerative and erythematous and began as small pustules. These lesions were painful and originally believed to represent either bacterial cellulitis or rosacea.

■ CENTRAL NERVOUS SYSTEM AND EYE INFECTIONS

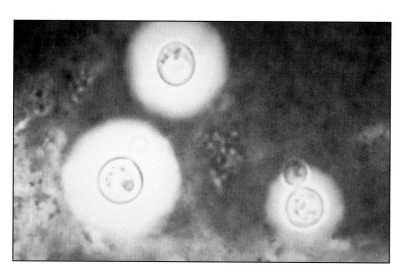

FIGURE 7-42.

Cryptococcal meningitis. India ink preparation of CSF sediment demonstrates the prominent capsule of *Cryptococcus neoformans*. Note the highly refractile cell wall and internal structure of the yeast. The India ink test is positive in 50% to 75% of patients with cryptococcal meningitis; this yield increases up to 88% in patients with AIDS. (*From* Farrar *et al.* [22]; *courtesy of* AE Prevost.)

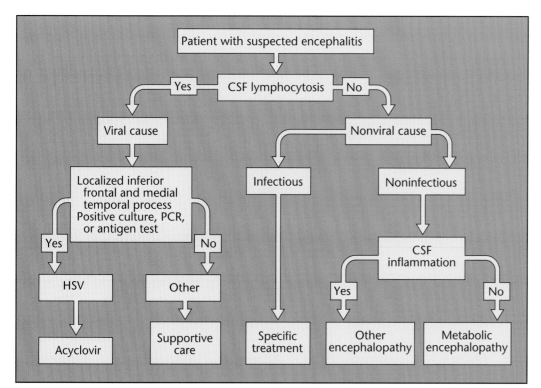

FIGURE 7-43.
General approach to the patient with suspected encephalitis. In the febrile patient with depressed mental status, nonviral causes of encephalitis must first be considered and excluded, as treatment is available for many. Epidemiologic, clinical, and laboratory data are important in the differential diagnosis. If a viral encephalitis is suspected, a diagnosis of HSV encephalitis should next be considered. For HSV encephalitis, early treatment with acyclovir may be beneficial, whereas for most other viral encephalitides, treatment is supportive. CSF—cerebrospinal fluid; PCR—polymerase chain reaction.

Differential Diagnosis of Common Central Nervous System Complications of AIDS

Disorder	Clinical		Neuroimaging		
	Onset	Alertness	Lesions, n	Type of lesions	Location of lesions
Cerebral toxoplasmosis	Days	Reduced	Multiple	Spherical, enhancing, mass effect	Cortex, basal ganglia
Primary central nervous system lymphoma	Days to weeks	Variable	One or few	Diffuse enhancement, mass effect	Periventricular, white matter
Progressive multifocal leukoencephalopathy	Weeks	Preserved	Multiple	Nonenhancing, no mass effect	White matter, adjacent to cortex
AIDS dementia complex	Weeks to months	Preserved	None, multiple, or diffuse	Increased T2 signal, no enhancement or mass effect	White matter, basal ganglia

FIGURE 7-44.
Differential diagnosis of common central nervous system complications of AIDS. (*Adapted from* Price *et al.* [23].)

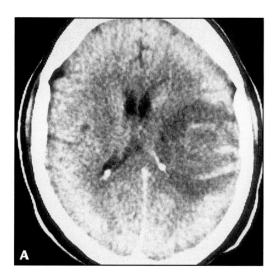
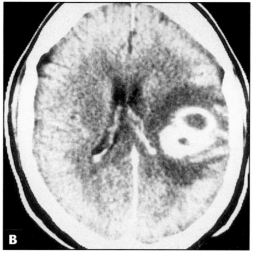

FIGURE 7-45.
Unenhanced and enhanced axial CT scans.
A, Unenhanced axial CT scan shows irregular areas of high and low attenuation producing effacement of the sylvian cistern and ipsilateral lateral ventricle on the left.
B, After contrast enhancement, somewhat thick, irregular, ring-enhancing lesions with multiple loculi are seen to be surrounded by an area of decreased attenuation, indicating cerebral edema. (*From* Wispelwey *et al.* [24]; with permission.)

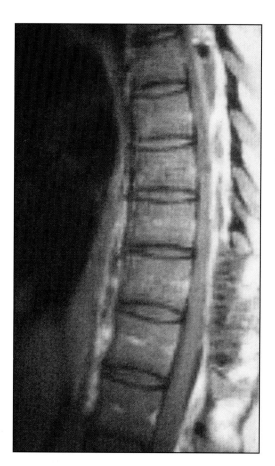

FIGURE 7-46.

Magnetic resonance (MR) evaluation of spinal epidural abscess. A sagittal T1-weighted MR image after gadolinium-DTPA contrast administration demonstrates a large spinal epidural abscess in a patient who developed fever and back pain after a motor vehicle accident. There is an irregular enhancing septate lesion extending the length of the epidural space. The patient has already had a partial decompressive laminectomy from T9–11. MRI is becoming the preferred imaging study for spinal infections because of its high resolution, ability to image the entire length of the cord, ability to both localize infection and identify contiguous infections, and noninvasiveness [25].

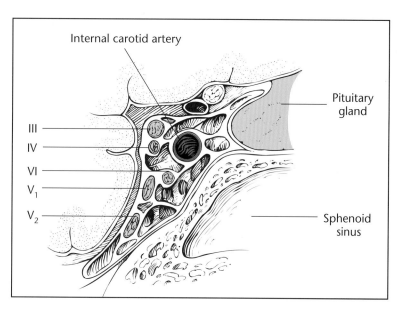

FIGURE 7-47.

The cavernous sinus in cross-section. Infection and occlusion of this sinus may follow sphenoid sinusitis or septic thrombophlebitis of the orbital veins. The neurovascular structures within the cavernous sinus may be involved in the inflammatory process, resulting in a number of clinical signs and symptoms. Spread of the inflammation into the internal carotid artery may lead to narrowing or occlusion of the artery, an event which may result in a cerebral infarction. Cranial nerves III, IV, and VI are frequently involved in cavernous sinus thrombophlebitis, resulting in varying degrees of ocular motility deficits. Symptoms of involvement of cranial nerves V_1 and V_2 (*ie*, facial numbness or pain) are possible but are not frequently observed.

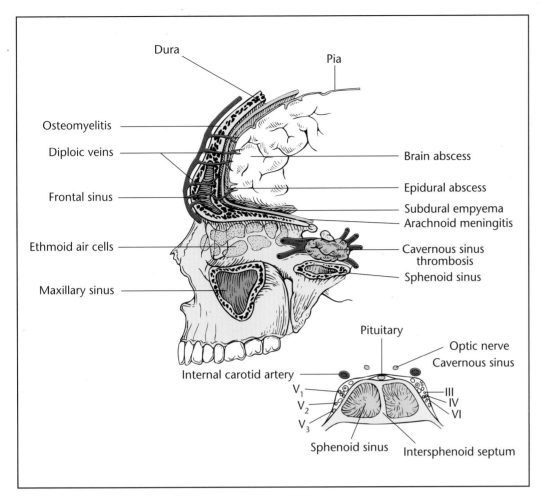

FIGURE 7-48.

Intracranial complications of sinusitis. The sagittal section shows the major routes for intracranial extension of infection, either directly or via the vascular supply. Note the proximity of the diploic veins to the frontal sinus and of the cavernous sinuses to the sphenoid sinus. The coronal section (*inset*) demonstrates the structures adjoining the sphenoid sinus. (*Adapted from* Vortel and Chow [26].)

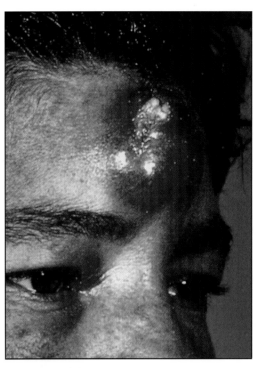

FIGURE 7-49.

Mucopyocele of the frontal sinus with perforation. Preoperative view.

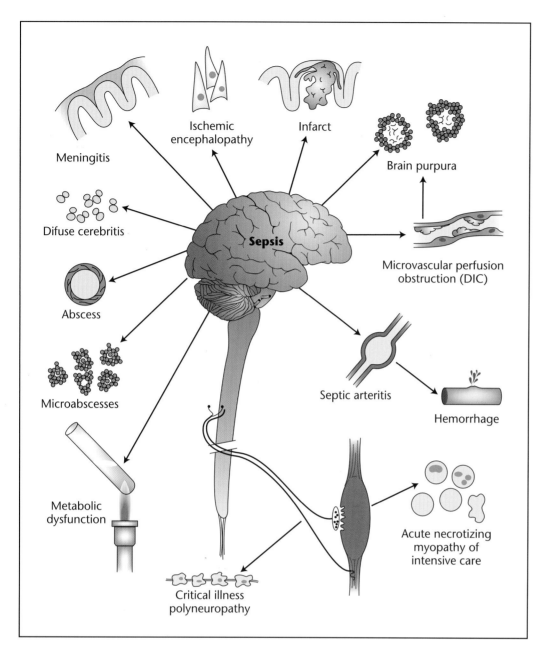

FIGURE 7-50.

The effects of sepsis on the nervous system. *Sepsis* is a term that implies the presence of microorganisms or their toxins in the blood or tissues of the body *and* a systemic response or effect on at least one organ system. It must be emphasized that the otherwise helpful localizing signs and symptoms that characterize some of these disorders are masked in critically ill, often comatose, septic patients, who are, owing to their attachment to ventilators, monitors, and various lines, difficult to assess neurologically. Accordingly, extensive investigation, including electroencephalography, neuroimaging, and cerebrospinal fluid and blood analysis, is usually necessary to identify which of these often diffuse or multifocal complications of sepsis are present. DIC—disseminated intravascular coagulation [27–30].

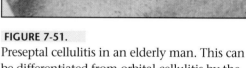

FIGURE 7-51.

Preseptal cellulitis in an elderly man. This can be differentiated from orbital cellulitis by the intense preseptal inflammatory reaction, the cellulitis extending over the entire face, and extension onto the contralateral eyelids. In the presence of any recent skin injury, *Staphylococcus aureus* is a common causative organism. In the absence of any recent wound, the list of possible causative organisms is similar to that in acute sinusitis (*Haemophilus influenzae*, pneumococcus, *Streptococcus* spp., and *S. aureus*).

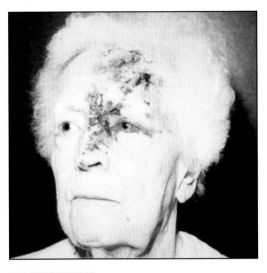

FIGURE 7-52.

Acute herpes zoster ophthalmicus. An elderly woman presented with tingling and subsequent pain on the left side of her forehead. She developed vesicular lesions over the distribution of the ophthalmic branch of the trigeminal nerve. The involvement of the tip of her nose (Hutchinson's sign) suggests involvement of the nasociliary nerve, a nerve that also supplies the cornea. In this case, the cornea has become inflamed, the eye is red, and there is a danger that glaucoma will develop. Patients with acute herpes zoster ophthalmicus should be treated with acyclovir, 800 mg five times a day for 5 days, beginning within 72 hours of the onset of symptoms; this reduces the incidence of ocular involvement, but it does not alter the course of postherpetic neuralgia.

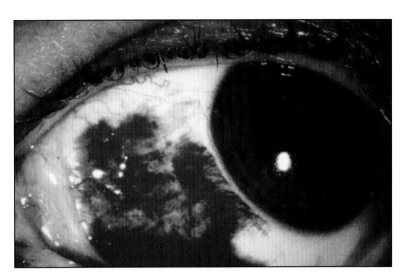

FIGURE 7-53.

Subconjunctival hemorrhage. This focal area of redness contrasts with the diffuse erythema associated with conjunctivitis. This lesion is caused by a broken blood vessel, is self-limiting, and will resolve spontaneously within 10 days.

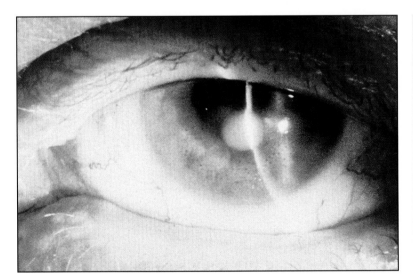

FIGURE 7-54.

Bacterial corneal ulcer under a soft contact lens. The patient had been wearing extended-wear contact lenses for 2 weeks between cleanings. She developed an acute onset of irritation of this eye and was found to have a deep infiltrate of the cornea. The most common organism in this setting is *Pseudomonas* and, when present, can lead to rapid perforation of the cornea and permanent loss of vision.

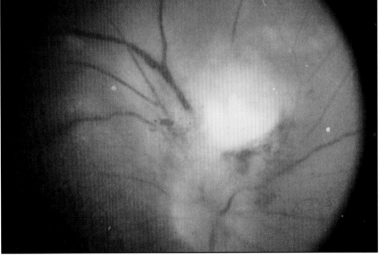

FIGURE 7-55.

Acute acquired toxoplasmosis. A middle-aged woman developed acute toxoplasmic retinochoroiditis in the area of the optic nerve following a systemic toxoplasmosis infection. This finding is unusual in immunocompetent patients but has been seen increasingly in patients who are immunocompromised either iatrogenically or because of an underlying condition. Note the hemorrhagic and necrotic appearance of the retina, which is markedly edematous surrounding the area of infection.

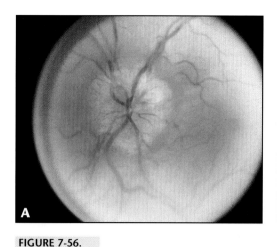

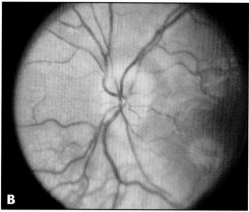

FIGURE 7-56.
Papilledema. This patient had acute elevation of her intracranial pressure secondary to an abscess. **A,** Note that the margins of the optic nerve are blurred, there is hyperemia, and there is edema of the surrounding retina. Papilledema appears to result from pressure on the nerve axons with resultant back-up of axoplasmic flow. **B,** Three weeks following drainage of the abscess, the edema of the optic nerve has markedly abated. There remains some gliosis of surrounding tissue, but the peripapillary retina has flattened. The term *papilledema* is reserved for optic nerve swelling that is associated with elevated intracranial pressure.

FIGURE 7-57.
Cytomegalovirus (CMV) retinitis. This is the acute appearance of CMV retinitis affecting the posterior fundus. There is necrosis and hemorrhage of the retina and CMV optic neuritis. Following treatment with intravenous ganciclovir, the lesions lost their acute appearance and the edema subsided. However, the retinal tissue which was involved in the inflammation never recovered nor did the patient's central vision.

■ UPPER RESPIRATORY AND HEAD AND NECK INFECTIONS

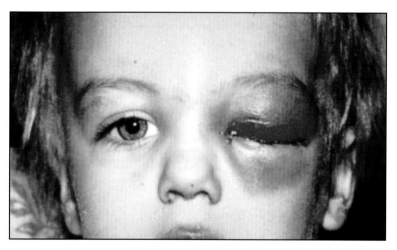

FIGURE 7-58.
Streptococcal bacterial cellulitis secondary to orbital trauma. A 2-year-old boy had nasal discharge, nasal congestion, and low-grade fever for about 10 days. The morning before presentation, he fell and sustained a 7-mm laceration just lateral to his left eye. Despite careful cleansing of the area, he developed dramatic periorbital swelling and erythema over the next 24 to 36 hours. His 9-year-old brother had had a "strep" throat the preceding week. Group A streptococcus was recovered from the culture of the wound. Bacterial cellulitis secondary to trauma is usually due to *Staphylococcus aureus* or *Streptococcus pyogenes* (group A streptococcus). Parenteral therapy was initiated with good response.

FIGURE 7-59.
Haemophilus influenzae type b bacteremic cellulitis. A 9-month-old boy had an upper respiratory tract infection for 3 days. On the morning of admission, he had a temperature of 40° C (104° F) and a small erythematous area under the medial portion of the lower lid. Within 6 hours, the erythema and swelling progressed to involve both upper and lower lids. The area was nontender. Eversion of the lids showed the globe to be normally placed with intact extraocular movements. The blood culture was positive for *H. influenzae* type b. Parenteral antibiotics were initiated and resolution was prompt. Within 24 hours, the erythema had receded partially, and the eye was approximately 25% open. In 48 hours, the eye was nearly completely open, and the cutaneous findings had resolved.

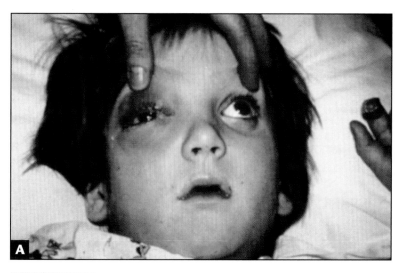

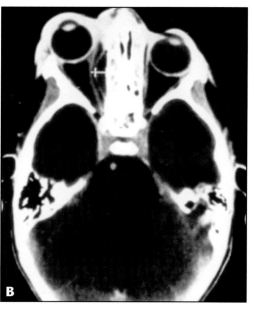

FIGURE 7-60.

Subperiosteal abscess. A 6-year-old boy had an upper respiratory tract infection for 5 days. He had been complaining of eye discomfort and headache behind his eye for 12 hours. On physical examination, he was afebrile. His eyelid was swollen and could not be opened spontaneously. When his lids were everted manually, the globe of his right eye was anteriorly displaced (proptotic). **A**, When moving his eyes up, there was an impairment of upward gaze. The remaining extraocular eye movements were within normal limits. The hallmark of a true orbital infection is 1) displacement of the globe, 2) impairment of extraocular eye movements, or 3) loss of visual acuity. **B**, Computed tomography (CT) scan shows that the ethmoid sinus is completely opacified. There is a subperiosteal abscess consequent to osteitis of the lateral wall of the ethmoid sinus (lamina papyracea), as evident in the coronal planes (*panel B*). This finding mandates surgical exploration and drainage of the abscess and the sinuses as well. In the axial view (not shown) there was a bilateral maxillary involvement: complete opacification on the right and mucosal thickening on the left. High-dose parenteral antibiotics are indicated. Culture of the subperiosteal abscess grew *Streptococcus pneumoniae*. (Panel B *from* Wald [31]; with permission.)

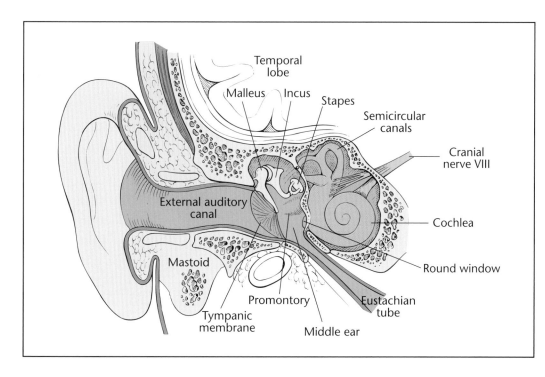

FIGURE 7-61.

Normal cross-sectional anatomy of the ear. The external, middle, and inner ear comprise a compact group of components situated in the temporal bone. Sound is funneled by the pinna into the external auditory canal, where it causes vibration of the tympanic membrane. Attached to the tympanic membrane is the malleus, which, with the incus, increases sound pressure by 30%. The stapes articulates with the long process of the incus, and the stapes footplate acts as a piston to transfer the sound vibrations to the cochlea, where the vibratory stimuli are transformed to nerve impulses. The inner ear also houses the semicircular canals, which, via a portion of the eighth cranial nerve, give dynamic and static information on the motion and position of the head.

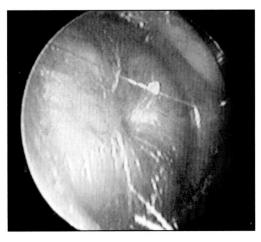

FIGURE 7-62.
Acute otitis media with bulging drum. An operative photograph of acute otitis media shows the drum to be inflamed with thickening and erythema, and the landmarks have been obliterated by the bulging drum. This acute process usually, though not invariably, is accompanied by fever and otalgia. Of note, bulging of the tympanic membrane may be seen in any acute inflammatory process of the ear, including acute mastoiditis, coalescent mastoiditis, and complicated mastoiditis. (*From* Bull [32]; with permission.)

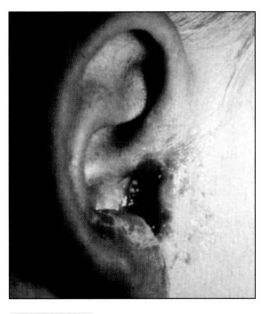

FIGURE 7-63.
Lateral view of the ear in acute diffuse otitis externa. External examination shows swelling of the ear canal and lymphadenopathy anterior to the tragus. A yellow, mucopurulent discharge may ooze from the ear opening, especially as the condition progresses. Movement of the tragus or auricle is extremely painful, which may limit or prevent otoscopic examination. (*Courtesy of* A. Willner.)

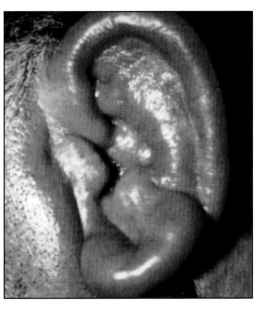

FIGURE 7-64.
Auricular erysipelas. Erysipelas is an acute, localized but spreading form of superficial cellulitis. It usually involves only the pinna in the ear and can spread to adjacent facial areas. It is caused mainly by group A β-hemolytic streptococci. The lesions are characteristically bright red, well demarcated, and tender, with an elevated and distinct advancing peripheral margin. Penicillin therapy brings a rapid response. (*Courtesy of* B. Benjamin.)

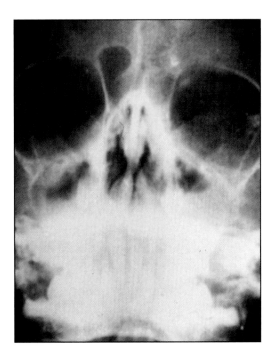

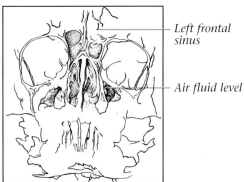

— *Left frontal sinus*

— *Air fluid level*

FIGURE 7-65.
Diagnostic radiographic findings. An occipitomental view demonstrates significant mucosal thickening in the right maxillary sinus. There is an air-fluid level in the left maxillary sinus, an unusual finding in children with acute sinusitis. The left frontal sinus, although rudimentary, is opacified.

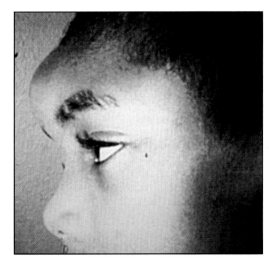

FIGURE 7-66.
Pott's puffy tumor. A 13-year-old boy presented with a 10-day history of respiratory symptoms and headache. His fever had been low-grade. The headache was not relieved by acetaminophen. During the last 3 days, his forehead had become tender to touch. On physical examination, the middle of his forehead was swollen, tender, and fluctuant. This is an example of Pott's puffy tumor—subperiosteal abscess of the frontal bone, secondary to frontal sinusitis.

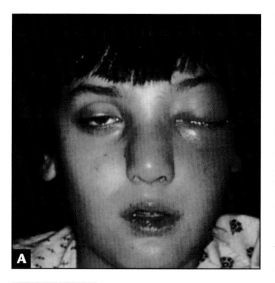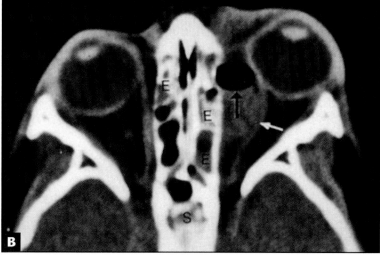

FIGURE 7-67.

Intra- and extraorbital suppurative complications of sinusitis. **A,** A 10-year-old boy had long-standing allergic symptoms, including chronic nasal discharge and congestion. For 3 days, he had left-sided facial pain and headache, with progressive swelling of his left eye. On physical examination, he was febrile to 38.4° C (101.2° F). When his lids were mechanically everted, his left globe was frozen and there was intense chemosis of the conjunctiva. **B,** An axial computed tomography (CT) scan shows anterior and lateral displacement of his left eye. There is an air-fluid level (*black arrow*) in the area between the lateral border of the left ethmoid and the medial rectus of his left eye (*white arrow*). E—ethmoid air cells; S—sphenoid sinus.

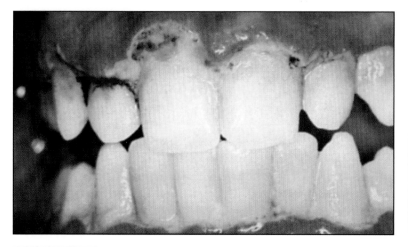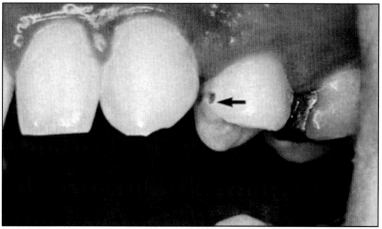

FIGURE 7-68.

Acute necrotizing ulcerative gingivitis (ANUG). Generalized severe view. Also termed *Vincent's infection* and *trench mouth*, ANUG is a severe form of gingivitis associated with infection by spirochetes, fusiform bacteria, and *Prevotella intermedia*. This rapidly progressing infection is characterized by acute fiery-red gingivitis, soft-tissue necrosis with formation of a necrotic surface layer (referred to as a pseudomembrane), severe pain, fetid odor, and, at times, malaise, lymphadenopathy, and low-grade fever. The hallmark sign of ANUG is necrosis and cratering of the interproximal papillae, referred to as "punched-out papillae." ANUG may be localized, generalized, or generalized severe (shown here) in its presentation.

FIGURE 7-69.

Dental caries. One of the most common bacterial infections in humans, dental caries is the process of decalcification of the inorganic portion of the tooth, followed by disintegration of the organic portion leading to cavitation. This disease is caused by the *Lactobacillus* and *Streptococcus mutans* class of acid-producing bacteria, which metabolize carbohydrates that have been ingested into the mouth and produce lactic acid, which in turn dissolves the mineralized portion of the tooth. Though this is considered a life-long disease, there are varying degrees of susceptibility within population groups. Some individuals remain at low risk for this disease whereas others are chronically affected. The use of systemic and topical fluorides, restricting the frequency of sucrose intake, and the removal of bacterial plaque are the major preventive measures used to control dental caries. Dental caries is subclassified principally by location, recurrence, and severity as coronal (smooth surface shown [dental caries, *arrow*] and fissure), cervical and root, recurrent (at the margins of dental restorations), and rampant caries. Root caries increases in prevalence with age due to gingival recession, which exposes the root surface and makes it susceptible to colonization by caries-producing organisms. The etiology of root caries is similar to coronal caries, with the addition of *Actinomyces* sp. as causative organisms. Rampant caries is seen principally in young individuals with high sucrose intake and high lactobacillus counts and in xerostomic individuals.

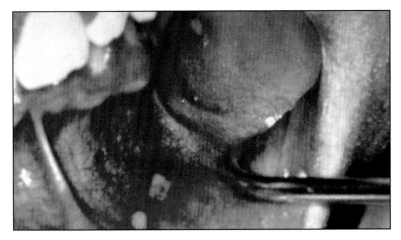

FIGURE 7-70.

Primary herpetic gingivostomatitis. Primary herpetic gingivostomatitis is a contagious disease caused by the herpes simplex virus type 1 and, less frequently, type 2. It may be subclinical or acute, affecting all of the soft tissues of the mouth including the gingiva, mucosa, tongue, lips, pharynx, and palate. Clinical signs include fiery red, swollen, and bleeding gingiva and formation of clusters of small vesicles that burst to form yellowish ulcers with a circumscribing red halo (*shown here*). The small ulcers may coalesce to form large ulcers. Symptoms include fever, malaise, and localized pain associated with ulceration. This phase of the infection usually regresses spontaneously in 10–14 days. Supportive treatment includes the use of a liquid diet, topical anesthetics, and acyclovir in severe cases. Following the primary infection, the patient continues to harbor the virus, which can later reactivate causing recurrent herpes simplex lesions. Primary herpetic gingivostomatitis should be clinically differentiated from erythema multiforme, which can produce similar-appearing oral lesions.

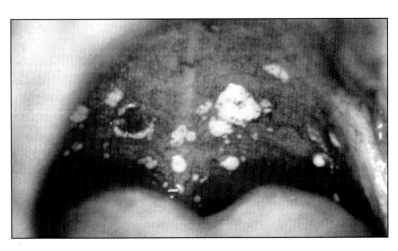

FIGURE 7-71.

Pseudomembranous candidiasis (thrush). Thrush presents clinically as white patches on the oral mucosa, which wipe off to reveal a red or ulcerated area. Diagnosis is made by clinical appearance and demonstration of the organism on a stained smear from the lesion.

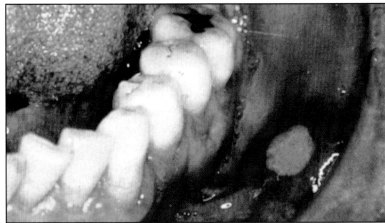

FIGURE 7-72.

Recurrent aphthous stomatitis. Recurrent aphthous stomatitis clinically presents as single or multiple painful ulcerations of the buccal and labial mucosa. It is considered to be an immune reaction to oral bacteria, particularly *Streptococcus sanguis* 2A. Up to six recurrences per year are common. Minor lesions (seen here) are 0.3–1.0 cm in diameter and heal within 10–14 days of onset. Major aphthae range in size from 1.0–5.0 cm (Sutton's disease, periadenitis mucosa necrotica recurrens) and can be disabling due to their frequent recurrences, severe pain, and prolonged duration of months. This disease may actually represent a spectrum of diseases that ranges from minor aphthae to major aphthae to Behçet's disease, which presents as ulcerative lesions of the oral cavity, eyes, and genitals. Treatment includes analgesics and topical corticosteroids for minor aphthae and topical tetracycline and steroid mouthrinse or lozenges in refractory cases of major aphthae.

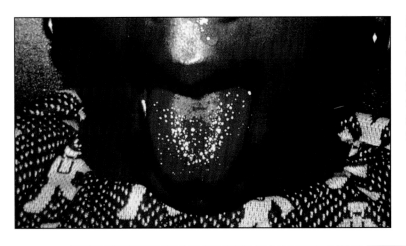

FIGURE 7-73.

Circumoral pallor and strawberry tongue in scarlet fever. Patients with streptococcal pharyngitis often have circumoral pallor and a strawberry tongue. The circumoral pallor is relative to the facial flushing and labial erythema often seen in this infection. The tongue is often erythematous with prominent papillation, giving a strawberry-like appearance. These features are often more noteworthy in patients with scarlet fever than those without.

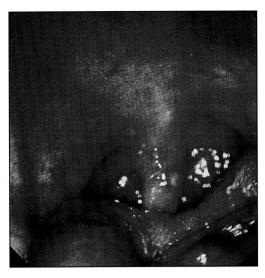

FIGURE 7-74.

Hand-foot-mouth syndrome (coxsackie A virus infection). A papulovesicular rash on the palms and soles is a rare clinical finding. When seen in association with pharyngitis, or pharyngostomatitis, especially in the summer or fall, the diagnosis of hand-foot-mouth syndrome, typically due to coxsackie A viruses, is strongly suggested. Oral lesions of hand-foot-mouth syndrome on the uvula and palate.

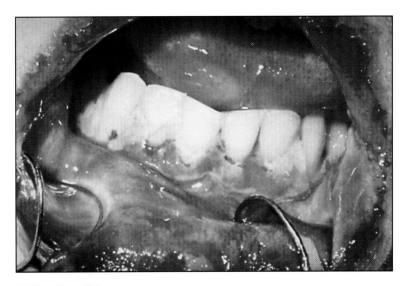

FIGURE 7-75.

Stevens-Johnson syndrome. Patients with erythema multiforme major (Stevens-Johnson syndrome) have both cutaneous and mucosal findings. The mucosal inflammation may include the oral and conjunctival mucosa, pharynx, and genitourinary and perineal mucosa. The pharyngitis is nonexudative, and tonsillar involvement is unusual. The syndrome is immunologically mediated, although some infectious agents, particularly *Mycoplasma pneumoniae* and herpes simplex virus, have been associated with recurrent cases. Therapy is largely supportive, although those with large areas of involved skin may be treated in a fashion similar to burned patients.

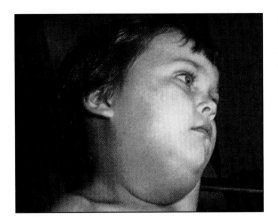

FIGURE 7-76.

Unilateral parotitis due to mumps virus infection in a 4-year-old girl. The angle of the jaw is obliterated, and the earlobe is tilted forward, hallmark findings of parotitis. (*Courtesy of the Centers for Disease Control and Prevention.*)

■ SEXUALLY TRANSMITTED DISEASES

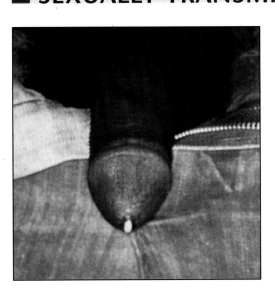

FIGURE 7-77.

Gonococcal urethritis with urethral discharge. On physical examination, a urethral discharge, which is usually purulent, is seen in 90% to 95% of men with gonococcal urethritis. The purulent discharge may appear spontaneously at the urethra, without urethral manipulation (stripping). Such appearance of discharge prior to stripping is more common in gonococcal than in nongonococcal urethritis. (*Courtesy of* M.F. Rein.)

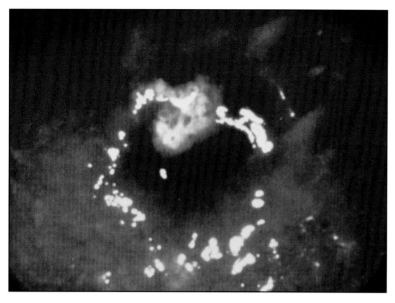

FIGURE 7-78.

Mucopurulent gonococcal cervicitis. On physical examination, the typical appearance of gonococcal infection in women includes cervical edema, erythema, and mucopurulent discharge, yielding mucopurulent cervicitis. The differential diagnosis of mucopurulent cervicitis includes gonococcal cervicitis, chlamydial cervicitis, herpetic cervicitis, chronic dysplastic changes due to human papillomavirus disease, and cervical inflammation due to chronic vaginitis.

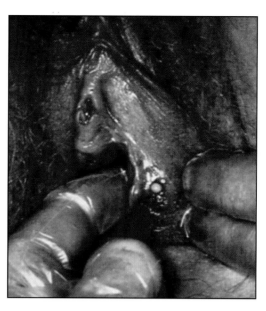

FIGURE 7-79.

Bartholinitis. Bartholinitis and inflammation of the labial glandular structures are occasionally seen in women with gonococcal infection. These conditions manifest as acute, painful swelling of the labial folds, and often, a discrete mass can be visualized on physical examination. In bartholinitis, purulent discharge can be expressed from the duct by applying pressure to the gland. The swollen gland itself is visible in this image, but normally Bartholin's glands are neither palpable nor visible.

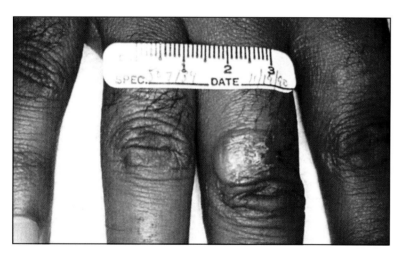

FIGURE 7-80.

Rash of disseminated gonococcal infection. The rash of disseminated gonococcal infection manifests as a sparse distribution of papular, vesicular, or pustular lesions, usually on the extensor surfaces of the extremities. Pustular lesion of disseminated gonococcal infection on the right middle finger is shown. Disseminated gonococcal infection is easily treated with appropriate antibiotics, such as quinolones or third-generation cephalosporins. Current recommendations call for a full week of antibiotic treatment.

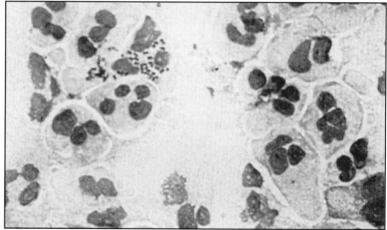

FIGURE 7-81.

Positive Gram stain of urethral smear. In the clinic setting, the Gram stain usually is used for presumptive diagnosis of gonococcal infection. Urethral Gram stain in symptomatic men has a sensitivity and specificity of > 95%. Gonococcal urethritis is demonstrated by the presence of > 5 leukocytes/oil-immersion field and observation of gram-negative intracellular diplococci. Some men, particularly those who have recently urinated, have smaller numbers of leukocytes.

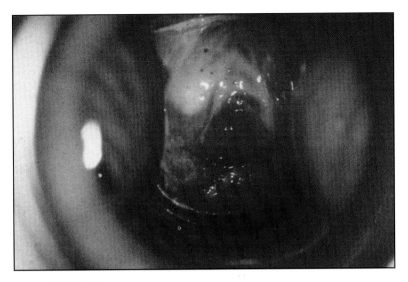

FIGURE 7-82.

Speculum examination of a woman with bacterial vaginosis showing adherent homogeneous discharge. Whereas the normal vaginal discharge is finely floccular, the discharge in bacterial vaginosis is homogeneous and often manifests small bubbles. The discharge is relatively thin, but, as here, it adheres to vaginal structures. An inflammatory response with erythema of the vaginal walls is usually absent. (*Courtesy of* H.L. Gardner.)

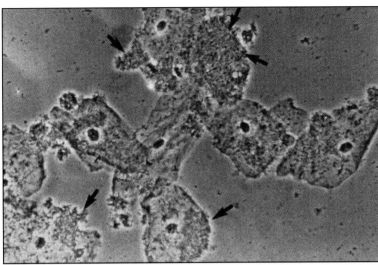

FIGURE 7-83.

Microscopic examination for clue cells in vaginal fluid from a woman with bacterial vaginosis. A second wet mount preparation of vaginal fluid is examined under high-power ($\times$ 400) microscopy for clue cells (*arrows*). Clue cells are squamous epithelial cells having a granular appearance and indistinct cell borders obscured by adherent microorganisms. Clue cells are the single best clinical indicator of bacterial vaginosis and result from the attachment of *Gardnerella vaginalis*, anaerobic gram-negative rods, and gram-positive cocci to the cells. If at least one in five epithelial cells in the vaginal fluid is a clue cell, the specimen is categorized as clue cell positive. A few clue cells may be present in the vaginal fluid of women without bacterial vaginosis, caused by lactobacilli that bind to vaginal epithelial cells.

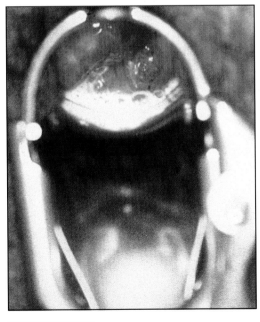

FIGURE 7-84.

Frothy vaginal discharge in trichomoniasis. Speculum examination of woman with trichomoniasis reveals a profuse, foul-smelling discharge containing bubbles. The discharge is loose and pools in the posterior fornix. Redness of the exocervix is also appreciated. Some investigators claim that the bubbles in trichomoniasis appear larger than those frequently accompanying bacterial vaginosis. The cervical discharge is seen to be mucoid; *Trichomonas vaginalis* causes vaginitis and exocervicitis but not endocervicitis; thus, a mucopurulent cervical discharge should raise suspicion of coincident gonococcal or chlamydial infection. (*From* Rein [33]; with permission.)

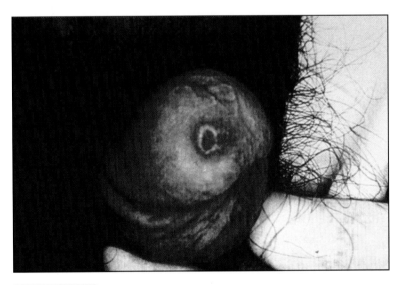

FIGURE 7-85.

Typical chancre of primary syphilis on glans penis. The typical appearance of the chancre is shown. Such lesions are usually indurated, indolent, and nontender. The ulcerations may be large or small but are always indurated and sharply demarcated. The chancre appears after an average of 3 weeks after infection, but the incubation period can range from 9 to 90 days. Intercurrent antibiotics can delay or dramatically modify the appearance of the chancre. Regional lymphadenopathy accompanies the chancre. Classically referred to as satellite bubo, involved nodes are moderately enlarged, discrete, and nontender. The inguinal nodes regularly enlarge because syphilis first spreads throughout the lymphatic vessels. The chancre heals spontaneously within about 3 to 6 weeks but may persist for up to 3 months and overlap the manifestations of secondary syphilis.

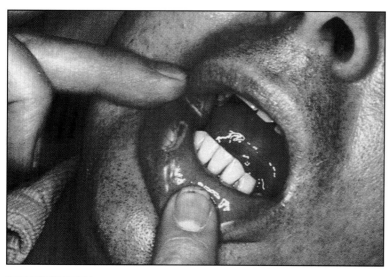

FIGURE 7-86.

Oral chancres in primary syphilis. A chancre developed on the lower lip of a man, caused by performing fellatio. Most chancres of the lip result from open-mouth or "wet" kisses and tend to occur on the upper lip in the man and the lower lip in the woman (due to the mechanics of kissing in our culture). The infecting partner is usually in the secondary stage of syphilis, with mucous patches in the mouth. Chancres resulting from fellatio are usually on the lower lip or at the commissure of the mouth. During preliminary sex play, whether kissing or fellatio, microscopic tears occur that become the portal of entry for the spirochete of syphilis. (*From* Fiumara [34]; with permission.)

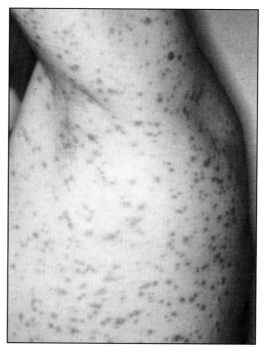

FIGURE 7-87.

Maculopapular rash of secondary syphilis on the trunk. The symptoms of secondary syphilis appear about a month after the onset of primary syphilis or about 8 weeks after the infectious exposure. This patient had flulike symptoms, rash, and generalized adenopathy. The rash may be macular, maculopapular, papular, or pustular. In this patient, the maculopapular rash also involved the midface, with mucous patches in the mouth, oval lesions in the lines of cleavage of the skin, which superficially resembled pityriasis rosea, and lesions on the palms and soles.

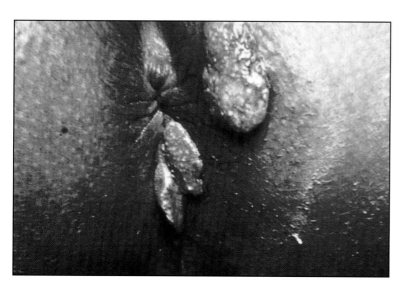

FIGURE 7-88.

Condyloma lata in the perianal region. Papular lesions on moist, intertriginous areas may coalesce to form broad, moist, highly infectious plaques called *condyloma lata*. These flat, wartlike lesions develop at sites to which *Treponema pallidum* has disseminated and are frequently seen around the anus, as in this image. They may also occur on the vulva or scrotum and are less commonly found in the axillae, under the breasts, or between the toes. Condyloma lata must be differentiated from condyloma acuminata, caused by human papillomavirus, which are generally more verrucous and exuberant.

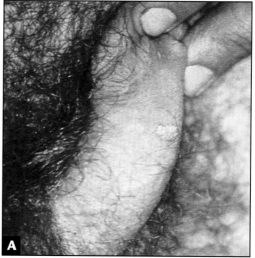

FIGURE 7-89.

Penile warts. **A,** Typical papilliferous wart of the penis in a healthy man. These exophytic lesions are initially soft and fleshy. They occur most frequently on the shaft and coronal sulcus and are commonly found under the prepuce. When lesions have the typical verrucous appearance seen here, a clinical diagnosis is made easily. The lesions may spread linearly or circumferentially. A smaller lesion is seen distally, just beneath the patient's fingers.

(Continued)

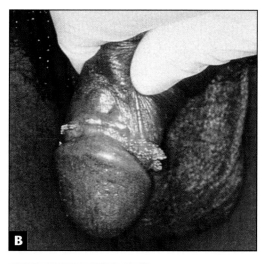
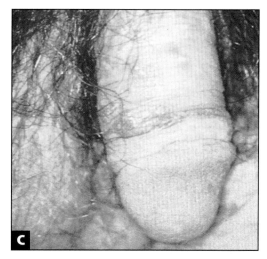
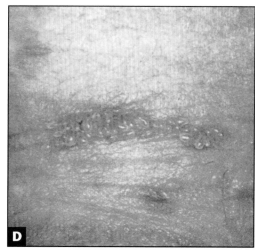

FIGURE 7-89. (CONTINUED)
B, Papilliferous warts of the penis involving the coronal sulcus. The coronal sulcus is a common site for condyloma acuminata in men, perhaps because of the susceptibility of this site to subclinical trauma during intercourse. Here, the warts have spread circumferentially, with the initial lesions to the patient's left. These older lesions have become hyperpigmented. **C,** Flatter, more chronic warts on the penis. These lesions were an incidental finding on a man who presented as an asymptomatic contact to a woman with chlamydial cervicitis. Chronic warts are likely to become keratinized.
D, Recurrent warts on the penile shaft. This patient had been treated 3 months previously, with complete resolution of visible lesions, but returned with recurrent, tiny lesions. A blush may be seen at the base of some of the individual lesions, which are highly vascular. The appearance of a tiny blood vessel running along the side of a lesion may assist in identifying it as a wart (as opposed to molluscum contagiosum) [35]. (*Courtesy of* M.F. Rein.)

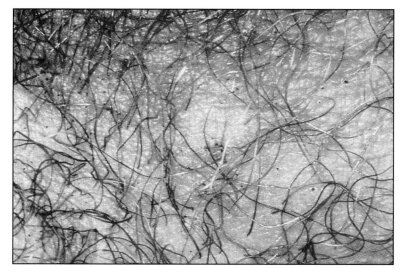

FIGURE 7-90.
Louse feces on skin. The feces are deposited after a blood meal and appear as reddish-brown dots on the affected skin. They may also be found in the underwear by the patient or examiner.

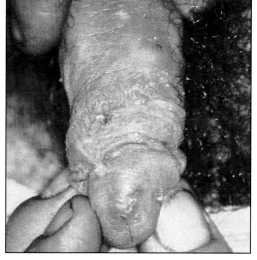

FIGURE 7-91.
Penile scabies with weeping lesions. Typically penile lesions are often weepy and crusted. Herpetic lesions also often heal with crusts but are far less pruritic at that stage; in addition, herpetic lesions are often clustered rather than scattered over the penis.

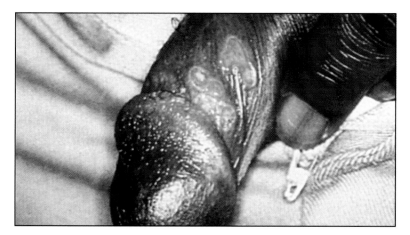

FIGURE 7-92.
Primary genital HSV infection in a man. Two clusters of large ulcers are seen on the left side of the penile shaft. Although these appear to be single lesions, each actually is formed from the coalescence of multiple ulcers. Such lesions are tender and nonindurated. Herpetic lesions tend all to be similar in size, whereas lesions of chancroid may vary in size. This patient also had bilateral tender lymphadenopathy of the inguinal nodes and was slightly febrile. He improved on oral acyclovir therapy. (*Courtesy of* M.F. Rein.)

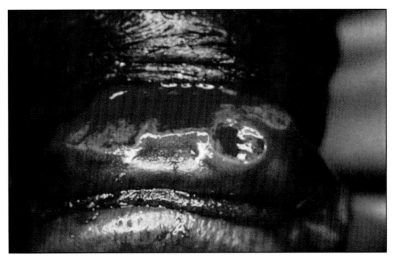

FIGURE 7-93.

Classic, purulent chancroid lesion on the distal penis. A purulent, bleeding lesion 2 cm in diameter is seen on the prepuce. This patient had two other smaller lesions on the shaft of the penis. The most common sites of involvement in men are the distal prepuce, the mucosal surface of the prepuce on the frenulum, and the coronal sulcus.

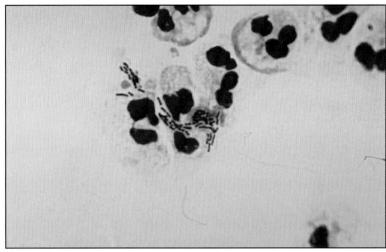

FIGURE 7-94 .

Classically, Gram stains of chancroid lesions are described as showing the organisms in "school-of-fish" patterns. These patterns are seen in only one third to one half of patients, and the finding is not specific for chancroid because other gram-negative rods can have similar arrangements. However, intracellular *H. ducreyi* is usually seen only in patients with chancroid, and Gram stain showing this finding can be a more specific, if insensitive, result from the chancroidal lesion. (*Courtesy of* E.J. Bottone.)

■ PLEUROPULMONARY AND BRONCHIAL INFECTIONS

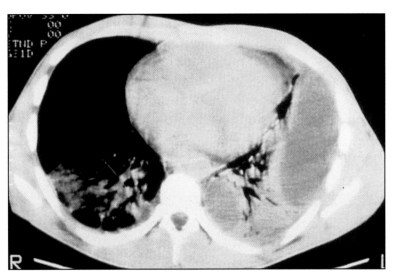

FIGURE 7-95.

Pneumococcal pneumonia with empyema. A previously healthy 25-year-old man, presumably HIV positive with a CD+ count of 21/mm^3, was hospitalized with a 4-day history of fever, productive cough, dyspnea, and pleuritic chest pain. Admission chest film revealed left lower, right lower, and right middle lobar consolidation with a left pleural effusion. Blood cultures were positive for type-14 *Streptococcus pneumoniae*. Six days after admission, computed tomography of the chest (shown here) revealed bibasilar infiltrates and a large loculated left pleural effusion. Radiographic-guided thoracentesis yielded 280 mL of cloudy fluid with a leukocyte count of 39,000/mm^3 with 99% polymorphonuclear leukocytes, protein of 4.0 mg/dL, and glucose of 5 mg/dL, which are consistent with empyema.

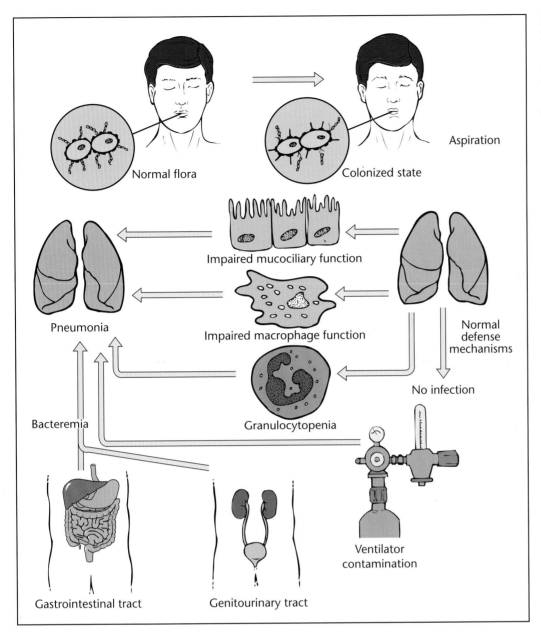

FIGURE 7-96.
Pathogenesis of gram-negative pneumonia.
Once gram-negative bacilli have established
colonization, multiplication results in high
bacterial concentrations in oral secretions.
Secretions are then aspirated in small liquid
boluses into the lungs. Pneumonia results if
the pulmonary defense mechanisms are
impaired by various mechanisms, including
alveolar hypoxia, decreased mucociliary
clearance, decreased phagocyte migration
associated with alcoholism, and neutrope-
nia. Other less frequent routes of infection
are bacteremic spread to the lung from
other foci of infection and aerosol contamination through respiratory equipment.

Normal flora

Colonized state

Aspiration

Impaired mucociliary function

Pneumonia

Impaired macrophage function

Normal
defense
mechanisms

Bacteremia

No infection

Granulocytopenia

Ventilator
contamination

Gastrointestinal tract

Genitourinary tract

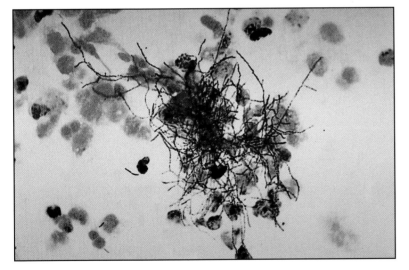

FIGURE 7-97.
Sputum Gram stain from a patient with *Nocardia asteroides* pneumonia. The organism appears as thin, weakly gram positive, branching,
often beaded filaments. *Nocardia* is a member of the order
Actinomycetales, along with *Actinomyces* and *Streptomyces*, and was
first described by Nocard in 1889 during an outbreak of bovine
farcy. Although *Nocardia* exhibits the fungal characteristic of aerial
hyphae, it is considered a higher bacterium because the cell wall
consists of peptidoglycans and lacks chitin and cellulose. *Nocardia* is
ubiquitous and is found primarily in soil and organic matter.

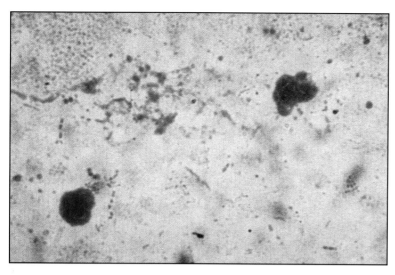

FIGURE 7-98.

Kinyoun stain of sputum demonstrating numerous acid-fast bacilli. Approximately 10,000 acid-fast bacilli are needed per milliliter of sputum to be detected microscopically. Sputum for culture must first be treated by decontamination and digestion to reduce bacterial overgrowth and release trapped mycobacterial cells from liquefied mucus. The specimen then undergoes high-speed centrifugation to concentrate the organisms in the sediment.

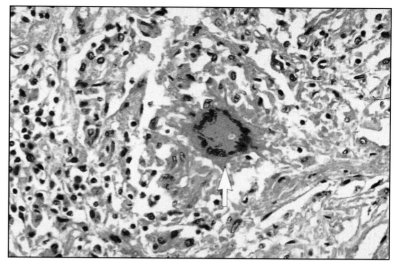

FIGURE 7-99.

Epithelioid cell granuloma containing Langhans' giant cells. Epithelioid cells are highly stimulated macrophages. The Langhans' giant cell (*arrow*) represents fused macrophages oriented around tuberculous antigen, with the multiple nuclei in a peripheral position. Activated macrophages secrete a fibroblast-stimulating substance that leads to collagen production and eventual fibrosis. This hard tubercle is able to contain infection and heals with fibrosis, encapsulation, and scar formation (*Courtesy of* G. Sidhu.)

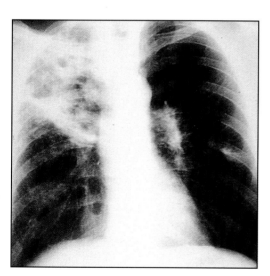

FIGURE 7-100.

Chest radiograph of a 39-year-old man with acute upper lobe tuberculosis demonstrating typical cavitary infiltrates. Apical localization of pulmonary tuberculosis is characteristic of adult infection. This localization has been attributed to the hyperoxic environment of the apices, but another theory proposes that lymph production is deficient at the apices, favoring retention of antigens at this location [36]. (*Courtesy of* N. Ettinger.)

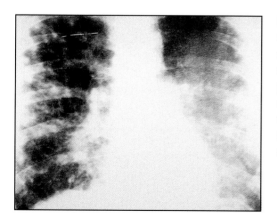

FIGURE 7-101.

Chest radiograph showing diffuse, bilateral micronodular infiltrates in inhalational histoplasmosis. A 32-year-old man was exposed to large concentrations of *Histoplasma capsulatum* spores in a closed space while cleaning an attic contaminated by large amounts of bat droppings. Exactly 2 weeks later, he presented with headache, cough, and fever. His chest radiograph showed diffuse micronodular infiltrates throughout both lung fields. Serologic tests were positive. An immunodiffusion test was positive for H and M bands, and the competent fixation test was positive at a titer of 1:64. The patient was febrile for almost 2 weeks but eventually made a complete recovery without any specific antifungal therapy.

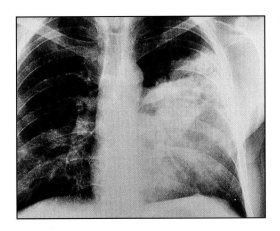

FIGURE 7-102.

Chest radiograph showing dense alveolar infiltrate in blastomycosis. A posteroanterior chest radiograph shows a large, dense alveolar infiltrate involving the left midlung in a 33-year-old intravenous drug user. Direct smears of sputum after potassium hydroxide digestion were positive for *Blastomyces dermatitidis*. Sputum cultures were also positive. The dense alveolar infiltrates can resemble infiltrates of pneumococcal or other bacterial pneumonia. This patient was initially started on oral ketoconazole therapy, but while receiving that therapy, he developed multiple skin lesions and blastomycotic meningitis. Therapy was switched to intravenous amphotericin B and he fully recovered. (*From* Bone *et al.* [37]; with permission.)

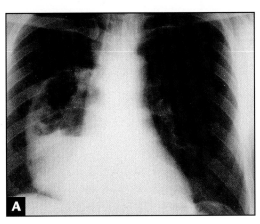

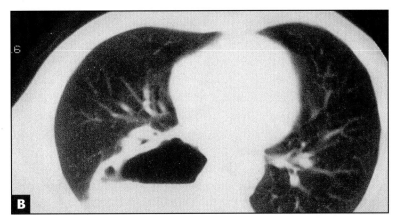

FIGURE 7-103.

A, Chest radiograph of right lower lobe abscess in a 60-year-old alcoholic. **B,** Computed tomography scan of the chest, demonstrating the extent of the abscess cavity. A consistent feature of anaerobic lung infections is tissue necrosis resulting in abscess formation, bronchopleural fistulae, and empyemas. Clinically, low-grade fever and foul-smelling sputum are generally present. Anemia and weight loss, as well as associated empyema, are also common. Although successful treatment for this patient involved lobectomy, clinical response is usually obtained with prolonged antimicrobial therapy and postural drainage. Indeed, surgical resection is relatively contraindicated, given the risks of spillage of abscess contents, and is usually reserved for patients with underlying neoplasms. Mortality of lung abscess in most series is 15% or less.

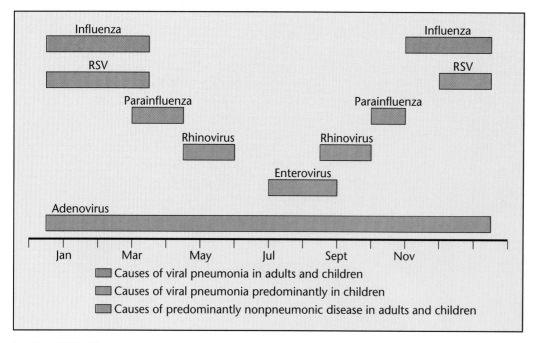

FIGURE 7-104.

Seasonal variation in respiratory virus infections. Viral pneumonia is caused by relatively few virus types. Not included in this graph are the viruses that cause primarily rashes (*eg,* measles and varicella) and are occasionally complicated by pneumonia, especially in adults. Each of the viruses has its own season, and outside that season, these viruses are seldom isolated. A concentration of cases of viral pneumonia occurs in the winter, with fewer cases in the spring and fall. Although viral pneumonia in adults is uncommon, it is an important clinical problem, and the clinical course can be severe. During the viral season, when a patient presents severely ill with acute pneumonia that is "atypical" (because no bacterial cause can be identified), the physician often concludes that it must be due to *Legionella pneumophila.* However, cultures of respiratory secretions for virus often will yield virus, usually influenza A or B virus. Although influenza causes pneumonia in children, most cases occur in very young infants. Respiratory syncytial virus (RSV) is more common than influenza and also affects a greater age range. Parainfluenza is also an important pathogen, especially in the immunocompromised child. In the summer, the only virus that causes pulmonary infiltration is the hantavirus (not shown). In contrast to the winter, many of the "atypical" cases of pneumonia in the summer are caused by *Legionella.* In truth, *Legionella* pneumonia really resembles typical pneumonia, except that a bacterial pathogen is not readily identified.

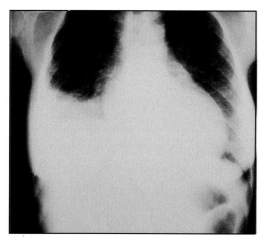

FIGURE 7-105.

Chest radiograph of a patient with amebic liver abscess showing elevation of the right hemidiaphragm with pleural effusion. The incidence of pulmonary involvement in *Entamoeba histolytica* liver abscess ranges from 3% to 30%. When the abscess is adjacent to the diaphragm, it leads to its elevation, secondary atelectasis, and reactive pleural transudate. Pleuritic pain referred to the shoulder is typical, and pulmonary symptoms may dominate the clinical presentation. Effective treatment of the liver abscess leads to prompt resolution of the lung disease [38].

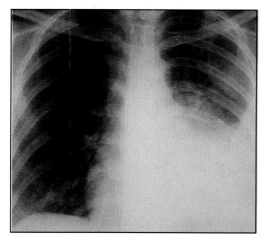

FIGURE 7-106.

Acute community-acquired pneumonia with complicated parapneumonic effusion. Posteroanterior chest radiograph of a 30-year-old woman with fever and cough shows a left lower lobe consolidation. The lateral aspect of the density has the appearance of a pleural effusion, forming a meniscus. Ultrasound study (not shown) was not helpful in delineating the effusion. A computed tomography (CT) scan (also not shown) reveals, however, the loculated pleural effusion and subjacent pulmonary consolidation. Pleural fluid was obtained by CT-guided diagnostic thoracentesis.

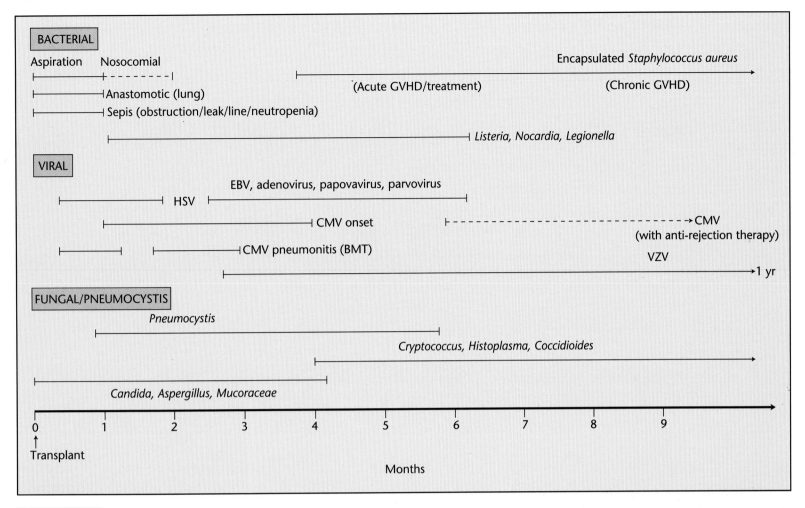

FIGURE 7-107.

Timetable for pulmonary infections following transplantation. Patients' greatest risk for specific infections occurs in a specified sequence after transplantation. Patients who deviate significantly from this pattern may represent increased epidemiologic exposure to a given pathogen or a unique susceptibility (*eg,* increased immune suppression or tissue injury). Technical problems, such as anastomotic leaks or infections of hematomas, are associated with infection in the first month following transplantation but become a source of recurrent disease if uncorrected. (BMT—bone marrow transplant; CMV—cytomegalovirus; EBV—Epstein-Barr virus; GVHD—graft-vs-host disease; HSV—herpes simplex virus; VZV—varicella-zoster virus.) (*Adapted from* Rubin *et al.* [39].)

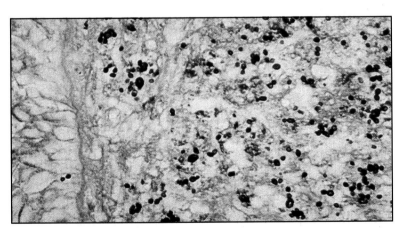

FIGURE 7-108.

Histopathologic specimen demonstrating *Histoplasma* tracheobronchitis. Transbronchial biopsy was performed on a Puerto Rican man with AIDS plus cough and shortness of breath. High-power view of the biopsy specimen stained with Gomori methenamine silver shows budding yeasts. Cultures grew *Histoplasma capsulatum.* (*Courtesy of* J. Jagirdar.)

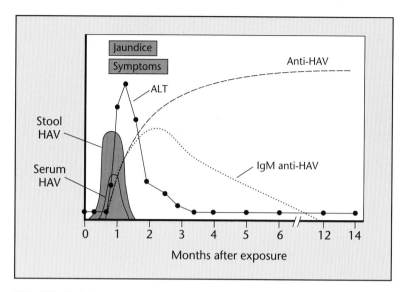
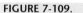

FIGURE 7-109.

Typical time course of hepatitis A with emphasis on serologic manifestations. Demonstration of IgM anti–hepatitis A virus (HAV) is diagnostic of
hepatitis A infection. IgM anti–HAV occurs at the time of onset of symptoms and may persist for months. (ALT—alanine aminotransferase.)

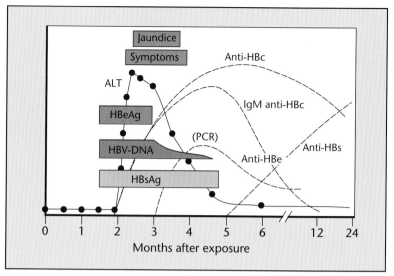

FIGURE 7-110.

Typical clinical, serologic, and virologic time course of hepatitis B. ALT—
alanine aminotransferase; HBc—hepatitis B core; HBeAg—hepatitis B e
antigen; HBsAg—hepatitis B surface antigen; HBV—hepatitis B virus;
PCR—polymerase chain reaction. (*Adapted from* Hsu *et al.* [40].)

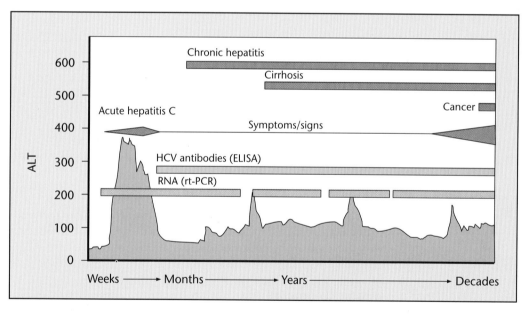

FIGURE 7-111.

Natural history of hepatitis C. Chronicity
may develop over months, years, or decades
and may lead to cirrhosis and an increased
risk for hepatocellular carcinoma. (ALT—
alanine aminotransferase; ELISA—enzyme-
linked immunoassay; HCV—hepatitis C
virus; rt-PCR—reverse transcriptase polymerase chain reaction.) (*Adapted from*
Lemon and Brown [41].)

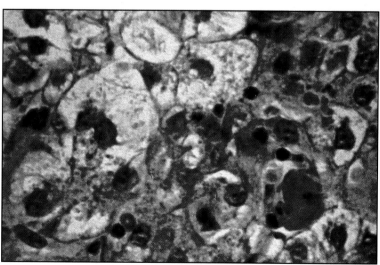

FIGURE 7-112.

Liver histology in acute viral hepatitis, with marked ballooning
degeneration of hepatocytes and acidophilic (apoptotic) body formation. Ballooned cells (whether singly, in groups, or diffusely) may
undergo necrosis by rupture or lysis. Acidophilic/apoptotic body formation is preceded by acidophilic degeneration characterized by cell
shrinkage, increased eosinophilia, increased angularity and loss of
attachment to neighboring cells, nuclear pyknosis, karyorrhexis or
karyolysis. Portions of a degenerating or dying hepatocyte may break
off, forming apoptotic bodies. Acidophilic/apoptotic bodies extruded
into sinusoids are eventually phagocytosed by Kupffer cells [42].
(Hematoxylin-eosin stain; original magnification, X 175.)

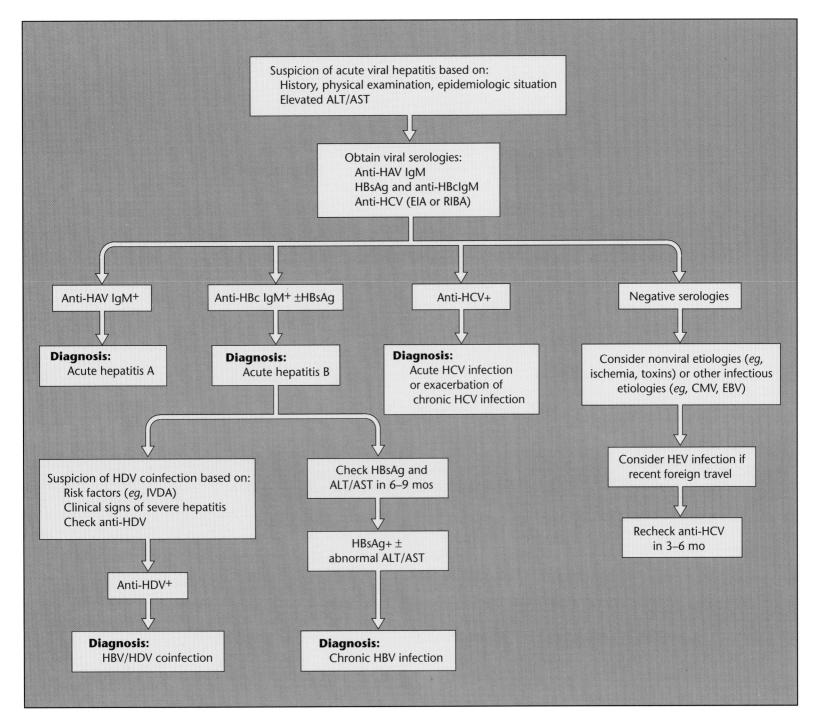

FIGURE 7-113.

Algorithm for diagnostic investigation of suspected viral hepatitis. The rate of possible coinfection, superinfection, or drug-induced etiologies must also be considered in cases with confusing or atypical clinical and serologic findings. ALT—alanine aminotransferase; AST—aspartate aminotransferase; CMV—cytomegalovirus; EBV—Epstein-Barr virus; EIA—enzyme immunoassay; HAV—hepatitis A virus; HBc—hepatitis B core; HBsAg—hepatitis B surface antigen; HBV—hepatitis B virus; HCV—hepatitis C virus; HDV—hepatitis D virus; HEV—hepatitis E virus; IVDA—intravenous drug abusers; RIBA—recombinant immunoblot assay. (*Adapted from* Hsu *et al.* [40].)

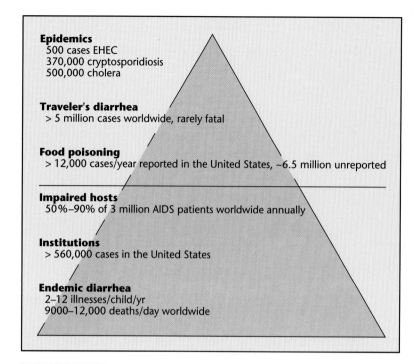

FIGURE 7-114.

Six types of microbial diarrhea. Worldwide, diarrheal diseases are second only to cardiovascular disease as a cause of death and are the leading cause of childhood death. Microbial diarrhea occurs in six settings. Reaching the greatest attention are occasional epidemics, such as those caused by enterohemorrhagic *Escherichia coli* (EHEC), water-borne cryptosporidiosis, and global spread of new cholera pandemics; traveler's diarrhea, which affects up to one third of 16 million international travelers each year; and food poisoning. Receiving considerably less attention but responsible for considerably more cases worldwide are diarrheal illnesses in impaired hosts (such as occurs in 50% to 90% of AIDS patients globally each year) and diarrhea in institutions (such as daycare centers, hospitals, and extended care facilities). Finally, there is endemic diarrhea, accounting for two to 12 illnesses per child per year and more than 9000 deaths each day globally [43].

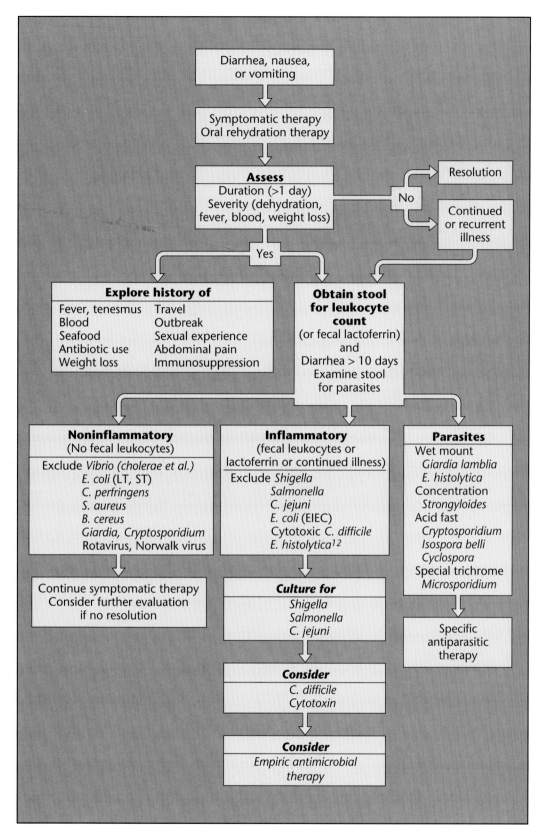

FIGURE 7-115.

Selective diagnostic and therapeutic approach to diarrhea, nausea, and vomiting. Although all patients with significant gastrointestinal illnesses should receive adequate rehydration, orally if possible, further diagnostic or more specific antimicrobial therapy should be directed by specific findings in the history or stool examination. Diarrhea lasting for > 1 day or associated with severe dehydration, bloody stool, fever, or weight loss warrants additional evaluation of history and stool examination for leukocytes or a leukocyte marker (such as lactoferrin). Diarrhea lasting for 10 days should prompt examination for parasites. EIEC—enteroinvasive *E. coli*; LT—heat-labile toxin; ST—heat-stable toxin. (*Adapted from* Guerrant and Bobak [44].)

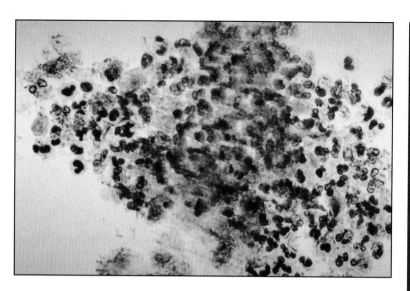

FIGURE 7-116.

Fecal leukocytes on wet mount of stool specimen stained with methylene blue. Clumps of numerous polymorphonuclear leukocytes can be seen in a patient with *Shigella* infection. Examination of fresh stool is a potentially helpful screen for colonic mucosal inflammation due to invasive bacteria, such as *Shigella* or *Campylobacter jejuni*, or idiopathic inflammatory disease. However, it requires that a skilled microscopist examine a freshly stained fecal specimen to avoid false-positive and false-negative readings.

Possible Casuses of Diarrhea in AIDS Patients

Pathogen	Diarrhea, % (*n* = 181)	No Diarrhea, % (*n* = 28)
Cytomegalovirus	12–45	15
Cryptosporidium	14–26	0
Microsporidium	7.5–33	0
Entamoeba histolytica	0–15	0
Giardia lamblia	2–15	5
Salmonella spp	0–15	0
Campylobacter spp	2–11	8
Shigella spp	5–10	0
Clostridium difficile toxin	6–7	0
Vibrio parahaemolyticus	4	0
Mycobacterium spp	2–25	0
Isospora belli	2–6	0
Blastocystis hominis	2–15	16
Candida albicans	6–53	24
Herpes simplex	5–18	40
Chlamydia trachomatis	11	13
Strongyloides	0–6	0
Intestinal spirochetes	11	11
One or more pathogens	55–86	39

FIGURE 7-117.

Possible causes of diarrhea in patients with AIDS. One or more identifiable pathogens can usually be identified in 65% to 86% of patients with diarrhea and AIDS. This list is led by cytomegalovirus, followed by *Cryptosporidium, Microsporidium*, and numerous other potential pathogens, some of which may respond to specific therapy and should be sought. This diagnosis usually can be accomplished by non-invasive special methods. (*Adapted from* Guerrant and Bobak [45].)

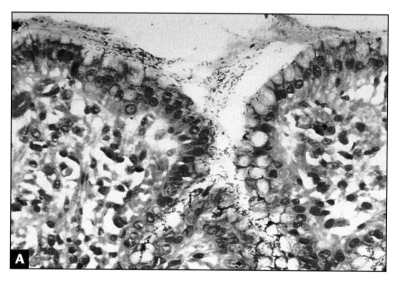

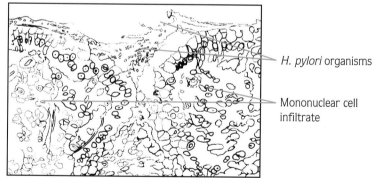

H. pylori organisms

Mononuclear cell infiltrate

FIGURE 7-118.

Heavy *Helicobacter pylori* infection of the gastric antrum. Large numbers of bacteria are seen within the mucus and foveolae. The surface epithelium has lost its orderly arrangement, and the mucin component of the superficial cells is greatly reduced. The inflammatory infiltrate in the lamina propria is predominantly mononuclear.

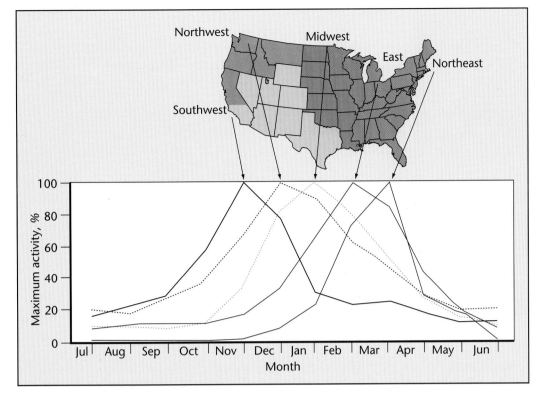

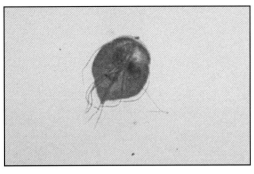

FIGURE 7-120.

Giardia lamblia trophozoite. Trophozoites are pear-shaped, bilaterally symmetrical bodies and measure 9 to 21 × 5 to 15 μm. Characteristic structures include four pairs of flagella and two nuclei in the area of the sucking disc. Trophozoites move by oscillating about the long axis, producing motion said to resemble a falling leaf. (Giemsa stain.) (*Courtesy of* M. Scaglia.)

FIGURE 7-119.

Regional rotavirus activity by month in the United States between 1984 and 1988. Data were collected in a 5-year retrospective survey of sentinel laboratories in the United States, covering the period 1984 to 1988. Results showed that rotavirus infections occur as epidemics predominantly in the winter months. The earliest outbreaks of each season tend to be in the western states in the fall months, with a wavelike progression across the continent toward the northeast, where the peak incidence of outbreaks is in the late winter and early spring [46].

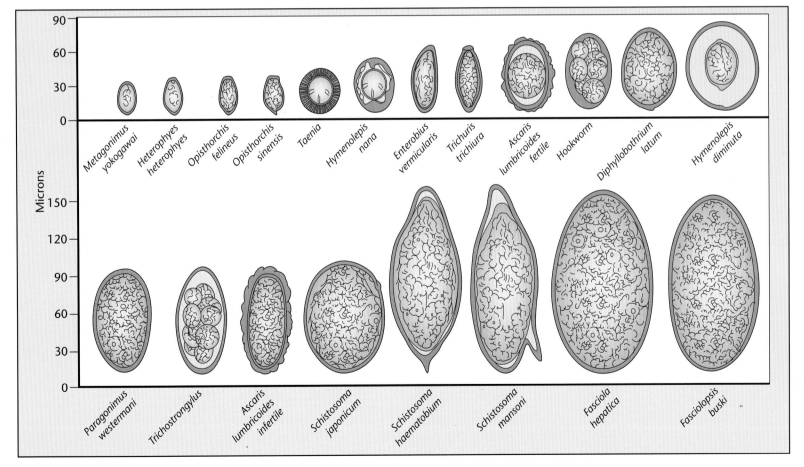

FIGURE 7-121.

Relative sizes of helminth eggs. Diagnosis of helminthic infection most commonly depends on careful examination of stool or urine for eggs [47].

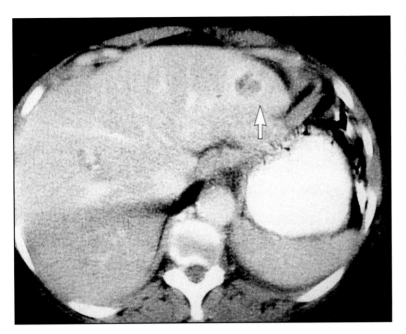

FIGURE 7-122.
Hepatic abscess. A computed tomography scan with oral and intravenous contrast material demonstrates a low-density lesion in the left lobe of the liver with an enhancing edge (*arrow*). This lesion proved to be a polymicrobial abscess in this patient with diverticulitis. Enhancement in the periphery of the abscess after intravenous injection of contrast material is a common finding in hepatic abscess, distinguishing it from a simple cyst or hepatic tumor.

■ EXTERNAL MANIFESTATIONS OF SYSTEMIC INFECTIONS

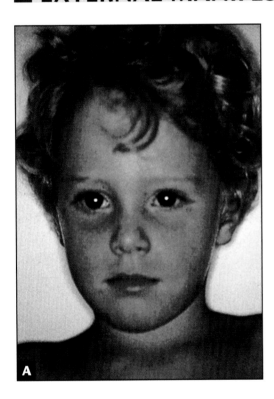

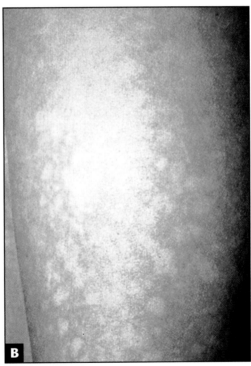

FIGURE 7-123.
Cutaneous rash of erythema infectiosum.
A, The initial cutaneous manifestation of erythema infectiosum, which occurs during the recovery phase of the infection and is thought to be immunologically mediated, is a malar flush, giving the characteristic appearance of "slapped cheeks" and circumoral pallor. **B,** The macular erythematous rash then spreads to the arms, trunk, and extremities, where it may fade with a reticulated or lacy pattern.

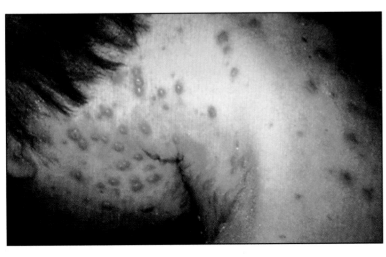

FIGURE 7-124.
Vesicular lesions of chickenpox. Chickenpox results from a patient's first infection with the varicella-zoster virus. The characteristic vesicular lesions on an erythematous base, resembling a dew drop on a rose petal, develop around the hair line and on the face.

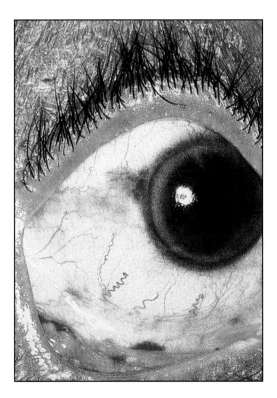

FIGURE 7-125.
Conjunctival hemorrhages in a patient with *Staphylococcus aureus* endocarditis.

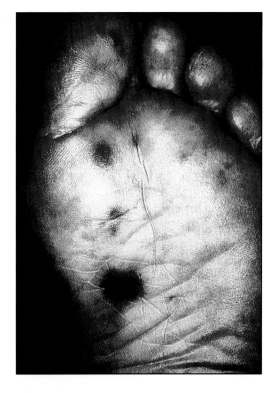

FIGURE 7-126.
Janeway lesions in a patient with *Staphylococcus aureus* endocarditis. Janeway lesions are generally painless, flat, and occasionally hemorrhagic, as in this case. Embolic in origin with microabscess formation in the dermis, they are almost pathognomonic of *S. aureus* endocarditis. (*From* Sande and Strausbaugh [48]; with permission.)

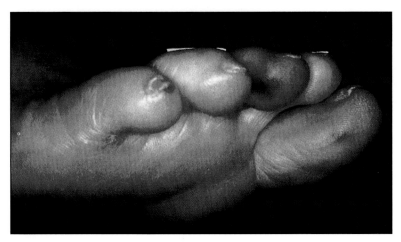

FIGURE 7-127.
Osler's nodes in patients with infective endocarditis. These lesions usually occur in the tufts of the fingers or toes and are painful and evanescent. They likely are mediated by immunopathologic factors.

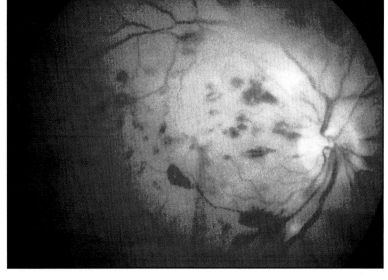

FIGURE 7-128.
Roth spots in infective endocarditis. Of uncertain pathogenesis, these lesions usually are characterized by a central clear area surrounded by hemorrhage.

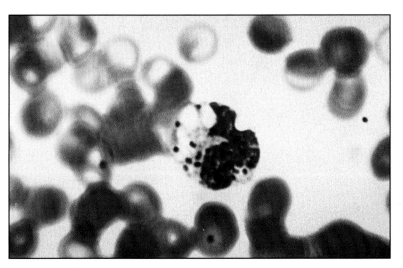

FIGURE 7-129.
Wright-stained smear of peripheral blood in fulminant *Neisseria meningitidis* bacteremia. Note the presence of extracellular and intracellular gram-negative diplococci. Direct visualization of meningococci on unspun peripheral blood is quite unusual. However, similar smears can be obtained by direct aspiration of necrotic skin lesions.

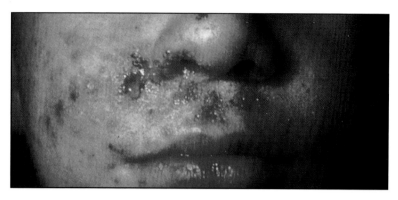

FIGURE 7-130.

Facial impetigo 3 days after onset. Serous, oozing, honey-yellow crusts with a "stuck-on" appearance below the nares and pustules below the lips are apparent in this child aged 5 years with classic impetigo. Culture yielded group A streptococci. (*Courtesy of* A.M. Margileth.)

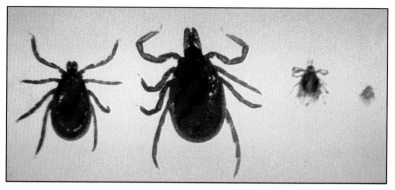

FIGURE 7-131.

Larva, nymph, and adult female and male *Ixodes dammini* ticks (from *right* to *left*). The larva (*far left*) is approximately 1 mm in diameter. *I. dammini* is the principal vector for transmission of Lyme disease in the eastern and midwestern United States. (*From* Rahn [51]; *courtesy of* Marge Anderson, Pfitzer Central Research, Groton, CT.)

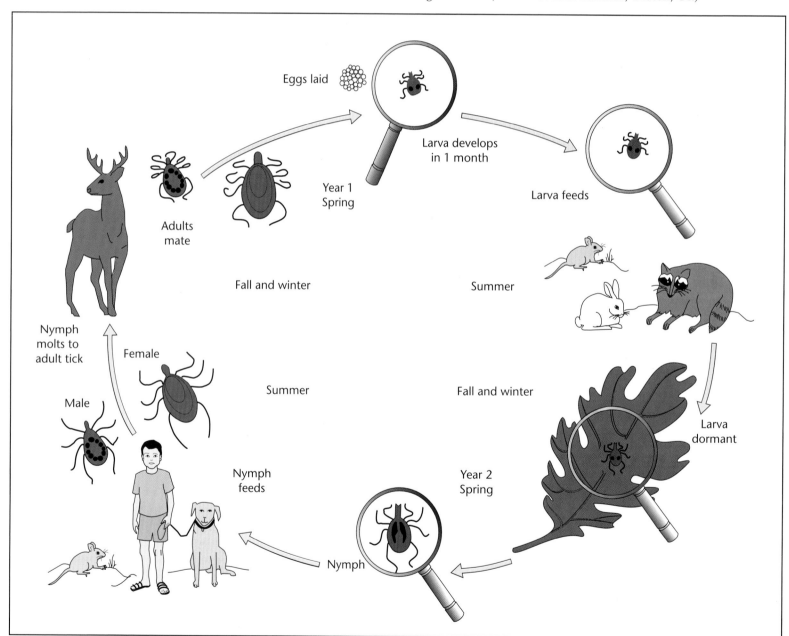

FIGURE 7-132.

Two-year life cycle of *Ixodes dammini* in the northeastern United States. Larvae are born in the spring uninfected and acquire *Borrelia burgdorferi* after feeding on their preferred host, the white-footed mouse. The following spring, larvae molt into nymphs that feed once again on small mammals (or occasionally humans), transmitting the infection to naive hosts. In the late summer and early fall, nymphs molt into adult male and female ticks. Adults mate in early fall, and eggs are laid. Humans and other animals are incidental hosts for *I. dammini* and not required for maintenance of the tick's life cycle. (*Adapted from* Rahn and Malawista [50].)

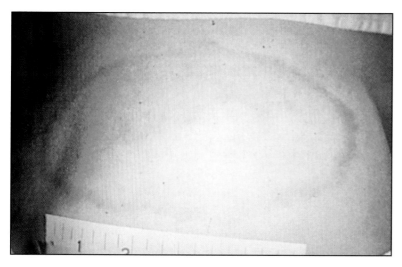

FIGURE 7-133.

Erythema (chronicum) migrans. Erythema migrans (EM), the pathognomonic skin lesion of Lyme disease, appears as an expanding erythematous lesion, often with central clearing, around the site of the tick bite. Rare lesions of EM can have erythematous and indurated centers resembling streptococcal cellulitis or vesicular and necrotic centers. EM is reported in 60% to 80% of patients. Common sites are the thigh, groin, trunk, and axilla. (*From* Steere *et al.* [51]; with permission.)

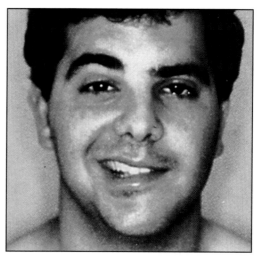

FIGURE 7-134.

Left facial palsy (Bell's palsy) in early Lyme disease. The left facial droop reflects a seventh nerve palsy (Bell's palsy), an early neurologic manifestation of Lyme disease, and one that may be bilateral. Other neurologic manifestations include lymphocytic meningitis or meningoencephalitis and other cranial or peripheral neuritis. They typically occur 2 to 8 weeks after infection. (*From* Klempner [52]; with permission.)

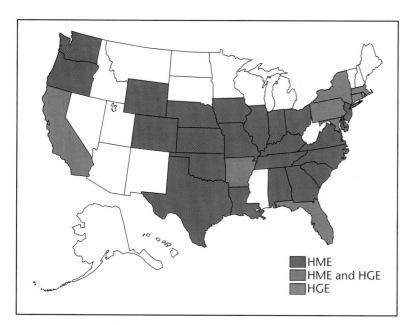

HME
HME and HGE
HGE

FIGURE 7-135.

Geographic distribution of recognized cases of human monocytic ehrlichiosis (*Ehrlichia chaffeensis* infection) and human granulocytic ehrlichiosis (*E. equi*–like agent) in the United States through 1994. Most cases of human monocytic ehrlichiosis (HME) occur in areas where Rocky Mountain spotted fever is frequently recognized, whereas human granulocytic ehrlichiosis (HGE) occurs mostly where Lyme borreliosis and deer ticks (*Ixodes* spp) are also frequent. The distribution of HME cases overlaps the geographic distribution of the Lone Star tick, *Amblyomma americanum*, the probable major vector of human monocytic ehrlichiosis in the United States. (HME data *courtesy of* J.E. Dawson.)

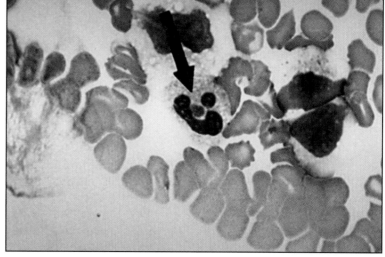

FIGURE 7-136.

Peripheral blood band neutrophil with a morula (*arrow*) from a patient with fatal granulocytic ehrlichiosis. The specific identity of this agent is not known, but it is very closely related to the granulocytic ehrlichiae *Ehrlichia phagocytophila* (in Europe) and *E. equi* (in the United States) only known to cause veterinary diseases. Unlike monocytic ehrlichiosis, ehrlichiae that infect granulocytes may appear in large numbers in peripheral blood. Infection is predominantly restricted to neutrophils and bands. Diagnosis is strongly suggested when morulae are observed only in peripheral blood neutrophils or bands. The diagnosis may be confirmed by polymerase chain reaction amplification of specific granulocytic ehrlichia nucleic acids from acute phase blood; by immunocytologic demonstration of granulocytic ehrlichiae with *E. equi* antibodies in peripheral blood, buffy coat smears, or tissues; or by the demonstration of a serologic reaction with *E. equi* in convalescence [53,54]. (Wright stain; original magnification, × 1200.)

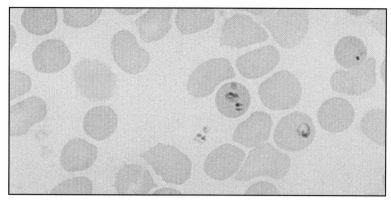

FIGURE 7-137.

Peripheral smear of human red blood cells infected with *Babesia microti*. The patient was a man aged 62 years from Minnesota with a several-week history of severe fatigue, malaise, weight loss, and night sweats [55].

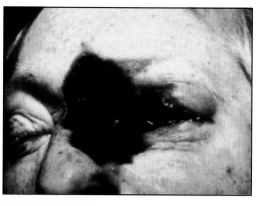

FIGURE 7-138.

Rapidly progressive rhinocerebral mucormycosis. A middle-aged man with insulin-dependent diabetes mellitus and recurrent ketoacidosis presented with rapidly progressive mucormycosis of the sinus, leading to cerebral infarction and death. (*Courtesy of* T. Walsh; *from* Walsh *et al.* [56].)

FIGURE 7-139.

American cutaneous leishmaniasis on a patient's cheek. Not all infections result in ulceration. Cutaneous leishmaniasis must be considered in the differential diagnosis of any chronic skin lesion in a person who has been exposed in an endemic area.

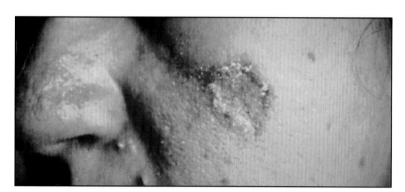

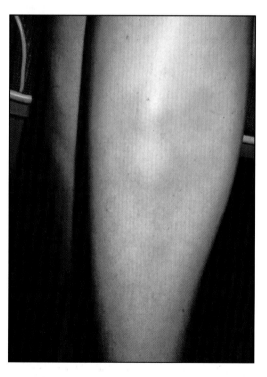

FIGURE 7-140.

Erythema nodosum in a patient with rheumatologic manifestations of histoplasmosis. The patient presented with pain in the knees and hips associated with mild swelling of the right knee. Although the patient denied pulmonary symptoms, her chest radiograph showed right paratracheal lymphadenopathy. Examination also showed erythema nodosum. A synovial fluid analysis was unremarkable. Although initially believed to have sarcoidosis, a diagnosis of histoplasmosis was considered because she presented during an outbreak, and serologic tests were positive for histoplasmosis with an M band by immunodiffusion and a complement fixation titer of 1:16 to the yeast and 1:8 to the mycelial antigen. Synovial fluid cultures were negative for fungus. She received 6 months of anti-inflammatory therapy with complete resolution of the arthritis and erythema nodosum. This manifestation of histoplasmosis represents a systemic immunologic reaction to acute pulmonary infection and not dissemination to the joints or skin [4–6]. Rarely, patients have exhibited bone or joint lesions as a manifestation of disseminated histoplasmosis.

URINARY TRACT INFECTIONS AND INFECTIONS OF THE FEMALE PELVIS

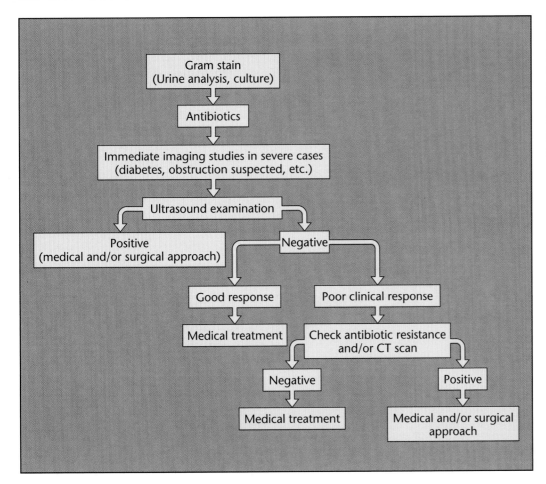

FIGURE 7-141.
Clinical management of complicated pyelonephritis. Complicated pyelonephritis usually necessitates hospitalization, thorough investigation of the urinary tract using imaging studies, and, when indicated depending on the underlying anomalies, aggressive medicosurgical procedures. CT—computed tomography.

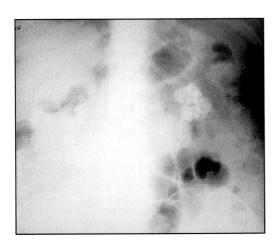

FIGURE 7-142.
Staghorn calculus seen on abdominal radiograph. Staghorn calculi are "infection stones" (struvite and calcium carbonate apatite), produced in association with infection with urease-producing organisms, primarily *Proteus mirabilis*. These are generally large calculi that follow the contours of the renal pelvis and may destroy the kidney. This abdominal film shows a staghorn calculus of the left kidney with associated calcification of the left upper ureter in a woman presenting with recurrent abdominal pain.

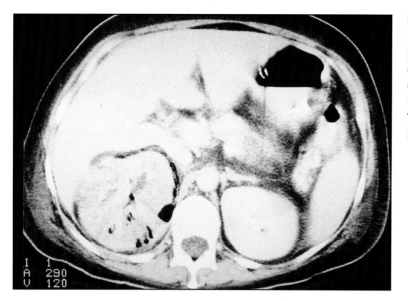

FIGURE 7-143.

Emphysematous pyelonephritis in a patient with diabetes. A rare presentation of urinary tract infection in diabetic patients is that of emphysematous pyelonephritis. This condition occurs in the presence of hyperglycemia with glucose excreted in the urine. Uropathogens may produce gas in the presence of elevated glucose. The computed tomography scan shows an enlarged, inflamed, right kidney with air within the parenchyma and subcapsular space.

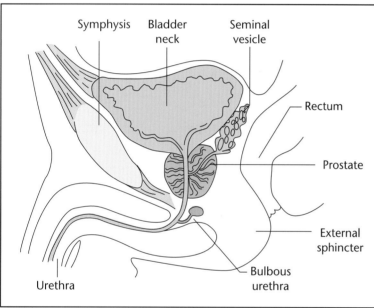

FIGURE 7-144.

Anatomy of the prostate. Coronal view.

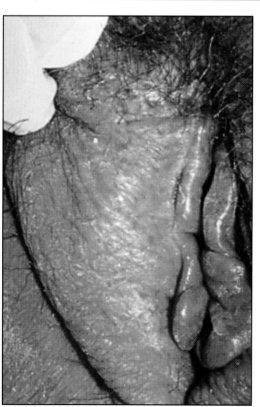

FIGURE 7-145.

Lichen simplex chronicus secondary to a candidal infection. Although the *Candida* infection had been treated successfully and cleared, the initial dermatitis led to a "itch-scratch-itch" cycle, which persisted. The pruritus, usually more intense at night, leads to scratching and results in lichenification, fissures, and even distinct papules and nodules called *prurigo nodularis*. Because of similar symptoms of chronic itching and burning, these patients are sometimes misdiagnosed as having recurrent chronic candidiasis. (*Courtesy of* L. Edwards.)

Differential Diagnostic Features of Vaginitis in Adult Women

Feature	Normal	Candida vaginitis	Bacterial vaginosis	Trichomonal vaginitis
Symptoms	None or physiologic leukorrhea	Vulvar pruritus, soreness, ↑ discharge, dysureia, dyspareunia	Moderate malodorous discharge	Profuse, purulent, offensive discharge; pruritus; dyspareunia
Discharge				
Amount	Scant to moderate	Scant to moderate	Moderate	Profuse
Color	Clear or white	White	White or gray	Yellow
Consistency	Floccular, nonhomogeneous	Clumped but variable	Homogeneous, uniformly coating walls	Homogenous
Bubbles	Absent	Absent	Present	Present
Appearance of vulva and vagina	Normal	Introital and vulvar erythema, edema, occasional pustules, vaginal erythema	No inflammation	Erythema and swelling of vulvar and vaginal epithelium, "strawberry" cervix
pH of vaginal fluid	< 4.5	< 4.5	> 4.7	5.0–6.0
Amine test (16% KOH)	Negative	Negative	Positive	Occasionally present
Saline microscopy	Normal epithelial cells, lactobacilli predominate	Normal flora, blastospores (yeast) 40%–50%, pseudohyphae	Clue cells, coccobacillary flora predominate, absence of leukocytes, motile curved rods	PMNs +++, motile trichomonads (80%–90%), no clue cells or abnormal flora
10% KOH microscopy	Negative	Positive (60%–90%)	Negative (except in mixed infections)	Negative

FIGURE 7-146.

Clinical and laboratory features of candidal, bacterial, and trichomonal vaginitis in adult women. Women who complain of abnormal discharge or vulvar discomfort should be evaluated for vaginitis. Vaginal discharge associated with vaginitis can act as an irritant to the vulva causing erythema and pain. (*Adapted from* Sobel [60].)

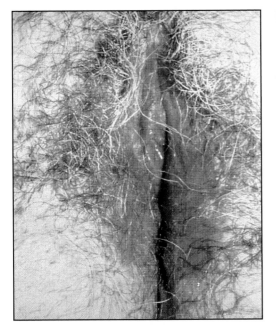

FIGURE 7-147.
Candidal infection causing "beefy" red appearance of the vulva. (*Courtesy of* L. Edwards.)

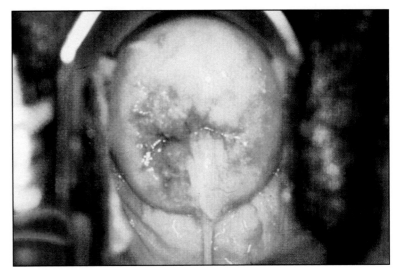

FIGURE 7-148.
Mucopurulent endocervical discharge in gonococcal endocervicitis. Note the thick, yellow exudate escaping from the endocervical canal.

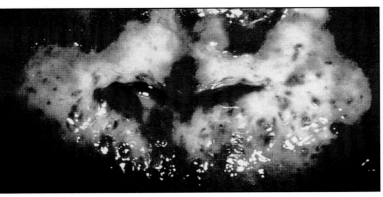

FIGURE 7-149.
Gross appearance of herpes cervicitis. Primary herpes cervicitis may also be characterized by increased surface vascularity and microulcerations without necrotic areas. (*Courtesy of* P. Wolner-Hanssen.)

■ CARDIOVASCULAR INFECTIONS

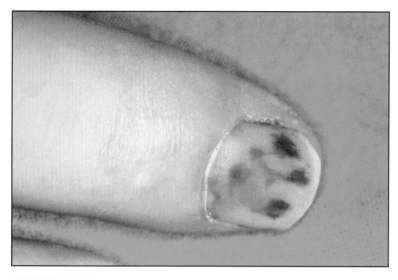

FIGURE 7-150.

Splinter hemorrhages in a fingernail. Splinter hemorrhages may be due to simple trauma, but when multiple nails are involved in a patient with infective endocarditis, they represent a vasculitic component of the infection.

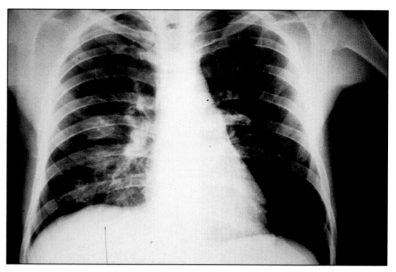

FIGURE 7-151.

Chest radiograph of a male intravenous heroin addict aged 25 years with right-sided endocarditis showing three infiltrates in the right lung secondary to septic pulmonary embolizations.

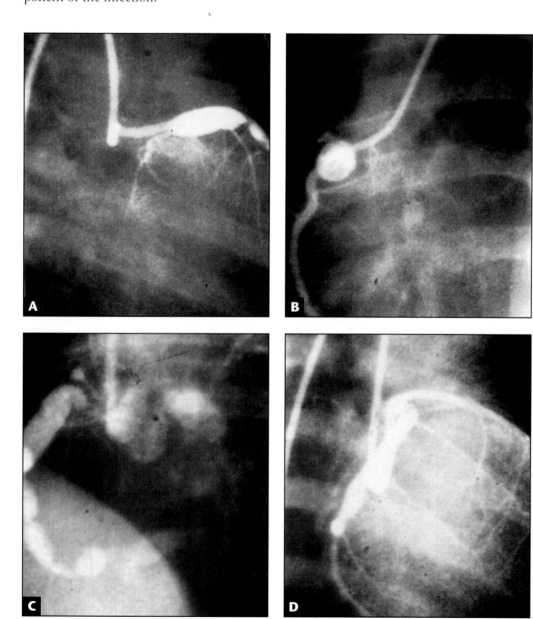

FIGURE 7-152.

A–D, Coronary angiograms of patients with Kawasaki disease demonstrating fusiform (**A**), saccular (**B**), and segmental (**C**) aneurysms and an ectatic coronary artery (**D**).

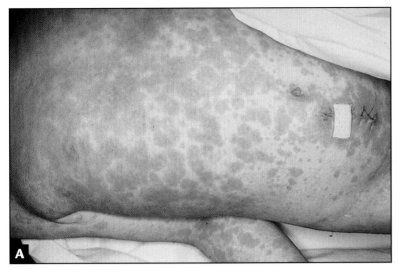

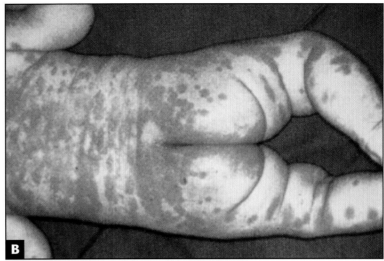

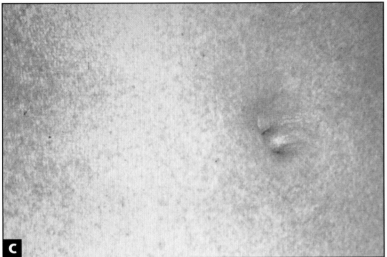

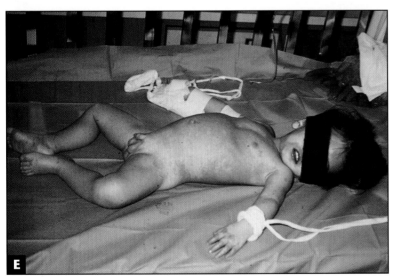

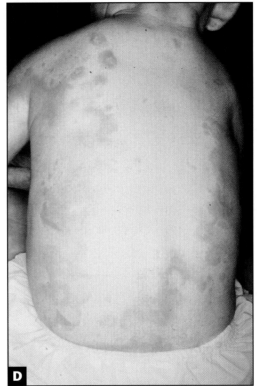

FIGURE 7-153.

Examples of rashes seen in patients with Kawasaki disease. The rash is typically polymorphous and appears within 5 days of the onset of fever. **A–D,** Such rashes may take various forms including an urticarial exanthem (**A**), a maculopapular morbilliform eruption (**B**), a scarlatiniform derma (**C**), or an erythema-multiforme–like rash (**D**). Bullous eruptions have not been described. **E,** The rash is usually extensive, involving the trunk and extremities with accentuation in the perineal region. (Panel B *from* Dajani *et al.* [61]; with permission.)

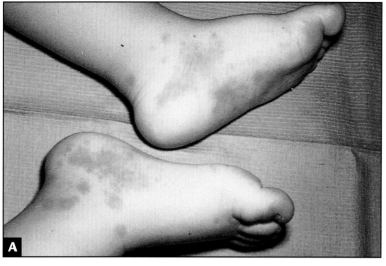

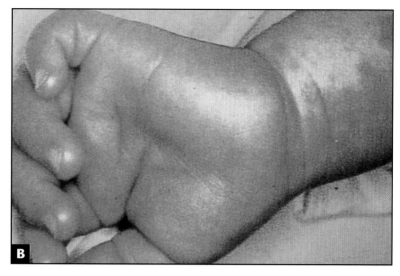

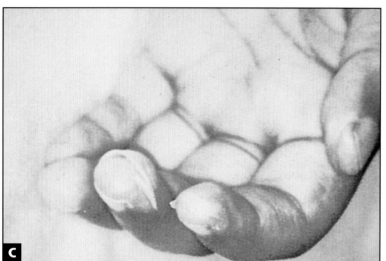

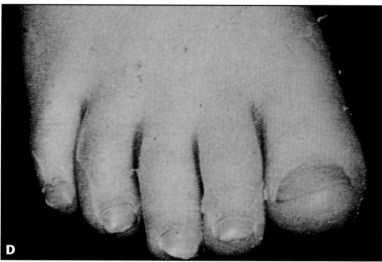

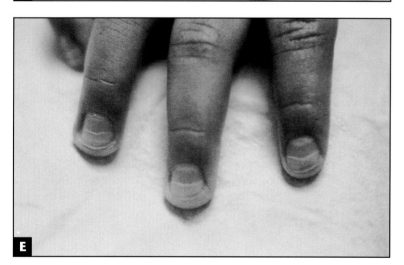

FIGURE 7-154.

Changes in the extremities are distinctive. **A** and **B**, Erythema of the palms and soles and/or firm, sometimes painful induration of the hands or feet often occurs in the early phase of the disease. **C** and **D**, Desquamation of the fingers and toes usually begins 1 to 3 weeks after onset of fever in the periungual region and may extend to the palms and toes. **E**, Approximately 1 to 2 months after the onset of fever, deep transverse grooves across the nails (Beau's lines) may appear. (Panels B and C *from* Dajani *et al.* [61]; with permission.)

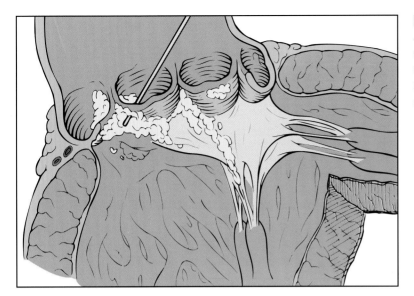

FIGURE 7-155.

Advanced aortic valve endocarditis. Perforation of the noncoronary cusp is shown with resultant jet lesion on the septal wall. Clearly shown is the ease with which the advanced infection can extend from the aortic valve onto the anterior cusp of the mitral valve and chordae tendineae. (*Adapted from* Netter [62].)

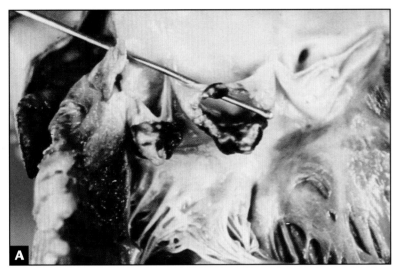

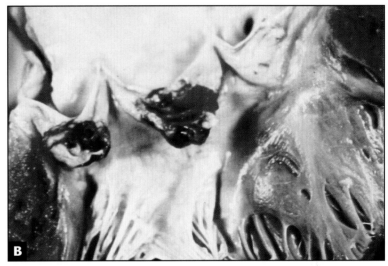

FIGURE 7-156.

Aortic valve with large hemorrhagic vegetations on both the left and noncoronary cusps. **A,** The metal probe highlights the large perforation of the noncoronary cusp on removal of the thrombus.

B, A similar perforation was present on the left coronary cusp. Small areas of calcification can be seen in the right coronary leaflet. (*Courtesy of* W.E. Dismukes.)

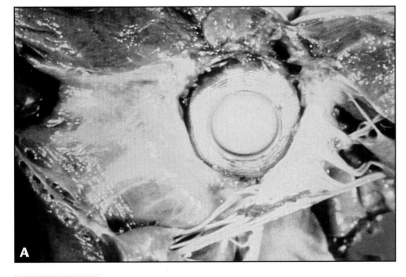

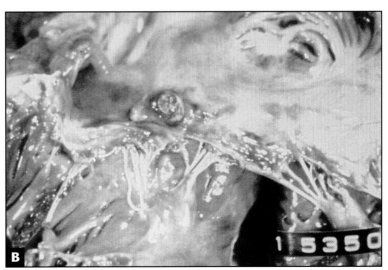

FIGURE 7-157.

Prosthetic valve endocarditis caused by *Enterococcus* species. The autopsy findings revealed that the infection had extended from the prosthetic valve to the noncoronary cusp and right atrium. **A,** The

closed valve from the left ventricular aspect with perivalvular dehiscence at its superior aspect is shown. **B,** The end of the fistulous tract entering the right atrium above the tricuspid valve is shown.

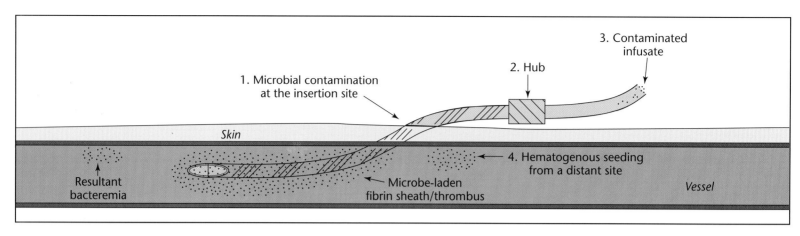

FIGURE 7-158.

Pathogenesis of catheter-related venous infection. Intravenous catheters are the most common source of device-related infections. In general, either (or both) of two mechanisms are considered to be the original source of the vast majority of catheter-related bloodstream infections: contamination at the insertion site (*1*), which usually occurs *during* the first week of catheterization, and contamination of the catheter hub (*2*) or from any of the various connections along the infusion line, which usually occurs *after* the first week of catheterization. Generally, microbes colonizing the patient's skin or attending healthcare worker's skin or gloves are responsible for contamination at the insertion site or the hub. Rarely, contaminated skin preparations or local wounds can cause contamination at the insertion site. Less common sources of catheter-related bloodstream infection include the infusate (*3*), such as large-volume parenteral solutions, blood products, total parenteral nutrition, and intravenous medicines, which may be associated with outbreaks of infusion-related bloodstream infections, and hematogenous seeding (*4*) of catheters, which occurs most commonly in patients in the intensive care unit. When a catheter-related thrombus becomes infected (suppurative thrombophlebitis), whether in a great central or peripheral vein, the vein can become a source of bacteremia or fungemia even though the insertion site might lack any sign of infection or inflammation in more than half the cases [65].

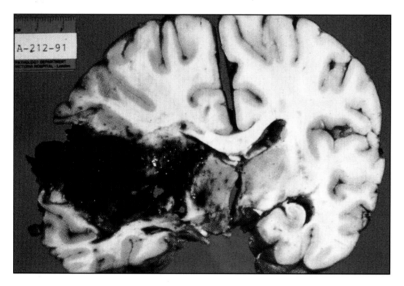

FIGURE 7-159.

Gross specimen showing endocarditic intracerebral hemorrhage. Intracerebral hemorrhage occurs in approximately 5% of patients with native-valve bacterial endocarditis, and in some cases it can be predicted by radiologic identification of "mycotic" aneurysms. Most of the cerebrovascular complications of bacterial endocarditis occur early, and the risk of these complications diminishes rapidly as the infection is controlled. (*Courtesy of* D.A. Ramsay and G.B. Young.)

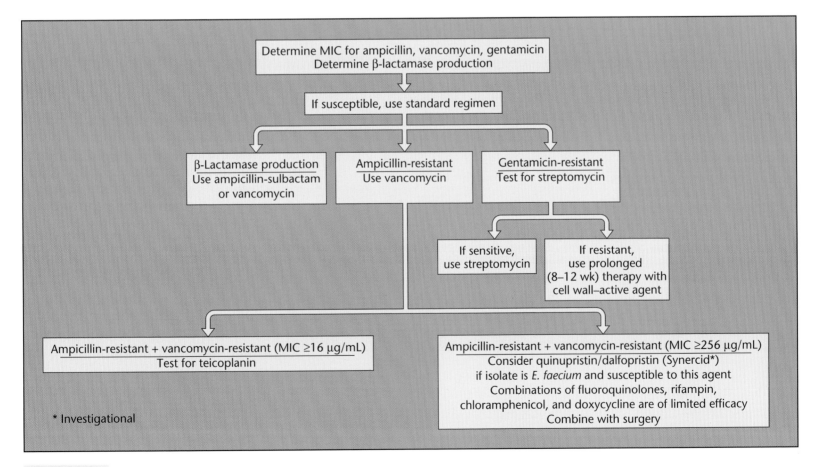

FIGURE 7-160.

Parasite cycle. Chagas' disease is caused by *Trypanosoma cruzi*, a protozoan present in sylvatic mammals of the Americas such as armadillos, rodents, and opossums, as well as in domestic animals. It has vertebrate and invertebrate cycles. Transmission to humans is by reduviid bugs while feeding, by fecal contamination rather than inoculation. After initial trypomastigote (flagellate form) parasitemia (*1*), the parasites penetrate cardiac muscle and other tissue cells where they transform into amastigotes (aflagellate form) (*2*). Intracellular parasite multiplication may lead to cell rupture with passage into the circulation or parasitism of other tissues including various ganglionic plexuses and segments of the alimentary tract. The cycle is completed when feeding bugs pick up blood trypomastigotes (*3*). The trypanosomes become epimastigotes in the insect midgut (*4*), and then multiply and migrate to the hindgut where they become metacyclic trypomastigotes (*5*), the infective form in humans. Continuous transmission is independent of human infection [64].

Determine MIC for ampicillin, vancomycin, gentamicin
Determine β-lactamase production

If susceptible, use standard regimen

β-Lactamase production
Use ampicillin-sulbactam or vancomycin

Ampicillin-resistant
Use vancomycin

Gentamicin-resistant
Test for streptomycin

If sensitive, use streptomycin

If resistant, use prolonged (8–12 wk) therapy with cell wall–active agent

Ampicillin-resistant + vancomycin-resistant (MIC ≥16 µg/mL)
Test for teicoplanin

Ampicillin-resistant + vancomycin-resistant (MIC ≥256 µg/mL)
Consider quinupristin/dalfopristin (Synercid*)
if isolate is *E. faecium* and susceptible to this agent
Combinations of fluoroquinolones, rifampin, chloramphenicol, and doxycycline are of limited efficacy
Combine with surgery

* Investigational

FIGURE 7-161.

Strategy for selection of an antimicrobial regimen when high-level resistance of enterococcus to components of the standard regimen is encountered. MIC—minimum inhibitory concentration.

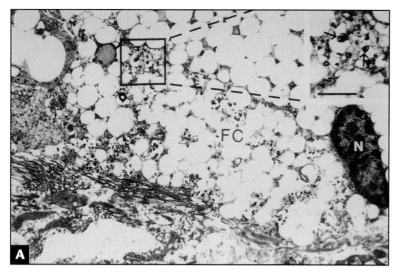
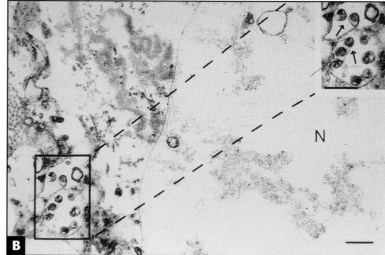

FIGURE 7-162.

Transmission electron micrographs of *Chlamydia pneumoniae* in atherectomy tissue. **A,** A foam cell (FC) within an atheromatous lesion. The nucleus (N) of the cell is also seen. The *boxed area* represents typical *C. pneumoniae* inclusions. The *inset* represents an enlargement of the boxed area and depicts the pear-shaped elemen-

tary bodies (*arrows*) of *C. pneumoniae*. *Bar*=1 μm. **B,** Endosomes within a foam cell of an atheromatous lesion with the pear-shaped elementary bodies of *C. pneumoniae* binding to the endosomal membranes. *Bar*=0.5 μm. (*From* Kuo *et al.* [65]; with permission.)

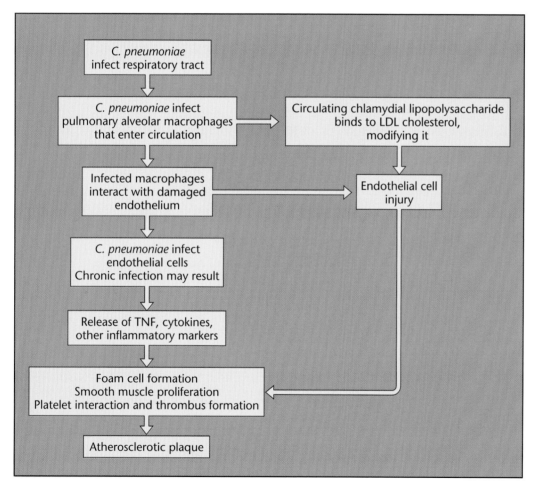

FIGURE 7-163.

Proposed pathogenetic mechanisms through which *Chlamydia pneumoniae* could induce atherosclerotic coronary artery disease. Chlamydiae are known for causing chronic infections, with resultant chronic inflammation. The development of atherosclerosis is known to be an ongoing inflammatory and fibroproliferative process. Chlamydiae have been shown to multiply within a variety of human cells, including macrophages, smooth muscle cells, and endothelial cells. These cell types are among those involved in atheroma formation according to the currently held response-to-injury hypothesis of atherosclerosis. This theory also proposes that circulating low-density lipoprotein (LDL) molecules may be modified and that the modified complex may be capable of inducing or promoting endothelial injury. Chlamydiae may bind to LDL, allowing it to be modified to cause such injury and to begin the cascade of events. Finally, chlamydiae are known inducers of tumor necrosis factor (TNF) and other cytokines. These compounds are also believed to play a role in the sequence of events that eventually can lead to atherosclerotic plaque formation [66,67].

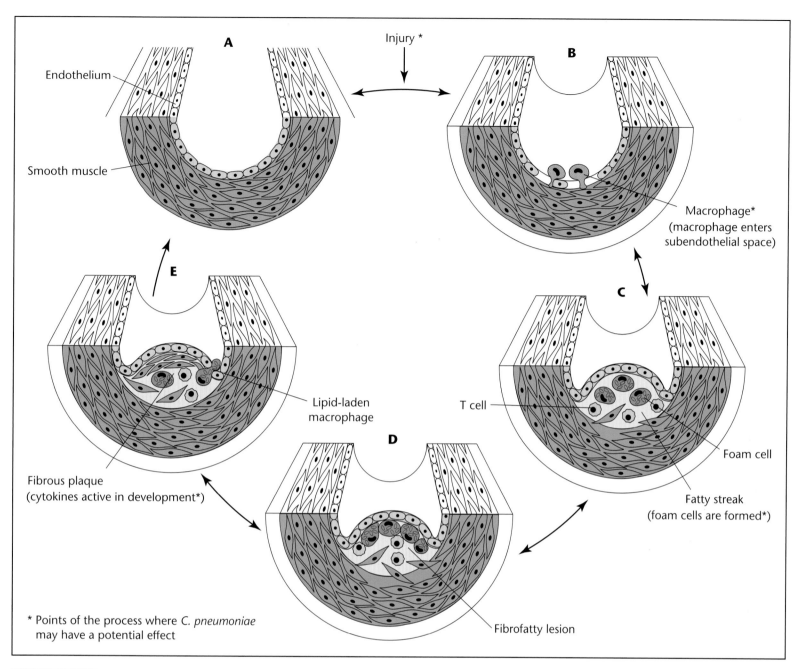

FIGURE 7-164.

Schematic illustrating the response-to-injury hypothesis of athero-sclerosis and the various points in the process where *Chlamydia pneumoniae* may play a role. Normal cross-section through a vessel wall is shown (*A*). With injury to the endothelium from a variety of sources, including chlamydial infection, comes increased adherence of monocytes, macrophages, and T lymphocytes (*B*). These cells can migrate through the endothelium and situate themselves within the subendothelial layer. Chlamydiae within the macrophages may gain access to the vessel wall in this way. Macrophages accumulate lipids and become large foam cells. Chlamydiae may contribute to foam cell formation (*C*). Foam cells, T cells, and smooth muscle cells eventually form the fatty streak. Chlamydiae may infect and replicate within all of these cells, potentially propagating the process. The fatty streak becomes a fibrofatty lesion (*D*). Fibrous plaque formation is complete (*E*). Cytokines are active here. Chlamydiae can activate cytokines. Some of the lipid-laden macrophages may return to the bloodstream, and when this occurs at sites of vessel branching, platelet mural thrombi may form. Each of the stages of lesion formation is potentially reversible. If the cause of injury is removed, or if the inflammatory or fibroprolifera-tive process is reversed, lesions may regress at any stage. (*Adapted from* Ross [67].)

■ REFERENCES

1. Cullen BR: Mechanism of action of regulatory proteins encoded by complex retro-viruses. *Microbiol Rev* 1992, 56:375–394.

2. Hahn BH: Viral genes and their products. In *Textbook of AIDS Medicine*. Edited by Broder S, Merigan TC, Bolognesi D. Baltimore: Williams & Wilkins; 1994:21–44.

3. Gaines H, von Sydow, Pehrson PO, *et al.*: Clinical picture of primary HIV infection presenting as a glandular-fever-like illness. *BMJ* 1988, 297:1363–1368.

4. Hulsebosch HJ, Claessen FAP, van Ginkel CJW, *et al.*: Human immunodeficiency virus exanthem. *J Am Acad Dermatol* 1990, 23:483–485.

5. Rosenberg PS, Biggar RJ: Trends in HIV incidence among young adults in the United States. *JAMA* 1998, 279:1894–1899.

6. Schwartz JJ, Myskowski PL: Molluscum contagiosum in patients with human immunodeficiency virus infection: A review of twenty-seven patients. *J Am Acad Dermatol* 1992, 27:583–588.

7. Mulligan K, Grunfeld C, Tai VW, *et al.*: Hyperlipidemia and insulin resistance are induced by protease inhibitors independent of changes in body composition in patients with HIV infection. *J Acquir Immune Defic Syndr* 2000, 25:35–43.

8. Spaide RF, Vitale AT, Toth IR, Oliver JM: Frosted branch angiitis associated with cytomegalovirus retinitis. *Am J Opthalmol* 1992, 113:522–528.

9. Deeks SG, Hecht FM, Swanson M, *et al.*: HIV-RNA and CD4 cell count response to protease inhibitor therapy in an urban AIDS clinic: response to both initial and salvage therapy. *AIDS* 1999, 13:F35–F43.

10. The Ocular Complications of AIDS Study Group: Mortality in patients with the acquired immunodeficiency syndrome treated with either foscarnet or ganciclovir for cytomegalovirus retinitis. *N Engl J Med* 1992, 326:213–220.

11. Jabs DA, Enger C, Haller J, de Bustros S: Retinal detachments in patients with cytomegalovirus retinitis. *Arch Opthalmol* 1991, 109:794–799.

12. Iannucci AA, Hart LL: Clindamycin in the treatment of toxoplasmosis in AIDS. *Ann Pharmacother* 1992, 26:645–647.

13. Kovacs JA: Efficacy of atovaquone in treatment of toxoplasmosis in patients with AIDS. The NIAID-Clinical Center Intramural AIDS Program. *Lancet* 1992, 340:637–638.

14. Connick E, Lederman MM, Kotzin B, *et al.*: Immune reconstitution in the first year of potent antiretroviral therapy and its relationship to virologic response. *J Infect Dis* 2000, 181:358–363.

15. Greenspan D, Greenspan JS, *et al.*: *AIDS and the Mouth*. Copenhagen, Munksgaard, 1990.

16. Masur H: Prevention and treatment of pneumocystis pneumonia. *N Engl J Med* 1992, 326:1853–1860.

17. Maxfield RA, Sorkin B, Fazzini EP, *et al.*: Respiratory failure in patients with acquired immunodeficiency syndrome and *Pneumocystis carnii* pneumonia. *Crit Care Med* 1986, 14:443–449.

18. Gao F, Bailes E, Robertson DL, *et al.*: Origin of HIV-1 in the chimpanzee *Pan troglodytes*. *Nature* 1999, 397:436–441.

19. Kemper CA, Meng TC, Nussbaum J, *et al.*: Treatment of *Mycobacterium avium* complex bacteremia in AIDS with a four-drug oral regimen: Rifampin, ethambutol, clofazimine, and ciprofloxacin. *Ann Intern Med* 1992, 116:466–472.

20. Johnson RD, McArthur JC, Narayano C: The neurobiology of human immunodeficiency virus infections. *FASEB J* 1988, 2:2970–2981.

21. Sampaio EP, Sarno EN, Galilly R, *et al.*: Thalidomide selectively inhibits tumor necrosis factor alpha production by stimulated human monocytes. *Exp Med* 1991, 173:669–703.

22. Farrar WE, Wood MJ, Innes JA, Tubbs H: *Infectious Diseases: Text and Color Atlas*, edn. 2. London: Gower Medical Publishing: an imprint of Times Mirror International Publishers Ltd; 1992.

23. Price RW, Brew BJ, Roke M: Central and peripheral nervous system complications of HIV-1 infections and AIDS. In *AIDS: Etiology, Diagnosis, Treatment, and Prevention*. Edited by DeVita VT Jr, Hellman S, Rosenberg SA, *et al.* Philadelphia: J.B. Lippincott; 1992:237–254.

24. Wispelwey B, Dacey R Jr, Scheld WM: Brain abscess. In *Infections of the Central Nervous System*. Edited by Scheld WM, Durack D, Whitley R. New York: Raven Press; 1991.

25. Post MJD, Sze G, Quencer RM, *et al.*: Gadolinium-enhanced MR in spinal infection. *J Comput Assist Tomogr* 1990, 14:721–725.

26. Vortel JJ, Chow AW: Infections of the sinuses and parameningeal structures. In *Infectious Diseases*. Edited by Gorbach SL, Bartlett JG, Blacklow NR. Philadelphia: W.B. Saunders; 1992:432.

27. Barton R, Cerra FB: The hypermetabolism–multiple organ failure syndrome. *Chest* 1989, 115:136–140.

28. Bone RC: Sepsis syndrome: New insights into its pathogenesis and treatment. *Intensive Care World* 1992, 4:50–59.

29. Nava E, Palmer RMF, Moncada S: Inhibition of nitric oxide synthesis in septic shock: How much is beneficial? *Lancet* 1991, 338:1557–1558.

30. Sprung C, Cerra FB, Freund HR, *et al.*: Plasma amino acids as predictors of the severity and outcome of sepsis. *Crit Care Med* 1991, 19:753–757.

31. Wald ER: Rhinitis and acute and chronic sinusitis. In *Pediatric Otolaryngology*, edn 2. Edited by Bluestone CB, Stool SE. Philadelphia: W.B. Saunders; 1990:736.

32. Bull TR: *A Color Atlas of E.N.T. Diagnosis*, edn 2. London: Wolfe Medical Publications; 1987:96.

33. Rein MF: In *Sexually Transmitted Diseases*. Edited by Holmes KK, *et al.* New York: McGraw-Hill; 1984.

34. Fiumara NJ: *Pictorial Guide to Sexually Transmitted Diseases*. New York: Cahners Publ.; 1989:42.

35. Oriel D: Genital human papillomavirus infection. In *Sexually Transmitted Diseases*, edn 2. Edited by Holmes KK, Mardh P-A, Sparling PF, *et al.* New York: McGraw Hill; 1990:435.

36. Goodwin RA, des Prez RM: Apical localization of pulmonary tuberculosis, chronic pulmonary histoplasmosis, and progressive massive fibrosis of the lung. *Chest* 1983, 83:801–805.

37. Bone RC, *et al.*: *Pulmonary and Critical Care Medicine. Care Volume*, vol. 2. St. Louis: Mosby; 1993.

38. Lyche KD, Jensen WA, Kirsch CM, *et al.*: Pleuropulmonary manifestations of hepatic amebiasis. *West J Med* 1990, 153:275–278.

39. Rubin RH, Wolfson JS, Cosimi AB, *et al.*: Infection in the renal transplant recipient. *Am J Med* 1981, 70:405–411.

40. Hsu HH, Feinstone SM, Hoofnagle JH: Acute viral hepatitis. In *Principles and Practice of Infectious Diseases*, 4th ed. Edited by Mandell GL, Bennett JE, Dolin R. New York: Churchill Livingstone; 1995:1136–1153.

41. Lemon SM, Brown EA: Hepatitis C virus. In *Principles and Practice of Infectious Diseases*, edn 4. Edited by Mandell GL, Bennett JE, Dolin R. New York: Churchill Livingstone: 1995:1474–1486.

42. Ueda N, Shah SV: Apoptosis. *J Lab Clin Med* 1994, 124:169–177.

43. Guerrant RL: Lessons from diarrheal diseases: Demography to molecular pharmacology. *J Infect Dis* 1994, 169:1206–1218.

44. Guerrant RL, Bobak DA: Bacterial and protozoal gastroenteritis. *N Engl J Med* 1991, 325:327–340.

45. Guerrant RL, Bobak DA: Nausea, vomiting, and noninflammatory diarrhea. In *Principles and Practice of Infectious Diseases*, edn 4. Edited by Mandell GL, Bennett JE, Dolin R. New York: Churchill Livingstone; 1995:965–978.

46. LeBaron CW, Lew J, Glass RI, *et al.*: Annual rotavirus epidemic patterns in North America: Results of a 5-year retrospective survey of 88 centers in Canada, Mexico, and the United States. Rotavirus Study Group. *JAMA* 1990, 264:983.

47. Brooke MM, Melvin DM: Morphology and Diagnostic Stages of Intestinal Parasites of Man. Atlanta: Centers for Disease Control and Prevention; 1972. [DHEW publication no. (PHS) 72-H116.]

48. Sande MA, Strausbaugh LJ: Infective endocarditis. In *Current Concepts in Infectious Diseases*. Edited by Hook EW, Mandell GL, Gwaltney JM Jr, *et al.* New York: Wiley: 1977.

49. Rahn D:L Lyme disease: Clinical manifestations, diagnosis, and treatment. *Semin Arthirtis Rheum* 1991, 20:201–218.

50. Rahn D, Malawista SE: Clinical judgement in Lyme disease. *Hosp Pract* 1990, 25(Mar 30):39–56.

51. Steere AC, *et al.*: The early clinical manifestations of Lyme disease. *Ann Intern Med* 1983, 99:76–82.

52. Klempner MS: Lyme disease [images in clinical medicine]. *N Engl J Med* 1992, 327:1793.

53. Chen SM, Dumler JS, Bakken JS, Walker DH: Identification of a granulocytotropic *Ehrlichia* species as the etiologic agent of human disease. *J Clin Microbiol* 1994, 32:589–595.

54. Bakken JS, Dumler JS, Chen SM, *et al.*: Human granulocytic ehrlichiosis in the upper Midwest United States: A new species emerging? *JAMA* 1994, 272:212–218.

55. Pruthi RK, Marshall WF, Wiltsie JC, Persing DH: Human babesiosis. *Mayo Clin Proc* 1995, 70:853–862.

56. Walsh T, Rinaldi M, Pizzo PA: Zygomycosis of the respiratory tract. In *Fungal Diseases of the Lung*. Edited by Saro GA, Davies SF. New York: Raven Press; 1993.

57. Ozols H, Wheat LJ: Erythema nodosum in an epidemic of histoplasmosis in Indianapolis. *Arch Dermatol* 1981, 117:709–712.

58. Thornberry DK, Wheat LJ, Brandt KD, Rosenthal J: Histoplasmosis presenting with joint pain and hilar adenopathy: pseudosarcoidosis. *Arthritis Rheum* 1982, 25:1396–1402.

59. Rosenthal J, Brandt KD, Wheat LJ, Slama TG: Rheumatologic manifestations of histoplasmosis in the recent Indianapolis epidemic. *Arthritis Rheum* 1983, 26:1065–1070.

60. Sobel JD: Vaginal infections in adult women. *Med Clin North Am* 1990, 74:1576.

61. Dajani AS, Bisno AL, Chung KJ, *et al.* for the Committee on Rheumatic Fever, Endocarditis, and Kawasaki Disease: *Diagnostic Guidelines for Kawasaki Disease*. Dallas: American Heart Association; 1989.

62. Netter FH: *The Ciba Collection of Medical Illustrations*, vol. 5. Edited by Yonkman FF. Summit, NJ: Ciba Pharmaceutical Products; 1969.

63. Maki DG: Infections due to infusion therapy. In *Hospital Infections*, edn 3. Edited by Bennett JV, Brachman PS. Boston: Little, Brown and Company; 1992:849–898.

64. Brener Z: O parasito: Relacoes hospedeiro-parasito. In *Trypanosoma cruzi e Doenca de Chagas*. Edited by Brener Z, Andrade A: Rio de Janeiro: Editora Guanabara Koogan SA: 1979:1–41.

65. Kuo C, Shor A, Campbell LA, *et al.*: Demonstration of *Chalmydia pneumoniae* in atherosclerotic lesions of coronary arteries. *J Infect Dis* 1993, 167:841–849.

66. Gaydos CA, Summersgill JT, Sahney NN, *et al.*: Replication of *Chlamydia pneumoniae* in vitro in human macrophages, endothelial cells, and aortic artery muscle cells. *Infect Immun* 1996, 64:1614–1620.

67. Ross R: The pathogenesis of atherosclerosis: A perspective for the 1990s. *Nature* 1993, 362:801–809.

■ ACKNOWLEDGMENT

The author wishes to thank the following colleagues who contributed figures to this chapter: Gregory J. Dore and David A. Cooper (Figs. 7-2 and 7-3); Alvin E. Friedman-Kien (Figs. 7-5 to 7-10); Janet L. Davis and Alan G. Palestine (Figs. 7-11 to 7-13); Deborah Greenspan and John S. Greenspan (Figs. 7-14 and 7-15); Mark J. Rosen (Fig. 7-16); Harold A. Kessler (Fig. 7-19); Judith Feinberg (Fig. 7-20); Jan Hirschmann (Figs. 7-21 to 7-26); Dennis L. Stevens (Figs. 7-27 and 7-28); Ellie J.C. Goldstein (Fig. 7-29); E. Dale Everett (Figs. 7-30 and 7-31); Gregory J. Raugi (Figs. 7-32 to 7-36); Robert Gelber, Rodolfo M. Abalos, Roland V. Cellona, Tranquilino T. Fajardo, Gerald P. Walsh, and Ricardo S. Guinto (Fig. 7-39); Bruce C. Gilliland and Mark H. Wener (Fig. 7-40); Daniel F. Hanley, Jonathan D. Glass, Justin C. McArthur, and Richard T. Johnson (Fig. 7-43); David G. Brock (Fig. 7-46); Oren Sagher (Fig. 7-47); Hans-Walter Pfister and Eberhard Wilmes (Fig. 7-49); David A. Ramsay and G. Bryan Young (Fig. 7-50); Thomas A. Deutsch (Figs. 7-51 to 7-57); Ellen R. Wald (Figs. 7-58 to 7-60A and 7-65 to 7-67); Ayal Willner, Kenneth M. Grundfast, and Rande H. Lazar (Fig. 7-61); Marlin E. Gher, Jr., and George Quintero (Figs. 7-68 to 7-72); Harris R. Stutman (Figs. 7-73 to 7-75); Jonathan M. Zenilman (Figs. 7-78 to 7-81); Sharon L. Hillier (Fig. 7-83); Nicholas J. Fiumara (Figs. 7-85, 7-87, and 7-88); Navjeet K. Sidhu-Malik and Michael F. Rein (Figs. 7-90 and 7-91); Allan Ronald (Fig. 7-93); Richard B. Roberts (Fig. 7-95); Melanie J. Maslow (Figs. 7-96 to 7-98); Jaishree Jagirdar (Fig. 7-97); Scott F. Davies and George A. Sarosi (Fig. 7-101); Howard L. Leaf (Fig. 7-103); Robert F. Betts, Ann R. Falsey, Caroline B. Hall, and John J. Treanor (Fig. 7-104); John Froude (Fig. 7-105); Christopher J. Salmon and Richard E. Bryant (Fig. 7-106); Lionel Rabin (Figs. 7-109 and 7-112); Richard L. Guerrant (Figs. 7-114 and 7-116); David Y. Graham and Robert M. Genta (Fig. 7-118); Robert D. Shaw (Fig. 7-119); Rosemary Soave (Fig. 7-121); Robert A. Gatenby (Fig. 7-122); Janet R. Gilsdorf and Thomas Shope (Figs. 7-123 and 7-124); W. Michael Scheld (Figs. 7-125, 7-127, and 7-128); Steven M. Opal and Stephen H. Zinner (Fig. 7-129); J. Stephen Dumler and David H. Persing (Fig. 7-136); Anastacio de Q. Sousa, Thomas G. Evans, and Richard D. Pearson (Fig. 7-139); Michel G. Bergeron, Dominique Giroux, and Claude Delage (Fig. 7-141); Lindsay E. Nicolle (Figs. 7-142 and 7-143); Edward D. Kim and Anthony J. Schaeffer (Fig. 7-144); David E. Soper (Fig. 7-148); José M. Miró and Walter R. Wilson (Fig. 7-150); Adnan S. Dajani and Kathryn A. Taubert (Fig. 7-152); Cathal O'Sullivan and C. Glenn Cobbs (Fig. 7-157); William J. Lewis and Robert J. Sherertz (Fig. 7-158); Harry Acquatella (Fig. 7-160); Oksana M. Korzeniowski (Fig. 7-161); and Judith A. O'Donnell (Fig. 7-163).

Neurology

ROGER N. ROSENBERG

The Decade of the Brain of the 1990s enacted by the United States Congress in 1989 to call attention to and to promote research into neurologic diseases has been concluded and with considerable success. It is clear that great progress has been made in the neurobiologic understanding of many neurologic diseases in this decade and also an appreciation of how much more there is to do. We all know that neurology is a highly visual specialty. Seeing the patient with a neurologic disorder may be sufficient to make the diagnosis by clinical inspection. The neurologic examination, magnetic resonance imaging, electroencephalography, positron-emission tomographic (PET) and functional magnetic resonance (fMRI) scanning, and light and electron microscopy are examples of visual images that define neurologic disease and normal brain functions. This chapter includes a pictorial comprehensive visual exposition and integration of all aspects of neurologic disease, including clinical syndromes and related neuropathology, neuroradiology, neurophysiology, neuropharmacology, neurochemistry, and aspects of molecular neurobiology. The goal of this chapter is to provide a holistic visual concept of neurologic disease to allow the internist an overall image of a specific neurologic disorder. Quality patient care requires the good judgment and factual knowledge of an experienced internist. This chapter is intended to provide essential information about neurologic disease in an immediate and integrated manner to facilitate the internist in the primary function of providing excellence in patient management.

There has been great progress in the past decade in our understanding of the cellular and molecular bases of many neurologic disorders. New therapies have been developed as a result of this recent knowledge. Thrombolytic therapy for stroke, pallidotomy for Parkinson's disease, new classes of anticonvulsants, and effective immune therapy for multiple sclerosis represent examples of recent significant therapeutic advances in neurology. Of great importance to the understanding of gene structure and function in the nervous system has been the discovery of DNA triplet repeat expansions in autosomal dominant neurogenetic diseases, including Huntington's disease, olivopontocerebellar atrophy (SCA1), Machado-Joseph disease, dentatorubropallidoluysian atrophy (DRPLA), fragile-X disease, myotonic muscular dystropy, and most recently, Friedreich's ataxia, which has the triplet repeat (GAA) within the first intron, a noncoding region of the gene. Alzheimer's disease, the leading cause of dementia in our society, affecting more than 4 million Americans and countless millions more around the world, has been shown to be a clinical syndrome due to specific different genetic mutations in selected families with dominantly inherited disease. Mutations in the amyloid precursor protein gene (chromosome 21), the presenilin 1 gene (chromosome 14), and the presenilin 2 gene (chromosome 1) result in dominantly inherited Alzheimer's disease. A major risk factor for Alzheimer's disease is the presence of the E4 allele of apolipoprotein E (chromosome 19). These clinical-molecular correlations, all less than 10 years old, attest to the scientific vigor of current neuroscientific research. It is my view that in the near future, these new data will lead to effective new therapy for Alzheimer's disease that will slow its rate of progress and significantly reduce the incidence of this major debilitating disease. PET and fMRI brain scanning have effectively defined regional brain areas for behaviors. The clarity of insights into heterogeneous brain functions shown by PET and fMRI is literally revolutionizing our concepts about how our brain thinks.

The topics covered in this chapter represent the most common and important neurologic diseases. The descriptive text for each disease sets the stage for the use of the detailed image and CD-ROM material, which is intended both for self-instruction and for lecture presentations. Images, algorithms, tables, and schematic drawings have been selected carefully for their clarity in conveying the essence of a partic-

ular disorder. The collection of figures for a specific disease is intended to provide a thorough and comprehensive description that enables the internist to generate a clear concept of current thinking about the pathogenesis of that disorder and finally a framework for rational therapy.

It is my hope that this chapter will be of value to internists in caring for patients with neurologic disorders by providing useful insights into disease mechanisms and information to improve the care of patients with disorders of the nervous system.

■ GENETIC DISEASES OF THE NERVOUS SYSTEM

ALZHEIMER'S DISEASE

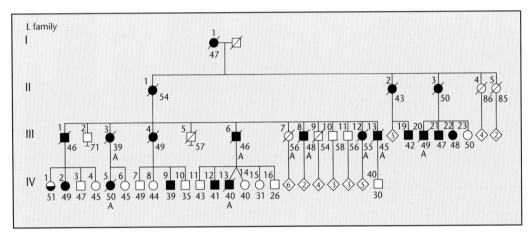

FIGURE 8-1.

The pedigree of a kindred with early-onset familial Alzheimer's disease (FAD) [1]. The disorder has affected male and female family members over four generations in an autosomal dominant pattern. The mean age of onset of dementia in this family is 41 years, and the typical duration of disease is approximately 8 years. The *numbers beneath each symbol* indicate the present age or age at death. The letter *A* indicates persons who have had an autopsy. The *closed symbols* represent persons who are affected with dementia, *open symbols* represent those without dementia, and *half-closed symbols* represent those with probable dementia. The *circles* represent females, and the *squares* represent males; a *slash through a symbol* indicates death, a *number above a symbol* indicates the position in that generation of pedigree, and a *number within a symbol* indicates the number of children. The neuropathology in this family demonstrates the typical findings of Alzheimer's disease, including neuritic amyloid plaques, neurofibrillary tangles, and amyloid angiopathy. This family has a mutation in the Alzheimer's disease gene on the long arm of chromosome 14. (*Courtesy of Thomas D. Bird and S. Mark Sumi.*)

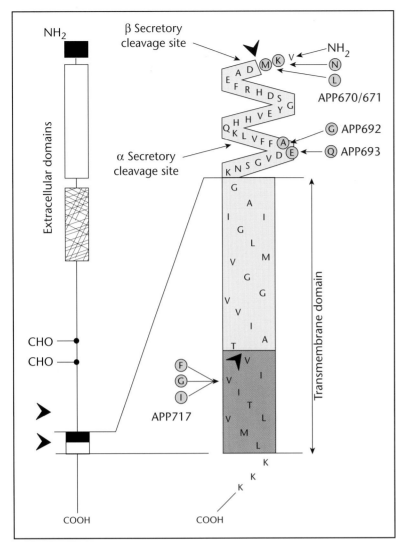

FIGURE 8-2.

The amyloid precursor protein (APP) coded for by a gene on chromosome 21. The *region between the black arrowheads* indicates where the APP protein is clipped to produce the Aβ amyloid that is deposited in the brains of individuals with Alzheimer's disease. The *right side* of the diagram shows the location of various mutations that have been discovered in cerebral amyloid disorders. For example, most families with early-onset familial Alzheimer's disease (FAD) and APP mutations have substitution of some other amino acid (usually isoleucine) for valine at position 717. Mutations at positions 692 and 693 result in hereditary cerebral amyloidosis of the Dutch type [2]. The double amino acid substitutions at positions APP 670/671 have caused early-onset FAD in a Swedish kindred. A *closed box* represents signal sequence; an *open box* represents cysteine-rich domain; a *hatched box* represents highly negatively charged domain (45% aspartic acid and glutamic acid residues). (*Adapted from* Van Broeckhoven [2].)

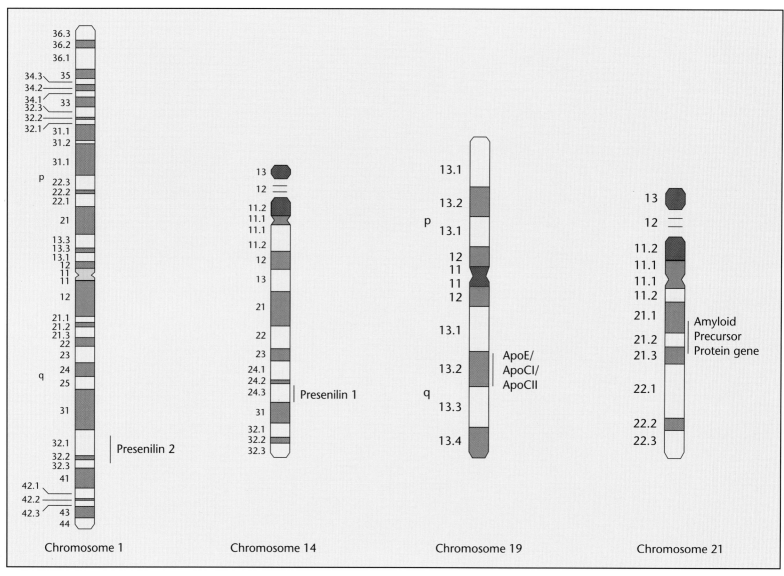

FIGURE 8-3.

Four different chromosomes that contain genes influencing the development of Alzheimer's disease. The amyloid precursor protein (APP) gene is on chromosome 21. Several mutations in this gene result in a form of early-onset, familial Alzheimer's disease (FAD). The presence of the APP gene in triplicate is responsible for the frequent occurrence of Alzheimer's disease in individuals with Down syndrome (trisomy 21). Mutations in a gene called *S182*, or presenilin 1, are responsible for early-onset FAD in families showing linkage to chromosome 14, such as the kindred in Figure 8-1 [3].

A gene on chromosome 1 called *STM2*, or presenilin 2, is responsible for FAD in Volga German kindreds as well as families of other ethnic backgrounds [4]. Finally, the apolipoprotein E (APO E) gene is on chromosome 19. The ε4 allele of APO E shows a strong association with late-onset familial Alzheimer's disease and sporadic cases of Alzheimer's disease. The ε4 allele of APO E apparently promotes earlier onset of the disease, which is especially true in individuals who are homozygous ε4/4 [5]. (*Courtesy of* Thomas D. Bird and S. Mark Sumi.)

DOWN SYNDROME (TRISOMY 21)

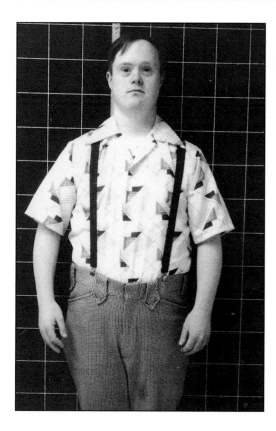

FIGURE 8-4.
Many typical physical features of Down syndrome. These features include short stature, frontal balding, thin hair, epicanthal folds, thick neck, and mild truncal obesity. This young man is moderately mentally retarded but able to perform in a sheltered workshop. (*Courtesy of* Thomas D. Bird and S. Mark Sumi.)

GENETIC DISEASES OF THE BASAL GANGLIA

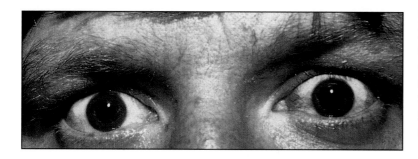

FIGURE 8-5.
Kayser-Fleischer ring. Wilson's disease is an autosomal recessive disorder of copper metabolism that can present with hepatic failure, psychiatric or personality disorder, or neurologic signs, including dysarthria, dystonia, rigidity, and tremor. Serum ceruloplasmin and urinary copper levels are elevated, and hepatic copper level is increased. The abnormality is the golden brown ring contrasted against the blue-gray iris bilaterally. (*From* Finelli [6]; with permission.)

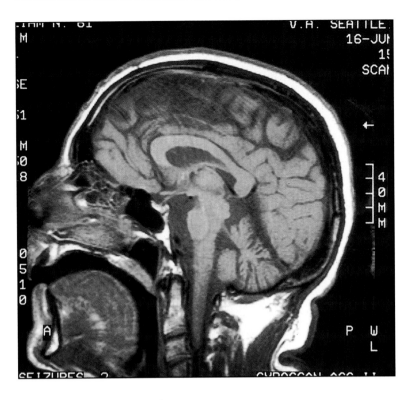

FIGURE 8-6.

A midline sagittal magnetic resonance imaging scan of a 61-year-old man with slowly progressive ataxia and dysarthria demonstrating atrophy of the cerebellum and pons. His clinical diagnosis is probable olivopontocerebellar atrophy (OPCA). Some cases of OPCA are sporadic and of unknown cause; others are clearly genetic. (*Courtesy of* Thomas D. Bird and S. Mark Sumi.)

GENETIC DISORDERS OF THE BRAIN STEM AND SPINAL CORD

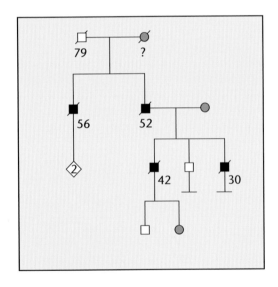

FIGURE 8-7.

Pedigree of a family with early-onset rapidly progressive amyotrophic lateral sclerosis (ALS). ALS is usually a sporadic disease without an obvious hereditary component. However, 5% to 10% of patients with ALS have a similarly affected relative. The inheritance is typical of an autosomal dominant disease, with male-to-male transmission. Affected members of the family have had a combination of both upper and lower motor neuron signs, including weakness, muscle atrophy, fasciculations, and hyperactive tendon reflexes. This family has been found to have a point mutation in exon 1 of the superoxide dismutase (SOD) gene on chromosome 21. Mutations in exon 1 have been associated with an especially aggressive, rapidly progressive form of ALS. Affected members of this family usually survive less than 2 years. Some but not all kindreds with familial ALS have been discovered to have mutations in the SOD gene [7]. The closed symbols represent persons who are affected with ALS; open symbols are persons without ALS. The circles represent females, and the squares represent males; a slash through a symbol indicates death, a number above a symbol is the position in that generation of pedigree, and numbers within a symbol indicate the number of children. (DNA finding *courtesy of* R.H. Brown; figure *courtesy of* Thomas D. Bird and S. Mark Sumi.)

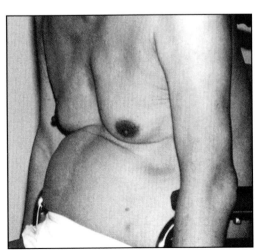

FIGURE 8-8.

Kennedy's spinobulbar muscular atrophy. This X-linked recessive disorder affects lower motor neurons in the brain stem and spinal cord. Affected males have onset of weakness and atrophy beginning in adulthood, which is usually slowly progressive and compatible with several decades of life. Fasciculations of tongue and perioral muscles are common. Upper motor neuron signs are absent. Gynecomastia is a frequent feature. Carrier females are asymptomatic and there is no male-to-male transmission of the disease. (*From* Nagashima *et al.* [8]; with permission.)

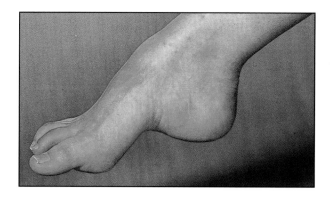

FIGURE 8-9.

Physical manifestations of Charcot-Marie-Tooth 1 (CMT 1) disease. The typical high arch, contracted heel cord, and foot drop posture of CMT. CMT 1A is associated with a DNA duplication at chromosome 17p11.2, which includes the PMP22 (peripheral myelin protein) gene. (*Courtesy of* Thomas D. Bird and S. Mark Sumi.)

GENETIC DISEASES OF MUSCLE

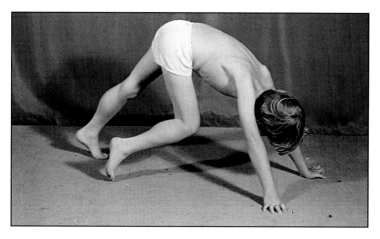

FIGURE 8-10.

A boy with Duchenne muscular dystrophy (DMD) demonstrating pseudohypertrophy of his calves and a positive Gower's maneuver ("climbing" from a sitting position because of proximal muscle weakness). DMD is the most common inherited form of muscle disease. It is transmitted in an X-linked recessive fashion. The disease presents as a slowly progressive weakness of the proximal lower extremities typically beginning between ages 3 and 5. The disease is associated with highly elevated serum creatine kinase levels, wheelchair dependence by age 12, and death usually in the third decade from pneumonia or cardiomyopathy. Female carriers of the gene rarely have symptoms of muscle disease. However, because of random inactivation of the X chromosome, female carriers often have an elevated serum creatine kinase level (about 70% of carriers) and occasionally have enlarged calves and mild muscle weakness. (*Courtesy of* Thomas D. Bird and S. Mark Sumi.)

MULTIFACTORIAL DISORDERS

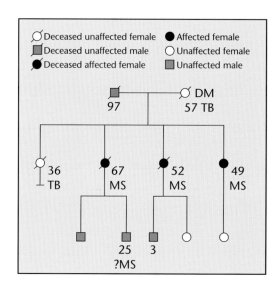

FIGURE 8-11.

Pedigree of familial multiple sclerosis (MS). MS is a remitting and relapsing demyelinating disorder that is relatively common in the northern latitudes of the western hemisphere. Its cause is unknown and cases are usually sporadic, without a positive family history. Approximately 10% to 20% of MS patients will have another affected family member. Less commonly, there may be three or more family members with MS, as demonstrated in this kindred. It is assumed that this phenomenon of multiplex MS families represents multifactorial inheritance. That is, some unknown environmental agent (such as a virus) is provoking the disease in a genetically predisposed host (such as an individual with a certain vulnerable HLA type). In persons with MS, the risks for developing the disease in first-degree relatives is approximately 2% to 3% [9]. Although this is a relatively small risk, it should be noted that the lifetime age-corrected risk for the sibling of a patient with MS to develop MS represents more than a 25-fold increase over the lifetime risk for the general population. DM—diabetes mellitus; TB—tuberculosis. (*Courtesy of* Thomas D. Bird and S. Mark Sumi.)

■ NEUROENDOCRINE DISORDERS

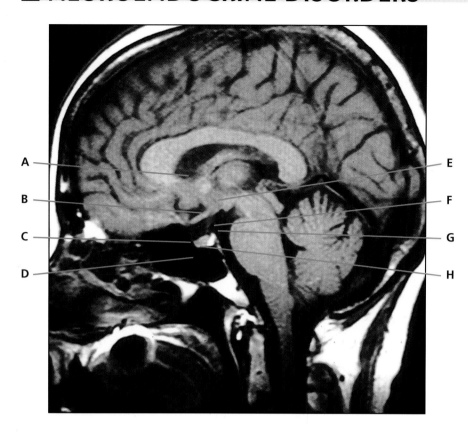

A
B
C
D
E
F
G
H

FIGURE 8-12.
Clinical presentations of pituitary and parapituitary lesions. **A,** Hydrocephalus is caused by the tumor blocking the foramen of Monro. **B,** There is a loss of visual acuity due to the optic nerve being affected or a visual field defect due to a disturbance of the optic chiasm. **C,** Cavernous sinus syndrome affecting cranial nerves V_1, III, IV, and VI due to bleeding into the adenoma (pituitary apoplexy). **D,** Cerebrospinal fluid rhinorrhea and possibly the tumor extending into the nose due to erosion of the floor of the sella into the sphenoidal sinus. **E,** Hypothalamic symptoms: hypopituitarism, hyperprolactinemia, and diabetes insipidus. **F,** Hypopituitarism due to disruption of the pituitary stalk by trauma, surgery, or tumor. **G,** Retro-orbital headache due to pressure on the diaphragm sella. **H,** Anterior pituitary failure. (*Courtesy of* Earl A. Zimmerman.)

■ COMA AND INTENSIVE CARE NEUROLOGY

ALTERED CONSCIOUSNESS AND SEDATION

Modified Ramsey Sedation Scale

Scale	Level Criteria
1	Patient anxious, agitated, and restless
2	Patient cooperative, oriented, and tranquil
3	Patient drowsy but responds to commands
4	Patient asleep and exhibits a brisk response to light glabellar tap or loud auditory stimulus
5	Patient asleep and exhibits a sluggish response to light glabellar tap or loud auditory stimulus
6	Patient asleep; no response

FIGURE 8-13.
Modified Ramsey sedation scale. Patients with critical illness often benefit from the use of sedation to optimize their management in an intensive care unit (ICU) environment. Preservation of the neurologic examination is paramount in documenting clinical improvement or deterioration in the critically ill neurologic patient. Pharmacologic sedation in this unique population of acute care patients requires careful consideration of the underlying neurophysiologic disturbances and potential adverse effects introduced by sedative drugs. To maintain patients at an ideal level of sedation, careful monitoring is required. One of the most widely used sedation scales was developed by Ramsey and coworkers and includes six levels of cognitive neurologic functioning. (*Adapted from* Ramsay *et al.* [10].)

Neurologic Conditions That Produce Unresponsiveness

Condition	Self-awareness	Sleep-wake Cycles	Motor Function	Experiences Suffering	Respiratory Function	Electroen-cephalogram	Prognosis for Neurologic Recovery
Persistent vegetative state*	Absent	Intact	No purposeful movement; no visual tracking	No	Normal	Polymorphic delta and theta; sometimes slow alpha	Traumatic PVS (1-y outcome): PVS, 15% of patients; dead, 33%; GR, 7%; MD, 17%; SD, 28%
							Nontraumatic PVS (1-y outcome): PVS, 32% of patients; dead, 53%; GR, 1%; MD, 3%; SD, 11%
Brain death	Absent	Absent	None or only reflex spinal movements	No	Absent	Electrocerebral silence	None
Locked-in syndrome	Present	Intact	Quadriplegia; pseudobulbar palsy; preserved vertical eye movements	Yes	Normal	Normal or mildly abnormal	Recovery unlikely; patients remain quadriplegic; prolonged survival possible
Akinetic mutism	Present	Intact	Paucity of movement	Yes	Normal	Nonspecific slowing	Recovery very unlikely and depends on cause

*Adults only

FIGURE 8-14.

Neurologic conditions that produce unresponsiveness. Due to the overlap of clinical and laboratory findings, these generalizations do not apply to every patient. Magnetic resonance imaging or computed tomography may be able to further differentiate the above conditions. GR—good recovery; MD—moderately disabled; PVS—persistent vegetative state; SD—severely disabled. (*Adapted from* Wijdicks [11].)

Metabolic Coma

Etiology	Specific Neurologic Signs	Diagnostic Steps
Hypoxia	Flaccid muscle tone, myoclonus	Preceding cardiac disease, polytrauma, resuscitation, attempted suicide
Hyperosmolar diabetic coma	Frequently: coma, seizures (20%–25%), focal signs	Blood glucose > 1100 mg %, high serum osmolarity
Diabetic ketoacidosis	Clouding of consciousness but rarely coma	Ketonuria, blood glucose > 400 mg %
Hypoglycemia	High variability, including coma, seizures, focal signs	Blood glucose < 30 mg %
Hepatic encephalopathy	Tremor, asterixis (wing beating); final stage: severe clouding of consciousness	Ammonia
Uremia	Delirium, seizures, myoclonus, asterixis; final stage: clouding of consciousness	Serum creatinine, urea, potassium
Dysequilibrium syndrome	Muscle cramps, seizures, coma	Postdialysis, urea, sodium, osmolarity
Hyponatremia	Clouding of consciousness; seizures and coma only in case of rapid change of serum sodium level	Serum sodium < 126 mmol
Hypernatremia	Delirium, "muscle weakness", coma only in case of rapid change	Serum sodium > 156 mmol, reduced urinary sodium excretion
Hypercalcemia	Delirium, headache, "muscle weakness"	Calcium and phosphate in serum and urine, parathormone
Hypocalcemia	Tetanic syndrome, delirium, pseudopsychotic behavior, seizures	Calcium and phosphate in serum and urine, parathormone
Thiamine deficiency	Wernicke encephalopathy; rarely coma	Vitamin B_1 level, 100 mg vitamin B_1 IV

FIGURE 8-15.

Causes, specific neurologic signs, and diagnostic tests in metabolic coma. Specific neurologic signs may be indicative of an etiologic cause of metabolic coma and diagnostic steps should be undertaken to confirm the diagnosis. IV—intravenous. (*Adapted from* Hacke [12].)

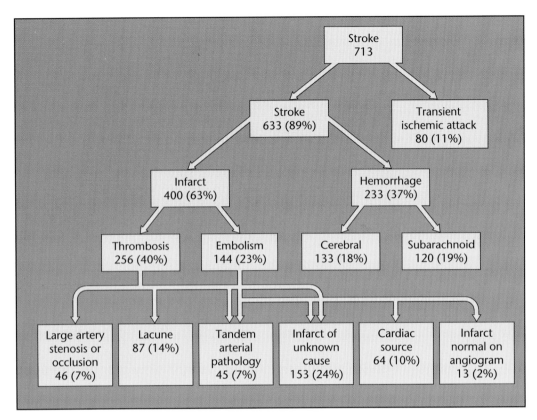

FIGURE 8-16.

Subtypes of ischemic stroke. Stroke is the leading cause of life-threatening neurologic disease and the third leading cause of death in the United States, with an incidence of 500,000 cases per year.

Stroke is a generic term for a clinical syndrome that includes infarction and hemorrhage (intracerebral, intraventricular, and subarachnoid). This term usually applies to any sort of cerebrovascular disease, either ischemic or hemorrhagic, with either permanent or transient symptoms. Intracranial hemorrhage can be subdivided into either subarachnoid or intracerebral, depending on the site and origin of the blood. The term *stable stroke* refers to a

patient with stroke who has shown little change in deficit over a specified period of time (*eg*, a new measurable neurologic deficit within the previous 24 hours that persisted for at least 24 hours) [13]. Anything less is considered a transient ischemic attack (TIA). Many TIA patients are actually found to have a stroke if a brain image is performed at an appropriate time. Therefore, shorter duration of symptoms (*eg*, 1 hour or 15 minutes) may be more pertinent for distinguishing between TIA and stroke.

With cerebral infarction, the differentiation of several clinical, pathophysiologic, and etiologic subtypes may be crucial to rational treatment and prediction of outcome. With the use of computed tomography, magnetic resonance imaging, and lumbar puncture, bleeding into and around the brain can be diagnosed, and these types of strokes can be separated from the more common ischemic stroke. The classification of ischemic stroke is difficult. Ischemic strokes classically are divided into thrombotic (two thirds) and embolic (one third) [14]. Ischemic infarction can be classified by the mechanism of ischemia (hemodynamic or thromboembolic) and the pathology of the vascular lesion: atherosclerotic, lacunar, cardioembolic, or indeterminate. Although the two subtypes can present in the same way, thrombotic infarcts more frequently have progressive onset, as opposed to the sudden onset of embolic strokes. (*Adapted from* Mohr *et al.* [14].)

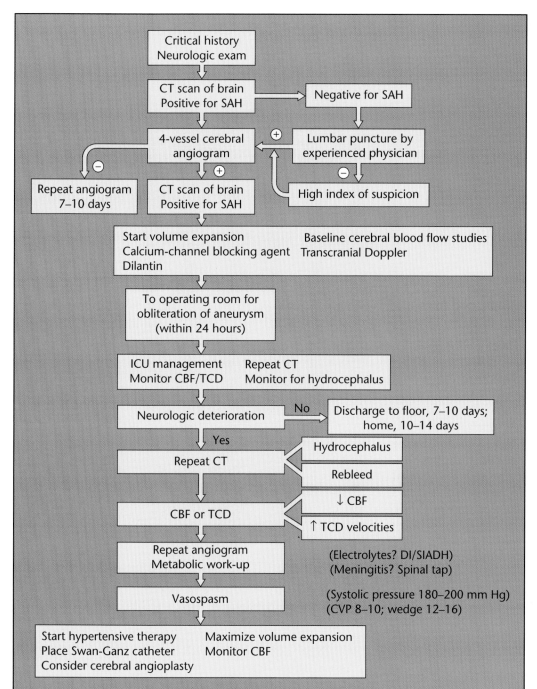

FIGURE 8-17.

Management of patients with subarachnoid hemorrhage (SAH). The management of SAH requires the integration of clinical diagnosis in the emergency room, urgent neuroimaging evaluation, special operative and anesthetic considerations, conventional intensive care, and unit-based critical care. The rational and intelligent approach to intensive care, therefore, requires an appreciation of the overall management protocol. CBF—cerebral blood flow; CT—computed tomography; CVP—central venous pressure; DI—diabetes insipidus; ICU—intensive care unit; SIADH—syndrome of inappropriate antidiuretic hormone; TCD—transcranial Doppler. (*Adapted from* Origitano [15].)

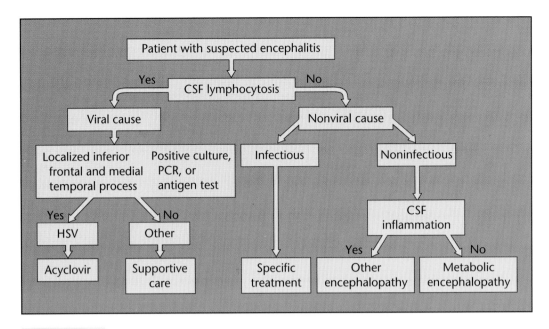

FIGURE 8-18.

General approach to the patient with suspected encephalitis. In the febrile patient with depressed mental status, nonviral causes of encephalitis must first be considered and excluded because treatment is available for many. Epidemiologic, clinical, and laboratory data are important in the differential diagnosis. If a viral encephalitis is suspected, a diagnosis of herpes simplex virus (HSV) encephalitis should next be considered. For HSV encephalitis, early treatment with acyclovir may be beneficial, whereas for most other viral encephalitides, treatment is supportive. A range of diagnostic tests is available to help in the evaluation of the patient with suspected encephalitis, and their use is guided by the clinical situation. Cerebrospinal fluid (CSF) examination is a key part of the evaluation of every patient, and assays for CSF virus–specific IgM (enzyme-linked immunosorbent assay) can aid in the rapid diagnosis of arbovirus infection. CSF cultures usually are negative for viruses but may be positive in bacterial infection. Serologic studies are useful in selected infections. Brain biopsy is usually necessary to diagnose herpes simplex virus encephalitis definitively, although polymerase chain reaction holds promise as a substitute for biopsy. Computed tomography, magnetic resonance imaging, and electroencephalography are used to identify or help exclude alternative diagnoses and to help establish the presence of a focal encephalitic process. PCR—polymerase chain reaction. (*Adapted from* Hanley *et al.* [16].)

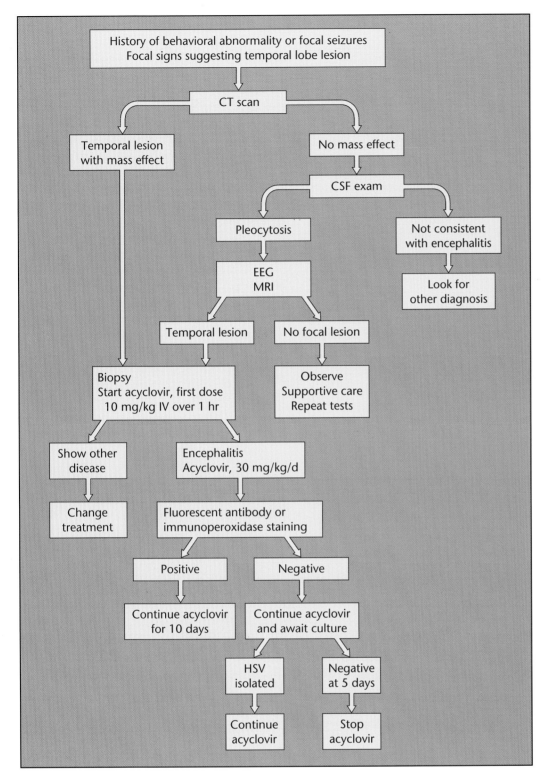

FIGURE 8-19.

Steps in the management of suspected herpes simplex virus encephalitis. CSF—cerebrospinal fluid; CT—computed tomography; EEG—electroencephalogram; HSV—herpes simplex virus; IV—intravenous; MRI—magnetic resonance imaging. (*Adapted from* Johnson [17].)

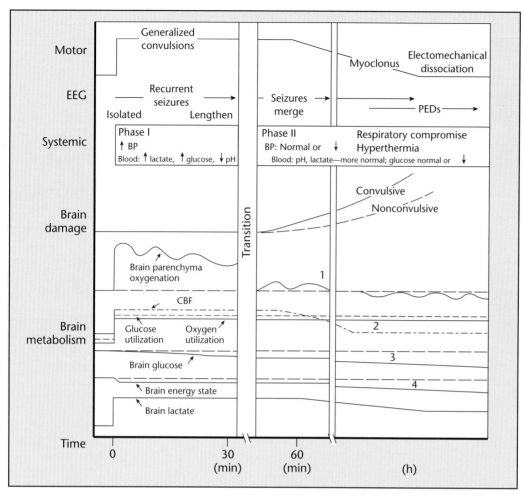

sive SE insofar that two distinct pathophysiologic periods during the evolution of seizures have been identified. In the first phase, typically lasting about 30 minutes, motor seizures steadily intensify and lengthen in duration, with shorter and shorter interictal periods. A rise in both cerebral blood flow and systemic hemodynamic parameters, such as blood pressure (BP) and tachycardia, reflects the high energy demand by the cerebral cortex. Systemic and cerebral lactate production are observed with a fall in blood pH. As the seizures merge and become continuous, the second phase begins, marked by a normalization or fall in hemodynamic indices. Tissue lactate normalizes, and there is a general fall in cerebral metabolism. Initial studies investigating SE-induced brain injury suggested that a mismatch between cerebral metabolism and blood flow resulted in ischemia. Further elaborate experiments controlling for systemic hemodynamics and oxygenation demonstrated only modest declines in cerebral glucose concentrations and normal cerebral blood flow, supporting the hypothesis that a lack of energy substrate is not the etiology of subsequent brain injury. Recent work has identified the excitatory amino acids such as glutamate as probable prime culprits in SE-induced neuronal injury. CBF—cerebral blood flow; EEG—electroencephalogram; PED—periodic epilepiform discharges. (*Adapted from* Lothman [18].)

FIGURE 8-20.

Summary of systemic alterations and brain metabolism in status epilepticus (SE). There is general agreement between the clinical progression of SE and experimental models of convul-

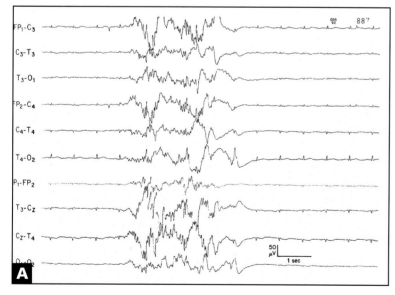

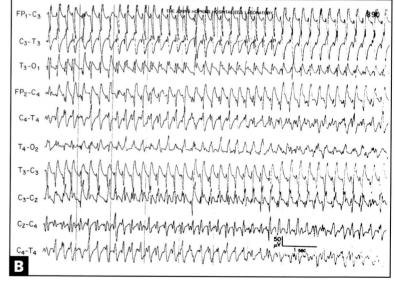

FIGURE 8-21.

Electroencephalograms (EEGs) in status epilepticus (SE) assessment. **A,** The objective of pharmacologic coma is to terminate status epilepticus (SE), as shown here in an 18-year-old man with encephalitis of unclear etiology. This does not usually require electrocerebral silence, as may be the goal when treating intractable elevated intracranial pressure. The therapeutic endpoint is to arrive at an EEG pattern demonstrating no overt epileptiform activity, or to establish a burst suppression pattern as shown in **B.** This EEG pattern is maintained for several hours before attempts are made to wean pharmacologic coma therapy. During this time, optimization of serum levels of selected anticonvulsant agents, such as phenytoin, is performed to provide chronic seizure protection. In unusual cases, it may be necessary to extend the barbiturate coma for several or more days before weaning from the barbiturate infusion. In this case, pharmacologic coma was maintained for 53 days before successful withdrawal was accomplished, with no return of SE. (*From* Mirski *et al.* [19]; with permission.)

CEREBROVASCULAR DISEASE

LARGE VESSEL ATHEROTHROMBOTIC CEREBROVASCULAR DISEASE

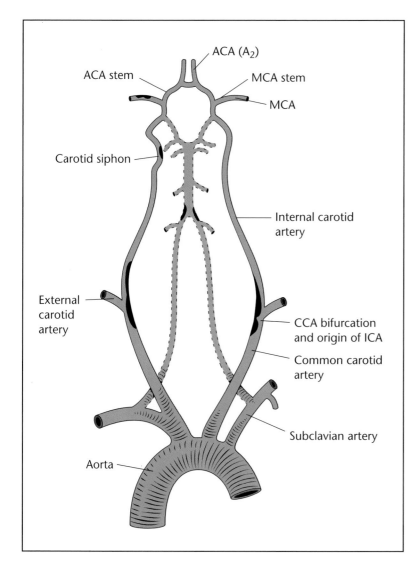

ACA (A₂)
ACA stem
MCA stem
MCA
Carotid siphon
Internal carotid artery
External carotid artery
CCA bifurcation and origin of ICA
Common carotid artery
Subclavian artery
Aorta

FIGURE 8-22.

Common locations of atherosclerotic plaques in the anterior circulation. Although atherosclerosis is a generalized disease, atherosclerotic plaque deposition tends to be a strategically focal process. Plaques are predominantly located at arterial branch points and bifurcations. Furthermore, certain arteries, such as carotid and coronary arteries and those of the lower extremities, are particularly susceptible to plaque formation, while others, such as those of the upper extremities, are rarely affected. The reasons for the focal location and selective distribution of atheroma formation is uncertain. Many believe that it is related to local hemodynamic conditions. Atherothrombotic disease of the internal carotid system that most often leads to stroke tends to occur at four specific sites, listed in order of frequency: 1) the bifurcation of the common carotid artery (CCA) and the origin of the internal carotid artery (ICA) [20]; 2) the distal internal carotid artery (siphon or petrous portion); 3) the middle cerebral artery (MCA) stem; and 4) the proximal anterior cerebral artery (ACA) stem and the origin of the proximal branches of the middle and anterior cerebral arteries. Atheroma of the bifurcation of more distal branches of the middle and anterior cerebral arteries are rare.

At the bifurcation of the common carotid artery–internal carotid artery origin, atherothrombotic occlusion is by far the most common cause of occlusion. Embolic occlusion is rare, as is primary thrombosis in the absence of atheromatous disease. In the distal portion of the internal carotid artery, however, embolic occlusion is more common, although less so than atherothrombotic cause. By contrast, in the middle cerebral artery (MCA) and anterior cerebral artery stems (M_1 and A_1 segments), primary embolic occlusion is the most common mechanism. When arterial occlusion occurs proximal to an adequate circle of Willis, the most common pathophysiologic mechanism of stroke is embolism rather than low flow. Only when collateral flow is limited do low-flow ischemia and infarction ensue. (*Adapted from* Kistler [21].)

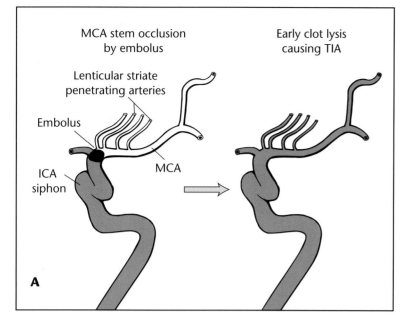

A

MCA stem occlusion by embolus — Early clot lysis causing TIA

Lenticular striate penetrating arteries

Embolus

ICA siphon

MCA

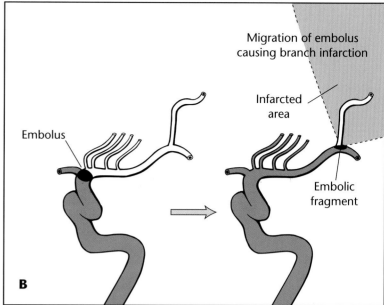

B

Migration of embolus causing branch infarction

Infarcted area

Embolus

Embolic fragment

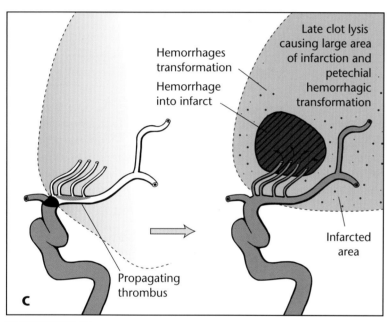

C

Hemorrhages transformation

Hemorrhage into infarct

Late clot lysis causing large area of infarction and petechial hemorrhagic transformation

Infarcted area

Propagating thrombus

FIGURE 8-23.

Carotid artery-to-artery embolic stroke. An embolus arising from a thrombus formed at the site of an atheromatous lesion may occlude the middle cerebral artery (MCA) stem or a more distal branch. Migration and lysis occur spontaneously. Reperfusion into an infarcted territory due to embolus lysis is thought to be the cause of hemorrhagic conversion of a blind infarct [22]. Migration, lysis, and dispersion of emboli as part of their natural evolution may result in fluctuating symptoms and signs. **A**, Clot lysis, if it occurs early enough, can lead to reversible ischemia. The deficit may resolve completely or in part. When emboli lyse and the symptoms resolve within 24 hours, a clinical diagnosis of transient ischemic attack (TIA) is customary. If the symptoms last only a few hours, however, an area of clinically silent infarction often is present and can be demonstrated by imaging studies. Thus, a better term, as proposed by Fisher, might be an *acceptable minor embolism*. Therefore, we generally refer to transient cerebral ischemia in the territory of the large vessel as either embolic or low flow. **B**, In some cases of proximal MCA stem embolism, the embolus may not completely block flow, allowing some distal MCA territory antegrade flow. If this embolus then migrates and lyses, it may block a distal branch, causing a distal branch territory infarct. **C**, On occasion, however, it may not lyse and becomes the nidus for further thrombus formation. Often the embolic MCA occlusion with propagated thrombi will eventually lyse, leading to recirculation in the infarcted brain. Petechial hemorrhagic transformation will likely ensue. Hemorrhage into infarct occurs less often. This is usually located in the territory supplied by the lenticular striate penetrating arteries. When this occurs, a complete MCA territory stroke that involves not only the deep white matter but also the cortical surface territory can ensue. (*Courtesy of* J. Philip Kistler.)

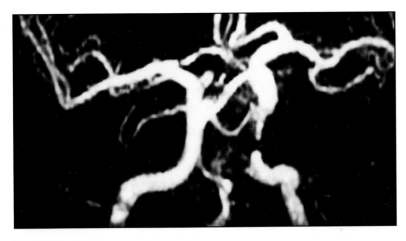

FIGURE 8-24.
Atherothrombotic disease of the siphon portion of the internal carotid artery. Distal (postophthalmic) internal carotid artery stenosis presents as an embolic stroke or transient ischemic attack (TIA), with the circle of Willis intact, or as a low-flow stroke or TIA, with the circle of Willis incomplete. We subscribe to the theory of a low-flow, as opposed to an embolic, cause of the ipsilateral hemispheric symptoms, that is, the availability of adequate collateral flow through the circle of Willis [23].

Magnetic resonance image (MRI) of a patient who presented with recurrent stereotypic episodes of right hand weakness associated with aphasia. Each episode lasted about 1 to 2 minutes, and the patient reported up to 20 spells per day for at least 1 week. Carotid duplex ultrasonography showed a wide open carotid bifurcation, but Doppler examination identified low diastolic flow velocity and a sharp systolic upstroke. A significant stenosis of the petrous part of the left carotid artery is seen. Diffusion-weighted MRI (not shown) of the brain between attacks showed a clinically relevant lesion in the right frontal cortex. Atherosclerosis of the carotid siphon is not as common as proximal internal carotid artery disease. Increased incidence of stroke is found when the lesions become large enough to produce a stenosis of more than 50% [24]. Clinically, stroke or TIA secondary to intracranial carotid stenosis is indistinguishable from the bifurcation stenosis. Noninvasive carotid examination and transcranial Doppler may help in diagnosis. High-resistance flow at the origin of the internal carotid artery, indicated by a very low diastolic velocity and sharp systolic upstroke, may suggest distal stenosis. Ophthalmic artery flow may be reduced or reversed if the siphon stenosis is proximal to its origin; but in contrast to common carotid bifurcation stenosis, it is usually normal. (*Courtesy of* J. Philip Kistler.)

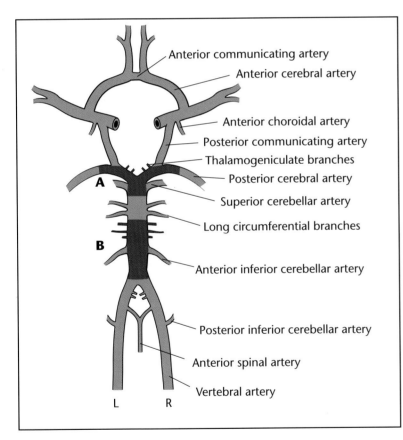

FIGURE 8-25.
Top of basilar syndrome and atherothrombotic disease. **A,** Stroke in the basilar artery territory may occur as a result of local thrombosis or secondary to an embolism. Embolic occlusion of the basilar artery tends to localize in the most distal part, where the basilar artery bifurcates into two posterior cerebral arteries. The resulting so-called top of basilar syndrome begins with loss of consciousness and quadriparesis. As it evolves, the patient often develops hyper-

somnia, bilateral ptosis, and impaired vertical gaze. When both distal posterior cerebral artery (PCA) territories are involved, cortical blindness may ensue. **B,** Atherothrombotic disease, on the other hand, commonly affects the proximal part of the artery, although it can affect any part of the vessel [25]. The clinical picture varies depending on the availability of retrograde collateral flow from the posterior communicating arteries. Among 18 cases of basilar artery occlusion studied by Kubik and Adams [25], 11 were atherothrombotic. The other eight were embolic. The locations of the arterial occlusion are shown.

In general, atherothrombotic occlusion of a branch of the basilar artery affects one side of the brain stem, causing unilateral symptoms and signs of motor, sensory, and cranial nerve dysfunction. Occlusion of a perforating branch that supplies the basis pontis causes unilateral weakness. Perforating branch infarction never crosses the midline except at the top of the basilar artery. There, the penetrating branches arising from the very top of the basilar artery as it bifurcates to each posterior cerebral artery stem may supply both sides of the brain stem. When the basilar artery is occluded, the infarction usually causes bilateral brain stem symptoms and signs. Basilar occlusion is often heralded by transient cerebral ischemia also involving both sides of the brain stem. The clinical findings of basilar artery occlusion may be progressive or may fluctuate for days before the fixed deficit occurs. When the basis pontis is involved bilaterally, a "locked-in" state may occur. In the complete locked-in syndrome, the midbrain is also involved, and the patient is quadriplegic with bilateral facial weakness and severe eye movement abnormality. Although consciousness is preserved owing to the sparing of the midbrain and pontine tegmentum, the patient is not able to respond owing to the lack of motor control of the eyes, face, mouth, tongue, or extremities. Some patients have been able to respond by blinking. When the particular activating system is involved in the midbrain tegmentum, stupor, and coma ensue. (*Courtesy of* J. Philip Kistler.)

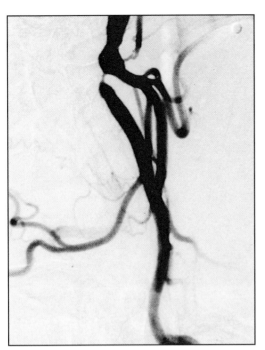

FIGURE 8-26.

Internal carotid artery (ICA) origin angioplasty. Angiogram showing the left ICA origin stenotic lesion in a 65-year-old man. The patient had recurrent episodes of speech difficulty and right arm weakness lasting 20 minutes or less. He was medically unable to have an endarterectomy. Transarterial angioplasty at the origin of the internal carotid artery and intracranially in the arteries at the base of the brain is now possible. The risk-to-benefit ratio of this procedure, however, has not been established, although several uncontrolled series have shown that, for the ICA origin, transarterial angioplasty is possible at low risk [26]. The benefits and potential long-term complications are unknown. Does rapid restenosis occur at the edge of the sheaths? What is the risk of endarterectomy after angioplasty, and can it even be done? At the least, because of the low risk of endarterectomy, a carefully controlled randomized trial is essential before this technique can be substituted for endarterectomy. We reserve angioplasty for the patient with symptoms in whom endarterectomy is medically contraindicated. Angioplasty of atheromatous lesions in the intracranial ICA, in the middle cerebral artery stem, and at the vertebrobasilar junction is possible as well. At these sites, however, safety data are lacking, and as at the ICA origin, the procedure must be considered innovative therapy. (*Courtesy of* J. Philip Kistler.)

LACUNAR DISEASE

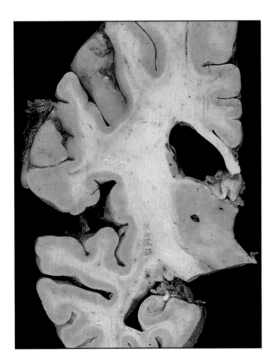

FIGURE 8-27.

Lacunar infarction. Lacunar strokes represent about 25% of all strokes [27]. This pathologic specimen shows a lacunar infarction in the basal ganglia, which is seen as a small fluid-filled cavity. This cavity formed after the infarcted tissue was removed by phagocytes. The majority of the lacunar infarcts are caused by occlusion of a single penetrating vessel that has a diameter of 100 to 400 μm, resulting in a small infarct with a diameter ranging from 0.3 to 2.0 mm [28]. The medial lenticulostriate branches have lumen diameters ranging from 100 to 200 μm, whereas the more lateral lenticulostriate arteries have larger lumen diameters (200 to 400 μm) [29]. The diameters of paramedian penetrating arteries that arise from the basilar artery vary from 40 to 500 μm [30]. (*Courtesy of* Jean-Paul Vonsattel.)

Lacunar Syndromes, Infarct Locations, and Clinical Findings

Lacunar Syndrome	Infarct Location	Clinical Findings
Pure sensory stroke	Thalamus (ventral posterior)	Sensory loss on one side of the body
	Pons	
	Deep white matter	
	(Cerebral cortex)	
Pure motor stroke	Posterior limb of the internal capsule	Severe motor weakness of the face, arm, and leg (weakness may be incomplete, affecting only the proximal part of the limbs)
	Basis pontis	
	Cerebral peduncle	Transient hypesthesia and paresthesias are compatible with the syndrome
	Medullary pyramid	
		Dysarthria is common
Ataxic hemiparesis	Upper pons	Weakness and cerebellar sign on the same side
	Posterior limb of the internal capsule	Slight hypesthesia may be found
	Thalamus	
	Middle and lower pons	
Dysarthria–clumsy hand syndrome	Basis pontis	Dysarthria and clumsiness of one hand
	Genu of the internal capsule	Often associated with ipsilateral lower facial paralysis, Babinski's sign (brisk deep tendon reflexes), deviation of the tongue, and dysphagia
	Corona radiata, cortical lesion	
Sensorimotor stroke	Thalamocapsular lacunes	Motor and sensory involvement
		The motor or sensory deficit may be incomplete

FIGURE 8-28.

Lacunar syndromes, infarct locations, and clinical findings. *Pure sensory stroke.* Pure sensory stroke syndrome was initially described by Fisher [31] in 1965. It is characterized by subjective numbness involving the face, arm, and leg without evidence of motor weakness, dysarthria, visual field defect, or neuropsychologic disturbances. Sensory symptoms are generally described as numbness, tingling, or being "asleep." Unpleasant and painful dysesthesia has also been reported. The neurologic examination may demonstrate a decrease in pain and cold sensation, but often joint position sensation and vibration are preserved. The sensory loss may be subtle and difficult to demonstrate by neurologic examination. The sensory symptoms may progress within seconds to hours [31]. They may start in the hand or foot and spread to the whole side of the body. In general, pure sensory lacunar syndrome is associated with infarction at the ventral posterior nuclei of the thalamus [32]. Rarely, cortical surface and deep white matter infarction or a pontine lesion may be responsible for pure sensory symptoms. According to Fisher's observation [33], when the abdomen is involved, thalamic lesion is much more likely. The prognosis of this syndrome is favorable. Marked improvement within weeks is common [33].

Pure motor hemiplegia and pure motor hemiparesis. Pure hemiplegia is one of the most common lacunar syndromes, accounting for 46% to 50% of the cases [34]. It is characterized by weakness of the face, arm, and leg on one side without sensory signs or visual field defect. Prodromal transient ischemic attacks were recorded in 16.1% to 57% of patients, usually within 48 hours [35]. We have seen cases with transient symptoms up to 10 days before developing the fixed deficits. The motor deficit is usually incomplete and often affects the proximal part of the extremity. In our experience, fine motor movement of the fingers and toes is usually present as well. There may be transient hypesthesia or paresthesia [29], and occasionally, the patient may refer to the onset of symptoms as a numbness. Dysarthria is also found. Lacunar infarction associated with pure motor hemiparesis has been reported in the posterior limb of the internal capsule, basis pontis, cerebral peduncle, and medulla [36]. An embolic infarct in an upper division of middle cerebral artery territory can sometimes mimic this type of lacunar syndrome. The deficit in the face, arm, and leg due to cortical infarction,

however, is usually disproportional. Moreover, in pure motor lacunar infarction, the tendon reflexes of the affected limbs often become brisker within the few hours of onset, which is faster than in most cases with similar deficit due to cortical infarction [35].

Ataxic hemiparesis. Ataxic hemiparesis is a syndrome in which pyramidal and cerebellar signs occur on the same side of the body. The weakness is mild, and the cerebellar ataxia is apparent in the least affected limb. Motor weakness is usually proportional in the face, arm, and leg, but it may be more severe in the leg or the arm. This syndrome was originally described by Fisher in 1965 [37] as "homolateral ataxia with crural paresis." The description was based on 14 patients who had weakness of the lower limb and Babinski's sign associated with dysmetria. In the ataxic hemiparesis syndrome, transient mild sensory symptoms, dysarthria, and nystagmus have been reported. Ataxic hemiparesis usually results from infarction at the junction of the upper third and inferior two thirds of the basis pontis [35]. Other locations, including internal capsule, thalamus, and lower pons, however, have been shown on imaging studies to cause hemiparesis and ataxia [35].

Dysarthria–clumsy hand syndrome. Dysarthria–clumsy hand syndrome is characterized by dysarthria, dysphagia, and slight weakness and clumsiness of the hand [38,39]. Several additional signs, including lower facial paralysis, ipsilateral brisk tendon reflexes, Babinski's sign, and deviation of the protruded tongue may be present. Fisher [35] stated that writing impairment is common when the dominant hand is affected. Sensory deficit is not a part of the syndrome. Fisher's pathologic study [35] suggests that dysarthria–clumsy hand syndrome is associated with a lacunar infarct at the genu of the internal capsule or at the junction of the upper one third and lower two thirds of the basis pontis. Occasionally, small cortical infarction can mimic this syndrome, but with cortical lesions, sensory deficit on the affected lips is usually present [28].

Sensorimotor stroke. Sensorimotor lacunar stroke syndrome is characterized by sensory loss and motor weakness on one side of the body without evidence of cortical involvement. Pathologically, it has been associated with an infarction in the posterolateral thalamus with extension into the adjacent posterior limb of the internal capsule [40]. (*Courtesy of* J. Philip Kistler.)

Classic Findings in Dominant and Nondominant Middle Cerebral Artery Occlusion

Dominant Stem Occlusion	Nondominant Stem Occlusion
Paralysis of contralateral face, arm, leg	Paralysis of contralateral face, arm, leg
Contralateral sensory impairment of face, arm, leg	Contralateral sensory impairment of face, arm, leg
Global aphasia	Contralateral neglect, anosognosia
Contralateral homonymous hemianopia	Contralateral homonymous hemianopia
Paralysis of conjugate gaze to the opposite side	Paralysis of conjugate gaze to the opposite side
Loss or impairment of optokinetic nystagmus	Loss or impairment of optokinetic nystagmus
Superior division occlusion	
Paralysis of contralateral face, arm, leg	Paralysis of contralateral face, arm, leg
Contralateral sensory impairment of face, arm, leg	Contralateral sensory impairment of face, arm, leg
Expressive aphasia, neglect	Neglect
Paralysis of conjugate gaze to the opposite side	Paralysis of conjugate gaze to the opposite side
Inferior division occlusion	
Minimal paralysis of contralateral face, arm, leg	Minimal paralysis of contralateral face, arm, leg
Receptive aphasia	Constructional apraxia
Minimal contralateral sensory impairment of face, arm, leg	Minimal contralateral sensory impairment of face, arm, leg
Homonymous hemianopia or upper quadrantopia	Homonymous hemianopia or upper quadrantopia

FIGURE 8-29.

Middle cerebral artery infarction. Cerebral embolism is the most common pathophysiologic cause of ischemic stroke, occurring in up to 60% of patients [41–43]. The refinement of extracranial and intracranial arterial ultrasound flow analysis, magnetic resonance imaging of the brain, and magnetic resonance angiography of the extracranial and intracranial circulation allow the physician to exclude reliably large vessel atherothrombotic stroke, lacunar stroke, or even dissection as a cause of cerebral infarction and thus to diagnose embolic stroke.

Clinical findings classically found in dominant and nondominant middle cerebral artery (MCA) stem or main branch occlusions. Cortical collateral flow from anastomotic vessels of the anterior and posterior cerebral arteries is responsible for the development of partial MCA syndromes. Partial MCA syndrome may also be due to an embolus that enters the MCA stem and moves distally, causing the recovery of ischemic noninfarcted tissue and its deficits. Partial syndromes resulting from embolic occlusion of the branches of MCA include hand weakness or arm and hand weakness (brachial syndrome) [44]. (*Adapted from* Adams *et al.* [45].)

Diagnostic Tests Used in the Evaluation of Embolic Stroke

Test	Reason
Cardiac	
Electrocardiogram	To diagnose atrial fibrillation and myocardial infarction
Transthoracic echocardiography	For visualization of left ventricular apex, left ventricular thrombus, and some aspects of prosthetic valves
Transesophageal echocardiography	More sensitive in detecting left atrial thrombus and smoke, interatrial septum, atrial aspect of mitral and tricuspid valves, vegetations less than 5 mm in size, endomyocardial abscess, ascending aortic atheromatous disease, and spontaneous echo contrast
Holter monitoring	To detect paroxysmal atrial fibrillation or sick sinus syndrome
Cerebral (brain and arteries)	
Carotid duplex ultrasound	To rule out carotid bifurcation atherosclerotic disease
Transcranial Doppler ultrasound	To rule out evidence of middle cerebral artery stem stenosis or siphon disease, to show if there is an occlusion of intracranial vessels or if they are open (embolus lysed)
MRI or MRA of the head and neck	To rule out lacunar stroke and atherosclerosis of large vessels and to evaluate intracranial collateral flow
Cerebral angiography	In the acute phase, to evaluate for intraarterial thrombolysis
Coagulation	
Hypercoagulable state evaluation, proteins C and S, fibrinogen, D-dimer, anticardiolipin Ab, F_{1+2}	To identify hypercoagulable conditions as a source of thromboembolism

FIGURE 8-30.

Diagnostic tests used in the evaluation of embolic stroke. These diagnostic tests are used to establish that embolism is the underlying pathophysiology of the ischemic stroke and to determine the precise source of the embolism for preventive therapy. The indications for transesophageal echocardiography (TEE) in the evaluation of a stroke and transient ischemic attacks depends on the severity of the stroke and the need to document all suspected sources of emboli precisely. The decision to order a transesophageal study should be based on the therapeutic implications of the information that might be gained. TEE is superior to transthoracic echocardiography in identifying left atrial thrombi, spontaneous left atrial contrast, aortic debris, intracardiac tumors, atrial septal aneurysms, patent foramen ovale or atrial septal defects, native valve vegetations or strands, and prosthetic valves [46]. Many physicians favor antithrombotic therapy when these entities are noted in a patient with embolic stroke. The National Institutes of Health–sponsored Warfarin Aspirin Recurrent Stroke Study (WARSS) [47] and a substudy of it using TEE to identify potential cardioaortic sources may provide some valuable information regarding the efficacy of antithrombotic versus antiplatelet therapy. The cerebral tests are needed to document the extent and location of the infarct and to rule out large artery atherothrombotic disease as the cause. The coagulation evaluation may identify a coagulation defect that leads to an overly active hemostatic system. In that case, anticoagulation may be an effective therapeutic strategy for stroke prevention. The Hemostatic System Activation Substudy of WARSS is examining the level of activity of the hemostatic system in WARSS patients and may find an association with increased clotting in a particular cardioembolic stroke–prone group of patients. MRA—magnetic resonance angiogram; MRI—magnetic resonance imaging. (*Courtesy of* J. Philip Kistler.)

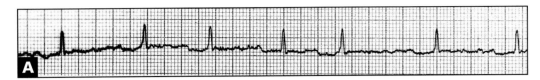

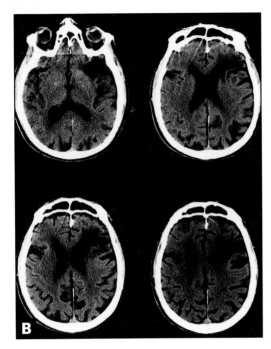

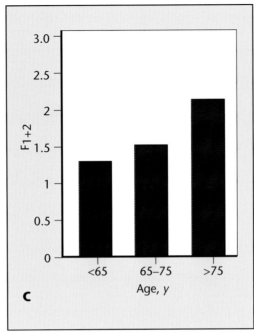

FIGURE 8-31.

Atrial fibrillation (AF). **A,** Electrocardiogram of a patient with AF. **B,** Computed tomography scans of an 89-year-old man who had chronic AF for 15 years and was on no medication. This scan was done in the first hour after the patient presented with a right middle cerebral artery territory stroke. The new infarct is not yet visible but an old infarct in the territory of the left middle cerebral artery is noted. The Framingham study showed that, after the age of 50 years, AF is the strongest independent risk factor for stroke. The overall attributable risk for stroke in patients with atrial fibrillation who are 50 to 59 years of age (1.5%) increased to 23% for those older than 80 years of age [48,49]. Five randomized trials studying the safety and efficacy of warfarin in the prevention of primary ischemic stroke among patients with AF have demonstrated that warfarin dramatically reduced the rate of stroke in patients 65 years and older [50–55]. Patients younger than 65 years also had significant benefit if they had diabetes, hypertension, or previous stroke as risk factors. The risk of intracranial hemorrhage was less than 0.25% per year. The highest rate of intracranial hemorrhage among the five trials was 0.89% per year [51]. In the two largest trials [52,53], the intensity of anticoagulation was low, prothrombin time ratio of 1.2 to 1.5, corresponding to an International Normalized Ratio (INR) of 1.5 to 2.7, and use of warfarin was safe. INRs above 3 have been associated with an increased risk of intracranial hemorrhage, especially in elderly patients [56]. Guidelines recommend a target INR of 2 to 3 in the treatment of patients with chronic atrial fibrillation [57,58]. **C,** Age-related increase in the rate of thrombin generation (the plasma level of F_{1+2}) among control patients in the Boston Area Anticoagulation Trial for Atrial Fibrillation [59]. Half of the patients in the control group were taking aspirin, and their mean F_{1+2} was the same as those not taking aspirin [59]. The age-related increase in the level of activity of the hemostatic system may suggest a mechanism to explain the age-related increase in stroke rate among patients with atrial fibrillation [59,60]. Similarly, the lack of effect of aspirin in reducing the level of activity of the hemostatic system may explain its relative lack of stroke-protective effect compared with warfarin in the atrial fibrillation trials [56,60]. (*Courtesy of* J. Philip Kistler.)

DISSECTION OF THE CERVICOCEREBRAL ARTERIES

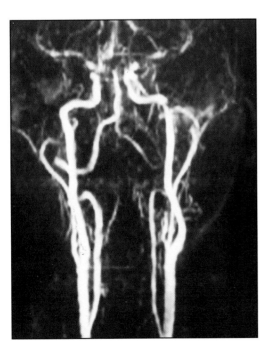

FIGURE 8-32.

Carotid dissection. A 54-year-old man presented with headache described as a sharp band from the forehead to the right ear and involving the right side of the neck. Twelve hours after the onset of headache, he noticed that his voice became hoarse. When he licked ice cream, he found it to be bitter. He also reported pulsatile tinnitus, which started 2 weeks before the headache. On examination, a right-sided Horner's syndrome was noted. Loss of taste sensation on the anterior part of the tongue was also demonstrated. The remainder of the examination was normal. No evidence of a cerebral infarct was seen on the magnetic resonance image performed on the day of admission. Cerebral angiography showed narrowing of right internal carotid artery from its origin at the bifurcation of the common carotid artery to the base of the skull. (*Courtesy of* J. Philip Kistler.)

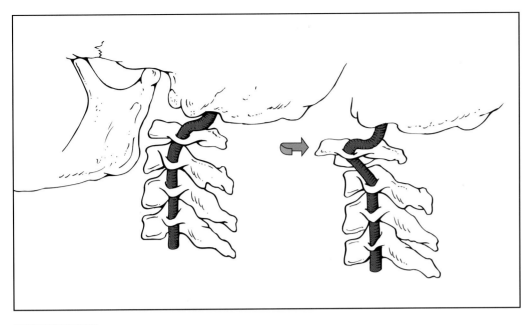

FIGURE 8-33.

Vertebral artery dissections are increasingly recognized as a cause of ischemic stroke and less commonly as a cause of subarachnoid hemorrhage. Dissection of the cervical vertebral artery usually occurs spontaneously or is associated with sudden mechanical injury of the artery from rotational forces [61–66]. Most cases have been associated with chiropractic or other neck manipulation, minor falls, automobile accidents, sudden head turning, or extensive coughing [66]. Spontaneous dissections associated with cystic medial degenera-

tion, arteritis, fibromuscular dysplasia, Marfan syndrome, and migraine have been reported [66]. Symptoms are usually characterized by the sudden onset of severe pain localized to the craniocervical region. The onset of ischemic symptoms may begin hours to weeks after the pain. The most common ischemic presentation is a partial or complete lateral medullary syndrome [67]. Isolated intracranial dissections arising in the vertebral artery between the posterior internal carotid artery and the basilar artery more frequently present with subarachnoid hemorrhage, but this is uncommon. The most common sight of origin of vertebral dissection is at C1 and C2. The vertebral artery is most mobile and thus most susceptible to mechanical injury at the C1 and C2 level as it leaves the transverse foramen and abruptly turns to enter the intracranial cavity [68]. Dissections at this site are more common in women, whereas intracranial dissections are more common in men. Either can occur throughout life from the first through the eighth decades. (*Courtesy of* J. Philip Kistler.)

ACUTE STROKE EVALUATION AND MANAGEMENT

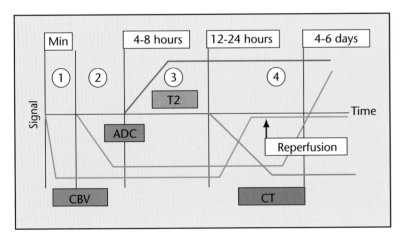

FIGURE 8-34.

Staging acute stroke patients with magnetic resonance imaging (MRI). In addition to new therapies, exciting new methods are being developed to detect and follow ischemic brain injury. Their use will revolutionize care of the acute stroke patient. Standard imaging techniques are unable to detect ischemic tissue consistently in the first 6 to 12 hours of stroke. Most neuroprotective strategies require that treatment begin before 6 hours. Advanced

diffusion or perfusion MRI is much more sensitive to ischemic injury in the first hours of stroke. Perfusion imaging detects brain regions that are less accessible to a bolus injection of intravenous contrast than normally perfused brain tissue. Diffusion imaging detects ischemic brain regions with lowered diffusibility of water. Water moves intracellularly when adenosine triphosphate (ATP) levels fall and ion gradients deteriorate. Intracellular water is ordered in a colloid matrix and is less diffusible. In addition, movement of water inside cells is dependent in large part on ATP. For these reasons, the apparent diffusion coefficient becomes less when ATP levels fall in ischemic brain. Diffusion imaging detects this change as increased signal intensity within minutes in animal models of stroke. Increased total water is detected as increased T2 signal. Computed tomography (CT) scan is less sensitive but also detects increased total water in stroke after a number of hours. The radiologic signature can be used to stage the progression of ischemic injury. Because the pathologic stage of the injury, and not time from onset of deficit, influences the potential for a positive response to therapy, we expect that magnetic resonance staging will determine future treatment decisions. ADC—apparent diffusion coefficients; CBV—cerebral blood volume. (*Courtesy of* J. Philip Kistler.)

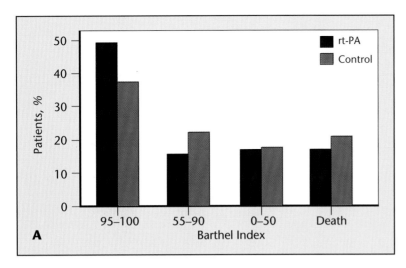
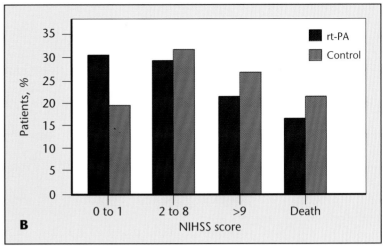

FIGURE 8-35.

National Institute of Neurological Disorders and Stroke (NINDS) trial of reteplase tissue plasminogen activator (rt-PA). **A** and **B**, The NINDS trial of rt-PA, a fibrinolytic agent, is the first study to show positive effect on outcome as measured by functional outcome (Barthel Index) with hyperacute treatment of the stroke patient. A controlled trial from Hong Kong has also shown benefit on outcome after treatment with low molecular weight heparin in the days after stroke [69]. Patients in the NINDS trial were selected according to strict criteria and managed according to protocol. Emphasis was directed at very early treatment; all patients were treated within 3 hours, and half were treated within 90 minutes of stroke onset. NIHSS—National Institutes of Health Stroke Service. (*Courtesy of* J. Philip Kistler.)

STROKE RECOVERY

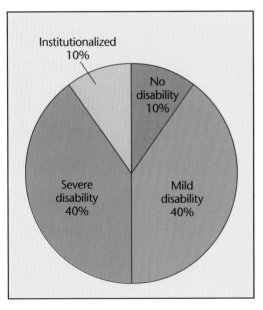

FIGURE 8-36.

Range of disability after stroke. About 400,000 patients survive stroke each year, surviving an average of 7 years. The range of recovery for these patients is broad. Stallones and coworkers [70] concluded that as many patients were institutionalized after stroke (10%) as were free of disability (10%). Most stroke patients were left with mild (40%) or severe (40%) disability. As a rule, however, the more severe the deficit at onset, the more substantial is the residual neurologic dysfunction. This relation holds for dysfunction as measured both in neurologic and in functional terms. (*Adapted from* Stallones *et al.* [70].)

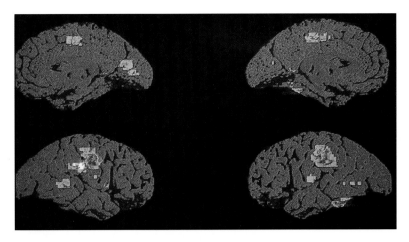

FIGURE 8-37.

Positron-emission tomography (PET) studies of the post-stroke recovered state. Studies using PET have confirmed the activity of several mechanisms in patients who have recovered from stroke. Weiller and coworkers [71] measured regional cerebral blood flow (CBF) in patients who recovered from a single, small, deep stroke. A regional increase in CBF reflects enhanced neural activity in a given brain area.

Using PET to measure regional CBF during movement of the recovered hand, the brain areas of each patient were identified that exhibited an increase in blood flow significantly greater than that seen in control subjects. Although the pattern of functional reorganization varied among individual patients, all patients showed significantly more activation of bilateral brain structures than did control subjects.

The PET scan from patient 1 from this study is shown here. There are four views of the brain: right medial view (*top left*), left medial view (*top right*), right lateral view (*bottom left*), and left lateral view (*bottom right*). The recovered hand was on the right. The highlighted pixels represent significantly activated pixels; the scale is arbitrary and thresholded to the level of statistical significance. Areas activated with movement of the recovered hand in this patient include the face area of the sensorimotor cortex in the infarcted hemisphere, consistent with cortical map reorganization. The contribution to recovery of the undamaged hemisphere was highlighted by significant activation in the primary sensorimotor and premotor cortices. The supplementary motor area, here projected onto the medial surface of the brain, is activated. This is consistent with the role of secondary motor areas in achieving restitution of function. (*From* Weiller *et al.* [71]; with permission.)

HYPERTENSIVE INTRACEREBRAL HEMORRHAGE

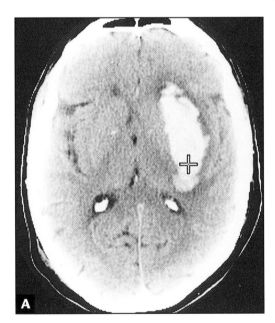 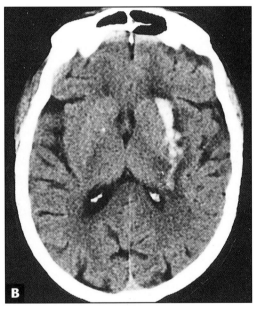

FIGURE 8-38.

Computed tomography scan showing a large left putamen hemorrhage (**A**) in a 68-year-old woman who collapsed at the dinner table, becoming aphasic and hemiplegic on the right side. She had a history of hypertension. She was taken emergently to the operating room, where a stereotactic aspiration of the hematoma was performed. The postoperative CT scan (**B**) is shown. At the time of discharge, the patient was able to ambulate and had only moderate residual expressive aphasia. In this case, the patient was seen in the emergency room within 1 hour of her ictus and was taken for emergent clot removal within 2 hours. Whether this contributed to her ultimate improvement and outcome has yet to be determined.

Putamen hemorrhage is characterized by progressive onset in almost two thirds of patients. Small hemorrhages cause moderate contralateral motor and sensory deficits. Moderate-sized hemorrhages can present with flaccid hemiplegia, hemisensory deficit, conjugate eye deviation toward the side of the lesion, and aphasia if the dominant hemisphere is involved. Large hemorrhages produce almost immediate coma [72].

Hypertensive cerebrovascular disease accounts for 70% to 90% of cases of spontaneous intracerebral hemorrhage [73]. The most common sources of hemorrhage are small penetrating arteries (less than 300 μm), including the thalamoperforating and lenticulostriate arteries and paramedian branches of the basilar artery [74]. There appears to be hypertension-induced degeneration of the media of the arterial wall, resulting in progressive development of microaneurysms [74]. This pathoanatomic factor accounts for the characteristic locations of hypertensive hemorrhages: basal ganglia (35% to 45%), subcortical white matter (25%), thalamus (20%), cerebellum (15%), and pons (5%) [75,76]. (*Courtesy of* J. Philip Kistler.)

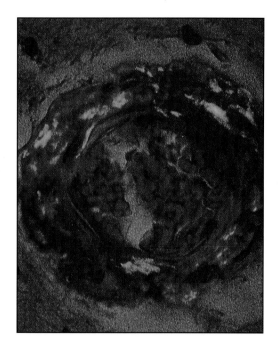

FIGURE 8-39.

Cerebral amyloid angiopathy (CAA). The term *amyloid* refers to protein deposits that, because of their physical structure, possess specific staining properties, such as the green birefringence to polarized light. Amyloid in this vessel has largely replaced the media layer, resulting in thickening of the vessel wall. Vascular amyloid in CAA is almost entirely restricted to the cortex, largely sparing the penetrating vessels of the white and deep gray matter. CAA is an important cause of spontaneous intracerebral hemorrhage in the elderly [77,78]. The presence of at least some cerebrovascular amyloid in the elderly is common, occurring in 20% or more of patients older than 70 years [77]. In most of these patients, the amyloid deposits have no evident effect on the patency of the vessel or integrity of the vessel wall. In a subset of patients, however, CAA initiates a cascade of steps that includes death of vascular smooth muscle cells (perhaps due to direct toxic properties of beta-amyloid [79]), cracking and necrosis of cerebral vessel walls [80–82], and ultimately intracerebral hemorrhage. (*Courtesy of* Jean Paul Vonsattel.)

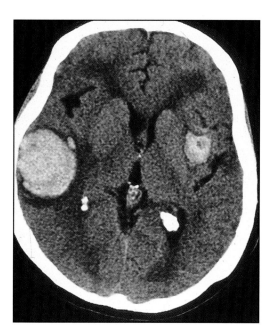

FIGURE 8-40.

Unenhanced computed tomography image from a 69-year-old woman who presented with hemorrhages in the right parietotemporal and left temporal lobes. Pathologic examination of cortical tissue obtained from evacuation of the right-sided hematoma demonstrated severe amyloid angiopathy. The hemorrhages in this patient illustrate the characteristic lobar location and multifocality of cerebral amyloid angiopathy (CAA)-related hemorrhage. The cause for *concurrent* hemorrhages in this patient is unknown. The interval between hemorrhages in patients with CAA appears to be highly variable, with some patients having no recurrence until years after their initial CAA-related hemorrhage [83].

Although concerns have been raised about the risk of surgical trauma provoking further hemorrhage from the amyloid-laden vasculature, surgical experience with CAA has generally been good [84]. Surgical indications for CAA-related hemorrhage (*eg*, acute neurologic deterioration of an otherwise stable patient) are thus similar to those for other types of hemorrhage. Examination of vessels in the wall of the hematoma or within the hematoma itself can provide important diagnostic information in support of CAA.

There are no known treatments to prevent CAA-related hemorrhage other than avoiding precipitants of hemorrhage such as anticoagulants. Indications for surgical treatment of CAA-related hemorrhages appear to be similar to those for surgical treatment of other types of cerebral hemorrhage. (*Courtesy of* J. Philip Kistler.)

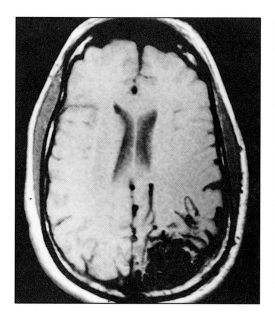

FIGURE 8-41.

Hemispheric arteriovenous malformation. A 44-year-old man had a seizure and was found to have a large left occipitoparietal arteriovenous malformation (AVM). T1-weighted magnetic resonance image shows the typical flow voids associated with AVMs. The flow voids are low density on the T1-weighted images. The lesion can be seen extending about 4 cm into the parietal cortex. The lesion was drained by the superior sagittal sinus. The risk with resection of AVMs is known to be associated with the size of the lesion, the eloquence of involved brain tissue, and whether the venous drainage is superficial or deep. AVM can present with hemorrhage, seizure, or progressive neurologic deficit. The lesions typically present in patients between 20 and 50 years old. When deciding whether to treat an AVM, the risks of treatment have to be carefully weighed against the natural history of the disease. AVMs have the potential for hemorrhage at a rate of about 4% per year [85]. Other risk factors can modify the actual hemorrhage rate, however, including intranidal aneurysms, deep venous drainage, paraventricular location, and single draining vein. AVM accounts for 6% to 13% of spontaneous intracerebral hematomas [86]. They are congenital abnormalities that develop between the 4th and 8th weeks of embryonic life [87]. AVMs are located predominantly in the cerebral hemispheres (70% to 93%) and most commonly involve branches of the middle cerebral artery. (*Courtesy of* J. Philip Kistler.)

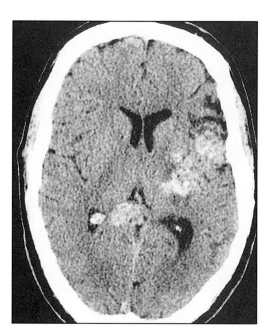

FIGURE 8-42.

Cavernous malformations. Cavernous malformations are blood vessel malformations of the central nervous system that can occur anywhere in the cerebrum, brain stem, or spinal cord. The lesions consist of thin-walled channeled vessels that have no muscular layer and that can hypertrophy with time. With the advent of magnetic resonance imaging (MRI), diagnosis of angiographically occult lesions has led to a clearer understanding of the natural history of the disease [88,89]. These lesions most commonly present with headache, seizures, or focal neurologic deficit [88,89]. Although MRI usually shows evidence of occult bleeding, overt hemorrhage is infrequent. The actual incidence of cavernous malformation hemorrhage is not known. Several series in the literature have documented hemorrhage rates from 07.5% to 20% per year. Once the lesion hemorrhages, the potential for future hemorrhage appears to be greater. The estimated risk of clinically significant hemorrhage is 0.25% to 0.7% per person-year of exposure [88,89].

Unenhanced computed tomography (CT) scan of a patient who had a significant parietal hemorrhage at the age of 1 year. By the age of 19 years, when this CT scan was obtained, he had had several more hemorrhages, rendering his contralateral arm plegic. The patient also began to have as many as eight simple partial seizures a day. Surgery is indicated in such lesions for seizure control and prevention of future bleeding. This patient had multiple lesions, as can be seen on the CT scan, with a right lesion posterior to the pulvinar on the right side. (*Courtesy of* J. Philip Kistler.)

■ DEMENTIAS

EVALUATION OF DEMENTIAS

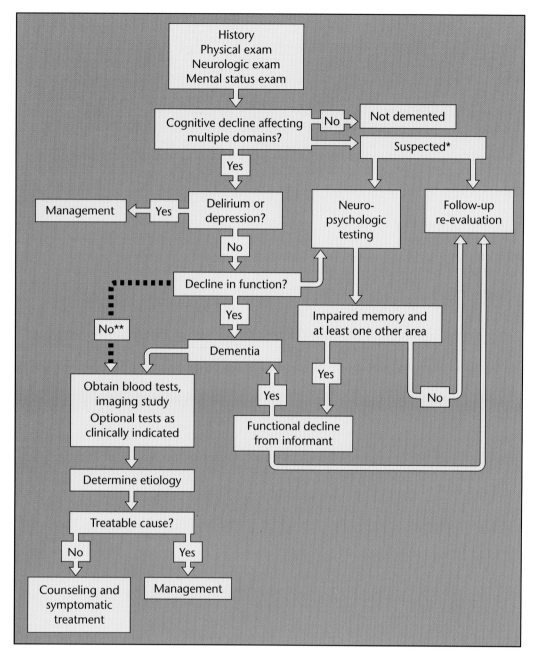

FIGURE 8-43

The clinical evaluation of dementia. The American Academy of Neurology has suggested this algorithm for the clinical evaluation and diagnosis of dementia [90,91]. Note that despite the absence of detection of abnormalities with office mental status testing (*eg*, Folstein Mini-Mental Status Exam) [92,93], dementia may be suspected (*) on the basis of the history or a threat to employment. In these cases, neuropsychologic evaluation is especially helpful. Note also that some neurologists do not recommend neuropsychologic testing in patients without functional decline (**). (*Adapted from* Corey-Bloom *et al.* [91].)

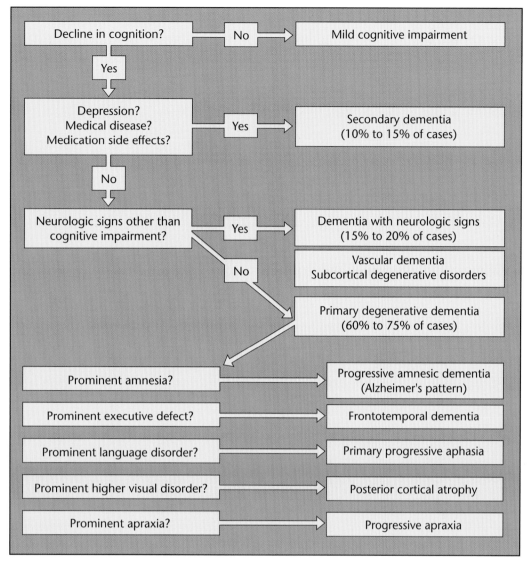

FIGURE 8-44.

Clinical classification of dementia. A useful clinical classification of dementia distinguishes mild cognitive impairment, secondary dementia, dementia with neurologic signs (or "dementia plus"), and primary degenerative dementia. Patients who complain of memory decline but have normal neuropsychologic test results may have mild cognitive impairment [94] (MCI). The clinician may reassure these patients that dementia has not been detected. However, because some patients prove to have incipient dementia, follow-up evaluation for a year or more is advised. Cases of secondary dementia are frequently "treatable." Cases of primary degenerative dementia are characterized by a prominent impairment in cognitive function in the absence of defects in primary sensory and motor function [95]. Aside from mental status, the neurologic examination is normal. This is the most common category of dementia, and usually is the result of degenerative disease. The diagnosis in progressive amnesic dementia is usually Alzheimer's disease (AD), and this profile is sometimes referred to as dementia of the Alzheimer type. These patients can often be managed exclusively by the primary caregiver, although as specific therapies become available, the involvement of a specialist may be useful. Syndromes of primary degenerative dementia, which depart from the usual Alzheimer's pattern, are distinctly unusual. These syndromes may have a different natural history than AD, raise special clinical issues, and are best handled with the assistance of a specialist. The presence of noncognitive neurologic signs in patients with dementia often indicates the presence of significant subcortical structural pathology or involvement of parts of the cortex that are usually spared in primary degenerative dementia. Often, a "subcortical" pattern of dementia is present [96,97]. Such cases of dementia with neurologic signs call for comprehensive neurologic evaluation and generally require the assistance of a specialist.

Relative Frequency of Causes of Dementia

Very common (about 50% of cases)
Alzheimer's disease
Common (10%–20% of cases)
Vascular dementia or mixed Alzheimer/vascular dementia
Less common (about 10% of cases)
Treatable medical or psychiatric conditions
Cortical or subcortical Lewy body disease
Uncommon (< 5% of cases)
Other primary degenerative dementias (Pick's disease and others)
Hydrocephalic dementia
Spongiform encephalopathy
Dementias lacking distinctive histology and many others

FIGURE 8-45.

Relative frequency of causes of dementia, by category. The relative frequencies of the leading causes of dementia in the general population have not been studied definitively [98]. Hospital-based studies and autopsy series indicate the approximate prevalences shown in the figure. The most prevalent cause of dementia by far is Alzheimer's disease, which probably accounts for at least half of all cases. The vascular dementias account collectively for 10% to 20% of cases, and constitute the second most common cause. The substantial proportion of patients who present with both vascular disease *and* Alzheimer's pathology poses a diagnostic challenge to the clinician. Dementia secondary to medical or psychiatric illness, despite its clinical importance, is apparently less common [99], although hospital-based studies may underestimate its incidence. Dementia complicating idiopathic Parkinson's disease (IPD) and dementia with cortical Lewy bodies (DLB) constitute the other important cluster. DLB and AD frequently occur concomitantly. All other causes of dementia, most of them degenerative, are quite uncommon. Among these, Pick's disease, hydrocephalic dementia, and spongiform encephalopathy have distinctive presentations. (*Courtesy of* Thomas J. Grabowski.)

ALZHEIMER'S DISEASE

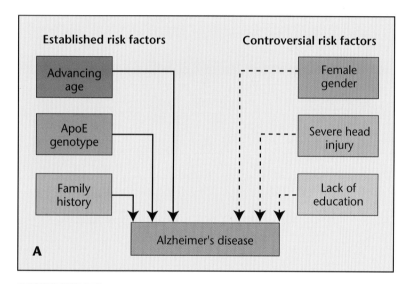

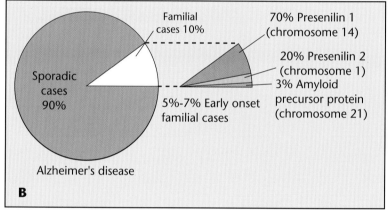

FIGURE 8-46.

Epidemiology of Alzheimer's disease. **A,** Among the established risk factors [100] for the development of Alzheimer's disease (AD), the most important is advancing age. The prevalence of AD at age 65 is approximately 0.5% of the population. The prevalence approximately doubles in each subsequent 5-year increment, reaching about 10% by age 85 [101]. On the basis of the limited data available, it appears that the incidence tends to level off after age 85 [102]. Following age, the most important risk factors are genetic. Up to 10% of AD cases are transmitted genetically in an autosomal dominant manner. An international combined analysis of case control studies found that patients with a first-degree rela-

tive with AD had a relative risk (RR) of 3.5 for developing AD. This risk was highest when the relative had onset of dementia before age 70. The presence of two first-degree relatives imparted a RR of 7.5 [103]. **B,** Three genes accounting for much of familial early onset AD have now been identified. A defect in the amyloid precursor protein gene on chromosome 21 was the first to be delineated, accounting for a small proportion (3%) of cases [104]. Most recently discovered were the presenilin genes, which appear to encode proteins that participate in intracellular transport. Defects in presenilin 1 may account for the majority (50% to 70%) of cases of early onset familial AD [105,106]. Weaker and controversial risk factors for the development of AD include past head injury, female gender [107], and limited degree of education. Estrogen replacement may be a protective factor in postmenopausal women [108]. (*Courtesy of* Thomas J. Grabowski.)

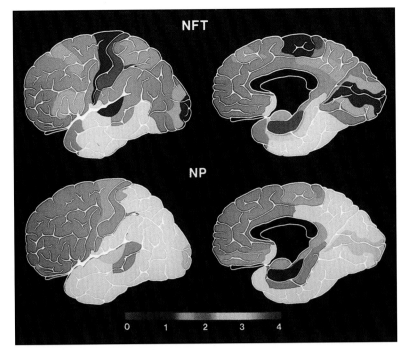

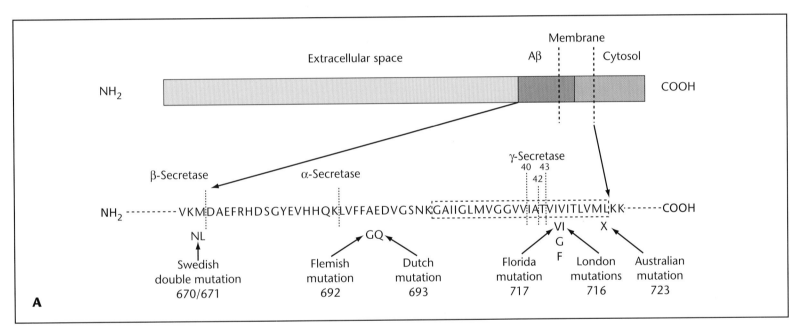

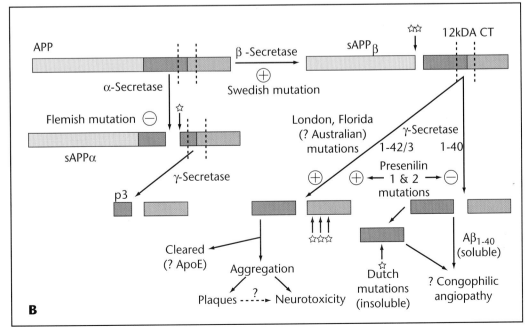

FIGURE 8-47.

Distribution of Alzheimer's pathology. The pathologic distinction between Alzheimer's disease (AD) and normal aging is based on quantitative criteria [109,110]. Neurofibrillary tangles (NFTs) occur first in highly characteristic locations, specifically the entorhinal cortex, the perirhinal cortex, the hippocampal sector CA1, and the amygdala. They also occur frequently in the nucleus basalis of Meynert, temporal isocortex (Brodmann's areas 20 and 21), hippocampal sectors CA3 and CA4, the dentate gyrus, and the presubiculum. Arnold *et al.* [111] surveyed the distribution of NFTs (*top*), finding the greatest numbers in the limbic periallocortex and allocortex. Tangles become progressively less numerous in the nonlimbic periallocortex, the nonprimary association cortex, and the primary association cortex. The smallest extent of NFTs that has been correlated with dementia encompasses areas 28, CA1, and the inferotemporal neocortex [112,113]. Neuritic plaques (NPs), on the other hand, have a somewhat different distribution (*bottom*) than NFTs. For example, they are relatively uncommon in the limbic periallocortex and the allocortex and they tend to be distributed more evenly throughout the cortex than are tangles. Most investigators have reported that NPs have less specific regional and laminar distributions. (*From* Arnold *et al.* [111]; with permission.)

FIGURE 8-48.

Amyloid precursor protein (APP) processing. **A,** APP is processed in neurons by three proteases, known as *secretases* [114]. Cleavage by α-secretase produces sAPPα, a peptide whose normal function remains obscure, while precluding production of the amyloidogenic peptide Aβ42. Mutations of the APP gene near the α-secretase cleavage site (Flemish and Dutch mutations) have been associated with hereditary cerebral amyloid angiopathy. In normal cells, not all APP is cleaved at the alpha site; action of β-secretase and γ-secretase produces Aβ40 and/or Aβ42. **B,** Mutations near the β (Swedish mutation) or γ (London, Florida, and Australian mutations) cleavage sites are associated with familial Alzheimer's disease (AD), presumably because of altered APP proteolysis.

(Continued)

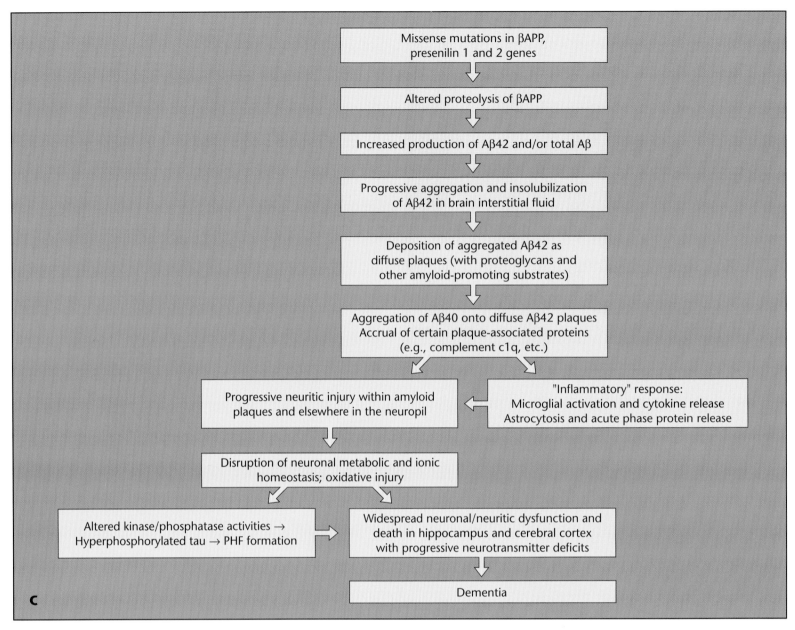

FIGURE 8-48. (CONTINUED)

Aβ42 is relatively insoluble and becomes the major component of senile plaques, primarily as diffuse plaques. Aβ40 is incorporated in mature plaques and is the chief form of Aβ in amyloid-laden vessel walls [115].

The relationship between neurofibrillary and amyloid pathology in AD has not yet been fully explained. The specificity of plaques for AD, the alterations in amyloid metabolism that arise from mutations of the APP and presenilin genes, and data from the transgenic mouse model have focused attention on amyloid deposition as the inciting

event [116], while neurofibrillary tangles (NFTs) mark dysfunctional neural systems that correlate with cognitive manifestations of the disease. C, The amyloid cascade hypothesis of Alzheimer pathogenesis suggests that altered amyloidogenesis leads to neurotoxicity, characterized by astrogliosis, activation of microglia, and the appearance of dystrophic neurites. A cascade of events follows that culminates in hyperphosphorylation of tau, NFT formation, and, ultimately, neural degeneration. (Panels A and B *adapted from* Storey *et al.* [114]; panel C *adapted from* Selkoe [115].)

VASCULAR DEMENTIAS

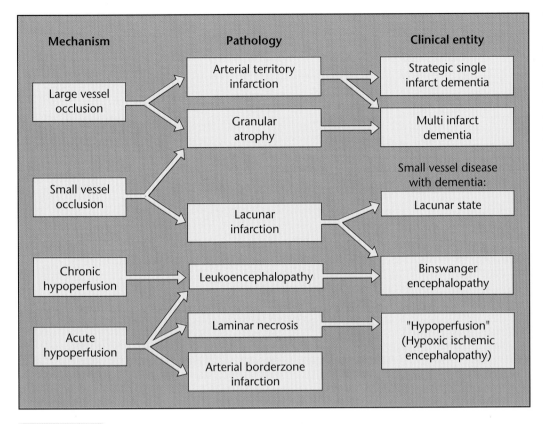

FIGURE 8-49.
Subtypes of ischemic vascular dementia (VaD). The National Institute of Neurological Disorders and Stroke—Association Internationale pour la Recherche et l'Enseignement en Neurosciences workshop recognized four subtypes of ischemic VaD as well as hemorrhagic dementia [117]. The relationships between the ischemic subtypes, the underlying mechanisms of injury, and their histopathologic correlates are illustrated.

Although one or a few strategic infarcts may cause dementia, VaD commonly results from an accumulation of infarcts [114–119]. These infarcts may affect the territories of large cere-bral vessels, a condition referred to as "multi-infarct dementia." Large vessel thromboembolism, however, may not be the dominant mechanism of VaD. A more common scenario is cumulative infarction of the territories of small penetrating arterioles. Such small vessel infarcts tend to complicate poorly controlled hypertension and diabetes. A less frequent presentation of VaD is Binswanger's encephalopathy, which is associated with diffuse leukoencephalopathy and ventriculomegaly and is thought to occur by an ischemic mechanism. Other cerebrovascular mechanisms leading to dementia are hypoxic-ischemic encephalopathy and cerebral hemorrhage.

The natural history of VaD is difficult to summarize, because the precise mechanisms of infarction and the topographic pattern of infarct accumulation vary among cases. The rate of progression is often uneven, punctuated by datable events, rebounds, and fluctuations [120]. The overall course in many cases, however, may be more rapid than that of AD. Ischemic VaD may have predominantly "subcortical" features: impaired executive function, impaired speed of thought, depression, and apathy. Spotty or mild impairment of classic "cortical" faculties, such as language, praxis, and visuospatial function, is the rule. Gait impairment and urinary incontinence are common. (*Courtesy of* Thomas J. Grabowski.)

DEGENERATIVE DEMENTIAS OF NON-ALZHEIMER'S TYPE

Principal Causes of Non-Alzheimer's Degenerative Dementia

Frontotemporal lobar degeneration
  Pick's disease
  Corticobasal degeneration
  Dementia lacking distinctive histopathologic features
  Frontotemporal dementia with parkinsonism linked to chromosome 17
Degenerative conditions with parkinsonism
  Dementia with Lewy bodies
  Idiopathic Parkinson's disease
  Progressive supranuclear palsy
  Corticobasal degeneration
Spongiform encephalopathies
  Creutzfeldt-Jakob disease

FIGURE 8-50.
Principal classes of non-Alzheimer's degenerative dementia. A significant number of cases of degenerative dementia are atypical by virtue of the unusual profile of cognitive impairment, the presence of motor signs, or the rapid rate of decline. Many such cases, along with 10% to 15% of typical cases (those that meet National Institute of Neurological and Communicative Disorders and Stroke—Alzheimer's Disease and Related Disorders Association criteria for probable Alzheimer's disease) are associated with non-Alzheimer's histopathologic features. Diagnostically, such cases are challenging, and surprises at autopsy are not infrequent.

Clinical Criteria for Frontotemporal Dementia

Core Diagnostic Features

Insidious and slowly progressive behavior disorder

Early loss of personal and social awareness

Disinhibition, impulsivity, utilization behavior, hyperorality

Mental rigidity and inflexibility

Stereotyped and perseverative behavior

Distractibility, motor impersistence

Affective symptoms

Depression, anxiety, excessive sentimentality, hypochondriasis, bizarre somatic preoccupation, emotional unconcern, inertia, aspontaneity

Speech disorder

Progressive reduction in speech; late mutism

Stereotypy, echolalia and perserveration

Preserved spatial orientation and praxis

Physical signs

    Early primitive reflexes

    Early incontinence

    Late akinesia, rigidity, tremor

    Low and labile blood pressure

Investigations

Normal electroencephalogram

Brain imaging: predominant frontal and/or anterior temporal abnormality

Neuropsychology: profound defect on tests of executive function

Features Supporting Diagnosis of Frontotemporal Dementia

Onset before age 65

Family history of similar disorder in a first-degree relative

Signs of motor neuron disease

Features Against Diagnosis of Frontotemporal Dementia

Abrupt onset, ictal events

Head trauma related to onset

Early severe amnesia, spatial disorientation, or apraxia

Myoclonus, cerebellar ataxia, choreoathetosis

Early, severe, pathologic electroencephalogram

FIGURE 8-51.

Clinical manifestations of frontotemporal dementia. Summary of the consensus clinical criteria for the diagnosis of frontotemporal dementia published by the Lund and Manchester centers [121,122]. Frontotemporal dementia is the syndrome of primary degenerative dementia with an early and prominent disorder of executive function and social behavior. Patients with pathologic diagnoses of Pick's disease, frontal lobe degeneration [123], and motor neuron disease [124] may present with this syndrome. In the Manchester series of 150 patients, the usual age at onset was 45 to 60 years; no difference in incidence occurred between men and women. The median duration of illness was 8 years. About 40% of the patients had a first-degree relative with dementia, mostly in dominant kindreds [125].

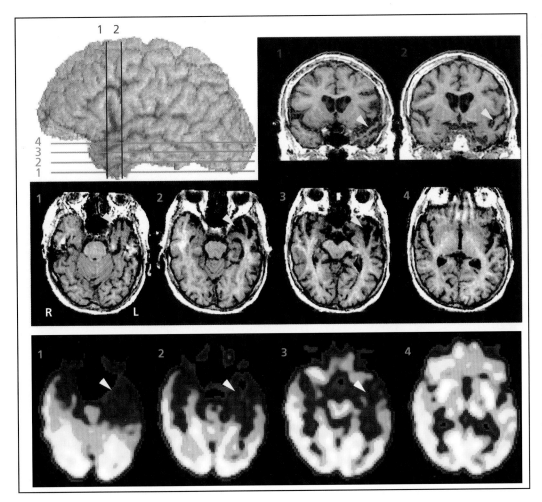

FIGURE 8-52.

Neuroimages of primary progressive aphasia. Magnetic resonance images (*top tiers*) and coregistered ^{18}F-fluorodeoxyglucose positron-emission tomograms (*bottom tier*) of the brain of a 73-year-old woman with primary progressive aphasia (PPA). Note the circumscribed atrophy of the left temporal and perisylvian areas (*arrowheads*) and the accompanying hypometabolism in these regions. The bilateral posterior temporoparietal metabolic deficits characteristic of Alzheimer's disease are absent.

Arnold Pick, in 1892, in the initial report of Pick's disease, concluded that "a more or less circumscribed type of aphasia could result from a single circumscribed atrophic process." Contemporary interest in this phenomenon began in 1982, with Mesulam's report of six cases of slowly progressive language disorder with preserved intellect, visually-mediated abilities, and insight [126]. Despite many case reports, PPA is rare. The Manchester group estimates the relative frequencies of progressive aphasia and dementia of Alzheimer's type at a ratio of 1 to 40 (versus a ratio of 1 to 5 for frontotemporal dementia and dementia of Alzheimer's type) [127]. The early disturbance is often characterized by anomia, word-finding difficulties in running speech, dysfluency, and frustration. As the disease progresses, apraxia is common, and depression is likely. Other cognitive deficits eventually emerge, but perhaps not always. An even less common variant of PPA, termed *semantic dementia*, has also been described, in which the salient defects are defective access to the meaning of words and visual agnosia [128].

In most cases, the pathologic findings are those of Pick's disease, Pick-spectrum pathology lacking Pick bodies, or nonspecific histopathologic findings characterized by neuronal loss, cortical gliosis, and spongiform change in the superficial cortical layers [129–131]. (*Courtesy of* Laboratory of Human Neuroanatomy and Neuroimaging, Department of Neurology, The University of Iowa.)

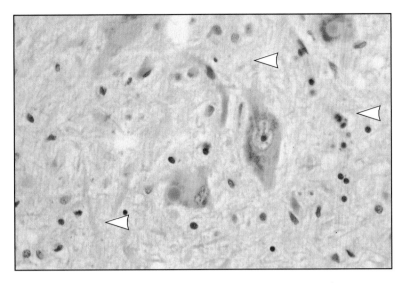

FIGURE 8-53.

Histopathologic changes in dementia with Lewy bodies (DLB). When they occur in cortical neurons, the eosinophilic cytoplasmic inclusions called Lewy bodies are much less conspicuous than those occurring in classic subcortical locations. Midbrain section (hematoxylin and eosin stain) from a patient with DLB, showing three classic Lewy bodies. In contrast, cortical Lewy bodies (*arrowheads*) may not be detected with standard stains because they lack the pale halo and are sparsely distributed. They are detectable after immunostaining with antibodies to ubiquitin. Cortical Lewy bodies occur most frequently in the anterior cingulate gyrus, anterior frontal, anterior temporal, and insular cortices [132]. Another characteristic pathologic feature of DLB is the presence of dystrophic neurites in sectors CA2 and CA3 of the hippocampus [133–135]. (*Courtesy of* Lee Reed, MD, Department of Pathology, The University of Iowa.)

Criteria for Dementia with Lewy Bodies

Dementia and

Probable DLB: two of three cardinal features (Possible DLB: one of three)
- Fluctuating sensorium/cognition
- Parkinsonism
- Visual hallucinations

Supporting features
- Repeated falls
- Syncope
- Transient LOC
- Neuroleptic sensitivity
- Systematized delusions
- Hallucinations in other modalities

Other reported associations
- REM sleep behavior disorder
- Depression
- Slow EEG

FIGURE 8-54.

Consensus criteria for dementia with Lewy bodies (DLB). The formal criteria for DLB presented here incorporated retrospective analysis of case records. These criteria have good specificity (90%) but limited sensitivity (50% to 75%). However, sensitivity is better in prospective than in retrospective ones; the primary difficulty in retrospective analysis is in defining and quantifying fluctuation. DLB is commonly misdiagnosed as vascular dementia [136–143]. EEG—electroencephalograph; LOC—loss of consciousness; REM—rapid eye movement.

BEHAVIORAL NEUROLOGY

AGNOSIA

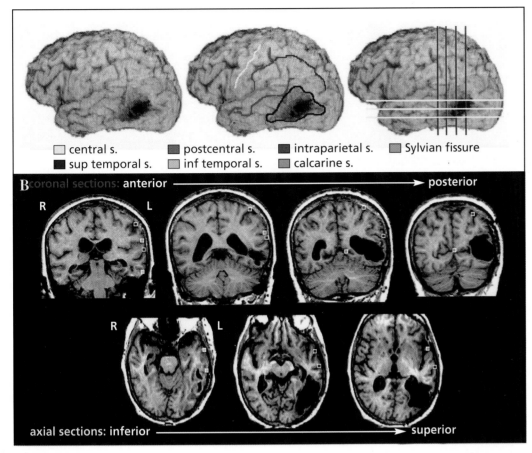

central s. | postcentral s. | intraparietal s. | Sylvian fissure
sup temporal s. | inf temporal s. | calcarine s.

B coronal sections: anterior → posterior

R L

axial sections: inferior → superior

FIGURE 8-55.

Visual object agnosia. Three-dimensional brain reconstruction of a patient with visual object agnosia. Magnetic resonance imaging (MRI) data from a subject with a left occipitotemporal lesion and visual object agnosia. The MRI data are reconstructed in three dimensions in the pictures in the top row. The first image in the top row shows the left lateral view of a three-dimensional reconstruction of contiguous coronal MRIs, after digital deletion of extracerebral structures, using Brainvox (a three-dimensional visualization and analysis system developed in the Human Neuroanatomy and Neuroimaging Laboratory at The University of Iowa) [133,134]. The surface extent of the lesion in the region of the left occipitotemporal junction is apparent. In the middle image, major cerebral sulci have been marked with traces that are color-coded, according to the key provided. The right image in the top row shows the orientations of the four coronal (*red*) and three axial (*yellow*) cuts depicted in the bottom two thirds of the figure, corresponding to the images in the middle and lower rows, respectively. (Coronal sections are displayed in anterior to posterior order, *left* to *right*. Axial [transverse] sections are displayed in inferior to superior order, *left* to *right*.) The colored traces of the sulci have been transferred (automatically) to coronal and axial sections (*middle* and *lower rows*). These images make the extent and location of the lesion apparent. In this case, the lesion extends from the cortical surface to the ventricular surface, beginning at the mid-portion of the middle and inferior temporal gyri, and continuing to the lateral occipital region, sparing the calcarine cortex, the superior temporal gyrus, and the parietal lobe. The full extent of the lesion was traced on the two-dimensional slices and then projected to the surface. The surface projection of the lesion is outlined with a black trace in the middle image of the upper row, to give some idea of its subcortical extent.

Visual object agnosia is a disorder of recognition confined to the visual realm, in which a patient cannot arrive at the meaning of some or all categories of previously known nonverbal visual stimuli, despite normal or near-normal visual perception and intact alertness, attention, intelligence, and language. Most patients also have an impairment in learning new visual stimuli. The condition is associated with bilateral or, rarely, unilateral occipitotemporal lesions. The profile of this patient with a left-sided lesion includes impaired recognition of tools and utensils and normal recognition of animals. (*Courtesy of* Laboratory of Human Neuroanatomy and Neuroimaging, Department of Neurology, The University of Iowa.)

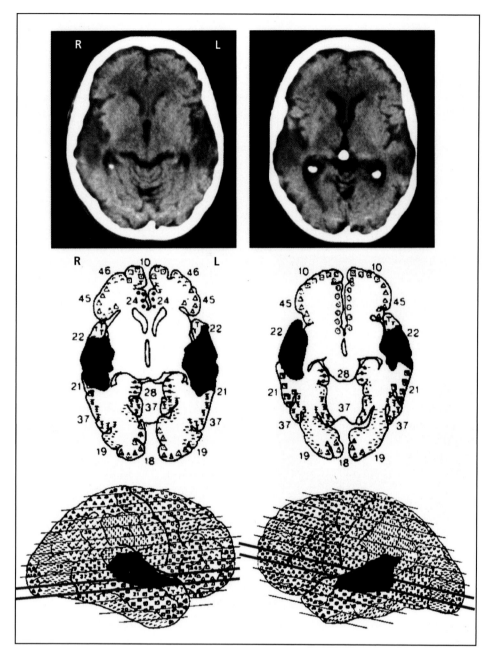

FIGURE 8-56.

Auditory agnosia. A 37-year-old right-handed woman had bilateral lesions in the posterior portion of the superior temporal gyrus, which produced the condition of auditory agnosia. The top row shows two transverse computed tomographic cuts, and the lesions are indicated by hypointense signal. The lesions are plotted on standard brain templates in the middle and bottom rows.

Auditory agnosia is a disorder of recognition confined to the auditory realm, in which a patient cannot arrive at the meaning of some or all categories of previously known auditory stimuli, despite normal or near-normal auditory acuity and intact alertness, attention, and intelligence. Strictly speaking, the term should be reserved for an inability to recognize nonverbal sounds, such as environmental sounds, melodies, and timbres, and the term *aphasia* should apply to the verbal component of auditory agnosia. In fact, some degree of aphasia (related to the left temporal lobe lesion) is virtually always present. This patient had a fluent aphasia, but language capacities through the visual modality were preserved, and she remained capable of reading and writing. The defining characteristic of auditory agnosia is a defect in the recognition of common environmental sounds. The patient could not determine the meaning of sounds such as knocking on the door, a telephone ringing, a baby crying, or a bird chirping. The defect is modality specific, and the patient had normal recognition of entities presented visually, even though the sounds of those stimuli were unrecognized. (*Courtesy of* Laboratory of Human Neuroanatomy and Neuroimaging, Department of Neurology, The University of Iowa.)

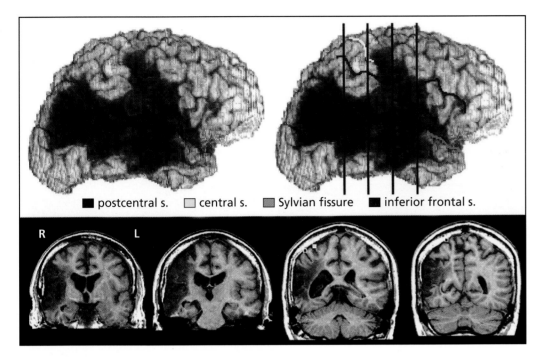

■ postcentral s.   □ central s.   ■ Sylvian fissure   ■ inferior frontal s.

FIGURE 8-57.

Anosognosia. A lesion in the right hemisphere involving a significant portion of the inferior parietal lobule (areas 39 and 40), shown in lateral three-dimensional brain reconstructions (*top*) and in coronal T1-weighted magnetic resonance imaging (MRI) cuts (*bottom*) in a patient with anosognosia. The patient, a 34-year-old right-handed woman, sustained an infarct in the territory of the right middle cerebral artery and developed severe anosognosia in connection with this lesion.

Anosognosia denotes a condition in which patients lose the ability to recognize disease states in themselves, and the term was first applied to a patient who denied a left hemiplegia [135]. The condition is in essence a disturbance of recognition, and in that sense, it conforms to the designation of agnosia. In the most extreme and paradigmatic examples, patients fail to recognize major disabilities such as a complete hemiplegia or hemianesthesia; marked pain may be ignored; the gravity of heart disease or cancer may go unacknowledged. Anosognosia also occurs in relation to cognitive and behavioral deficits. Patients give little indication of understanding that their cognition and behavior are compromised and fail to appreciate the ramifications of their disabilities. The term anosognosia can be applied whenever there is a significant discrepancy between the patient's report of his or her disabilities and the objective evidence regarding the patient's level of functioning. (*Courtesy of* Laboratory of Human Neuroanatomy and Neuroimaging, Department of Neurology, The University of Iowa.)

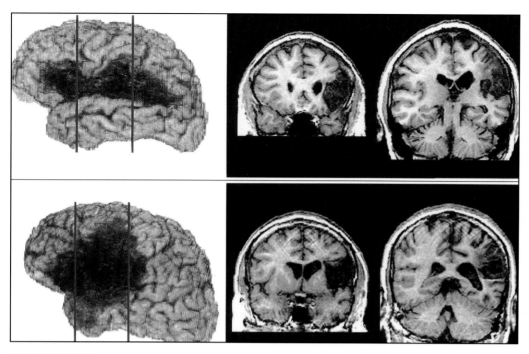

FIGURE 8-58.

Global aphasia. Three-dimensional magnetic resonance imaging reconstructions of two patients with global aphasia. The top row depicts a 74-year-old right-handed man who suffered a large infarct in the territory of the left middle cerebral artery, which damaged all language-related regions in the perisylvian sector, including Broca's area, Wernicke's area, and the parietal opercular region. The other patient, a 68-year-old right-handed man, is shown in the bottom row. The patient had a similar presentation; virtually all of the regions in the immediate vicinity of the sylvian fissure are damaged, although there is some sparing of the more posterior aspects of the region. Both lesions are shown in lateral (*left*) and coronal (*right*) orientations. As is typical of global aphasia, these patients had right hemiplegia affecting face, arm,

and leg, right hemisensory impairment, and right homonymous hemianopia.

As the term implies, global aphasia involves virtually complete dilapidation of speech and linguistic capacities. The patient is rendered incapable of both comprehending and producing verbal messages. Verbatim repetition, naming, reading, and writing are all severely impaired. The patient may, however, retain the capacity for singing, and it is worth testing for this, because the production of fluent singing can be highly encouraging in a patient who is otherwise virtually mute. The syndrome is related to two main patterns of lesion: extensive destruction of the perisylvian region, including Broca's area, the inferior parietal cortices, Wernicke's area, and underlying white matter and subcortical structures (as seen in both these patients); or two noncontiguous lesions, one involving Broca's area and the other involving Wernicke's area. In the latter presentation, the patient does *not* have a right hemiparesis, owing to the sparing of motor cortex between the two lesions, and the prognosis for recovery of some linguistic abilities is considerably better [143]. Otherwise, global aphasia has a worse prognosis for recovery than any of the other aphasia syndromes. (*Courtesy of Laboratory of Human Neuroanatomy and Neuroimaging, The University of Iowa.*)

■ NEURO-ONCOLOGY

EPIDEMIOLOGY OF BRAIN TUMORS

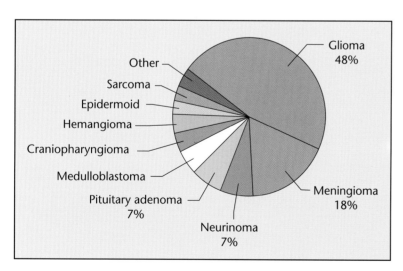

FIGURE 8-59.

Relative frequency of primary intracranial tumors and gliomas. Gliomas are the most common primary intracranial neoplasm, comprising 48% of all primary intracranial tumors when all age groups are considered. Meningiomas are the second most common primary intracranial tumor. Medulloblastomas are the most common nongliomatous intracranial tumor in children, and thus account for a significant proportion of intracranial tumors when all ages are considered. Other types of intracranial tumors occur less frequently. When gliomas are considered alone, tumors derived from astrocytes are most common. Astrocytic tumors, which include astrocytomas and glioblastomas, account for 71% of all gliomas. Oligodendroglial and ependymal tumors are less common.

This chart includes only primary brain tumors, not intracranial metastases. In some series, intracranial metastases are the most frequent intracranial tumor, and can account for 50% of all intracranial tumors [144]. In autopsied patients with cancer, 20% to 40% have intracranial metastases [145,146]. (*Adapted from* Evans [147].)

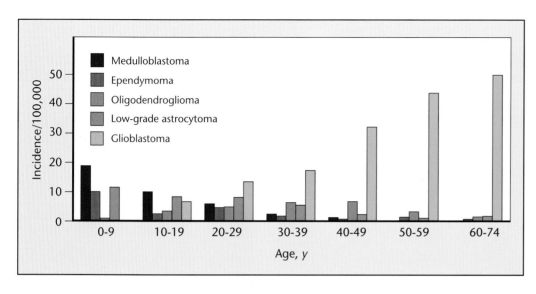

FIGURE 8-60.

Incidence of several types of primary brain tumors in different age groups. Although the overall incidence of brain tumors increases with age, different histologic types have different age distributions. Medulloblastomas are most common in early childhood, and are rare in adulthood. Ependymomas are also more common in childhood. Oligodendrogliomas are most frequently diagnosed in young adults. Low grade astrocytomas are common in young adults, but become less frequent with age, when glioblastoma multiforme becomes the most common astrocytic tumor. The high incidence of glioblastomas in older adults accounts for the overall increase in brain tumors with age. (*Adapted from* Evans [147]; and Levin *et al.* [148].)

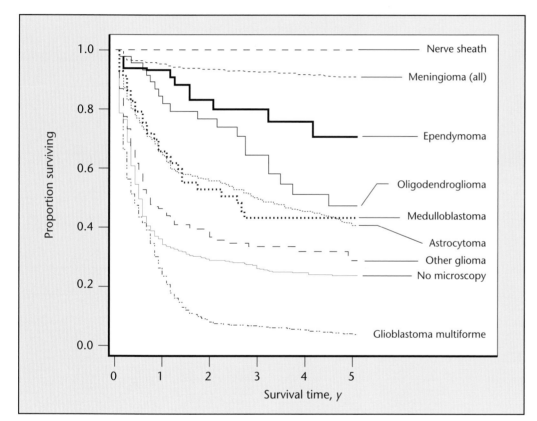

FIGURE 8-61.

Kaplan-Meier survival curves for patients with various types of central nervous system tumors. The data are from the Victorian Cancer Registry in Victoria, Australia, from 1982 to 1991 [149]. As the survival curves show, glioblastoma multiforme is almost invariably lethal, and survival time is short, with less than 5% of patients surviving 5 years. Meningioma, on the other hand, has little effect on the survival of the patient. (This curve includes both benign and malignant meningiomas.) Patients with ependymoma, low-grade astrocytoma, or oligodendroglioma have intermediate survival curves and can live for years after their initial diagnosis. The astrocytoma curve includes anaplastic and well-differentiated tumors. The curve indicating "no microscopy" refers to tumors that were identified on clinical and radiologic study only. (*Courtesy of* Karen L. Fink and S. Clifford Schold, Jr.)

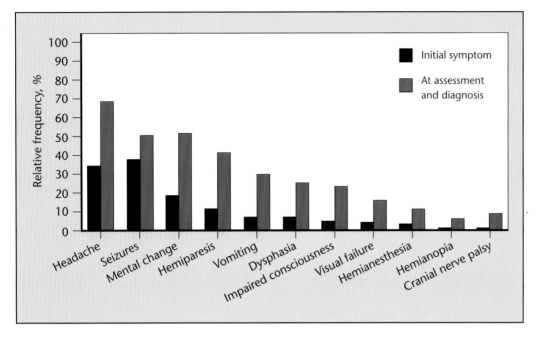

time a diagnosis is made [150,151].

Brain tumor patients who present with seizures may have a better prognosis than those who present with other signs and symptoms. Tumors that cause seizures tend to be located peripherally and supratentorially, and are thus more surgically accessible. In addition, seizures occur more often in patients with low-grade gliomas than in patients with high-grade tumors [152]. The onset of seizures after 25 years of age should be investigated with magnetic resonance imaging (MRI). Up to 60% of patients presenting with new seizures after age 25 will have an abnormality detected on MRI, and 13% to 18% of these patients will have a brain tumor [153].

This information was collected from a series of 653 patients with cerebral gliomas seen at the National Hospital in London from 1955 to 1975 [150,151]. Therefore most of these patients received their diagnosis before computed tomography or MRI became available. (*Courtesy of* Karen L. Fink and S. Clifford Schold, Jr.)

FIGURE 8-62.

Initial symptoms and symptoms at diagnosis in patients with brain tumors. The most common initial symptoms in patients with primary malignant gliomas are headaches (35%) and seizures (38%). Patients with brain tumors usually develop additional symptoms before definitive diagnosis. Many patients have noticeable mental status changes (52%) or hemiparesis (43%) by the

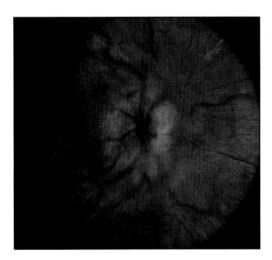

FIGURE 8-63.

Funduscopic photo showing a patient's well-developed papilledema. The funduscopic examination is important in any patient with headache, and can be an important indicator of the presence of a brain tumor. This patient presented at age 11 with retro-orbital headaches, nausea, and vomiting. Her general examination and neurologic examination were normal except for papilledema and enlargement of her blind spot. The optic disc seen here is blurred and elevated. Exudates are present in the retina, and the nerve fiber layer is visible in the right eye, as yellow streaks directed from the optic disc toward the macula. (*Courtesy of* Karen L. Fink and S. Clifford Schold, Jr.)

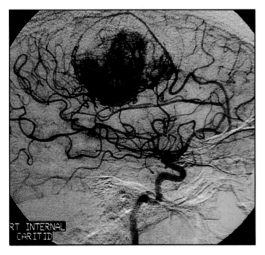

FIGURE 8-64.

Arterial phase angiogram with a tumor blush following injection of the right internal carotid artery. Before the availability of computed tomography and magnetic resonance scanning, angiography was the only way to directly visualize intracranial tumors. The most helpful findings on angiography are abnormal vessels feeding a tumor, or a "tumor blush" of contrast indicating a hypervascular tumor. This patient had a very vascular tumor, a hemangiopericytoma. The tumor was fed by both internal carotid arteries, by the posterior circulation, and by the left external carotid artery. In some patients, the arterial phase of the angiogram is normal, but a tumor blush appears during the venous phase. (*Courtesy of* Karen L. Fink and S. Clifford Schold, Jr.)

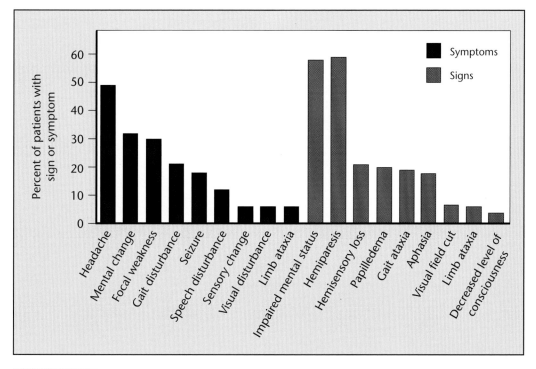

FIGURE 8-65.

Initial signs and symptoms in patients with intracranial metastases. Headache is the most frequent complaint in patients with intracranial metastatic disease, and occurs in 49% of patients. When a focal headache is present, it has localizing value, but usually the headache is generalized. The classic "brain tumor headache," which is worst in the morning, is present in only a minority of cases. The most common presenting symptoms experienced by patients with intracranial metastases are depicted in this bar graph, and include changes in mentation (32%), focal weakness (30%), gait ataxia (21%), and seizures (18%). Visual and sensory symptoms are unusual as a presenting complaint.

The most frequent signs on neurologic examination in patients with brain metastases are impaired mental status, which occurs in 58% of patients, and hemiparesis, which occurs in 59% of patients. Mental status changes in patients with brain metastases may be subtle, so the mental status examination is important in patients with a history of cancer who present with headache. Only 32% of patients with intracranial metastases complain of focal weakness, but 60% have hemiparesis on examination. Similarly, hemisensory loss can be demonstrated on examination in 21% of patients with brain metastases, yet only 6% of patients complain of sensory symptoms. Other neurologic signs such as papilledema (20%), gait ataxia (19%), aphasia (18%), visual field cuts (7%), and limb ataxia (6%) occur less frequently. When mental status changes, progressive headache, or focal neurologic signs are seen in a patient with a history of cancer, a contrast-enhanced computed tomography or magnetic resonance imaging scan of the head is indicated. (Data *from* Posner [154]; originally published in Cairncross *et al.* [155] and Young *et al.* [156].)

■ MOVEMENT DISORDERS

PARKINSONISM

Characteristics of Parkinsonism

Major Features	Variable Features			
	Motor	Autonomic	Cognitive	Other
Rest tremor	Freezing of gait	Urinary frequency	Slowness in thinking	Glabellar, palmomental, snout reflexes (frontal release signs)
Rigidity	Dystonia	Constipation	Dementia	
Bradykinesia	Muscle ache	Impotence in men	Depression	Limitation of upgaze
Loss of postural reflexes	Kyphosis			Interruption of smooth ocular pursuit
				Seborrhea

FIGURE 8-66.

Characteristics of parkinsonism. The term *parkinsonism* is applied to neurologic syndromes in which patients exhibit some combination of rest tremor, rigidity, bradykinesia, and loss of postural reflexes. Patients with all these clinical features are likely to have a disturbance of the nigrostriatal dopamine system. In patients who lack one or two of these major features, the presence of dopaminergic dysfunction is less certain. Many patients with parkinsonism may also have other characteristic signs and symptoms. For example, in the "freezing" phenomenon, patients experience sudden transient inability to move one or both feet. This may happen on gait initiation, during turning, encountering boundaries (*eg*, curbs and doorways), upon reaching a destination, when startled, or under emotional pressure. Severe episodes of freezing can lead to frequent falls and are a major source of disability. Some patients who experience freezing in the lower extremities also have a similar phenomenon during speaking, or in the upper extremities while writing or performing other fine motor movements. (*Courtesy of* Stanley Fahn.)

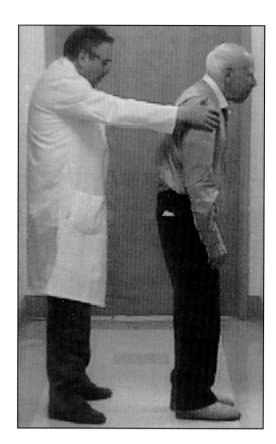

FIGURE 8-67.

Demonstration of the pull test. The examiner stands behind the patient and pulls the patient backwards. After explaining that the patient should take a step backwards to prevent falling, the examiner gives a quick pull on the shoulders and tests for retropulsion. On the first attempt, it is advisable to use only mild to moderate force when pulling. If the patient recovers well, then a stronger pull is used. The patient may require a practice with a mild pull to appreciate what is expected of him. The examiner needs to be prepared to catch the patient should he not recover his balance. If the patient is larger than the examiner, it is wise to have a wall behind the examiner to keep both the patient and examiner from falling. (*Courtesy of* Stanley Fahn.)

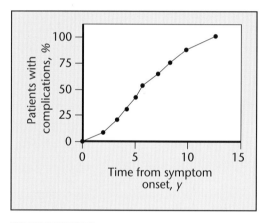

FIGURE 8-68.

Time course for developing motor response complications in patients with Parkinson's disease (PD) treated with levodopa. In most patients with PD, symptoms of the disease respond well to levodopa, but the response becomes increasingly complex with time. Most commonly, the benefits of levodopa wear off—gradually or suddenly—a few hours after taking the med-

ication. This can be circumvented by taking more frequent doses of levodopa. However, when dyskinesia becomes severe, the amount of levodopa taken at each dose must be decreased. To titrate the dose more accurately, levodopa can be given without carbidopa, or carbidopa/levodopa can be dissolved in water acidified with vitamin C. Sometimes, each dose of levodopa becomes so small that no benefit results. Some patients may do better using longer-acting agents, such as time-release carbidopa/levodopa or dopamine agonists. Patients with intolerable "off" periods may achieve a rapid response from the injectable medication apomorphine, or by crushing the pill and taking it with liquid to speed up entry into the small intestine. Since levodopa is not absorbed from the stomach, delay in gastric emptying may produce an apparent failure to respond to a dose of levodopa in a patient who otherwise does well, and this also may improve when the pill is dissolved in liquid. When patients do develop severe dyskinesias or dystonia, adding dopamine agonists and reducing the dose of levodopa often provide a smoother response and less severe involuntary movements than giving levodopa alone. When this fails, the atypical neuroleptic clozapine sometimes reduces dyskinesia without worsening PD symptoms. Surgical pallidotomy also may reduce levodopa-induced involuntary movements. The freezing phenomenon usually improves with increased medication, but occasionally it persists in someone who is otherwise adequately treated, and sometimes even worsens as medication is increased. Rarely, antiparkinsonian medications such as amantadine and levodopa may produce myoclonus severe enough to interfere with function. Patients with PD may have myoclonus even in the absence of medication, but these patients often have dementia as well, and the diagnosis of PD may be incorrect. (*Adapted from* Chase *et al.* [157].)

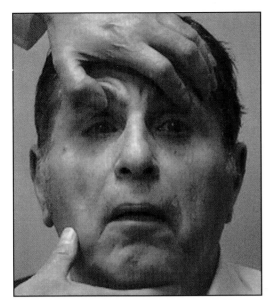

FIGURE 8-69.

A patient with progressive supranuclear palsy (PSP) who is having his oculocephalic reflexes (doll's eyes) tested to determine whether the origin of the gaze palsy is supranuclear. The patient, who is unable to look down voluntarily, is asked to look straight ahead at an object while the examiner tilts the patient's head backwards and keeps the eyelids apart to look for downward movement of the eyes. If the eyes move downward, the origin of the gaze palsy is supranuclear.

The defining description of PSP appeared in 1964 in an article by Steele *et al.* [158]. The prevalence of PSP has been estimated at 1.39 per 100,000. The mean age at onset is about 65 years, with a male preponderance in most series. Symptoms are steadily progressive, and death usually occurs 5 to 10 years after onset from aspiration or from the sequelae of multiple falls or bed sores. When supranuclear palsy (especially the loss of downgaze) appears early in the course of an akinetic-rigid syndrome, the diagnosis of PSP is likely.

PSP may be suspected in the absence of supranuclear palsy when other typical features are present. Frequent or continuous square wave jerks (small saccades alternately to the left and right in the horizontal plane) are often present. Patients with PSP lose postural reflexes early in the course of the disorder, and falling is an early feature. While walking, patients often assume a broad base, abduct the upper extremities at the shoulder and flex at the elbows, producing a characteristic gait that suggests PSP. Freezing (abrupt, transient interruption of motor activity) may be severe, and in some cases may be the major manifestation of PSP. Facial dystonia (deep nasolabial folds and furrowed brow) may create an angry or puzzled look when combined with a wide-eyed, unblinking stare. Axial rigidity is often more prominent than rigidity of the extremities, and in some cases, the limbs may have normal or reduced tone. Patients may be unable to open their lids even in the absence of orbicularis oculi spasms. This has been termed "apraxia of eyelid opening," but the phenomenon does not represent true apraxia; it might be the result of inappropriate inhibition of the levator palpebrae [159]. (*Courtesy of* Stanley Fahn.)

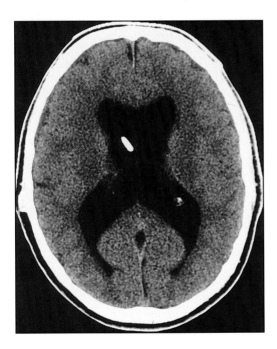

FIGURE 8-70.

Computed tomography scan of a patient with normal-pressure hydrocephalus, which shows dilated ventricles. The patient had an excellent response to ventriculopleural shunting. In 1965, Hakim and Adams described patients with gait disturbance, dementia, and urinary incontinence caused by communicating hydrocephalus (large ventricles) with normal cerebrospinal fluid (CSF) pressure [160]. In some patients, trauma or subarachnoid hemorrhage preceded the development of symptoms, but others had no apparent cause. Patients with this condition of normal pressure hydrocephalus (NPH) may improve temporarily after lumbar puncture and permanently after surgical diversion of CSF (*eg*, after ventriculoperitoneal shunting). Some patients with NPH seem to have their feet stuck to the ground, producing a "magnetic" gait, but other forms of gait disorder have also been observed. Patients with NPH may have facial masking, hypophonia, or other features of mild parkinsonism, so that NPH should be considered whenever gait disturbance is out of proportion to the other signs of parkinsonism. Enlarged ventricles and gait disorder, however, are not pathognomonic of NPH, and some patients with this combination do not improve after shunting. To identify patients who are candidates for surgical shunting, some clinicians have measured improvement after multiple daily lumbar punctures. Attempts to establish other radiologic or laboratory criteria for identifying good candidates for shunting have not been successful. (*Courtesy of* Stanley Fahn.)

HUNTINGTON'S DISEASE

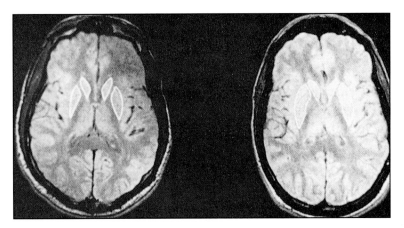

FIGURE 8-71.

Magnetic resonance imaging scan showing putaminal volume loss in a patient with early Huntington's disease (*left*) while the caudate appears normal when compared with the normal subject on the right. With disease progression caudate atrophy will be evident on computed tomography (CT) scan; detection of glucose hypometabolism on positron-emission tomography may even precede that of caudate atrophy on CT. None of these imaging techniques, however, reliably detects asymptomatic gene carriers, which requires DNA testing. (*From* Harris *et al.* [161]; with permission.)

TICS

Drugs Used to Treat Tic Disorders

Tics	Obsessive-Compulsive Disorder	Attention-Deficit Disorder
Clonazepam	Imipramine	Clonidine
Clonidine	Fluoxetine	Imipramine
Baclofen	Sertraline	Desipramine
Tetrabenazine	Clomipramine	Selegiline
Risperidol	Clonazepam	Guanfacine
Fluphenazine	Carbamazepine	Methylphenidate
Pimozide		Pemoline
Haloperidol		
Trifluoperazine		
Thiothixene		
Botulinum toxin may be helpful for dystonic tics such as blinking or blepharospasm and neck jerks		

FIGURE 8-72.

Drugs used to treat tic disorders. The decision to treat tics is based on the degree to which the abnormal movements and sounds disrupt the patient's daily function. The benefits of tic suppression must be weighed against the risk of the medication's adverse effects. The magnitude of the tic's effect on the patient's school, work, and social life and whether the major problem is posed by the tics, attention deficit, or obsessions and compulsions must be considered.

If medication is prescribed, a drug that does not produce a tardive dyskinesia syndrome, although usually less effective, is appropriate. If this is not effective, a dopamine-receptor blocker may be necessary. All drugs should be started with a small dosage that is increased slowly, while monitoring for side effects. An adequate duration of drug trial on a sufficient dosage is necessary before deciding on efficacy—tics wax and wane and it is difficult to separate therapeutic effect from the natural history in a single patient. Changes should be made as a sequence of single steps and should always be tapered slowly. This is especially true for dopamine-receptor blockers—abrupt withdrawal can produce a withdrawal emergent syndrome. (*Courtesy of* Stanley Fahn.)

Pharmacologic Treatment of Myoclonus

Medication	Dose range	Indication
ACTH	150 units/m²/d	Infantile spasms, opsoclonus
Clonazepam	0.5 to 20 mg/d	Most forms of myoclonus
5-Hydroxytryptophan	25 mg qid to 500 mg qid	Post-hypoxic myoclonus
Piracetam	400 mg tid to 16 g/d	Cortical myoclonus
Tetrabenazine	25 mg/d to 300 mg/d	Segmental myoclonus
Valproic acid	15 mg/kg/d to 2000 mg/d	Most forms of myoclonus
Gabapentin	100 mg tid to 600 mg tid	Most forms of myoclonus
Topiramate	200 mg bid	Most forms of myoclonus

FIGURE 8-73.

Pharmacologic treatment of myoclonus. The pharmacologic treatment of myoclonus includes a variety of agents that are listed here with suggested dose ranges and indications. Doses are calculated for adults, except for adenocorticotropic hormone (ACTH). (*Courtesy of* Stanley Fahn.)

DRUG-INDUCED MOVEMENT DISORDERS

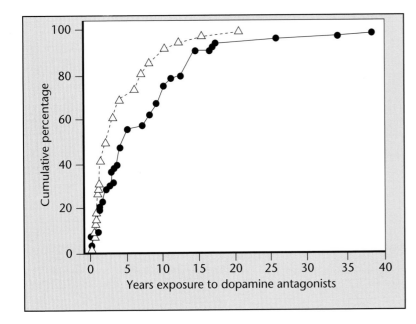

FIGURE 8-74.

Relationship between exposure to neuroleptics and development of tardive dystonia. The cumulative percentage of patients with tardive dystonia is shown in relation to years of exposure to dopamine receptor antagonists in two different series of patients. The first series (*black circles*) comprises 67 patients followed at Columbia-Presbyterian Medical Center, and the second group (*open triangles*) consists of 43 patients reported in the literature before 1986. In both groups, cases of tardive dystonia developed shortly after exposure to neuroleptics, and no minimum safe duration of exposure was detected. (*Adapted from* Kang *et al.* [162].)

Seizure Classification

Simple Partial Seizures

With motor signs
  Focal motor without march
  Focal motor with march (Jacksonian)
  Versive
  Postural
  Phonatory (vocalization or speech arrest)
With somatosensory or special sensory symptoms (simple
  hallucinations)
  Somatosensory
  Visual
  Auditory
  Olfactory
  Gustatory
  Vertiginous

With autonomic symptoms or signs
  Epigastric sensation
  Pallor
  Sweating
  Flushing
  Piloerection
  Pupillary dilation
  Cardiac arrhythmia
With psychic symptoms (rare without impairment of consciousness)
  Dysphasic
  Dysmnesic (*eg*, déjà vu)
  Cognitive (*eg*, dreamy states, distortion of time sense)
  Affective (fear, anger, etc.)
  Illusions (*eg*, macropsia)
  Structured hallucinations (*eg*, music, scenes)

Complex Partial Seizures

Simple partial onset followed by impairment of consciousness
  With simple partial features only prior to impaired consciousness
  With automatisms

With impairment of consciousness at onset
  Impairment of consciousness only
  With automatisms

Partial Seizures Evolving to Secondarily Generalized Tonic-clonic Convulsions

Simple partial seizures to generalized tonic-clonic convulsions
Complex partial seizures to generalized tonic-clonic convulsions
Simple partial seizures to complex partial seizures to generalized tonic-clonic convulsions

FIGURE 8-75.

Seizure classification. Seizures and epilepsy are not synonymous. Seizures are clinical manifestations of a paroxysmal, abnormal, excessive or hypersynchronous, usually self-limited, cerebral cortical neuronal discharge. Epilepsy is a chronic neurologic condition that is characterized by recurrent epileptic seizures, which are unprovoked by any known proximate insult [163,164]. Based on epidemiologic studies in Rochester, Minnesota, Hauser estimated that about 10% of the population have a seizure by age 74; 3% develop epilepsy, a condition with recurring epileptic seizures; and 4.1% have unprovoked seizures [165]. Most seizures and epilepsies develop in the very young and very old, because a variety of disorders damage or affect the brain in these age groups [166].

To properly classify the type of epilepsy the patient has, it is usually necessary to understand what type of seizures occur. Seizures are divided into partial (focal, localized) seizures and generalized seizures.

Simple partial seizures are seizures in which consciousness is not lost. Simple partial seizures may have motor signs, sensory signs, autonomic symptoms or signs, and even psychic or cognitive effects, depending in which region of the brain they start.

Complex partial seizures are partial seizures that involve alteration of consciousness. Consciousness is a very difficult term to define and some patients are quite reactive and may even be able to speak during the seizure, but they are amnestic for everything that happens. Therefore, most epileptologists define loss of consciousness as a lack of memory for the event, confusion, or disorientation.

Seizures can evolve to secondarily generalized tonic-clonic seizures. It is important to note the initial focal findings to properly classify these patients and differentiate them from patients with generalized seizures only. (*Adapted from* Commission on Classification and Terminology of the International League Against Epilepsy [167].)

Genetic Localization-related Epilepsies

Syndrome (nomenclature)	Gene locus	Gene product
AD nocturnal frontal lobe epilepsy (ADNFLE type 1): ENFL1 (75% penetrant)	20q13.2–q13.3 [168]	Alpha-4 subunit of the nicotinic acetylcholine receptor CHRNA4 [169]
AD nocturnal frontal lobe epilepsy (ADNFLE type 2): ENFL2	15q24 [170]	?
AD partial epilepsy with variable foci	22q11–q12 [171,172]	?
AD rolandic epilepsy with speech dyspraxia	? Possible triplet repeat [173]	?
Familial temporal lobe epilepsy (autosomal dominant, 60% penetrant)	? [174], 10q [175]	?
Benign occipital epilepsy (BOE)	? [176]	?
Benign rolandic epilepsy	?	?
Periventricular nodular heterotopia	Xq28 [177]	Filamin-1 [178]
Benign familial neonatal convulsions (EBN1)	20q13.2–13.3 [179,180]	Potassium voltage-gated channel (KCNQ2)
Benign familial neonatal convulsions (EBN2)	8q24 [181,182]	KCNQ3
Benign familial infantile convulsions (BFIC) (onset 3–12 months, AD)	19q [183]	?
Familial infantile convulsions with paroxysmal choreoathetosis (ICCA syndrome)	16p12–q12 [184,185]	?
Febrile convulsions (FEB1) (AD)	8q13–21 [186]	?
Febrile convulsions (FEB2) (AD)	19p13.3 [187]	?
Febrile convulsions (FEB3) (AD)	2q23–24 [188]	?
Febrile convulsions (FEB4)	5q14–q15 [189]	?
Generalized epilepsy with febrile seizures plus (GEFS+)	19q13 [190] SCN1 gene	Sodium channel, voltage-gated, type I, alpha polypeptide
Generalized epilepsy with febrile seizures plus, type 2 (GEFSP2)	2q24	SCN1A gene
Childhood absence epilepsy	Possible 1p	?
Juvenile absence epilepsy (ECA1)	8q24 [191]	?
Juvenile myoclonic epilepsy, 1 (EJM1)	6p11 [192,193]	?
Juvenile myoclonic epilepsy, 2 (EJM2)	15q14 [194]	Possibly alpha-7 subunit of nAChR (CHRNA7)
Epilepsy with generalized tonic clonic seizures on awakening	6p	?
Lafora's disease (EPM2A)	6q24 [195,196]	Laforin
Epilepsy, progressive, with mental retardation (EPMR) (Northern epilepsy syndrome)	8p [197]	?
Unverricht-Lundborg disease (Baltic myoclonic epilepsy) (EPM1)	21q22.3 [198–200]	Cystatin B [201]
Benign adult familial myoclonic epilepsy (BAFME)	8q23.3–q24.11 [202]	?
Myoclonic epilepsy with ragged red fibers (MERRF)	Mitochondrial DNA	t-RNA lysine [203,204]
Angelman syndrome (AS)	15q11–q13 [205]	UBE3A [206]

FIGURE 8-76.

Etiologies of genetic localization-related and generalized epilepsies. As of October 2000, McKusick [207] listed 194 genetic disorders with epilepsy as part of the syndrome. Genetic epilepsies are growing in number and many more entities await discovery. Most genetic epilepsies are known from the study of a few informative families and linkage analysis. Only a few gene products are known, such as the t-RNA lysine defect in myoclonic with ragged red fibers (MERRF) [203,204]. This is an area of intense research interest because understanding the genetics of epilepsies may lead to effective and disease-specific therapies. AD—autosomal dominant.

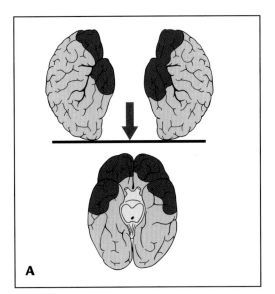

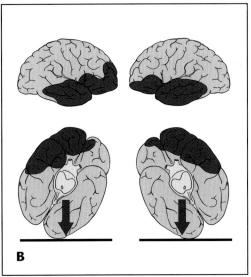

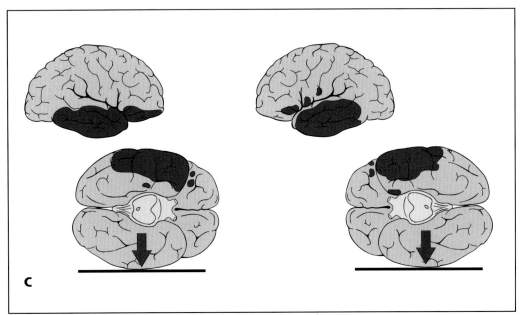

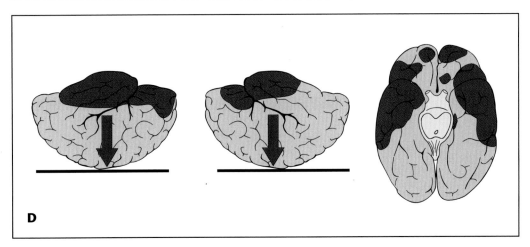

FIGURE 8-77.

Epilepsy caused by head trauma. Head trauma is a frequent cause of epilepsy, but usually the injuries are quite severe, often involving penetration of the dura and intracranial bleeding [208]. Concussions are very common, and many patients recall having a head injury before seizures, although these are likely unrelated. Early seizures, occurring less than 1 week after trauma, confer a significant risk factor for chronic epilepsy to develop, probably within 1 to 4 years [209]. Late seizures, occurring 1 week after the trauma, are an ominous predictor of chronic epilepsy, with about half of the cases developing seizures within the first post-injury year. Electroencephalogram may not be a

good predictor of late epilepsy after trauma [210]. Courville studied head trauma victims in a large series of autopsied cases to correlate contusion location and the direction of impact [211]. No matter what the direction of impact, the frontal and temporal lobes seem to bear the brunt of contusions, which may explain why posttraumatic epilepsy often involves the frontal or temporal lobes when there is closed head injury. **A,** Contusions of the temporal lobe from a posterior impact. **B,** Contusions of the temporal lobe from posterolateral impact. **C,** Contusions of the temporal lobe from lateral impact; **D,** Contusions of the temporal lobe from vertical impact.

Differential Diagnosis of Non-epileptic Seizures

Syncope
Hyperventilation
Breath holding spell
Sleep disorder
    Narcolepsy/cataplexy
    Sleep apnea
    Parasomnia
Migraine
Cerebrovascular disease movement disorders
Transient global amnesia
Toxic/metabolic encephalopathy
Movement disorders
Vertigo
Psychiatric/behavioral
    Psychogenic seizures
        Conversion disorder
        Malingering
    Episodic lack of control
    Panic disorder
    Obsessive-compulsive behavior
    Stereotypy
    Dissociative states
        Psychogenic fugue
        Multiple personality
        Psychogenic amnesia
        Depersonalization disorder
    Normal daydreaming

FIGURE 8-78.

Differential diagnosis of non-epileptic seizures. A wide variety of disorders can mimic epilepsy and be misdiagnosed as epileptic seizures. These include syncope, hyperventilation, breath holding spells, and sleep disorders. Certainly vascular disease movement disorders, vertigo, and migraine are also considerations in the differential diagnosis. Usually electroencephalogram and a good clinical history are able to separate the nonepileptic events from the epileptic. Psychogenic seizures are particularly disturbing aspects that neurologists encounter frequently. Patients who are susceptible to psychogenic seizures usually have a history of physical or sexual abuse, and the most common etiology is conversion disorder, however, malingering and other dissociative states may also be present.

Laboratory Investigation of Seizures

Blood work
Routine EEG
    Timing
    Activation procedures
        Photic, hyperventilation, sleep
Sleep deprived EEG
Video-EEG monitoring
Cognitive testing
Neuroimaging structure and function
    MRI, CT
    PET, SPECT
    MR Spectroscopy, functional MRI
    Angiography, MR angiography
    MEG

FIGURE 8-79.

Laboratory investigation of seizures. A variety of tests have been used to determine the causes of seizures or epilepsy, as treatment may be needed for an underlying disorder. Blood chemistries and other blood work occasionally identify an underlying metabolic disturbance responsible for seizures. Electroencephalogram (EEG) is the single most useful test, but it is best if recording is done during a seizure or just after it, when spiking is more prevalent. Before specific epileptiform discharges can be identified, several EEGs are often necessary, including an EEG done during sleep or after sleep deprivation. When the diagnosis is unclear, video EEG is the best way to confirm a diagnosis of epilepsy or nonepileptic seizures. Cognitive testing is useful in patients with complaints of memory problems or who display psychiatric symptoms or signs, because depression is common in epilepsy and cognitive training or psychiatric intervention may help minimize disability. Neuroimaging is as important as EEG in the diagnosis of epilepsy etiology. Computed tomography (CT) scan is rarely useful and even if an abnormality is detected, magnetic resonance imaging (MRI) almost always shows it better. MRI is the procedure of choice, and epilepsy protocols exist to look for hippocampal sclerosis and migrational disturbances, which are common causes of partial epilepsy. The remaining tests listed here are not routine, but in select cases they may be helpful in planning epilepsy surgery. Magnetic resonance (MR) spectroscopy, functional MRI, and magnetoencephalography (MEG) currently are under investigation for their usefulness as neuroimaging tools for localization of the epileptogenic zone. PET—positron-emission tomography; SPECT—single photon emission computed tomography.

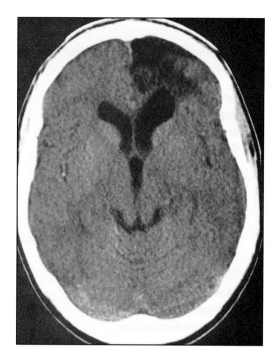

FIGURE 8-80.
Computed tomography (CT) scan showing a large area of encephalomalacia in the left frontal lobe with dilation of the left frontal horn of the lateral ventricle. The CT scan is from a 21-year-old male who was in a motor vehicle accident at age 16. He suffered a right-sided skull fracture and early seizures and was in a coma for 3 weeks. He has simple partial adversive seizures that secondarily generalize but are well controlled with phenytoin and gabapentin. (*Courtesy of* Paul C. Van Ness.)

TREATMENT OF EPILEPSY

Drugs Used in the Treatment of Epilepsy

Drugs for Partial Epilepsies

First line
- Phenytoin
- Carbamazepine
- Oxcarbazepine
- Gabapentin
- Levetiracetam
- Divalproex sodium or valproic acid

Second line
- Lamotrigine
- Topiramate
- Tiagabine
- Zonisamide
- Felbamate
- Primidone
- Phenobarbital
- Benzodiazepines

Drugs for Generalized Epilepsies

For absence seizures only
- Ethosuximide

For all generalized seizures

First line
- Divalproex sodium or valproic acid
- Lamotrigine
- Topiramate

Second line
- Primidone
- Phenobarbital
- Clonazepam
- Felbamate

Possible
- Levetiracetam
- Zonisamide

FIGURE 8-81.
Drugs used in the treatment of epilepsy. The goals of epilepsy treatment include freedom from seizures without side effects, maximal quality of life, minimal disability, simple monotherapy regimens, and the use of antiepileptic drugs without drug interactions. If seizures are provoked, it is reasonable to eliminate the provocative factors and expect a good outcome without treatment. If seizures are unprovoked and it is a first seizure, it still may not be necessary to treat, because many patients have a single seizure in their lifetime, and it may not be possible to identify the provocative factors [212,213]. However, if the history is highly suggestive of focal onset, the neuroimaging studies are abnormal, the neurologic exam is abnormal, and the electroencephalogram (EEG) shows epileptiform abnormalities indicating a high risk of seizure recurrence, it would be reasonable to begin treatment after a single seizure. A good example of this would be a patient with a brain tumor, stroke, or other obvious structural lesion; the EEG may show slowing or spiking and the clinical exam fits with the neuroimaging studies. These patients may be harmed by additional seizures while they are acutely ill, and it is reasonable to treat them to prevent further seizures. If more than one unprovoked seizure occurs, the patient has epilepsy, and by classifying the seizure and epilepsy type, an appropriate antiepileptic drug (AED) can be chosen. Most patients should begin treatment with first-line antiepileptic drugs. Drugs are considered first line owing to their ease of use or low toxicity or second line owing to their slow titration to effective dose, higher risk for toxicity, or need for more intensive laboratory monitoring. With numerous new antiepileptic drugs available in recent years, and no comparative studies to decide the appropriate order of medication trials, the designation of drugs as first line or second line is an approximation and will likely change as new data become available. Individual patient characteristics will influence dose, timing, compliance, need for polypharmacy, and the type of formulation (tablet, liquid, capsule). Individual pharmacokinetic variables can increase or decrease the daily dosage necessary. Patient compliance is improved if the physician allows the patient to choose the formulation of the drug.

■ NEUROMUSCULAR DISEASE

DIAGNOSTIC STUDIES

Diagnostic Immunologic, Biochemical, and Molecular Blood Studies in Neuromuscular Diseases

Lyme Western and PCR	Lyme neuritis
Anti-Hu titer	Paraneoplastic sensory neuropathy
Cryoglobulins	Cryoglobulinemic neuropathy
anti-MAG titer	MAG paraproteinemic sensory neuropathy
Phytanic acid	Refsum's disease
Long-chain fatty acids	Adrenoleukodystrophy
Arylsulfatase	Metachromatic leukodystrophy
Leukocyte DNA analysis for	
Chromosome 17 duplication	Charcot-Marie-Tooth disease type 1A
Chromosome 17 deletion	HNPP (tomaculous neuropathy)
Transthyretin mutations	Famillal amyloid neuropathy
Connexin 32 mutations	Charcot-Marie-Tooth disease type 1X
SOD mutations	Familial ALS
SMN mutations	Familial spinal muscular atrophy
Androgen receptor triplet repeat	Bulbospinal motor neutron disease

FIGURE 8-82.

Examples of immunologic, biochemical, and molecular blood studies that provide specific diagnostic information in neuro-muscular diseases. ALS—amyotrophic lateral sclerosis; HNPP—hereditary neuropathy with predisposition to pressure palsies; MAG—myelin-associated glycoprotein; PCR—polymerase chain reaction; SMN—survival motor neuron; SOD—superoxide dismutase. (*Courtesy of* David Pleasure.)

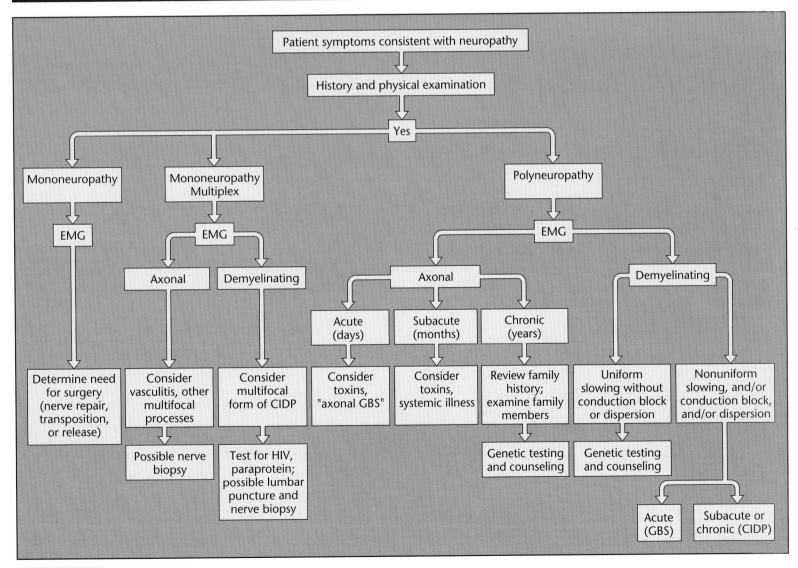

FIGURE 8-83.

Evaluation of patients with neuropathy. CIDP—chronic inflammatory demyelinating polyneuropathy; EMG—electromyogram; GBS—Guillain-Barré syndrome. (*Adapted from* Asbury [214].)

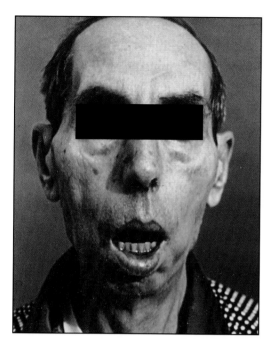

FIGURE 8-84.

A patient with myotonic dystrophy who has the typical symptoms of muscle wasting, ptosis, and frontal balding. Myotonic dystrophy is a relatively common form of muscular dystrophy. It can present in children and adults and is inherited as an autosomal dominant trait. The characteristic myotonic discharges correlate with clinical myotonia. Weakness is also a feature of myotonic dystrophy and often affects distal as well as proximal muscles. Other features common in adults with myotonic dystrophy include cataracts, testicular atrophy, and an organic mental syndrome. Skeletal muscle biopsy usually shows nonspecific myopathic changes. Affected family members demonstrate a triplet repeat (CTG) expansion in the 3' untranslated region of the myotonic dystrophy gene, and, as in other triplet repeat–associated neural degenerative disorders (*eg,* X-linked spinal and bulbar muscular atrophy, Huntington's disease, Machado-Joseph disease, and fragile X syndrome), clinical severity tends to be worse in the affected children of an adult with myotonic dystrophy [215,216]. (*Courtesy of* David Pleasure.)

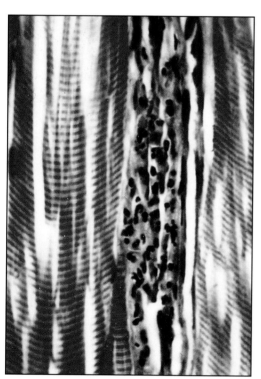

FIGURE 8-85.

Dermatomyositis. Dermatomyositis is an inflammatory disorder involving skeletal muscle and the skin. Patients with dermatomyositis generally have an elevated serum creatine kinase and a myopathic electromyogram. In adults, but not children, dermatomyositis can occur in conjunction with carcinoma [217]. Skeletal muscle biopsy, modified Gomori trichrome, showing a necrotic muscle fiber. Although fibers frequently show this pathology in dermatomyositis, this specific example is from the biopsy of a patient with rhabdomyolysis due to myophosphorylase deficiency. (*Courtesy of* David Pleasure.)

BACTERIAL INFECTIONS

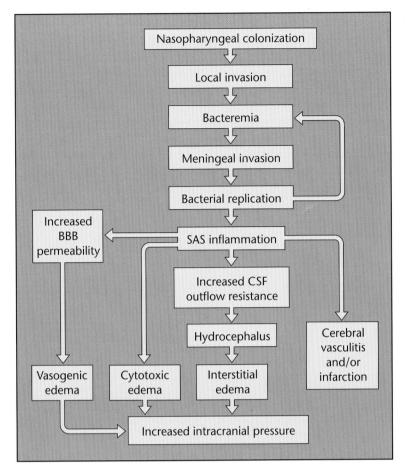

FIGURE 8-86.

Pathogenesis of meningitis. For bacterial meningitis to occur, the host usually acquires a new organism by colonization of the nasopharynx. This may lead to direct seeding of cerebral spinal fluid (CSF) spaces, but more likely causes local spread to the sinuses or the lungs (pneumonia) or bacteremia, which then results in meningeal invasion. BBB—blood-brain barrier; SAS—subarachnoid space. (*Adapted from* Roos *et al.* [218].)

Causative Organisms of Bacterial Meningitis (Percentage of Cases by Age)

Organism	<1 mo	1–23 mo	2–29 y	30–59 y	≥60 y
Haemophilus influenzae	0	0.7	5.4	12.1	2.5
Neisseria meningitidis	0	30.8	59.8	18.2	3.6
Streptococcus pneumoniae	8.7	45.2	27.2	60.6	68.6
Streptococci group B	69.5	19.2	5.4	3	3.6
Listeria monocytogenes	21.8	0	2.2	0.1	21.7

FIGURE 8-87.

Causative organisms of bacterial meningitis by age-related relative frequency. *Haemophilus influenzae* type b was the leading cause of meningitis until widespread use of vaccine. Now *H. influenzae* is not a significant cause of bacterial meninigits in the vaccinated population [219]. Meningococcal meninigitis caused by *Neisseria meningitidis* affects mostly children and young adults. As of 1995, *N. meningitidi* had replaced *H. influenzae* as the leading cause of bacterial meningitis in these age groups in the United States [220]. Congenital terminal complement deficiencies (C5-C8) predispose to meningococcemia. Pneumococcal meningitis caused by *Streptococcus pneumoniae* is the most common cause of bacterial meninigits in adults. Predisposing factors include pneumonia, otitis media, sinusitis, head trauma, CSF leaks, sickle cell disease, splenectomy, diabetes and alcoholism. (*Adapted from* Schuchat *et al.* [221].)

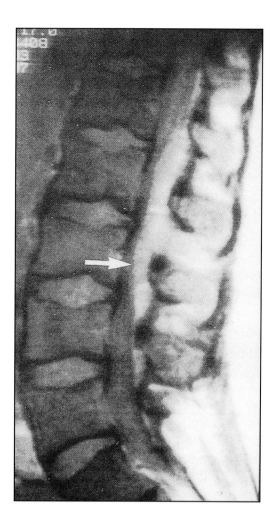

FIGURE 8-88.

Contrast-enhanced T1-weighted magnetic resonance image (MRI) done as part of a diagnostic work-up for spinal epidural abscess. This scan reveals an epidural mass (*arrow*) extending from the lower part of the L1 vertebral body to the upper part of the L4 vertebral body. Patients with acute spinal epidural abscess have a high peripheral leukocytic count from 12,000 to 15,000 cells per mm^3. If the process is chronic, the peripheral leukocyte count may be normal. Cerebrospinal fluid (CSF) examination is consistent with parameningeal infection, with an elevated cell count, elevated protein level, normal glucose level, and negative cultures. When the process is acute, usually polymorphonuclear leukocytes predominate, with up to 100 to 200 cells per mm^3; in chronic cases, mononuclear cells predominate, usually with fewer than 50 cells per mm^3. CSF cultures are negative unless the organism has spread to the CSF and subsequently caused meningitis. Blood cultures are positive 60% to 70% of the time. The definitive diagnostic studies, however, are computed tomography myelograms and MRI scans, with MRI the study of choice. MRI scans directly visualize the extent of the abscess and should include T1-weighted images before and after contrast enhancement and a T2-weighted image. (*From* Gelfand *et al.* [222]; with permission.)

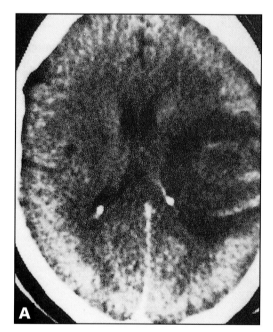

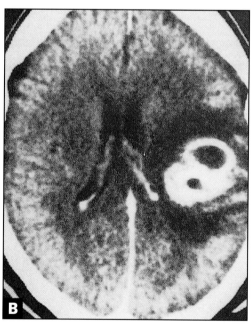

FIGURE 8-89.

Computed tomography (CT) imaging studies for brain abscess. Routine laboratory studies are usually not helpful; they may show peripheral leukocytosis and increased erythrocyte sedimentation rate, but these findings are nonspecific. In addition to complete blood count, chest radiograph, electrocardiogram, and echocardiogram as needed, blood cultures should also be obtained. Lumbar puncture may reveal a parameningeal response, but the procedure is usually contraindicated until an imaging study of the brain has been performed. CT plain imaging and with contrast should be performed. Magnetic resonance imaging is even more sensitive, and reveals abscess or cerebritis at earlier stages of development than CT. **A,** Plain axial CT reveals mass effect in the left hemisphere with effacement of the sylvian fissure and the ipsolateral ventricle. **B,** With contrast, CT reveals a multiloculated ring enhanced lesion. The surrounding area of decreased attenuation represents cerebral edema. (*From* Wispelwey *et al.* [223]; with permission. *See also* Falcone *et al.* [266].)

Virologic and Serologic Studies for Acute CNS Viral Syndromes

Agent	Specimens for Virus Detection	Serologic Studies
Enteroviruses		
Polio	Throat washing, stool, and CSF (culture and PCR)	Acute or convalescent sera
Coxsackie		
Echo virus		
Lymphocytic choriomeningitis virus	Blood, CSF	Acute or convalescent sera
Mumps	Saliva, throat washing, CSF, urine	Acute or convalescent sera
Measles	Throat washing, urine, conjunctival secretions	Acute or convalescent sera
		IgM ELISA of serum
Arboviruses	Blood, CSF	IgM antibody ELISA of CSF or serum
		Acute or convalescent sera
Herpesviruses		
Herpes simplex (HSV)		
Type 1	Brain biopsy, PCR of CSF	CSF antibody detection after day 10
		Acute or convalescent sera (±)
Type 2	CSF, genital and vesicle fluid, blood	Acute or convalescent sera
Varicella-zoster	Vesicle fluid, CSF	Acute or convalescent sera
Cytomegalovirus	Urine, saliva, blood (circulating leukocytes), CSF	Acute or convalescent sera
	PCR amplification	
Epstein-Barr virus	Rarely cultured	Acute sera for antibody profile
Rabies	Saliva, CSF, neck skin biopsy, brain biopsy	Serum after day 15
Adenovirus	Nasal or conjunctival swab, urine, stool	Acute or convalescent sera
Influenza	Throat washing	Acute or convalescent sera

FIGURE 8-90.
Specific virologic and serologic studies for the diagnosis of acute central nervous system (CNS) viral syndromes. Viruses may be isolated from extraneural sites. For most infections, except reactivated infections such as with herpes simplex virus type 1 (HSV-1) or herpes zoster, extraneural isolation is usually diagnostic. Obviously if virus can be isolated from the cerebrospinal fluid (CSF), that is preferred. Detection of virus-specific nucleic acid by polymerase chain reaction (PCR) is only in limited use and is still experimental in most cases. Serologic studies require a fourfold increase between the acute and convalescent specimen to be considered positive. Acute phase sera should be obtained immediately or as soon as infection is suspected. If the acute phase sera is not obtained until the end of the first week of the disease, the chances of seeing a fourfold rise drops to 50%. Most viral infections of the CNS result in the intrathecal synthesis of specific antibody. When analyzing CSF antibody synthesis one looks for an increased CSF to serum antibody ratio. Therefore, paired CSF and serum samples are required. A correction should also be used for blood brain barrier breakdown, which results in serum to CSF antibody leakage. This can be done by using CSF to serum albumin or other viral antibody ratios. Unfortunately, most antibody studies are not positive until at least 1 week after the onset of infection. ELISA—enzyme-linked immunosorbent assay. (*Adapted from* Jubelt [225].)

Approved Anti-HIV Agents—2000

Agent	Mechanism of action	Limiting side effects	Indication
Zidovudine (ZDV) (Retrovir, Glaxo Wellcome, Research Triangle Park, NC)	nRTI	Anemia Neutropenia Myopathy Hepatitis (hepatic steatosis with lactic acidosis)	Initial therapy when <500 CD4+ T cells/μl
Didanosine (DDI) (Videx, Bristol-Myers Squibb, Princeton, NJ)	nRTI	Painful sensory neuropathy Pancreatitis	Progressive disease while on ZDV, as monotherapy or with ZDV
Zalcitabine (ddC) (Hivid, Roche Laboratories, Nutley, NJ)	nRTI	Same as DDI	Only in combination with ZDV
Stavudine (d4T) (Zerit, Bristol-Myers Squibb, Princeton, NJ)	nRTI	Painful sensory neuropathy Hepatitis (hepatic steatosis with lactic acidosis)	Intolerance or failure of ZDV or DDI
Lamivudine (3TC) (Epivir, Glaxo Wellcome, Research Triangle Park, NC)	nRTI	Nausea, vomiting, diarrhea Leukopenia/anemia Painful sensory neuropathy	Failure or intolerance of other drugs
Abacavir (Ziagan, Glaxo Wellcome, Research Triangle Park, NC)	nRTI	Hypersensitivity reactions	Initial regimens, naïve patients
ZDV + 3TC (Combivir, Glaxo Wellcome, Research Triangle Park, NC)	nRTI	See ZDV and 3TC above	Reduces "pill burden overload" in combination therapy
Saquinavir (Inverase, Fortovase, Glaxo Wellcome, Research Triangle Park, NC)	PI	Diarrhea Abdominal pain	Combination therapy
Ritonavir (Norvir, Abbott, North Chicago, IL)	PI	Diarrhea, nausea, vomiting	Combination therapy
Indinavir (Crixivan, Merck & Co., West Point, PA)	PI	Same as Ritonavir Hyperbilirubinemia Nephrolithiasis	Combination therapy
Nelfinavir (Viracept, Agouron, La Jolla, CA)	PI	Diarrhea	Combination therapy
Amprenavir (Agenerase, Glaxo Wellcome, Research Triangle Park, NC)	PI	Nausea, vomiting, diarrhea Rash including Stevens-Johnson Perioral paresthesias	Combination therapy
Nevirapine (Viramune, Roxane, Columbus, OH)	NNRTI	Hepatitis Rash	Combination therapy
Delaviradine (Pharmacia & Upjohn, Kalamazoo, MI)	NNRTI	Rash	Combination therapy
Efavirenz (Sustiva, DuPont Pharmaceuticals, Wilmington, DE)	NNRTI	Hepatitis Encephalopathy Transient 25% Limiting 3% Rash	Combination therapy

FIGURE 8-91.

Treatment of HIV encephalopathy and other syndromes caused by the direct effects of HIV infection. Specific antiretroviral agents can be used for all syndromes caused directly by HIV. Symptomatic treatment such as antidepressants or antipsychotics for HIV encephalopathy may be useful. For the painful sensory neuropathy, analgesics, antidepressants (especially tricyclics), anticonvulsants (carbamazepine, phenytoin), and topical capsaicin ointment may be helpful. Specific agents for the treatment of HIV infections include nucleoside reverse transcriptase inhibitors (nRTI), protease inhibitors (PI), and nonnucleoside reverse transcriptase inhibitors (NNRTI). Therapy is recommended for all patients with symptomatic established HIV infection. Combination therapy is used but definitive data regarding the superiority of one regimen over another is not yet available. Initial regimens of two nRTIs plus a PI (or two PIs) or two nRTIs plus a NNRTI is recommended [226]. Both CD4+ cell and HIV RNA levels are used to decide when to start and change therapy [226]. Triple combination therapies with RTIs and PIs have been referred to as highly active antiretroviral therapy (HAART) [227]. When prescribing anti-HIV therapy, it is important to know the interactions between these agents as well as the interactions between these agents and other medication classes (antihistamines, antifungals, antimycobacterials, oral contraceptives, cytochrome P450 metabolized drugs, benzodiazepines, antibiotics, methadone, anticonvulsants, antiarrhythmics, calcium channel blockers, and ergot alkaloids).

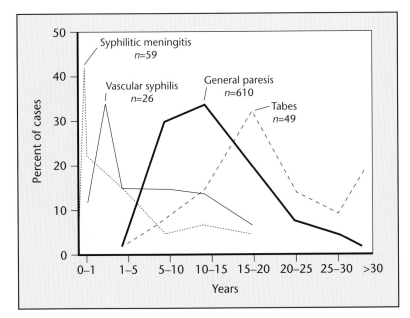

FIGURE 8-92.

Time course for the appearance of neurosyphilic manifestations. Starting with the onset of the primary syphilitic infection of skin chancre, usually on the penis or perineum, the development of neurosyphilitic syndromes over three decades is shown. Syphilitic meningitis occurs with either secondary or tertiary syphilis. All other syndromes of neurosyphilis occur during the tertiary stage. All forms of syphilis of the central nervous system ultimately result from active meningeal inflammation. When the meningeal inflammation extends to the cerebral blood vessels, cerebrovascular neurosyphilis results, usually within 5 years after the primary infection. The parenchymal forms of neurosyphilis—general paresis (dementia) and tabes dorsalis—occur after 5 years. Although each syndrome has a predictable time course, appearances often overlap, and several syndromes may occur at the same time. (*Adapted from* Simon [228].)

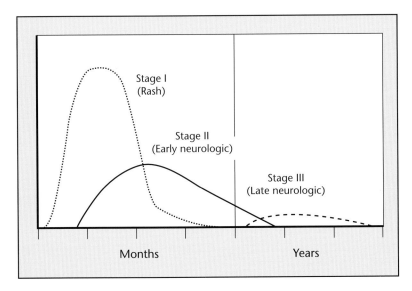

FIGURE 8-93.

Clinical stages of Lyme disease. Lyme disease results from infection by the spirochete *Borrelia burgdorferi*, which is transmitted by ticks. Lyme disease may develop into a chronic persistent infection in a fashion somewhat similar to syphilis. For this reason, Lyme disease has been divided into stages. The nervous system is involved clinically in 10% to 15% of patients. Stage I, the acute stage, is characterized by a rash—erythema chronicum migrans (ECM)—which is an erythematous ring that develops around the tick bite site about 8 to 9 days (range, 3 to 32 days) after exposure. Smaller secondary (migratory) rings may occur later. Neurologic manifestations may occur in stage I concurrently with ECM, but they are more frequent in stage II. Stage II, the subacute

stage, is characterized by prominent cardiac and neurologic manifestations. This stage usually begins several months after the bite and the onset of ECM. Stage III, the chronic stage, is characterized by chronic arthritis. Neurologic manifestations also occur in stage III but they are less prominent than those of stage II. Stage III usually begins about 1 year after onset.

In the acute stage I, a systemic flu-like syndrome with fever, chills, and malaise may occur. Neurologic manifestations include headache and neck stiffness but normal cerebrospinal fluid (CSF) parameters. Stage II is also referred to as the "early neurologic stage" because dissemination of the organism to the central nervous system begins. During this stage, aseptic meningitis with complications of cranial nerve palsies, especially facial (Bell's palsy), and radiculoneuritis are most prominent. The facial or Bell's palsy is usually bilateral. The radiculoneuritis may take the form of a Guillain-Barré–like syndrome, but the CSF shows pleocytosis; sometimes the radiculoneuritis is focal. Occasionally, mild meningoencephalitis along with irritability, emotional lability, decreased concentration and memory, and sleep abnormalities may occur.

Stage III or the chronic stage is also referred to as the "late neurologic stage." This stage is characterized by chronic or late persistent infection of the nervous system. Syndromes included in this stage are encephalopathy, encephalomyelopathy, and polyneuropathy. The encephalopathy is characterized by memory and other cognitive dysfunction. The encephalomyelopathic signs are combined with progressive long tract signs and optic nerve involvement. White matter lesions may be visible on magnetic resonance imaging of the brain. The late polyneuropathy is primarily sensory. (*Adapted from* Davis [229].)

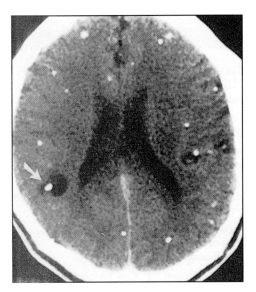

FIGURE 8-94.

Noncontrast computed tomography (CT) scan showing numerous calcified (inactive) cysticerci and an active cyst with scolex (*arrow*) with contrast ring enhancement of active cysts in a patient with neurocysticercosis. The diagnosis of cysticercosis should be considered in patients who reside in endemic areas and have seizures, meningitis, or papilledema (increased intracranial pressure). CT and magnetic resonance imaging are especially useful, as they may demonstrate live parenchymal cysts with enhancement (diffuse or ring pattern), calcified dead cysts, hydrocephalus, and intraventricular and subarachnoid cysts with enhancement. Usually the cerebrospinal fluid (CSF) shows mild pleocytosis, but may be normal or show severe pleocytosis due to meningitis when subarachnoid or intraventricular cysts die. There may be up to several thousand leukocytes (usually mononuclear), a low glucose level, and an elevated protein level. CSF and serum antibody tests are usually positive (80% to 98% sensitivity depending on the test). (*From* Cameron *et al.* [230]; with permission.)

■ NEUROIMMUNOLOGY

MULTIPLE SCLEROSIS

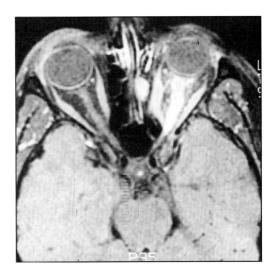

FIGURE 8-95.

Magnetic resonance image showing optic neuritis in a patient with multiple sclerosis (MS). Optic neuritis, internuclear ophthalmoplegia, and various patterns of nystagmus are the most common ophthalmologic declarations of MS. Optic neuritis causes relatively acute impairment of vision, progressing over hours to days, reaching a nadir in about 1 week. During the acute phase, orbital pain, brow pain, and pain with eye movement occur. Depression of vision affects the whole field of one eye, sometimes both [231]. The disc is spared with retrobulbar neuritis: "The patient sees nothing—neither does the doctor." Optic neuritis is the presenting feature in 25% of MS cases and occurs at some stage of the illness in 73%. Conversely, 50% to 75% of patients with isolated optic neuritis later develop definite MS within 12 to 15 years [232]. Bilateral optic neuritis, occurring acutely in the company of transverse myelitis, is termed *neuromyelitis optica* or *Devic's disease*. This form of MS attack occurs most often in young people and carries a poorer prognosis [233]. (*Courtesy of* Michael R. Swenson.)

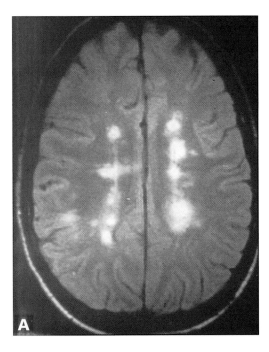

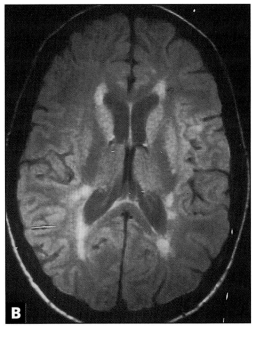

FIGURE 8-96.

Periventricular plaques. The utility of magnetic resonance imaging (MRI) is seen most dramatically in images of the brain of patients with multiple sclerosis (MS). The periventricular white matter is typically involved, demonstrating multiple lesions with characteristically prominent T1 prolongation (**A**) and high T2-weighted signal density (**B**). Elliptical lesions deep in the white matter directed toward the ventricular margin appear in the corona radiata and tend to point toward the ventricular margin—a morphology known as *Dawson's finger* [234]. Subependymal lesions may be nodular or confluent. Subcortical–cortical junction lesions and callosal lesions distinguish MS from vascular diseases. Brain MRI is abnormal in more than 95% of patients with MS [235]. (*Courtesy of* Michael R. Swenson.)

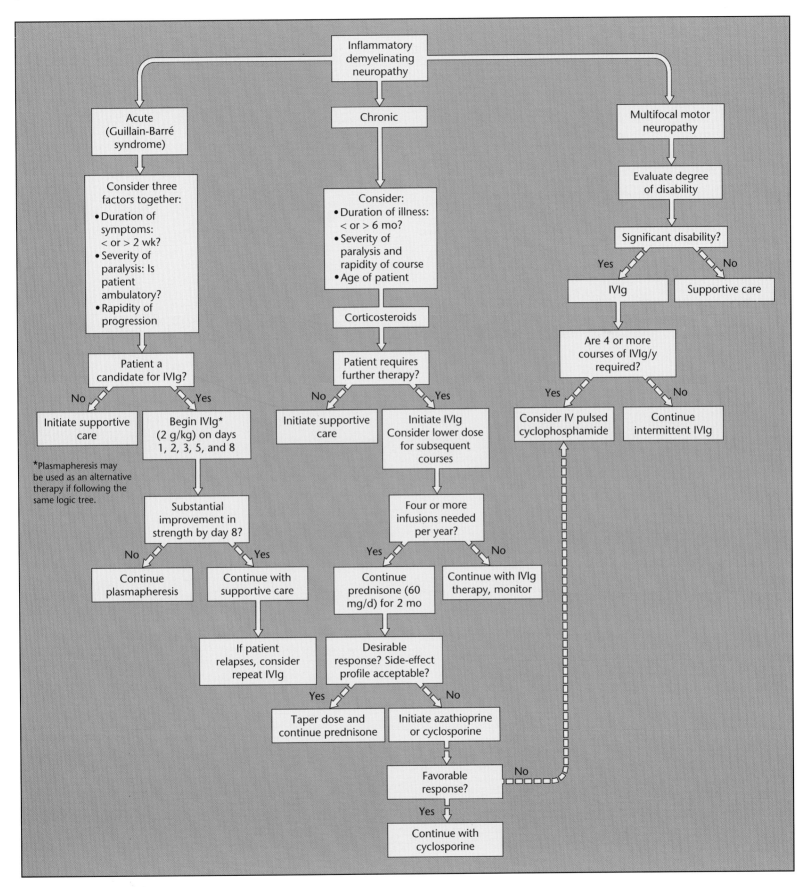

FIGURE 8-97.

Suggested clinical algorithm for treatment of inflammatory demyelinating polyradiculoneuropathy [236]. This algorithm favors early use of intravenous immunoglobulin (IVIg). In centers where plasma exchange is easily available, either option could be exercised. (*Adapted from* Parry [236].)

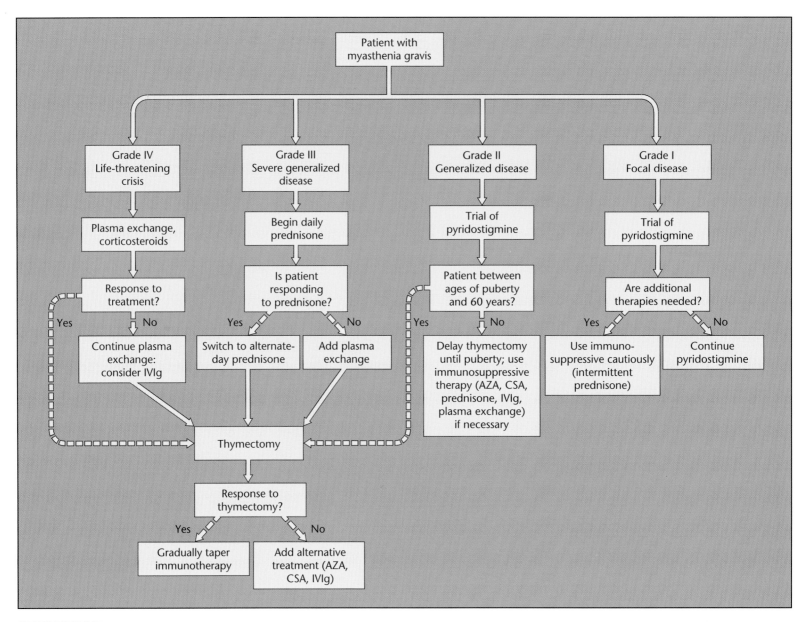

FIGURE 8-98.

Clinical algorithm for the treatment of myasthenia gravis. Treatment strategies in myasthenia gravis include the use of pharmacologic agents directed at the function of the neuromuscular junction; immunosuppressant and immunomodulating techniques; surgical thymectomy. AZA—azathioprine; CSA—cyclosporine; IVIg—intravenous immunoglobulin. (*Adapted from* Mendell [237].)

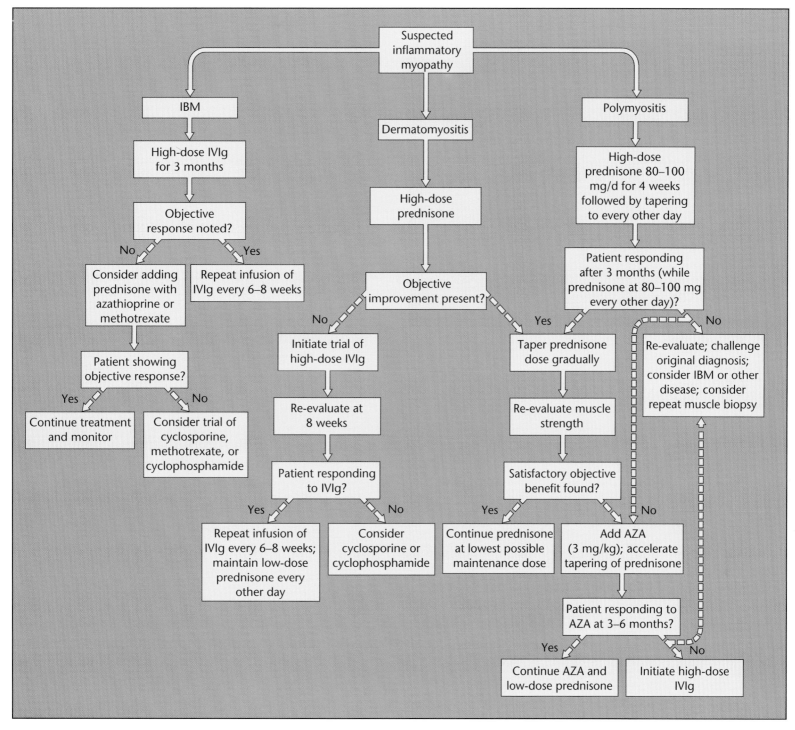

FIGURE 8-99.

Clinical algorithm for the treatment of inflammatory myopathies. AZA—azathioprine; IBM—inclusion body myositis; IVIg—intravenous immunoglobulin. (*Adapted from* Dalakas [238].)

■ NEUROTOXIC DISORDERS

SOURCES OF HUMAN TOXICANTS

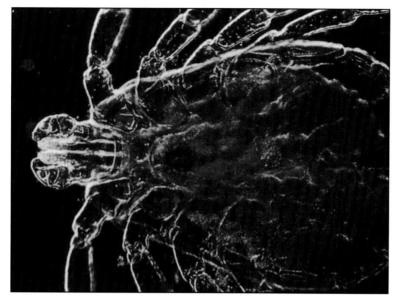

FIGURE 8-100.

Tick neurotoxicity. *Dermancentor andersoni* is the tick most frequently implicated in the northwest United States with human neurologic illness. Other neurologically affected hosts are deer, llama, and sheep. Tick infestation precedes symptoms by several days. Anorexia, diarrhea, and irritability are noted first and are followed by weakness and atonia. Removal of the tick at this stage prevents the onset of true paralysis. Retained mouth parts should be excised and a thorough search instituted for other ticks. Improvement commences immediately and is often complete by 48 hours. Most cases of tick bite occur in the months of April to June, particularly in the northwest United States. Weakness usually begins about 5 days after attachment of the tick and is preceded by fatigue, irritability, and distal paresthesias. Flaccid weakness begins in the legs and ascends to the torso, arms, and face and may involve the bulbar and respiratory muscles. The paralysis may develop rapidly and resembles the Guillan-Barré syndrome. Diplopia and pupillary dilatation are common. Sensory deficits are absent. Death follows involvement of respiratory centers. (*From* Villee *et al.* [239]; with permission.)

CHRONIC ALCOHOLISM

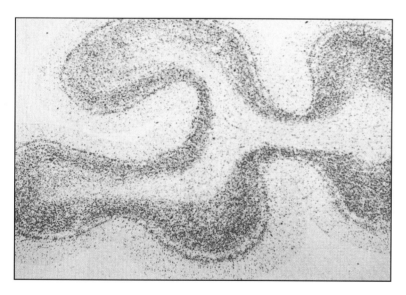

FIGURE 8-101.

Chronic alcoholism. Cerebellar degeneration is seen in adults with impaired nutrition and a long history of excessive alcohol consumption. The cerebellar syndrome, which may be accompanied by peripheral neuropathy, sometimes appears abruptly but more commonly evolves over a period of several weeks or months, after which it remains unchanged for several years. Shown is a light microscopic section demonstrating severe involvement of the vermian cortex (cresyl violet stain). The molecular layer is narrow; Purkinje cells are absent, and the Bergmann glia are greatly increased; the granule cell layer is thinned. Gliosis of the molecular layer is apparent. Alcoholic women have a significantly smaller cross-sectional corpus callosum area than alcoholic men or control subjects of either gender. (*From* Lieber [240]; with permission.)

Classification and Diagnostic Criteria for Headache Disorders, Cranial Neuralgias, and Facial Pain

1 Migraine
1.1 Migraine without aura
1.2 Migraine with aura
1.3 Ophthalmoplegic migraine
1.4 Retinal migraine
1.5 Childhood periodic syndromes that may be precursor to or associated with migraine
1.6 Complications of migraine
1.7 Migrainous disorder not fulfilling above criteria
2 Tension-type headache
2.1 Episodic tension-type headache
2.2 Chronic tension-type headache
2.3 Tension-type headache not fulfilling above criteria
3 Cluster headache and chronic paroxysmal hemicrania
3.1 Cluster headache
3.2 Chronic paroxysmal hemicrania
3.3 Cluster headache-like disorder not fulfilling above criteria
4 Miscellaneous headaches unassociated with structural lesion
4.1 Idiopathic stabbing headache
4.2 External compression headache
4.3 Cold stimulus headache
4.4 Benign cough headache
4.5 Benign exertional headache
4.6 Headache associated with sexual activity
5 Headache associated with head trauma
5.1 Acute post-traumatic headache
5.2 Chronic post-traumatic headache
6 Headache associated with vascular disorder
6.1 Acute ischemic cerebrovascular disease
6.2 Intracranial hematoma
6.3 Subarachnoid hemorrhage
6.4 Unruptured vascular malformation
6.5 Arteritis
6.6 Carotid or vertebral artery pain
6.7 Venous thrombosis
6.8 Arterial hypertension
6.9 Headache associated with other vascular disorder
7 Headache associated with non-vascular intracranial disorder
7.1 High cerebrospinal fluid pressure
7.2 Low cerebrospinal fluid pressure
7.3 Intracranial infection
7.4 Intracranial sarcoidosis and other noninfectious inflammatory diseases
7.5 Headache associated with intrathecal injections

7.6 Intracranial neoplasm
7.7 Headache associated with other intracranial disorder
8 Headache associated with substances or their withdrawal
8.1 Headache induced by acute substance use or exposure
8.2 Headache induced by chronic substance use or exposure
8.3 Headache from substance withdrawal (acute use)
8.4 Headache from substance withdrawal (chronic use)
8.5 Headache associated with substances but with uncertain mechanism
9 Headache associated with noncephalic infection
9.1 Viral infection
9.2 Bacterial infection
9.3 Headache related to other infection
10 Headache associated with metabolic disorder
10.1 Hypoxia
10.2 Hypercapnia
10.3 Mixed hypoxia and hypercapnia
10.4 Hypoglycemia
10.5 Dialysis
10.6 Headache related to other metabolic abnormality
11 Headache or facial pain associated with disorder of cranium, neck, eyes, ears, nose, sinuses, teeth, mouth, or other facial or cranial structures
11.1 Cranial bone
11.2 Neck
11.3 Eyes
11.4 Ears
11.5 Nose and sinuses
11.6 Teeth, jaws, and related structures
11.7 Temporomandibular joint disease
12 Cranial neuralgias, nerve trunk pain, and deafferentation pain
12.1 Persistent pain of cranial origin
12.2 Trigeminal neuralgia
12.3 Glossopharyngeal neuralgia
12.4 Nervus intermedius neuralgia
12.5 Superior laryngeal neuralgia
12.6 Occipital neuralgia
12.7 Central causes of head and facial pain other than tic douloureux
12.8 Facial pain not fulfilling criteria in groups 11 or 12
13 Headache not classifiable

FIGURE 8-102.

Classification and diagnostic criteria for headache disorders, cranial neuralgias, and facial pain. In 1988, a panel of international experts created a comprehensive classification of all headache types divided into 13 categories [241].

International Headache Society Criteria for the Migraine Syndrome

Migraine without aura

At least five attacks fulfilling the following three criteria:

- Headache attacks lasting 4–72 hours
- Headache with at least two of the following characteristics:

  Unilateral location

  Pulsating quality

  Moderate or severe intensity

  Aggravation by physical activity
- Patient experiences at least one of the following during headache:

  Nausea and/or vomiting

  Photophobia and phonophobia

At least one of the following applies:

  Patient's history, physical, and neurologic examination do not suggest a disorder with secondary headache

  Such a disorder is suggested but ruled out by appropriate investigations

  Such a disorder is present but first incidence of migraine does not occur in close temporal relation with the disorder

Migraine with aura

At least two attacks fulfilling the following criterion:

  Headache has at least three of the following characteristics:

- One or more fully reversible aura symptom indicating focal cerebral, cortical, and/or brainstem dysfunction
- At least one aura symptom develops gradually over more than 4 minutes, or two or more symptoms occur in succession
- No individual aura symptom lasts more than 60 minutes.
- Headache follows aura with a free interval of less than 60 minutes (it can also begin before or simultaneously with the aura)

At least one of the following:

- History and physical and neurologic examinations do not suggest a disorder with secondary headache
- Such a disorder is suggested but ruled out by appropriate investigations
- Such a disorder is present but migraine attacks do not occur for the first time in close temporal relation with the disorder.

Other migraine syndromes

FIGURE 8-103.

International Headache Society (IHS) criteria for the migraine syndrome. In the IHS system, migraine is divided into migraine without aura, migraine with aura, and other migraine syndromes. All neurologic symptoms associated with migraine are termed aura, because of the presumption that the majority of neurologic phenomena occur immediately prior to a migraine headache. The IHS criteria are an extremely useful research tool, allowing studies on migraine to be done across cultural and language boundaries. Their specificity is high but, because patients who do not fit all the criteria can still have migraine, the sensitivity is lower.

Components of the Migraine Syndrome

Pain	Location: unilateral, bilateral, retro-orbital, occipital/suboccipital, parietal, or central facial
	Quality: throbbing, steady, aching, burning, boring, superficial, or deep
	Intensity: variable from mild to extremely severe and disabling
General irritability	Photophobia, phonophobia, osmophobia, kinesiophobia
Gastrointestinal symptoms	Anorexia, nausea, vomiting, diarrhea
Neurologic symptoms	Cortical symptoms
	Visual: spots, lines, grids, heat waves, fortification of spectra, lightning streak, "rope of light," "rockets" (can be positive with bright colors or lights or negative with black spots)
	Hemiparesis
	Hemisensory loss
	Aphasia (expressive or receptive), confusional states, transient global amnesia
	Brainstem symptoms
	Vertigo, loss of consciousness, forelimb weakness or numbness
Mood symptoms	Depression, euphoria, (hypo)mania, irritability, increased energy level

FIGURE 8-104.

Components of the migraine syndrome. Migraine is very frequent; studies point to a previous underestimation although some experts believe the prevalence is increasing. Women share a higher burden, approximately 33% as opposed to 13% for men, especially during the reproductive years, mainly because of hormonal influences [242]. Patients usually begin the manifestations of migraine early in life [243]. The prevalence of migraine decreases from whites to blacks to Asians [244]. Fewer than a third of migraine patients report being very satisfied with their acute treatment [245]. Lost productivity secondary to migraine is approximately $13 million per year [246]. A high proportion of patients are not diagnosed, and many would benefit from therapeutic treatment. The burden on personal, familial, and professional life as well as on society as a whole is enormous [247].

Migraine, like the other primary headaches, is a syndrome and not a specific disease. It has a wide spectrum of manifestations, intensity, and symptoms [248]. Migraine also has comorbidities with other medical and psychiatric illnesses [249,250], and patients with migraine report a significantly worse quality of life than patients without migraine [247].

While migraine pain is classically described as throbbing, the pain can be steady, aching, or burning; the intensity of migraine pain is highly variable and can range from mild to extremely severe pain. The quality of migraine pain is also highly variable. There can be no pain at all, but other components of the migraine syndrome can be present. Symptoms of general irritability are an important part of the migraine syndrome. Photophobia, phonophobia, and aggravation by movement occur very commonly. Osmophobia is less common but still a major symptom for many migraine patients. The gastrointestinal symptoms associated with migraine are the second most common cause of disability in migraine. There is a continuum from anorexia to vomiting. Nausea is present in 90% of migraine patients, and 60% of these patients experience vomiting. Diarrhea is seen in up to 25% of migraine patients. The intensity of these symptoms correlates with the head pain. There is comorbidity between migraine and irritable bowel syndrome, although this has not been studied in detail. The brainstem symptoms of vertigo, loss of consciousness, and forelimb numbness or weakness are less common. These features would typically occur with basilar artery migraine. The origin of the brainstem symptoms is unclear. The cortical symptoms are thought to relate to spreading depression occurring in the cortex, producing transient cortical dysfunction.

Mood changes, including increased energy and productiveness, euphoria, increased sex drive and appetite, irritability or depression, are often associated with migraine. While typically thought of as part of the prodrome, they can occur before, during, or after the headache.

Nonspecific and Semispecific Drug Therapies for Migraine

Non-specific	Usual Dosage	Maximum Dosage/d
NSAIDs		
Ibuprofen	400 mg–800 mg	3200 mg
Naproxen	250 mg–550 mg	1100 mg
Fenoprofen	300 mg–600 mg	2400 mg
Meclofenamate	100 mg	300 mg
Tolmetin	200 mg–400 mg	1800 mg
Aspirin	650 mg–1000 mg	4000 mg
Analgesics		
Acetaminophen	650 mg–1000 mg	4000 mg
Tramadol	50 mg	400 mg
Minor narcotics		
Codeine	30 mg–60 mg	360 mg
Hydrocodone	5 mg–75 mg	375 mg
Oxycodone	5 mg	30 mg
Semi-specific		
Isometheptene	65 mg	6 capsules/d
Butalbital	50 mg	200 mg–400 mg
Sodium valproate IV	500 mg	1500 mg

FIGURE 8-105.
Nonspecific and semispecific drug therapies for migraine. Nonspecific therapies, such as nonsteroidal anti-inflammatory drugs (NSAIDs), analgesics, narcotics, and non-narcotics, relieve pain but do not attack the specific mechanism of migraine. For many patients with intermittent acute migraine, use of 800 mg ibuprofen, 500 mg naproxen, or another NSAID or acetaminophen can be sufficient. The addition of an antihistamine with antiemetic action (hydroxyzine 25 mg–50 mg) or dopamine antagonist (promethazine 25 mg–50 mg) can enhance the potential of this approach significantly. Codeine, oxycodone, and hydrocodone are effective for some patients but must be used carefully. If the patient requires more than 10 tablets per month, habituation should be suspected and alternative therapy sought. These minor narcotics can be used as individual agents or combined with an antihistamine or dopamine antagonist. Isometheptene or butalbital compounds are effective for some patients with migraine, but their mechanism of action is not fully elucidated. If the patient requires as many as 10 butalbital doses per month, habituation and rebound withdrawal headache should be considered and the use of butalbital discontinued. Slow intravenous (IV) injections of 500 mg sodium valproate have proven efficient in aborting a migraine attack [251].

A. Migraine Treatment: Triptans

Generic	Strength, mg	Max mg/24 h	1/2 life, h	T max, h	Efficacy,* %
First-generation triptans					
Sumatriptan PO	25, 50, 100	200	2.5	2	62/33
Sumatriptan NS	5, 20	40	2		64/31
Sumatriptan SC	6	12	2	12	80/40
Second-generation triptans					
Naratriptan	1, 2.5	5	6	1.5–3	58/27
Zolmitriptan	2.5, 5	10	3	2.5	67/33
Rizatriptan	5, 10	30	3	1.5	72/41

*Meta-analysis of patients at 2 hours: first number = improvement from moderate or severe headache to mild or none; second number = pain free.

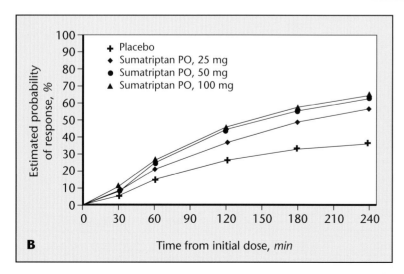

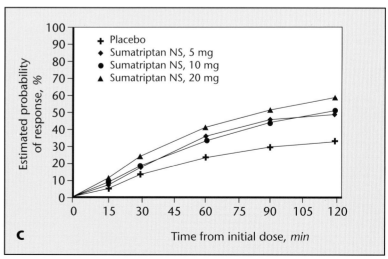

FIGURE 8-106. (CONTINUED)

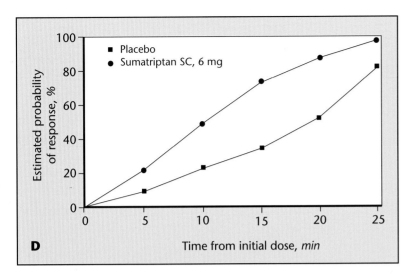

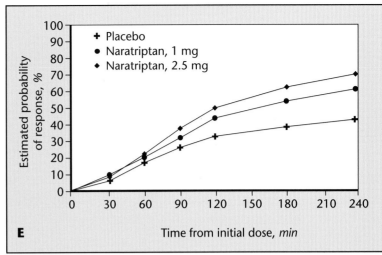

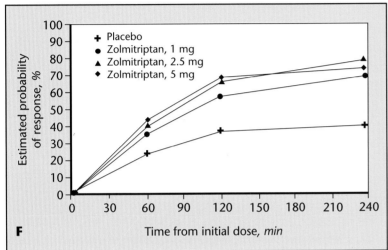

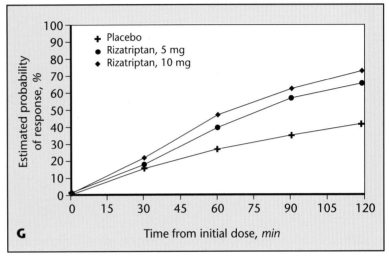

FIGURE 8-106. (CONTINUED)

Specific migraine treatment: first- and second-generation triptans. Triptans represent one of the most dramatic advances in migraine therapy of the last century. Since the development of sumatriptan newer triptans have been designed in an attempt to improve efficacy and decrease side effects. A main pharmacologic difference is their central nervous system penetration. They act on 5-HT1B/D receptors on meningeal and brain vessels, on presynaptic perivascular trigeminal nerve endings, and on the central projections of trigeminal fibers conveying pain [252–254]. Individual patient sensitivity to each triptan seems to vary. **A**, Dosing schedules for the first- and second-generation triptans. For most migraine patients, the triptans produce rapid and complete relief of the headache with relatively early return to functional status. **B**, Estimated probability of achieving initial headache response within 240 minutes with sumatriptan PO. **C**, Estimated probability of achieving initial headache response within 120 minutes with sumatriptan NS. **D**, Time to relief from time of injection with sumatriptan SC. **E**, Estimated probability of achieving initial headache response within 240 minutes with naratriptan. **F**, Estimated probability of achieving initial headache response within 240 minutes with zolmitriptan. **G**, Estimated probability of achieving initial headache response within 120 minutes with rizatriptan. In general, for uncomplicated intermittent migraine, 60% to 70% of patients will have good relief within 2 hours and more than 80% will have good relief within 4 hours [255–260]. Evidence suggests that even milder migraine headaches can be effectively treated by a triptan [261,262]. Recurrence within 24 hours typically is 25% to 35%, but often recurrences are mild and will respond well to a second dose of

triptan. In general, the triptans have onset of effect within 30 to 60 minutes, achieving peak effect at approximately 4 hours. About 50% of patients will maintain a response for 24 hours without recurrence or having to take supplementary medication. There do appear to be idiosyncratic differences between patients in response to the triptans. Patients who fail to respond to the one triptan can respond to one of the others. Consequently, it is worth trying all of the currently available triptans before assuming that the patient is "triptan-unresponsive." A simplistic approach to triptan usage is that patients can take a dose of the medication and then repeat that dose once within 24 hours if necessary. For most of the triptans, repeating 2 doses within 24 hours is usually tolerated well. Of the available dose forms, most patients prefer tablets. Sumatriptan is available by both nasal spray and injection. The nasal spray at times produces an unpleasant taste for the patient and this can preclude usage. Patients with very rapidly progressing headache can prefer the subcutaneous injection to achieve relief as rapidly as possible. Between 30% and 40% of patients will have adverse events, typically mild but occasionally severe. Adverse events reported by more than 5% of patients include somnolence or fatigue, dizziness, paresthesia or sensation of chest/throat pressure, or nausea. These events tend to rarefy over time and are similar although more frequent or severe than those reported for dihydroergotamine. There is concern over the coronary arteries where ergots or triptans can produce up to a 20% constriction; however, this is not clinically significant in healthy individuals. Patients with coronary artery disease should not receive these drugs.

Differential Diagnosis of Vascular Headache

Ischemic stroke
  Thrombotic
  Embolic
Vasculitis
  Arteritis
    Giant cell arteritis
      Temporal arteritis
      Takayasu's arteritis
    Polyarteritis nodosa
      Classic polyarteritis
      Allergic angiitis (Churg-Strauss syndrome)
      Systemic necrotizing vasculitis
    Isolated CNS angiitis
    Wegener's granulomatosis
    Hypersensitivity vasculitis
  Arteriolitis
    Systemic lupus erythematosus
    Behçet's disease
  Venous thrombosis
  Subarachnoid hemorrhage
  Intracerebral hemorrhage

FIGURE 8-107.

Differential diagnosis of vascular headaches. The most common causes of vascular headaches are listed.

Differential Diagnosis of Infectious Headache

Intracerebral infections
  Acute infectious processes (bacterial or viral)
    Meningitis (*Neisseria, Streptococcus*)
    Parenchymal brain infections
      Encephalitis (herpes simplex)
      Abscess (*Staphylococcus*)
  Chronic infectious processes (bacterial, fungal, or viral)
    Meningitis (atypical tubercle bacillus, cryptococcus)
    Parenchymal
      Encephalitis (mucor mycosis, syphilis, HIV)
      Abscess (*Nocardia, Cryptococcus*)
  Infectious vasculitis
    Syphilis
Extracranial infections
  Infections of endothelial-lined cavities
  Infectious vasculitis
  Abscess

FIGURE 8-108.

Differential diagnosis of infectious headache. The most frequent causes of infectious headaches are listed.

Differential Diagnosis of Metabolic Headache

Major organ failure
  Hepatic failure
  Renal failure
  Pulmonary failure with carbon dioxide retention
Endocrinopathies
  Hyperthyroidism
  Hypothyroidism
  Hypoparathyroidism
  Addison's disease
  Cushing's disease
Conditions producing headache associated with vascular changes
  Fever
  Anemia
  Carbon dioxide retention with vasodilatation

FIGURE 8-109.

Differential diagnosis of metabolic headache. The most frequent metabolic causes of headache are listed.

ACKNOWLEDGMENT

The author wishes to thank his colleagues who contributed to the *Atlas of Clinical Neurology* second edition for allowing the use of their figures in this chapter of the *Atlas of Internal Medicine*.

REFERENCES

1. Lampe T, Bird TD, Nochlin D, *et al*.: Phenotype of chromosome 14-linked familial Alzheimer's disease in a large kindred. *Ann Neurol* 1994, 36:368–378.

2. Van Broeckhoven CL: Molecular genetics of Alzheimer disease: identification of genes and gene mutations. *Eur Neurol* 1995, 35:8–19.

3. Sherrington R, Rogaev EI, Liang Y, *et al*.: Cloning of a gene bearing missense mutations in early-onset Alzheimer's disease. *Nature* 1995, 375:754–760.

4. Levy-Lahad E, Wasco W, Poorkaj P, *et al*.: Candidate gene for the chromosome 1 familial Alzheimer's disease locus. *Science* 1995, 26:973–977.

5. Roses AD: Apolipoprotein E genotyping in the differential diagnosis, not prediction, of Alzheimer's disease. *Ann Neurol* 1995, 18:6–14.

6. Finelli PF: Kayser-Fleischer ring: hepatolenticular degeneration (Wilson's disease). *Neurology* 1995, 1261–1262.

7. Rosen DR, Siddique T, Patterson D, *et al*.: Mutations in Cu/Zn superoxide dismutase gene are associated with familial amyotrophic lateral sclerosis. *Nature* 1993, 362:59–62.

8. Nagashima T, Seko K, Hirose K, *et al*.: Familial bulbo-spinal muscular atrophy associated with testicular atrophy and sensory neuropathy (Kennedy-Alter-Sung syndrome): autopsy case report of two brothers. *J Neurol Sci* 1988, 87:141–152.

9. Ebers GC: Genetics and multiple sclerosis: an overview. *Ann Neurol* 1994, 36:S12–S14.

10. Ramsay MAE, Savege TA, Simpson BRJ, Goodwin R: Controlled sedation with alphaxalone-alphadolone. *BMJ* 1974, 2:656–659.

11. Wijdicks EFM: *Neurology of Critical Illness*. Philadelphia: FA Davis, 1995.

12. Hacke W, ed: *Neurocritical Care*. Berlin: Springer-Verlag, 1994.

13. Classification of cerebrovascular disease III. Special report from the National Institute of Neurological Disorders and Stroke. *Stroke* 1990, 21:637–676.

14. Mohr JP, Barnett HJM: Classification of Ischemic Strokes. In *Stroke: Pathophysiology, Diagnosis and Management*. Edited by Barnett HJM, Mohr JP, Stein BM, Yatsu FM. New York: Churchill Livingstone; 1986:281–292.

15. Origitano TC: Treatment of Aneurysmal Subarachnoid Hemorrhage. In *Atlas of Cerebrovascular Disease*. Edited by Gorelick PB. Philadelphia: Current Medicine; 1996:19.1–19.11.

16. Hanley DF, Glass JD, McArthur JC, Johnson RT: Viral Encephalitis and Related Conditions. In *Atlas of Infectious Diseases* vol 3. Edited by Mandell GL, Bleck TP. Philadelphia: Current Medicine; 1995:3.1–3.36.

17. Johnson RT: *Current Therapy in Neurologic Disease* edn 2. Philadelphia: BC Decker; 1987.

18. Lothman E: The biochemical basis and pathophysiology of status epilepticus. *Neurology* 1990, 40(suppl 2):13–23.

19. Mirski MA, Williams MA, Hanley DF: Prolonged pentobarbital and phenobarbital coma for refractory generalized status epilepticus. *Crit Care Med* 1995, 23:400–403.

20. Fisher CM, Gore I, Okabe M, *et al*.: Atherosclerosis of the carotid and vertebral arteries: extracranial and intracranial. *J Neuropathol Exp Neurol* 1965, 24:455–476.

21. Kistler JP: Cerebrovascular Disease. In *Atherosclerosis and Coronary Artery Disease*. Edited by Fuster V, Ross R, Topol EJ. Philadelphia: Lippincott-Raven; 1996:463–474.

22. Adams RD, Sidman RL: Cerebrovascular Diseases. In *Introduction to Neuropathology*. New York: McGraw-Hill; 1968:197.

23. Kistler JP, Buonanno FS, Gress DR: Carotid endarterectomy—specific therapy based on pathophysiology. *N Engl J Med* 1991; 325:505–507.

24. Wechsler LR, Kistler JP, Davis KR, *et al*.: The prognosis of carotid siphon stenosis. *Stroke* 1986, 17:714–718.

25. Kubik CS, Adams RD: Occlusion of the basilar artery: a clinical and pathological study. *Brain* 1946, 69:73–121.

26. Beebe HG, Archie JP, Baker WH, *et al*.: Concern about safety of carotid angioplasty. *Stroke* 1996, 27:197–198.

27. Mohr JP, Kase CS, Wolf PA: Lacunes in the NINCDS pilot stroke data bank [abstract]. *Ann Neurol* 1982, 12:84.

28. Fisher CM: Lacunar stroke and infarcts: a review. *Neurology* 1982, 32:871–876.

29. Fisher CM: Capsular infarcts; the underlying vascular lesion. *Arch Neurol* 1979, 36:65–73.

30. Mohr JP: Lacunes. *Stroke* 1982, 13:3–11.

31. Fisher CM: Pure sensory stroke involving face, arm, and leg. *Neurology* 1965, 15:76–80.

32. Fisher CM: Thalamic pure sensory stroke: a pathological study. *Neurology* 1978, 28:1141–1144.

33. Fisher CM: Pure sensory stroke and allied conditions. *Stroke* 1982, 13:434–447.

34. Orgogozo JM, Bogousslavsky J: Lacunar Syndromes. In *Handbook of Clinical Neurology*. Edited by Toole JF. New York: Elsevier Science Publishers; 1989:235–269.

35. Besson G, Hommel M: Lacunar Syndrome. In *Advances in Neurology*, vol 62. Cerebral Small Artery Disease. Edited by Pullicino PM, Caplan LR, Hommel M. New York: Raven Press; 1993:141–159.

36. Ropper AH, Fisher CM, Kleinman GM: Pyramidal infarction in the medulla: a cause of pure motor hemiplegia sparing face. *Neurology* 1979, 29:91–95.

37. Fisher CM, Cole M: Homolateral ataxia with crural paresis: a vascular syndrome. *J Neurol Neurosurg Psychiatry* 1965, 28:48–55.

38. Fisher CM: A lacunar syndrome: the dysarthria-clumsy hand syndrome. *Neurology* 1967, 17:614–617.

39. Fisher CM: Ataxic hemiparesis: a pathologic study. *Arch Neurol* 1978, 35:126–128.

40. Mohr JP, Kase CS, Meckler RJ, *et al*.: Sensorimotor stroke due to thalamocapsular ischemia. *Arch Neurol* 1977, 34:739–741.

41. Kistler JP, Ropper AH, Martin JB: Cerebrovascular Diseases. In *Harrison's Principles of Internal Medicine* edn 13. Edited by Isselbacher KJ, Martin JB, Braunwald E, *et al*.: New York: McGraw-Hill; 1994:2233–2256.

42. Kistler JP, Ropper AH, Heros RC: Therapy of ischemic cerebral vascular disease due to atherothrombosis. *N Engl J Med* 1984, 311:27–34, 100–105.

43. Sacco RL, Ellenberg JH, Mohr JP, *et al*.: Infarcts of undetermined cause: the NINCDS Stroke Data Bank. *Ann Neurol* 1989, 25:382–390.

44. Melo TP, Bogousslavsky J, Van Melle G, *et al*.: Pure motor stroke: a reappraisal. *Neurology* 1992, 42:789–798.

45. Adams RD, Victor M: Cerebrovascular Diseases. In *Principles of Neurology*. Edited by Adams RD, Victor M. New York: McGraw-Hill; 1993:669–748.

46. Orsinelli DA, Pearson AC: Detection of prosthetic valve strands by transesophageal echocardiography: clinical significance in patients with suspected cardiac source of embolism. *J Am Coll Cardiol* 1995, 26:1713–1718.

47. Bladin PF: A radiologic and pathologic study of embolism of the internal carotid-middle cerebral arterial axis. *Radiology* 1964, 82:615–625.

48. Wolf PA, Abbott RD, Kannel WB: Atrial fibrillation: a major contributor to stroke in the elderly. The Framingham study. *Arch Intern Med* 1987, 147:1561–1564.

49. Wolf PA, Abbott RD, Kannel WB: Atrial fibrillation as an independent risk factor for stroke: the Framingham study. *Stroke* 1991, 22:983–988.

50. Petersen P, Godtfredsen J, Boysen G, *et al*.: Placebo-controlled, randomized trial of warfarin and aspirin for prevention of thromboembolic complications in chronic atrial fibrillation: the Copenhagen AFASAK study. *Lancet* 1989, 1:175–179.

51. Stroke Prevention in Atrial Fibrillation Investigators: stroke prevention in atrial fibrillation study: final results. *Circulation* 1991, 89:527–539.

52. Boston Area Anticoagulation Trial for Atrial Fibrillation Investigators: The effect of low dose warfarin on the risk of stroke in patients with nonrheumatic atrial fibrillation. *N Engl J Med* 1990, 323:1505–1511.

53. CAFA Study Investigators: Canadian atrial fibrillation (CAFA) study. *J Am Coll Cardiol* 1991, 18:349–355.

54. Ezekowitz MD, Bridgers SL, James KE, *et al.*: Warfarin in the prevention of stroke associated with nonrheumatic atrial fibrillation. *N Engl J Med* 1992, 327:1406–1412.

55. Laupacis A, Boysen G, Connolly S, *et al.*: Atrial fibrillation: risk factors for embolization and efficacy of anti-thrombotic therapy. *Arch Intern Med* 1994, 154:1449–1457.

56. Turpie AGG, Gunstensen J, Hirsh J, *et al.*: Randomized comparison of two intensities of oral anticoagulant therapy after tissue heart valve replacement. *Lancet* 1988, 1:1242–1245.

57. Fourth ACCP Consensus Conference on Antithrombotic Therapy. Edited by Dalen JE, Hirsh J. *Chest* 1995, 108(suppl 4):225S–522S.

58. Becker RC, Ansell J: Antithrombotic therapy: an abbreviated reference for clinicians. *Arch Intern Med* 1995, 155:149–161.

59. Kistler JP, Singer DA, Millenson MM, *et al.*, for the BAATAF investigators: Effect of low intensity warfarin anticoagulation on level of activity of the hemostatic system in patients with atrial fibrillation. *Stroke* 1993, 24:1360–1365.

60. Kistler JP, Bauer KA: The Level of Activity of the Hemostatic System, the Rate of Embolic Stroke, and Age: Is There a Correlation? In *Cerebrovascular Diseases*. Edited by Moskowitz MA, Caplan LR. Boston: Butterworth-Heinemann; 1995:437–442.

61. Mas J-L, Henin D, Bousser MG, *et al.*: Dissecting aneurysm of the vertebral artery and cervical manipulation: a case report with autopsy. *Neurology* 1989, 39:512–515.

62. Nguyen Bui L, Brant-Zawadzki M, Verghese P, *et al.*: Magnetic resonance angiography of cervicocranial dissection. *Stroke* 1993, 24:126–131.

63. Frisoni GB, Anzola GP: Vertebrobasilar ischemia after neck motion. *Stroke* 1991, 22:1452–1460.

64. Frumkin LR, Baloh RW: Wallenberg's syndrome following neck manipulation. *Neurology* 1990, 40:1990:611–615.

65. Sherman DG, Hart RG, Easton JD: Abrupt change in head position and cerebral infarction. *Stroke* 1981, 12:2–6.

66. Saver JL, Easton JD, Hart RG: Dissections and Trauma of Cervicocerebral Arteries. In *Stroke: Pathophysiology, Diagnosis and Management* edn 2. Edited by Barnett HJM, Bennett MS, Mohr JP, *et al.* New York: Churchill Livingstone; 1992:671–688.

67. Caplan LR, Baquis GD, Pessin MS, *et al.*: Dissection of the intracranial vertebral artery. *Neurology* 1988, 38:868–877.

68. Barnett HJM: Progress towards stroke prevention. Robert Wartenberg Lecture. *Neurology* 1980, 30:1212–1225.

69. Kay R, Wong KS, Yu YL, *et al.*: Low molecular weight heparin for the treatment of acute ischemic stroke. *N Engl J Med* 1995, 333:1588–1593.

70. Stallones RA, Dyken ML, Fang HCH, *et al.*: Epidemiology for stroke facilities planning. *Stroke* 1972, 3:360–371.

71. Weiller C, Ramsay SC, Wise RJS, *et al.*: Individual patterns of functional reorganization in the human cerebral cortex after capsular infarction. *Ann Neurol* 1993, 33:181–189.

72. Ojeman R, Mohr J: Hypertensive brain hemorrhage. *Clin Neurosurg* 1975, 23:220.

73. Mohr J, Caplan L, Melski J, *et al.*: The Harvard Cooperative Stroke Registry: a prospective registry. *Neurology* 1978, 28:754–762.

74. Fisher C: Pathological observations in hypertensive cerebral hemorrhage. *J Neuropathol Exp Neurol* 1971, 30:536–550.

75. Freytag E: Fatal hypertensive intracerebral hematomas: a survey of the pathological anatomy in 393 cases. *J Neurol Neurosurg Psychiatry* 1968, 31:616–620.

76. Ojeman R, Mohr J: Hypertensive brain hemorrhage. *Clin Neurosurg* 1975, 23:220–244.

77. Kase CS: Cerebral Amyloid Angiopathy. In *Intracerebral Hemorrhage*. Edited by Kase CS, Caplan LR. Boston: Butterworth-Heinemann; 1994:179–200.

78. Vinters HV: Cerebral amyloid angiopathy: a critical review. *Stroke* 1987, 18:311–324.

79. Yankner BA, Dawes LR, Fisher S, *et al.*: Neurotoxicity of a fragment of the amyloid precursor associated with Alzheimer's disease. *Science* 1989, 245:417–420.

80. Mandybur TI: Cerebral amyloid angiopathy: the vascular pathology and complications. *J Neuropathol Exp Neurol* 1986, 45:79–90.

81. Vonsattel JP, Myers RH, Hedley-Whyte ET, *et al.*: Cerebral amyloid angiopathy without and with cerebral hemorrhages: a comparative histological study. *Ann Neurol* 1991, 30:637–649.

82. Maeda A, Yamada M, Itoh Y, *et al.*: Computer-assisted three-dimensional image analysis of cerebral amyloid angiopathy. *Stroke* 1993, 24:1857–1864.

83. Yong WH, Robert ME, Secor DL, *et al.*: Cerebral hemorrhage with biopsy-proved amyloid angiopathy. *Arch Neurol* 1992, 49:51–58.

84. Greene GM, Godersky JC, Biller J, *et al.*: Surgical experience with cerebral amyloid angiopathy. *Stroke* 1990, 21:1545–1549.

85. Ondra S, Troupp H, George E, *et al.*: The natural history of symptomatic arteriovenous malformations. *J Neurosurg* 1990, 73:387–391.

86. Tsementzis S: Surgical management of intracerebral hematomas. *Neurosurgery* 1985, 16:562–572.

87. McCormick WF: The pathology of vascular ("arteriovenous") malformations. *J Neurosurg* 1966, 24:807–816.

88. Curling OJ, Kelly DJ, Elster A, *et al.*: An analysis of the natural history of the cavernous angioma. *Neurosurgery* 1991, 75:702.

89. Robinson J, Award I, Little J: Natural history of cavernous angioma. *J Neurosurg* 1991, 75:709–714.

90. Report of the Quality Standards Subcommittee of the American Academy of Neurology: Practice parameter for diagnosis and evaluation of dementia (summary statement). *Neurology* 1994, 44:2203–2206.

91. Corey-Bloom J, Thal LJ, Galasko D, *et al.*: Diagnosis and evaluation of dementia. *Neurology* 1995, 45:211–218.

92. Folstein MF, Folstein SE, McHugh PR: "Mini-Mental State." A practical method for grading the cognitive state of patients for the clinician. *J Psychiat Res* 1975, 12:189–198.

93. Tombaugh TN, McIntyre NJ: The mini-mental state examination: a comprehensive review. *JAGS* 1992, 40:922–935.

94. Petersen RC, Smith GE, Waring SC, *et al.*: Mild cognitive impairment: clinical characterization and outcome. *Arch Neurol* 1999, 56:303–308.

95. Marsden CD: Assessment of dementia. In *Handbook of Clinical Neurology*, vol 46. Edited by Frederiks JAM. Amsterdam: Elsevier Science Publishers; 1985:221–231.

96. Albert ML, Feldman RG, Willis AL: The 'subcortical dementia' of progressive supranuclear palsy. *J Neurol Neurosurg Psych* 1974, 37:121–130.

97. Cummings JL, Benson DF: Subcortical dementia. *Arch Neurol* 1984, 41:874–879.

98. van Duijn CM: Epidemiology of the dementias: recent developments and new approaches. *J Neurol Neurosurg Psych* 1996, 60:478–488.

99. Weytingh MD, Bossuyt PMM, van Crevel H: Reversible dementia: more than 10% or less than 1%? A quantitative review. *J Neurol* 1995, 242:446–471.

100. Katzman R, Kawas C: The epidemiology of dementia and Alzheimer disease. In *Alzheimer Disease*. Edited by Terry RD, Katzman R, Bick KL. New York: Raven Press; 1994:105–122.

101. Jorm AF, Korten E, Henderson AS: The prevalence of dementia: a quantitative integration of the literature. *Acta Psychiatr Scand* 1987, 76:465–479.

102. Hagnell O, Ojesjo L, Rorsman B: Incidence of dementia in the Lundby study. *Neuroepidemiology* 1992, 11:61–66.

103. van Duijn CM, Stijnen T, Hofman A: Risk factors for Alzheimer's disease: overview of the EURODEM collaborative re-analysis of case-control studies. *Int J Epidemiol* 1991, 20:S4–S12.

104. Goate A, Chartier-Harlin MC, Mullan M, *et al.*: Segregation of a missense mutation in the amyloid precursor protein gene with familial Alzheimer's disease. *Nature* 1991, 349:704–706.

105. Alzheimer's Disease Collaborative Group: The structure of the presenilin 1 (S182) gene and identification of six novel mutations in early onset AD families. *Nat Genet* 1995, 11:219–222.

106. Levy-Lahad E, Wijsman EM, Nemens E, *et al.*: A familial Alzheimer's disease locus on chromosome 1. *Science* 1995, 269:970–973.

107. Brayne C, Gill C, Huppert FA, *et al.*: Incidence of clinically diagnosed subtypes of dementia in an elderly population. *Br J Psychiatr* 1995, 167:255–262.

108. Tang M-X, Jacobs D, Stern Y, Marder K, *et al.*: Effect of estrogen during menopause on risk and age at onset of Alzheimer's disease. *Lancet* 1996, 348:429–432.

109. Khachaturian ZS: Diagnosis of Alzheimer's disease. *Arch Neurol* 1985, 42:1097–1105.

110. Mirra SS, Heyman A, McKeel D, *et al.*: The consortium to establish a registry for Alzheimer's disease (CERAD). Part II. Standardization of the neuropathologic assessment of Alzheimer's disease. *Neurology* 1991, 41:479–486.

111. Arnold SE, Hyman BT, Flory J, *et al.*: The topographical and neuroanatomical distribution of neurofibrillary tangles and neuritic plaques in the cerebral cortex of patients with Alzheimer's disease. *Cerebral Cortex* 1991, 1:103–116.

112. Hof PR, Bierer LM, Perl DP, *et al.*: Evidence for early vulnerability of the medial and inferior aspects of the temporal lobe in an 82-year-old patient with preclinical signs of dementia. *Arch Neurol* 1992, 49:946–953.

113. Hyman BT, Arriagada PV, McKee AC, *et al.*: The earliest symptoms of Alzheimer disease: anatomic correlates. *Soc Neurosci Abstr* 1991, 15:352.

114. Storey E, Cappai R: The amyloid precursor protein of Alzheimer's disease and the Ab peptide. *Neuropathol Appl Neurobiol* 1999, 25:81–97.

115. Selkoe DJ: Alzheimer's disease: a central role for amyloid. *J Neuropathol Exp Neurol* 1994, 53:438–447.

116. Selkoe DJ: The pathophysiology of Alzheimer's disease. In *Early Diagnosis of Alzheimer's Disease*. Edited by Scinto LFM, Daffner KR. Totowa, NJ: Humana Press; 2000:83–104.

117. Roman GC, Tatemichi TK, Erkinjuntti T, *et al.*: Vascular dementia: diagnostic criteria for research studies. Report of the NINDS-AIREN International Workshop. *Neurology* 1993, 43:250–260.

118. Erkinjuntti T, Hachinski VC: Rethinking vascular dementia. *Cerebrovasc Dis* 1993, 3:3–23.

119. Tatemichi TK: How acute brain failure becomes chronic: a view of the mechanisms of dementia related to stroke. *Neurology* 1990, 40:1652–1659.

120. Hershey LA, Modic MT, Jaffe DF, Greenough PG: Natural history of the vascular dementias: a prospective study of seven cases. *Can J Neurol Sci* 1986, 13:559–565.

121. The Lund and Manchester Groups: Clinical and neuropathological criteria for frontotemporal dementia. *J Neuro Neurosurg Psychiatry* 1994, 57:416–418.

122. Neary D, Snowden JS, Gustafson L, *et al.*: Frontotemporal lobar degeneration: a consensus on clinical diagnostic criteria. *Neurology* 1998, 51:1546–1554.

123. Brun A: Frontal lobe degeneration of non-Alzheimer type. I. Neuropathology. *Arch Gerontol Geriatr* 1987, 6:193–208.

124. Neary D, Snowden JS, Mann DMA, *et al.*: Frontal lobe dementia and motor neuron disease. *J Neurol Neurosurg Psychiatry* 1990, 53:23–32.

125. Chow TW, Miller BL, Hayashi VN, Geschwind DH: Inheritance of frontotemporal dementia. *Arch Neurol* 1999, 56(7):817–822.

126. Mesulam MM: Slowly progressive aphasia without generalized dementia. *Ann Neurol* 1982, 11:592–598.

127. Snowden JS, Neary D, Mann DMA: *Fronto-Temporal Lobar Degeneration: Fronto-Temporal Dementia, Progressive Aphasia, Semantic Dementia*. New York: Churchill Livingstone; 1996.

128. Hodges JR, Patterson K, Oxbury S, Funnell E: Semantic dementia. Progressive fluent aphasia with temporal lobe atrophy. *Brain* 1992, 115:1783–1806.

129. Graff-Radford NR, Damasio AR, Hyman BT, *et al.*: Progressive aphasia in a patient with Pick's disease: a neuropsychological, radiologic, and anatomic study. *Neurology* 1990, 40:620–626.

130. Kertesz A, Hudson L, Mackenzie IRA, Munoz DG: The pathology and nosology of primary progressive aphasia. *Neurology* 1994, 44:2065–2072.

131. Turner RS, Kenyon LC, Trojanowski JQ, *et al.*: Clinical, neuroimaging, and pathologic features of progressive nonfluent aphasia. *Ann Neurol* 1996, 39:166–173.

132. Perry E, McKeith I, Perry R, eds.: *Dementia with Lewy Bodies: Clinical, Pathologic, and Treatment Issues*. Cambridge: Cambridge University Press; 1996.

133. Damasio H, Frank RJ: Three-dimensional in vivo mapping of brain lesions in humans. *Arch Neurol* 1992, 49:137–143.

134. Frank RJ, Damasio H, Grabowski TJ: Brainvox: an interactive, multimodal visualization and analysis system for neuroanatomical imaging. *Neuroimage* 1997, 5:13–30.

135. Babinski J: Contribution a l'etude des troubles mentaux dans l'hemiplegie organique cerebrale (agnosognosie). *Rev Neurol* 1914, 27:845–847.

136. Ungerleider LG, Mishkin M: Two cortical visual systems. In *Analysis of Visual Behavior*. Edited by Ingle DJ, Goodale MA, Mansfield RJW. Cambridge, MA: MIT Press; 1982:549–586.

137. Newcombe F, Ratcliff G: Disorders of visuospatial analysis. In: *Handbook of Neuropsychology*, vol 2. Edited by Boller F, Grafman J. Amsterdam: Elsevier; 1989:333–356.

138. Rizzo M: "Balint's syndrome" and associated visuospatial disorders. In *Bailliere's International Practice and Research*. Edited by London KC. Philadelphia: WB Saunders; 1993:415–437.

139. Damasio AR, Tranel D, Damasio H: Face agnosia and the neural substrates of memory. *Annu Rev Neurosci* 1990, 13:89–109.

140. Zihl J, Von Cramon Z, Mai N: Selective disturbances of movement vision after bilateral brain damage. *Brain* 1983, 106:313–340.

141. Rizzo M, Hurtig R: Looking but not seeing: attention, perception, and eye movements in simultanagnosia. *Neurology* 1987, 37:1642–1648.

142. Damasio AR, Benton AL: Impairment of hand movements under visual guidance. *Neurology* 1979, 29:170–174.

143. Tranel D, Biller J, Damasio H, *et al.*: Global aphasia without hemiparesis. *Arch Neurol* 1987, 44:304–308.

144. Walker AE, Robins M, Weinfeld FD: Epidemiology of brain tumors: the national survey of intracranial neoplasms. *Neurology* 1985, 35:219–226.

145. Cairncross JG, Posner JB: The management of brain metastases. In *Oncology of the Nervous System*. Edited by Walker MD. Boston: Martinus Nijhoff; 1983:341–377.

146. Delattre JY, Krol G, Thaler HT, *et al.*: Distribution of brain metastases. *Arch Neurol* 1988, 45:741–744.

147. Evans RG: The role of radiation therapy in the treatment of brain tumors in children. In *Brain Tumors: A Comprehensive Text*. Edited by Morantz RA, Walsh JW. New York: Marcel Dekker; 1994: 659–677.

148. Levin VA, Sheline GE, Gutin PH: Neoplasms of the Central Nervous System. In *Cancer: Principles and Practice of Oncology* vol 2. Edited by DeVita VT Jr, Hellman S, Rosenberg SA. Philadelphia: JB Lippincott; 1989:1557–1611.

149. Giles GG, Gonzales MF: Epidemiology of Brain Tumors and Factors in Prognosis. In *Brain Tumors: An Encyclopedic Approach*. Edited by Kaye AH, Laws ER Jr. New York: Churchill Livingstone; 1994:47–67.

150. Pell MF, Thomas DGT: General Introduction to the Clinical Features of Malignant Brain Tumours. In *Malignant Brain Tumours*. Edited by Thomas DGT, Graham DI. London: Springer-Verlag; 1995:109–114.

151. McKeran RO, Thomas DGT: The clinical study of gliomas. In *Brain Tumours: Scientific Basis, Clinical Investigation and Current Therapy*. Edited by Thomas DGT, Graham DI. London: Butterworth; 1980:194–230.

152. Cascino GD: Epilepsy and brain tumours: implications for treatment. *Epilepsia* 1990, 31:537–544.

153. Henry C, Despland PA, Regli F: Initial epileptic crisis after the age of 60: aetiology, clinical aspect and EEG. *Schweiz Med Wochenschr* 1990, 120:787–792.

154. Posner JB: *Neurologic Complications of Cancer*. Philadelphia: FA Davis; 1995. Contemporary Neurology Series, vol 45.

155. Cairncross JG, Kim J-H, Posner JB: Radiation therapy for brain metastases. *Ann Neurol* 1980, 7:529–541.

156. Young DF, Posner JB, Chu F, *et al.*: Rapid-course radiation therapy of cerebral metastases: results and complications. *Cancer* 1974, 4:1069–1076.

157. Chase, TN, Mouradian MM, Engber TM: Motor response complications and the function of striatal efferent systems. *Neurology* 1993, 43(suppl 6):S23–S27.

158. Steele RC, Richardson JC, Olszewski J: Progressive supranuclear palsy: a heterogeneous degeneration involving the brain stem, basal ganglia and cerebellum with vertical gaze and pseudobulbar palsy, nuchal dystonia and dementia. *Arch Neurol* 1964, 10:333–359.

159. Lepore FE, Duvoisin RC: "Apraxia" of eyelid opening: an involuntary levator inhibition. *Neurology* 1985, 35:423–427.

160. Hakim S, Adams RD: The special clinical problem of symptomatic hydrocephalus with normal cerebrospinal fluid pressure: observations on cerebrospinal fluid hydrodynamics. *J Neurol Sci* 1965, 2:307–327.

161. Harris GJ, Pearlson GD, Peyser CE, *et al.*: Putamen volume reduction on magnetic resonance imaging exceeds caudate changes in mild Huntington's disease. *Ann Neurol* 1992, 31:69–75.

162. Kang UJ, Burke RE, Fahn S: Natural history and treatment of tardive dystonia. *Mov Disord* 1986, 1:193–208.

163. Hauser W, Hesdorffer D: *Epilepsy Frequency, Causes and Consequences*. New York: Demos; 1990.

164. Engel J Jr: *Seizures and Epilepsy*. Philadelphia: FA Davis, 1989.

165. Hauser WA, Annegers JF, Rocca WA: Descriptive epidemiology of epilepsy: contributions of population-based studies from Rochester, Minnesota. *Mayo Clin Proc* 1996, 71:576–586.

166. Camfield CS, Camfield PR, Gordon K, *et al.*: Incidence of epilepsy in childhood and adolescence: a population-based study in Nova Scotia from 1977 to 1985. *Epilepsia* 1996, 37:19–23.

167. Commission on Classification and Terminology of the International League Against Epilepsy. Proposal for revised clinical and electroencephalographic classification of epileptic seizures. *Epilepsia* 1981, 22:489–501.

168. Phillips HA, Scheffer IE, Berkovic SF, *et al.*: Localization of a gene for autosomal dominant nocturnal frontal lobe epilepsy to chromosome 20q 13.2 [letter] [see comments]. *Nat Genet* 1995, 10:117–118.

169. Steinlein OK: Neuronal nicotinic receptors in human epilepsy. *Eur J Pharmacol* 2000, 393:243–247.

170. Phillips HA, Scheffer IE, Crossland KM, *et al.*: Autosomal dominant nocturnal frontal-lobe epilepsy: genetic heterogeneity and evidence for a second locus at 15q24. *Am J Hum Genet* 1998, 63:1108–1116.

171. Scheffer I, Phillips H, Mulley J, *et al.*: Autosomal dominant partial epilepsy with variable foci is not allelic to autosomal dominant nocturnal frontal lobe epilepsy. *Epilepsia* 1995, 36:(suppl 3) S28.

172. Xiong L, Labuda M, Li DS, *et al.*: Mapping of a gene determining familial partial epilepsy with variable foci to chromosome 22q11-q12. *Am J Hum Genet* 1999, 65:1698–1710.

173. Scheffer IE, Jones L, Pozzebon M, *et al.*: Autosomal dominant rolandic epilepsy and speech dyspraxia: a new syndrome with anticipation. *Ann Neurol* 1995, 38:633–642.

174. Berkovic S, McIntosh A, Howell R, Hopper J: Familial temporal lobe epilepsy: a benign, unrecognized and common disorder. *Epilepsia* 1994, (suppl 8)35:109.

175. Ottman R, Risch N, Hauser WA, *et al.*: Localization of a gene for partial epilepsy to chromosome 10q [see comments]. *Nat Genet* 1995, 10:56–60.

176. Kuzniecky R, Rosenblatt B: Benign occipital epilepsy: a family study. *Epilepsia* 1987, 28:346–350.

177. Eksioglu YZ, Scheffer IE, Cardenas P, *et al.*: Periventricular heterotopia: an X-linked dominant epilepsy locus causing aberrant cerebral cortical development. *Neuron* 1996, 16:77–87.

178. Fox JW, Lamperti ED, Eksioglu YZ, *et al.*: Mutations in filamin 1 prevent migration of cerebral cortical neurons in human periventricular heterotopia. *Neuron* 1998, 21:1315–1325.

179. Leppert M, Anderson VE, Quattlebaum T, *et al.*: Benign familial neonatal convulsions linked to genetic markers on chromosome 20. *Nature* 1989, 337:647–648.

180. Singh NA, Charlier C, Stauffer D, *et al.*: A novel potassium channel gene, KCNQ2, is mutated in an inherited epilepsy of newborns. *Nat Genet* 1998, 18:25–29.

181. Lewis TB, Leach RJ, Warck K, *et al.*: Genetic heterogeneity in benign familial neonatal convulsions: identification of a new locus on chromosome 8q. *Am J Human Genet* 53:670–675.

182. Charlier C, Singh NA, Ryan SG, *et al.*: A pore mutation in a novel KQT-like potassium channel gene in an idiopathic epilepsy family. *Nat Genet* 1998, 18:53–55.

183. Guipponi M, Rivier F, Vigevano F, *et al.*: Linkage mapping of benign familial infantile convulsions (BFIC) to chromosome 19q. *Hum Mol Genet* 1997, 6:473–477.

184. Szepetowski P, Rochette J, Berquin P, *et al.*: Familial infantile convulsions and paroxysmal choreoathetosis: a new neurological syndrome linked to the pericentromeric region of human chromosome 16. *Am J Hum Genet* 1997, 61:889–898.

185. Lee WL, Tay A, Ong HT, *et al.*: Association of infantile convulsions with paroxysmal dyskinesias (ICCA syndrome): confirmation of linkage to human chromosome 16p12-q12 in a Chinese family. *Hum Genet* 1998, 103:608–612.

186. Wallace R, Berkovic S, Howell R, *et al.*: *J Med Genet* 1996, 33:308–312.

187. Johnson EW, Dubovsky J, Rich SS, *et al.*: Evidence for a novel gene for familial febrile convulsions, FEB2, linked to chromosome 19p in an extended family from the Midwest. *Hum Mol Genet* 1998, 7:63–67.

188. Peiffer A, Thompson J, Charlier C, *et al.*: A locus for febrile seizures (FEB3) maps to chromosome 2q23-24. *Ann Neurol* 1999, 46:671–678.

189. Nakayama J, Hamano K, Iwasaki N, *et al.*: Significant evidence for linkage of febrile seizures to chromosome 5q14-q15. *Hum Mol Genet* 2000, 9:87–91.

190. Wallace RH, Wang DW, Singh R, *et al.*: Febrile seizures and generalized epilepsy associated with a mutation in the Na(+)-channel beta-1 subunit gene SCN1B. *Nat Genet* 1998, 19:366–370.

191. Fong GCY, Shah PU, Gee MN, *et al.*: Childhood absence epilepsy with tonic-clonic seizures and electroencephalogram 3–4-Hz spike and multispike-slow wave complexes: linkage to chromosome 8q24. *Am J Hum Genet* 1998, 63:1117–1129.

192. Greenberg DA, Delgado-Escueta AV, Widelitz H, *et al.*: Juvenile myoclonic epilepsy (JME) may be linked to the BF and HLA loci on human chromosome 6. *Am J Med Genet* 1988, 31:185–192.

193. Liu AW, Delgado-Escueta AV, Serratosa JM, *et al.*: Juvenile myoclonic epilepsy locus in chromosome 6p21.2-p11: linkage to convulsions and electroencephalography trait. *Am J Hum Genet* 1995, 57:368–381.

194. Elmslie FV, Rees M, Williamson MP, *et al.*: Genetic mapping of a major susceptibility locus for juvenile myoclonic epilepsy on chromosome 15q. *Hum Mol Genet* 1997, 6:1329–1334.

195. Serratosa JM, Delgado-Escueta AV, Posada I, *et al.*: The gene for progressive myoclonus epilepsy of the Lafora type maps to chromosome 6q. *Hum Mol Genet* 1995, 4:1657–1663.

196. Minassian BA, Ianzano L, Meloche M, *et al.*: Mutation spectrum and predicted function of laforin in Lafora's progressive myoclonus epilepsy. *Neurology* 2000, 55:341–346.

197. Tahvanainen E, Ranta S, Hirvasniemi A, *et al.*: The gene for a recessively inherited human childhood progressive epilepsy with mental retardation maps to the distal short arm of chromosome 8. *Proc Natl Acad Sci U S A* 1994, 91:7267–7270.

198. Lehesjoki AE, Koskiniemi M, Norio R, *et al.*: Localization of the EPM1 gene for progressive myoclonus epilepsy on chromosome 21: linkage disequilibrium allows high resolution mapping. *Hum Mol Genet* 1993, 2:1229–1234.

199. Lehesjoki AE, Eldridge R, Eldridge J, *et al.*: Progressive myoclonus epilepsy of Unverricht-Lundborg type: a clinical and molecular genetic study of a family from the United States with four affected sibs. *Neurology* 1993, 43:2384–2386.

200. Alakurtti K, Virtaneva K, Joensuu T, *et al.*: Characterization of the cystatin B gene promoter harboring the dodecamer repeat expanded in progressive myoclonus epilepsy, EPM1. *Gene* 2000, 242:65–73.

201. Pennacchio LA, Lehesjoki AE, Stone NE, *et al.*: Mutations in the gene encoding cystatin B in progressive myoclonus epilepsy (EPM1) [see comments]. *Science* 1996, 271:1731–1734.

202. Mikami M, Yasuda T, Terao A, *et al.*: Localization of a gene for benign adult familial myoclonic epilepsy to chromosome 8q23.3-q24.1. *Am J Hum Genet* 1999, 65:745–751.

203. Chomyn A, Lai ST, Shakeley R, *et al.*: Platelet-mediated transformation of mtDNA-less human cells: analysis of phenotypic variability among clones from normal individuals—and complementation behavior of the tRNALys mutation causing myoclonic epilepsy and ragged red fibers. *Am J Hum Genet* 1994, 54:966–974.

204. Shoffner JM, Wallace DC: Mitochondrial genetics: principles and practice. *Am J Hum Genet* 1992, 51:1179–1186.

205. Minassian BA, DeLorey TM, Olsen RW, *et al.*: Angelman syndrome: correlations between epilepsy phenotypes and genotypes. *Ann Neurol* 1998, 43:485–493.

206. Jennett B: Epilepsy and acute traumatic intracranial haematoma. *J Neurol Neurosurg Psychiatry* 1975, 38:378–381.

207. McKusick VA, ed. Online Mendelian Inheritance in Man. Bethesda, MD: National Center for Biotechnology Information, National Library of Medicine; 2000. Available at: http://www.ncbi.nlm.nih.gov/omim/. Accessed October, 2000.

208. Jennett B: Epilepsy and acute traumatic intracranial haematoma. *J Neurol Neurosurg Psychiatry* 1975, 38:378–381.

209. Jennett B: Early traumatic epilepsy. Incidence and significance after nonmissile injuries. *Arch Neurol* 1974, 30:394–398.

210. Jennett B, Van De Sande J: EEG prediction of post-traumatic epilepsy. *Epilepsia* 1975, 16:251–256.

211. Courville CB: Traumatic Lesions of the Temporal Lobe as the Essential Cause of Psychomotor Epilepsy. In Temporal Lobe Epilepsy. Edited by Baldwin M, Bailey P. Springfield, IL: Charles C. Thomas; 1958:220–239.

212. Hauser WA, Anderson VE, Loewenson RB, McRoberts SM: Seizure recurrence after a first unprovoked seizure. *N Engl J Med* 1982, 307:522–528.

213. Hart RG, Easton JD: Seizure recurrence after a first, unprovoked seizure. *Arch Neurol* 1986, 43:1289–1290.

214. Asbury AK: New Aspects of Disease of the Peripheral Nervous System, In *Harrison's Principles of Internal Medicine with CME Examination, Update IV.* Edited by Isselbacher KJ, Adams RD, Braunwald E, *et al.* New York: McGraw-Hill; 1983:211–229.

215. Mahadevan M, Tsilfidis C, Sabourin L, *et al.*: Myotonic dystrophy mutation: an unstable CTG repeat in the 39 untranslated region of the gene. *Science* 1992, 255:1253–1255.

216. Paulson HL, Fischbeck KH: Trinucleotide repeats in neurogenetic disorders. *Annu Rev Neurosci* 1996, 19:79–107.

217. Sigurgeirsson B, Lindelof B, Edhag O, Allander E: Risk of cancer in patients with dermatomyositis or polymyositis: a population-based study. *N Engl J Med* 1992, 326:363–367.

218. Roos KL, Tunkel AR, Scheld WM: Acute Bacterial Meningitis in Children and Adults. In *Infections of the Central Nervous System* edn 2. Edited by Scheld WM, Whitley RJ, Durack PT. Philadelphia: Lippincott-Raven; 1997:335–401.

219. Gold R: Epidemiology of bacterial meningitis. *Infect Dis Clin North* Am 1999, 13:515–525.

220. Rosenstein NE, Perkins BA: Update on Haemophilus influenzae serotype b and meningococcal vaccines. *Pediatr Clin North Am* 2000, 47:337–352.

221. Schuchat A, Robinson K, Wenger JD, *et al.*: Bacterial meningitis in the United States in 1995. *N Engl J Med* 1997, 14:970–976.

222. Gelfand MS, Bakhtian BJ, Simmons BP: Spinal sepsis due to *Streptococcus milleri*: two cases and review. *Rev Infect Dis* 1991, 13:559–563.

223. Wispelwey B, Dacey RG Jr, Scheld WM: Brain Abscess. In *Infections of the Central Nervous System* edn 2. Edited by Scheld WM, Whitley RJ, Durack DT. Philadelphia: Lippincott-Raven; 1997:463–493.

224. Falcone S, Post MJ: Encephalitis, cerebritis, and brain abscess: pathophysiology and imaging findings. *Neuroimaging Clin North Am 2000*, 10:333–353.

225. Jubelt B: The Diagnosis of Viral Meningitis and Encephalitis. In *Neurology and Neurosurgery Update Series* vol 2, no 30. Edited by Scheinberg P, Davidoff RA, Arnason BGW. Princeton NJ: Education Center; 1981.

226. Carpenter CCJ, Cooper DA, Fischl MA, et al.: Antiretroviral therapy in adults: updated recommendations of the International AIDS Society–USA Panel. *JAMA* 2000, 283:381–390.

227. Blankson J, Siliciano RF: Interleukin 2 treatment for HIV infection. *JAMA* 2000, 284:236–238.

228. Simon RP: Neurosyphilis. *Arch Neurol* 1985, 42:606–613.

229. Davis E: Spirochetal Disease. In *Diseases of the Nervous System: Clinical Neurobiology* edn 2. Edited by Asbury AK, McKhann GM, McDonald WI. Philadelphia: WB Saunders; 1992:1359–1370.

230. Cameron ML, Durack DT: Helminthic infections. In *Infections of the Central Nervous System* edn 2. Edited by Scheld WM, Whitley RJ, Durack DT. New York: Raven Press; 1997:845–878.

231. Glaser JS: Topical diagnosis: Prechiasmal visual pathways. In *Neuroophthalmology* edn 2. Edited by Glaser JS. Philadelphia: JB Lippincott; 1990:123–128.

232. Francis DA, Compston DA, Batchelor JR, *et al.*: A reassessment of the risk of MS developing in patients with optic neuritis after extended follow-up. *J Neurol Neurosurg Psychiatry* 1987, 50:758–765.

233. Leys D, Petit H, Block AM, *et al.*: Neuromyelitis optica (Devic's disease): four cases. *Rev Neurol* (Paris) 1987, 143:722.

234. Yock DH: White Matter Disorders. In *Magnetic Resonance Imaging of CNS Disease*, Chap. 7. St. Louis: Mosby Year–Book; 1995.

235. Thorp JW, Miller DH: MRI: its application and impact. *Internat MS J* 1994,1:7–15.

236. Parry GJ: Inflammatory demyelinating polyneuropathies: new perspectives in treatment. *Adv Neuroimmunol* 1994, 1:9–15.

237. Mendell J: Neuromuscular junction disorders: A guide to diagnosis and treatment. *Adv Neuroimmunol* 1994, 1:9–16.

238. Dalakas MC: Polymyositis, dermatomyositis, and inclusion-body myositis. *N Engl J Med* 1991, 325:1487–1498.

239. Villee CA, Solomon EP, Martin CE, *et al.*: *Biology* edn 2. Philadelphia: WB Saunders; 1989.

240. Lieber CS: *Medical and Nutritional Complications of Alcoholism*. New York: Plenum; 1992.

241. Headache Classification Committee of the International Headache Society: Classification and diagnostic criteria for headache disorders, cranial neuralgias and facial pain. *Cephalalgia* 1988, 7:1–96.

242. Launer LJ, Terwindt GM, Ferrari MD: The prevalence and characteristics of migraine in a population-based cohort: the GEM study. *Neurology* 1999, 53(3):537–542.

243. Stewart WF, Linet MS, Celentano DD, *et al.*: Age- and sex-specific incidence rates of migraine with and without aura. *Am J Epidemiol* 1991, 134:1111–1120.

244. Stewart WF, Lipton RB, Liberman J: Variation in migraine prevalence by race. *Neurology* 1996, 47(1):52–59.

245. Lipton RB, Stewart WF: Acute migraine therapy. *Headache* 1999, 39:S20–S26.

246. Hu XH, Markson LE, Lipton RB, *et al.*: Burden of migraine in the United States: disability and economic costs. *Arch Intern Med* 1999, 159(8):813–818.

247. Terwindt GM, Ferrari MD, Tijhuis M, *et al.*: The impact of migraine on quality of life in the general population: the GEM study. *Neurology* 2000, 55:624–629.

248. Couch JR: Complexities of presentation and pathogenesis of migraine headache. In *Treating the Headache Patient*. Edited by Cady RK, Fox AW. New York: Marcel Dekker; 1995.

249. Lenaerts M: Migraine and epilepsy: comorbidity and temporal relationship. Paper presented at: Ninth Congress of the International Society; June 1999; Barcelona, Spain.

250. Merikangas KR, Merikangas JR, Angst J: Headache syndromes and psychiatric disorders: association and familial transmission. *J Psychiatr Res* 1993, 27:197–210.

251. Mathew NT, Kailasam J, Meadors L, *et al.*: Intravenous valproate sodium (depacon) aborts migraine rapidly: a preliminary report. *Headache* 2000, 40(9):720–723.

252. Goadsby PJ, Hargreaves RJ: Mechanisms of action of serotonin 5-HT1B/D agonists: insights into migraine pathophysiology using rizatriptan. *Neurology* 2000, 55:S8–S14.

253. Goadsby PJ: The scientific basis of medication choice in symptomatic migraine treatment. *Can J Neurol Sci* 1999, 26:20–26.

254. Humphrey PP, Feniuk W: Mode of action of the anti-migraine drug sumatriptan. *Trends Pharmacol Sci* 1991, 12:444–446.

255. Silberstein SD: Rizatriptan versus usual care in long-term treatment of migraine. *Neurology* 2000, 55:S25–S28.

256. Solomon GD, Cady RK, Klapper JA, *et al.*: Clinical efficacy and tolerability of 2.5 mg zolmitriptan for the acute treatment of migraine. *Neurology* 1997, 49:1219–1225.

257. Nappi G, Sicuteri F, Byrne M, *et al.*: Oral sumatriptan compared with placebo in the acute treatment of migraine. *J Neurol* 1994, 241:138–144.

258. Sargent J, Kirchner J, Davis R, Kirkhart B: Oral sumatriptan is effective and well tolerated for the acute treatment of migraine: results of a multicenter study. *Neurology* 1995, 45:S10–S14.

259. Tfelt-Hansen P, Ryan RE Jr: Oral therapy for migraine: comparisons between rizatriptan and sumatriptan. A review of four randomized, double-blind clinical trials. *Neurology* 2000, 55:S19–S24.

260. The International 311C90 Long-term Study Group: The long-term tolerability and efficacy of oral zolmitriptan (Zomig, 311C90) in the acute treatment of migraine. An international study. *Headache* 1998, 38:173–183.

261. Cady RK, Lipton RB, Hall C, *et al.*: Treatment of mild headache in disabled migraine sufferers: results of the Spectrum Study. *Headache* 2000, 40(10):792–797.

262. Lipton RB, Stewart WF, Cady R, *et al.*: Sumatriptan for the range of headaches in migraine sufferers: results of the Spectrum Study. *Headache* 2000, 40(10):1–9.

Oncology

DAVID S. ETTINGER

The field of oncology has grown rapidly, and this growth will continue because of the advances in molecular medicine. Advances have been seen in the areas of prevention, screening, diagnosis, treatment, and supportive care of a wide variety of cancers.

Oncology is a subspecialty that, in addition to subspecialty care, involves primary care of cancer patients. From the time a diagnosis of cancer is made, through the consideration and provision of the various available treatments, whether with palliative or curative intent, to possible cure, long-term treatment, or terminal care, the continuum of care that should be available to patients with cancer requires a seamless coordination among many health care providers.

It is important for primary care physicians to keep up with advances in order to care properly for their patients either by themselves or by referring their patients to an appropriate oncologic subspecialist.

This chapter provides the busy primary care physician with up-to-date, concise, easy-to-read, understandable, and useful information for preventing, diagnosing, staging, and treating various malignancies and their complications.

■ CANCER PREVENTION AND CONTROL

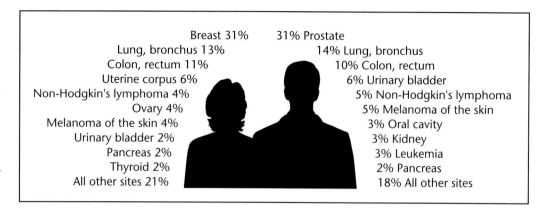

Breast 31%   31% Prostate
Lung, bronchus 13%   14% Lung, bronchus
Colon, rectum 11%   10% Colon, rectum
Uterine corpus 6%   6% Urinary bladder
Non-Hodgkin's lymphoma 4%   5% Non-Hodgkin's lymphoma
Ovary 4%   5% Melanoma of the skin
Melanoma of the skin 4%   3% Oral cavity
Urinary bladder 2%   3% Kidney
Pancreas 2%   3% Leukemia
Thyroid 2%   2% Pancreas
All other sites 21%   18% All other sites

FIGURE 9-1.

Estimated new cancer cases in the United States, 2001, by gender. Prostate cancer is the most prevalent cancer in men; there will be an estimated 198,100 new cases in the United States in 2001. The incidence of prostate cancer increases with age; more than 70% of all prostate cancers are diagnosed in men over 65. The incidence rates are higher for blacks than for whites. In women, breast cancer is most prevalent, with an estimated 192,200 new cases expected in the United States in 2001. Lung cancer is ranked second both for men and women with 169,500 estimated new cases in 2001 (90,700 in men, 78,800 in women). (*Adapted from* Greenlee [1].)

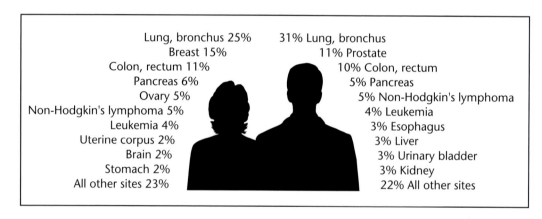

Lung, bronchus 25%   31% Lung, bronchus
Breast 15%   11% Prostate
Colon, rectum 11%   10% Colon, rectum
Pancreas 6%   5% Pancreas
Ovary 5%   5% Non-Hodgkin's lymphoma
Non-Hodgkin's lymphoma 5%   4% Leukemia
Leukemia 4%   3% Esophagus
Uterine corpus 2%   3% Liver
Brain 2%   3% Urinary bladder
Stomach 2%   3% Kidney
All other sites 23%   22% All other sites

FIGURE 9-2.

Estimated cancer deaths in the United States, 2001, by gender. In both men and women, lung cancer is ranked number one in deaths due to a malignancy. It is estimated that 157,400 (90,100 men, 67,300 women) people will die from lung cancer in 2001. For colorectal, breast, and prostate cancer, the estimated deaths in 2001 are 56,700, 40,600, and 31,500 respectively. (*Adapted from* Greenlee [1].)

Recommendations for Early Detection of Cancer for Normal Risk, Asymptomatic People

Cancer Site	Population	Test or Procedure	Frequency
Breast*	Women, age 20+	Breast self-exam	Monthly, age 20+
		Clinical breast exam	Every 3 years, age 20–39; annually, age 40+
		Mammography	Annually, age 40+
Colorectal‡	Men and women, age 50+	Fecal occult blood test (FOBT)	Annually
		Flexible sigmoidoscopy	Every 5 years
		Fecal occult blood test and flexible sigmoidoscopy§	Annually FOBT and flexible sigmoidoscopy every 5 years, beginning at age 50
		Double-contrast barium enema†	DCBE every 5–10 years, beginning at age 50
		Colonoscopy†	Colonoscopy every 10 years, beginning at age 50
Prostate¶	Men, age 50+	Digital rectal examination and prostate-specific antigen test	Annual digital rectal examination and prostate-specific antigen should be offered to men 50 years and older.
Cervix **	Female, age 18+	Pap test and pelvic examination	All women who are, or have been, sexually active, or have reached aged 18, should have annual Pap test and pelvic examination. After a woman has had > 3 consecutive satisfactory normal annual examinations, the Pap test may be performed less frequently at the discretion of her physician.
Cancer-related checkup	Men and women, age 20+	Examinations every 3 years between ages 20–39 years; annually, age 40+	The cancer-related checkup should include examination for cancers of the thyroid, testicles or ovaries, lymph nodes, oral cavity, and skin; and health counseling about tobacco, sun exposure, diet and nutrition, risk factors, sexual practices, and environmental and occupational exposures.

*The American Cancer Society (ACS), American College of Radiology (ACR), and American Medical Association (AMA) endorse the guidelines shown. The National Cancer Institute (NCI) recommends mammography every 1–2 years for women in their forties and mammography every 1–2 years for women aged 50 years and older. The United States Preventive Services Task Force (USPSTF) recommends mammography every 1–2 years for women aged 50–69 years.

†Beginning at age 40, annual clinical breast examination should be done prior to mammography.

‡The ACS, ACR, American College of Gastroenterology, American Gastroenterological Association, American Society of Colon and Rectal Surgeons, American Society for Gastrointestinal Endoscopy, Crohn's and Colitis Foundation of America, Oncology Nursing Society, and Society of American Gastrointestinal Endoscopic Surgeons have endorsed these guidelines for average risk adults. ACS guidelines do not include FOBT alone except under circumstances where flexible sigmoidoscopy is unavailable; ACS guidelines do not endorse flexible sigmoidoscopy alone. The USPSTF recommends screening for adults aged 50 years and older with annual FOBT or sigmoidoscopy (periodicity unspecified).

§Digital rectal exam should be done at the time of sigmoidoscopy, barium enema, and colonoscopy.

¶The ACS and the American College of Physicians have recommended that men should be made aware of the availability of prostate cancer screening, and that physicians should be prepared to discuss the benefits and limitations of screening and risks associated with treatment. The American Society of Internal Medicine, NCI, American Association of Family Physicians (AAFP), USPSTF, and American College of Preventive Medicine do not recommend that providers routinely offer prostate cancer screening to patients.

**This guideline represents a consensus between the ACS, NCI, AMA, AAFP, and the American College of Obstetricians and Gynecologists. The USPSTF recommends routine Pap testing for women who are or who have been sexually active, beginning with the onset of sexual activity and repeated at least every 3 years.

FIGURE 9-3.

Recommendations for early detection of cancer for normal risk, asymptomatic people. For the physician, screening begins with a thorough history and physical examination. The guidelines represent the recommendations of the various organizations interested in screening guidelines.

■ HEAD AND NECK CANCER

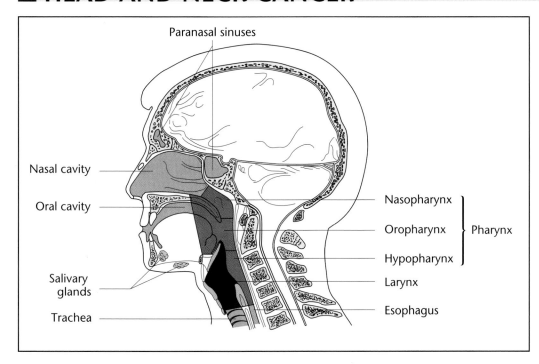

Paranasal sinuses
Nasal cavity
Oral cavity
Salivary glands
Trachea
Nasopharynx
Oropharynx ⎫ Pharynx
Hypopharynx ⎭
Larynx
Esophagus

FIGURE 9-4.

Anatomic regions of head and neck. Head and neck cancer includes malignancies arising from several different anatomic sites. Different staging principles are defined for each region. Squamous cell carcinoma is the most common histopathologic classification. Tobacco in all of its forms is the single most important risk factor. Tobacco-induced carcinogenesis is greatly enhanced in the presence of alcohol. (*Courtesy of* Everett E. Vokes.)

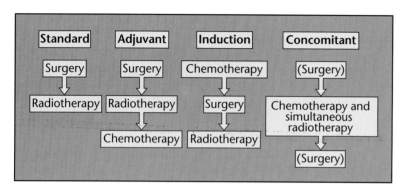

FIGURE 9-5.

Tumor stage classification for head and neck cancer. The natural history of head and neck cancer is characterized by local and regional disease progression. The staging system is based on a TNM classification, where *T* represents the size of the primary tumor, *N* describes the number and size of regionally enlarged lymph nodes, and *M* characterizes distant involvement most frequently in bone, lungs, or liver. The T and N stages are used to assign an overall stage (I through IV) to the tumor. More than 50% of patients with head and neck cancer present with locoregionally advanced disease (stage III or IV). (*Courtesy of* Everett E. Vokes.)

FIGURE 9-6.

Sequencing of multimodality therapy for head and neck cancer. *Parentheses* indicate optional use. Standard therapy focuses on local treatment modalities reflecting the locoregional predominance of the disease. Patients with stage I or II disease are treated with curative intent using either surgery or radiotherapy. A total of 60% to 80% of patients with such disease will be cured. However, the low cure rate following standard therapy for patients with stage III or IV disease has led to adjuvant induction and concomitant therapy. (*Courtesy of* Everett E. Vokes.)

■ THORACIC NEOPLASMS

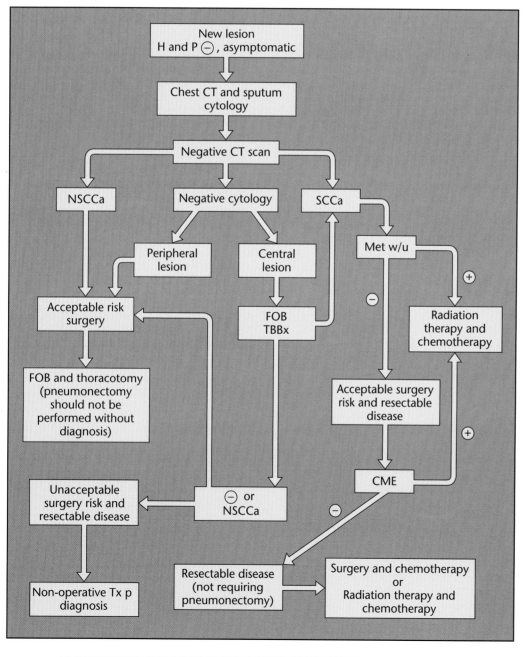

FIGURE 9-7.

Algorithm for patients with a suspicious new lung nodule and a negative chest computed tomography (CT) scan. The major pathologic types of lung cancer are adenocarcinoma, squamous cell carcinoma, large cell undifferentiated carcinoma, and small cell carcinoma. Adenocarcinoma is the most frequent histologic subtype of non–small cell cancer (NSCCa). The purpose of staging NSCCa is to determine the appropriate therapy and prognosis. In part, it is to differentiate disease that is lung cancer (SCCa) despite an early stage, is rarely a surgical disease. Adenocarcinoma accounts for less than 5% of patients diagnosed with SCCa. For early stage SCCa, the primary therapy is both radiation therapy and chemotherapy. CME—cervical mediastinoscopy; FOB—fiberoptic bronchoscopy; H and P—history and physical; Met w/u—metastatic work-up; TBBx—transbronchial biopsy; Tx p—therapy after. (*Adapted from* Nesbitt *et al.* [3].)

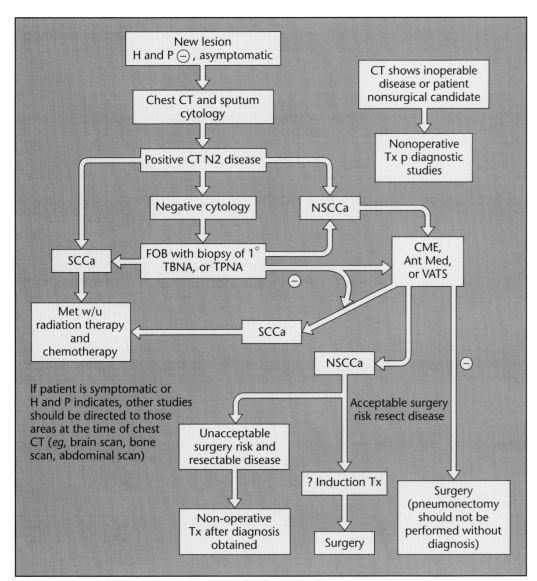

FIGURE 9-8.

Algorithm for patients with a suspicious new lung nodule and a chest computed tomography (CT) scan showing mediastinal lymphadenopathy. Patients with mediastinal lymph node disease have either stage IIIA or stage IIIB disease. Whereas the former may be resectable, the latter is not. If a patient has known mediastinal disease (stage IIIA), consideration could be given to induction chemotherapy ± radiation therapy (RT) or chemotherapy and RT prior to possibly resecting the disease. For unresectable stage IIIA disease, the treatment is usually a combination of chemotherapy and RT. Stage IIIB disease is usually treated with radiation therapy or a combination or radiation therapy and chemotherapy. Metastatic disease (stage IV) is treated with chemotherapy. Ant Med—anterior mediastinoscopy; CME—cervical mediastinoscopy; FOB—fiberoptic bronchoscopy; H and P—history and physical; Met w/u—metastatic work-up; N2—mediastinal lymph nodes; NSCCa—non–small cell carcinoma; SCCa—small cell carcinoma; TBNA—transbronchial needle aspiration; TPNA—transthoracic percutaneous needle aspiration; Tx—therapy; Tx p—therapy after; VATS—video-assisted thoracoscopy. (*Adapted from* Nesbitt *et al.* [3].)

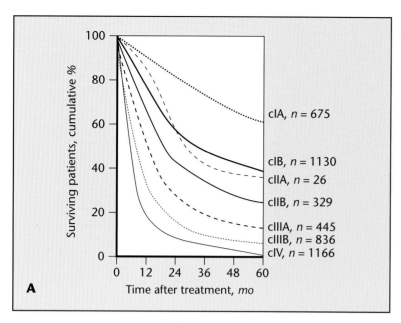

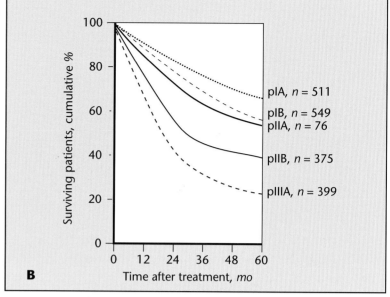

FIGURE 9-9.

Cumulative survival of patients with lung cancer according to (**A**) clinical stage and (**B**) surgical stage. **A**, Cumulative proportion of patients with non-small cell lung cancer expected to survive 5 years according to clinical stage of disease. Pairwise comparisons: cIA vs cIB, $P < 0.05$; cIB vs cIIA, $P > 0.05$; cIIA vs cIIB, $P < 0.05$; cIIB vs cIIIA, $P < 0.05$; cIIIB vs cIV, $P < 0.05$. **B**, Cumulative proportion of patients with non-small cell lung cancer expected to survive 5 years according to surgical pathologic stage. Pairwise comparisons: pIA vs pIB, $P < 0.05$; pIB vs pIIA, $P >$; pIIA vs pIIB, $P < 0.05$; pIIB vs pIIIA, $P < 0.05$. Surgical pathologic staging of lung cancer is more accurate than clinical staging. Based on clinical staging, approximately 10%

of lung cancer patients will have stage I disease (T_1N_0, T_2N_0) and has a 50% or greater 5-year survival rate. Stage II disease (T_1N_1, T_2N_1, T_3N_0) occurs in 20% of patients and has a 20% to 40% 5-year survival rate. Approximately 20% of patients will have stage III disease. Fifteen percent will have stage IIIa disease ($T_{1-3}N_2$, T_3N_1). This is considered a surgical disease in selected patients. The 5-year survival rate is 15% to 30%. Stage IIIB disease (T_4N_{0-3}, any TN_3) accounts for another 15% of patients and has a 5-year survival rate of 5%. Stage IV disease (M_1) accounts for 40% of non-small cell lung cancer and has a 2% 5-year survival rate. (*Adapted from* Mountain [4].)

■ MEDIASTINAL TUMORS

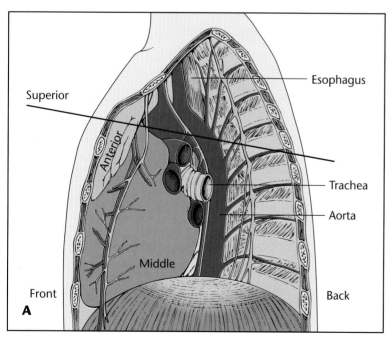

B. Occurrence of Tumors in the Mediastinal Divisions

Superior (30%)
  Lymphoma
  Thyroid tumors
  Bronchogenic cysts
  Thymoma and thymic cysts
  Parathyroid adenoma
Anterior (20%)
  Lymphoma
  Thymoma and thymic cysts
  Germ cell tumors*
  Thyroid tumors
  Pericardial cysts
  Lipoma

Middle (20%)
  Lymphoma
  Bronchogenic cysts
  Pericardial cysts
  Sarcoidosis
  Lung cancer
Posterior (30%)
  Neurogenic tumors
  Lymphoma
  Esophageal tumors and cysts
  Fibrosarcoma
  Spinal column tumors
  Pheochromocytoma
  Paraganglioma

*Germ cell tumors include malignant types and the more common seminomas and teratomas (dermoid cysts).

FIGURE 9-10.

Tumors of the mediastinum. **A**, The customary subdivisions of the mediastinum. **B**, A partial listing of mediastinal tumors and the relative frequency of occurrence of tumors in the various mediastinal

divisions. About 25% of mediastinal tumors are malignant. There is some overlap in cell types. (*Adapted from* Skarin [5].)

■ BREAST CANCER

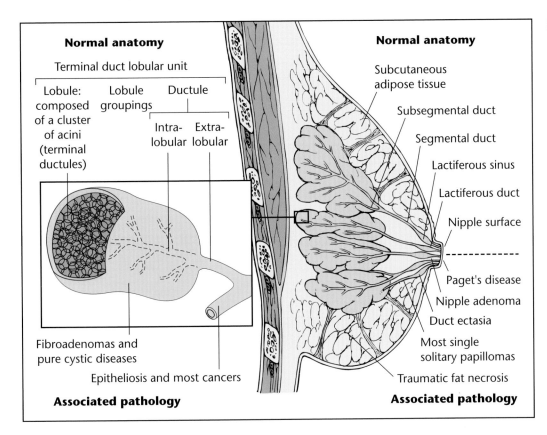

Normal anatomy

Terminal duct lobular unit

Lobule:
composed
of a cluster
of acini
(terminal
ductules)

Lobule
groupings

Ductule

Intra-
lobular

Extra-
lobular

Fibroadenomas and
pure cystic diseases

Epitheliosis and most cancers

Associated pathology

Normal anatomy

Subcutaneous
adipose tissue

Subsegmental duct

Segmental duct

Lactiferous sinus

Lactiferous duct

Nipple surface

Paget's disease

Nipple adenoma

Duct ectasia

Most single
solitary papillomas

Traumatic fat necrosis

Associated pathology

FIGURE 9-11.

Breast anatomy, normal and abnormal. Within the breast, the epithelial elements are organized into lobular units consisting of acini that feed into ductules. The latter in turn coalesce into larger ducts that form a reservoir, or lactiferous sinus, proximal to the nipple. These epithelial structures, supported by adipose and fibrous tissue, give rise to more than 95% of breast malignancies. Adenocarcinoma of the breast can be divided into invasive and noninvasive (carcinoma *in situ*) types. The most common type of invasive breast cancer is infiltrating ductal carcinoma, accounting for approximately 75% to 80% of cases. Carcinoma *in situ* is characterized by proliferation of malignant cells within the ducts or lobules of the breast without invasion of the stromal tissue on light microscopic examination. The major subtypes of noninvasive breast cancer care ductal carcinoma *in situ* (DCIS) and lobular carcinoma *in situ* (LCIS). DCIS now represents 10% to 15% of all breast cancers and 20% to 30% of those detected mammographically. (*Adapted from* Skarin [6].)

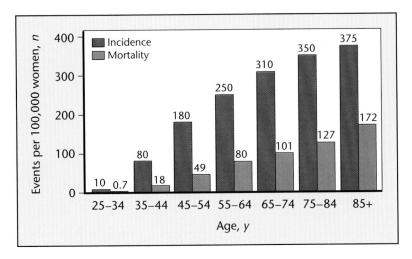

FIGURE 9-12.

Breast cancer incidence and mortality by age. The incidence of breast cancer has been increasing for the past 30 years, with an increase of 2% to 4% per year in the past decade. During this period, the mortality rate has remained essentially unchanged. The risks of developing and dying of breast cancer are age-related, with the greatest risk expressed in patients older than 45 years of age. It is estimated that 12% of American women will develop breast cancer during their lives and 3.5% will die of the disease. (*Courtesy of* James J. Perry and Hyman B. Muss.)

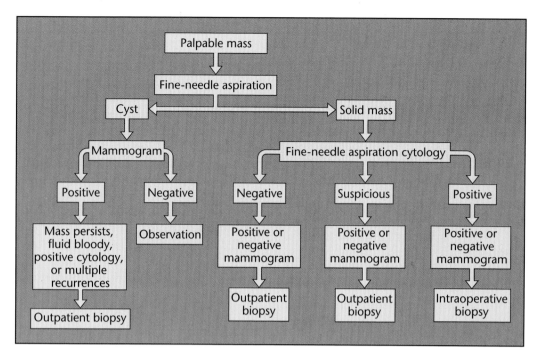

FIGURE 9-13.

Suggested management of palpable breast masses in women. Mammography is not used to evaluate adolescents, and subareolar masses are not removed from the developing breasts of pubertal girls. Whether observation is an appropriate alternative in the management of a palpable mass that is benign according to physical examination, mammography, and cytologic examination is controversial. For patients with a palpable breast mass, mammography may help to define the lesion but cannot substitute for a tissue diagnosis. Mammographic results are negative in 10% to 15% of women with breast cancer, particularly young premenopausal women with dense breast tissue. (*Adaped from* Donegan [7].)

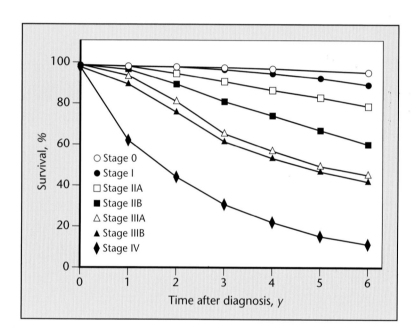

FIGURE 9-14.

Breast cancer survival rates according to the American Joint Committee on Cancer Stage. At diagnosis, more than 50% of patients have disease confined to the breast alone (stages 0, I), approximately 30% to 40% have ipsilateral regional lymph node involvement (stage II, III), and fewer than 10% present with disease (stage IV). (*Adapted from* Beahrs *et al.* [8].)

A. Risk Categories for Selection of Therapy in Early-stage Breast Cancer Patients

Factors	Minimal/Low Risk (Has All Listed Findings)	Intermediate Risk	High Risk (Has At Least One Factor)
Nodal status*	Negative	Negative	Positive
Tumor size*	≤ 1 cm	≥ 1–2 cm	≥ 2 cm
ER and/or PgR status	Positive	Positive	Negative
Grade[†]	Grade 1	Grade1–2	Grade 2–3
Age	≥ 35		< 35

*Determined pathologically.
[†] Histologic and/or nuclear grade.

B. Treatment Recommendations for Node-negative and Node-positive Patients

Patient Group	Minimal/Low Risk	Node-negative Patients Intermediate Risk	High Risk	Node-positive Patients
Premenopausal, ER, or PgR positive	None or tamoxifen	Chemotherapy + tamoxifen*,[†]	Chemotherapy + tamoxifen[†]	Chemotherapy + tamoxifen[†]
Premenopausal, ER, and PgR negative	Not applicable	NA	Chemotherapy	Chemotherapy
Postmenopausal, ER, or PgR positive	None or tamoxifen	Tamoxifen + chemotherapy*	Tamoxifen + chemotherapy	Tamoxifen + chemotherapy
Postmenopausal, ER, and PgR negative	Not applicable	NA	Chemotherapy	Chemotherapy

*Tamoxifen alone can be considered for certain patients depending on age, size of tumor, other medical problems, psychosocial issues, and personal assessment of risks and benefits of adjuvant therapy.
[†]The additional role of ovarian ablation (surgical, medical, or radiotherapeutic) is still under active investigation.

FIGURE 9-15.

Consensus treatment recommendations for patients with primary breast cancer. **A, B,** Minimal/low risk is defined as an estimated > 90% chance of remaining disease-free at 10 years; intermediate risk is defined as 80%–90% chance of remaining disease-free at 10 years; high risk is defined as < 70%–80% chance of being disease-free at 10 years. ER—estrogen receptor; NA—not applicable; PgR—progesterone receptor. (*Data from* Goldhirsch [9].)

■ COLORECTAL CANCER

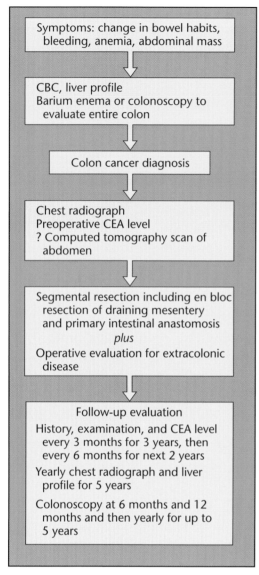

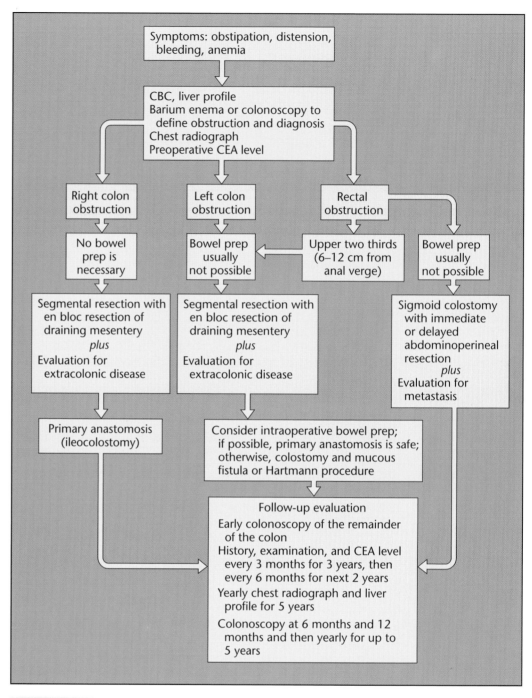

FIGURE 9-16.

Management of nonobstructing colon carcinomas. Colorectal carcinoma is the third most common carcinoma in both men and women in the United States. The average age at presentation is 60 to 65 years, but there appears to be an increase in younger patients. Right-sided lesions tend to grow into the bowel lumen and therefore are insidious at onset. Patients can present with vague abdominal pain, anemia, or blood in the stool. Others present with an abdominal mass on physical examination. Once colorectal carcinoma has been detected, it is necessary to complete surgical resection of all gross malignant disease and lymph node draining the primary area. CBC—complete blood count; CEA—carcinoembryonic antigen. (*Adapted from* Beart [10].)

FIGURE 9-17.

Management of obstructing colorectal carcinomas. Patients with left-sided colon lesions are more likely to present with partial obstruction; crampy, colicky pain; a change in bowel habits (*eg*, constipation alternating with diarrhea); or decreased stool caliber. For obstructing colon carcinoma, the primary treatment is surgical resection; for obstructing rectal carcinoma, a diverting procedure (*eg*, colostomy) may be the treatment choice. CBC—complete blood count; CEA—carcinoembryonic antigen. (*Adapted from* Beart [10].)

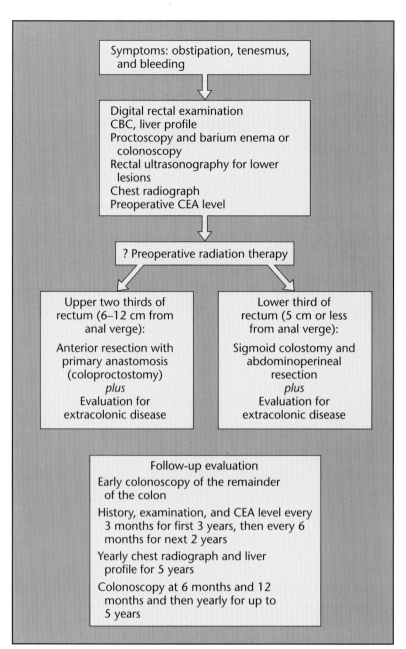

FIGURE 9-18.

Management of rectal carcinomas. Advanced rectal carcinoma is associated with symptoms such as tenesmus and pelvic pain, implying invasion into the local tissue and sacral nerve roots. Despite surgical resection of rectal carcinoma, the local recurrence rate is high. Therefore, the standard treatment after resection of a rectal tumor with positive lymph nodes (Duke's C) or rectal wall invasion (Duke's B) is chemotherapy and radiation. CBC—complete blood count; CEA—carcinoembryonic antigen. (*Adapted from* Beart [10].)

■ PANCREATIC CANCER

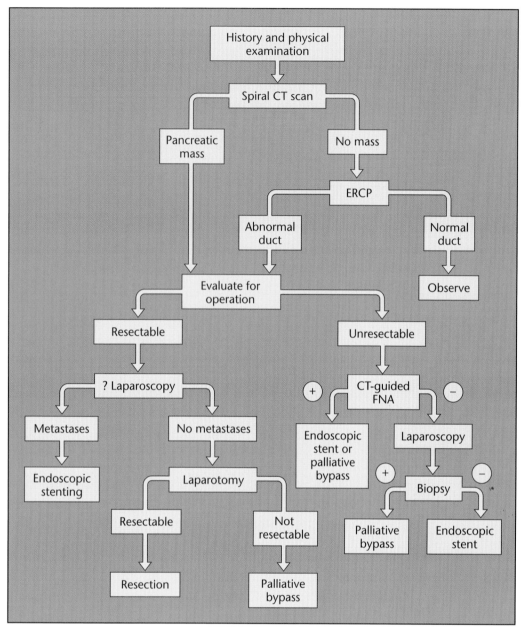

FIGURE 9-19.

When the history and physical examination suggest the possibility of pancreatic cancer, the first diagnostic test the authors use is a spiral computed tomography (CT) scan. If a pancreatic mass is detected, then the patient is evaluated for operation. If no mass is seen on CT scan, then the patient will undergo an endoscopic retrograde cholangiopancreatography (ERCP). If the ERCP demonstrates normal pancreatic and common bile ducts, then the patient may be observed with close follow-up. If the duct anatomy is abnormal, then the patient is evaluated for operation. Some endoscopists may also obtain endoscopic needle aspiration or duct brushings at this point as well.

Patients are evaluated for operation on the basis of CT evidence for resectability and presence of metastases. If the CT scan demonstrates metastases or definite involvement of the major vessels (*eg*, portal vein or superior mesenteric artery) by tumor, the patient's diseases are classified as unresectable. Other factors that may influence whether or not a patient is an operative candidate are their ages and general overall medical condition.

In patients determined to be candidates for operation, the use of laparoscopy as a first step is controversial. Advocates perform laparoscopy to determine if there are any peritoneal or liver metastases present that were not detected by the CT scan. If metastases are present, laparotomy is avoided and the patient may undergo endoscopic stenting. If no metastases are detected by laparoscopy, the patient will undergo laparotomy. Intraoperative determination of resectability will then determine whether or not the patient is a candidate for a resection of the tumor or a palliative bypass procedure. If a patient is not an operative candidate, tissue confirmation of pancreatic cancer is the next step; this is done using CT- or ultrasound-guided fine-needle aspiration (FNA). Endoscopic FNA, biopsy, or brushings are also options. If the biopsy is positive, then the patient can undergo endoscopic stenting or be reevaluated for a palliative bypass. If the biopsy is negative, the patient can undergo laparoscopy and biopsy.

■ LIVER CANCER (PRIMARY OR METASTATIC)

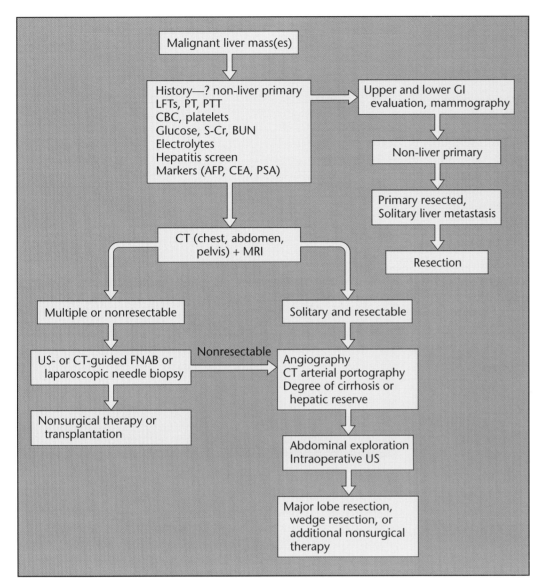

FIGURE 9-20.

Algorithm for evaluating solid liver lesions. The liver is the largest visceral organ in the human body. Since it is a frequent site for metastatic disease, it is important to determine whether or not a malignant liver mass is a primary liver cancer or metastatic. The frequency of hepatic metastases for the common primary carcinoma is as follows: 70% colorectal, 60% breast, 50% to 70% pancreas, 30% to 50% lung, and 35% to 40% renal. Resection of isolated hepatic metastases from colorectal carcinoma can produce a 30% 5-year survival rate. AFP—α-fetoprotein; BUN—blood urea nitrogen; CBC—complete blood count; CEA—carcinoembryonic antigen; CT—computed tomography; FNAB—fine-needle aspiration biopsy; GI—gastrointestinal; LFT—liver function test; MRI—magnetic resonance imaging; PSA—prostate-specific antigen; PT—prothrombin time; PTT—partial thromboplastin time; S-Cr—serum creatinine; US—ultrasonography. (*Adapted from* Niederhuber [11].)

■ OVARIAN CANCER

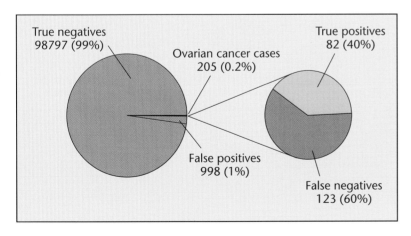

FIGURE 9-21.

Hypothetical example of an ovarian cancer screening program using the measurement of CA-125 as the screening test. To be of value, a screening test must be accurate (sensitivity and specificity), reliable, safe, relatively cheap, and accepted by both the individual patient and physician. For this example, specificity has been emphasized over sensitivity to avoid unnecessary diagnostic procedures. Considering a positive CA-125 test of more than 35 U/mL with a sensitivity and specificity of 40% and 99%, respectively, only 40% of women with ovarian cancer would test positive. The CA-125 value of 35 U/mL as being positive would not be effective in picking up early cases of ovarian cancer. (*Adapted from* Helzlsouer [12].)

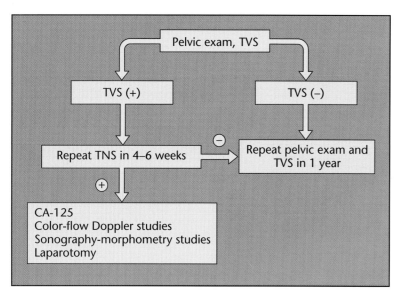

FIGURE 9-22.

Transvaginal sonography (TVS) is a screening tool for ovarian carcinoma in postmenopausal women older than 50 years or older than 30 years with positive family history (two or more relatives with ovarian cancer). For women who have two or more relatives with ovarian carcinoma, at least one of whom is a first-order relative, risk estimates as great as 80% or more have been reported. Specific hereditary syndromes have been described, including hereditary breast-ovarian cancer syndrome, hereditary ovarian cancer syndrome, and the Lynch II syndrome (associated with colon cancer). These syndromes appear in younger patients. (*Adapted from* Look [13].)

A. Staging Procedures for Ovarian Carcinoma

Appropriate surgeon
   Gynecologic oncologist or suitably trained surgeon with knowledge of the natural history of ovarian cancer
Appropriate incision
   Extended midline allowing access to upper abdomen and diaphragm
Cytology
   Ascites, washings from paracolic gutters and pelvis with warmed saline
Diaphragmatic scrapes
Careful laparotomy with clear documentation
Biopsies from adhesions and any suspicious areas
Random biopsies from peritoneum on pelvic side wall, paracolic gutters, and bowel
Bilateral salpingo-oophorectomy
Total abdominal hysterectomy
When unable to remove the uterus, perform an endometrial sample (dilatation and curettage)
Bilateral selective pelvic and paraaortic lymphadenectomy

B. 5-Year Survival According to Cancer Stage

Stage	5-Year Survival, %
All stages	35–42
Stage I	70–100
Stage II	55–63
Stage III	10–27
Stage IV	3–15

FIGURE 9-23.

Staging procedures for ovarian carcinoma (**A**) and 5-year survival according to stage (**B**). The most important prognostic factor for patients with ovarian carcinoma remains the stage of disease at diagnosis. That is why the staging procedures are important. Almost 70% of patients will have advanced disease (stage III or IV), most confined to the peritoneal cavity (stage III), reflecting intraperitoneal dissemination as the most common route of spread. (*Adapted from* Crawford and Shepherd [14].)

UTERINE CARCINOMA

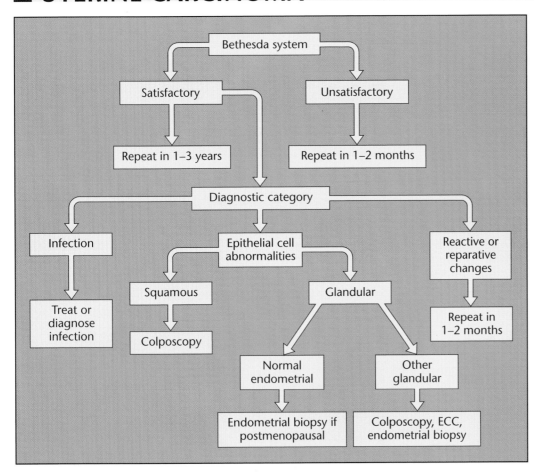

FIGURE 9-24.

The use of the Bethesda System for reporting cervical and vaginal cytologic diagnoses leading to clinical assessment of the patient. This system was introduced in 1988 by the National Cancer Institute (NCI) and revised in 1991 defining specific criteria for specimen adequacy. The premalignant state of carcinoma of the cervix is variously called *cervical intraepithelial neoplasia* or *squamous intraepithelial lesions*. These lesions can be detected by cervical cytology, the most effective screening test for cancer. The transition from mild disease to severe dysplasia and carcinoma *in situ* to frankly invasive cancer may take years, permitting early diagnosis and cure for most patients. (*Adapted from* Herman and Grosen [15].)

GENITOURINARY MALIGNANCIES

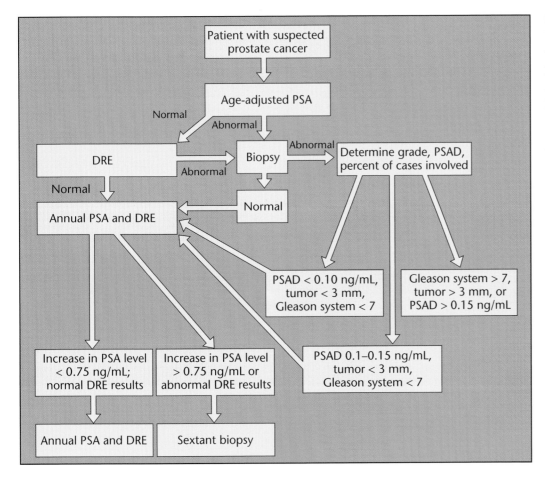

FIGURE 9-25.

Diagnosis of prostate cancer. It is important to diagnose prostate cancer early, since the prospects for cure are virtually nonexistent for approximately 60% of patients who present with tumors no longer confined to the prostate gland. The usual age at diagnosis for prostate cancer is between 60 and 70 years. The availability of serum markers has improved the ability to diagnose the disease. The most useful marker is the prostate-specific antigen (PSA). DRE—digital rectal examination; PSAD—prostate-specific antigen density. (*Adapted from* Scher *et al.* [16].)

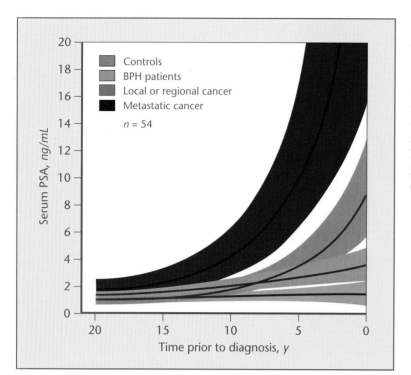

FIGURE 9-26.
Average curves (± 95% confidence intervals) of prostate-specific antigen (PSA) levels (µg/L) as a function of years before diagnosis for three diagnostic groups. The curves assume an age of diagnosis of 75 years. The curves reveal significant differences in the rate of change in PSA levels between all the groups, with levels increasing slowly in the control group, followed by patients with benign prostatic hypertrophy (BPH), followed by a significant increase in PSA levels in patients with prostate cancer. In this latter group, the rapid increase takes place at least 10 years before diagnosis. (*Adapted from* Carter *et al.* [17].)

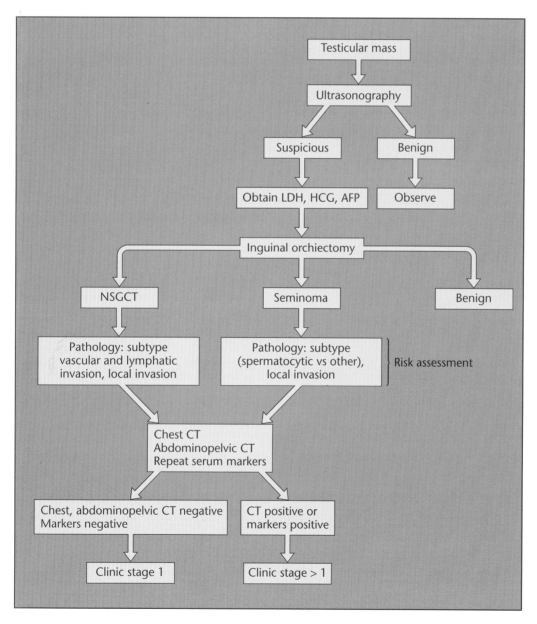

FIGURE 9-27.
Diagnosis, staging, and risk assessment of patients with testicular germ cell tumors. Testicular cancer is a rare disease, yet it is the most common malignancy in men between 15 and 35 years of age. More than 90% of testicular neoplasms are of germ cell origin, and most (40%) are seminomas. A scrotal mass is usually the initial presentation of testicular cancer; however, many times it is misdiagnosed as epididymitis. Testicular cancer is an excellent example for the clinical application of serum markers, such as α-fetoprotein (AFP) and β-HCG (human chorionic gonodotropin). CT—computed tomography; LDH—lactate dehydrogenase; NSGCT—nonseminomatous germ cell tumor. (*Adapted from* Small and Torti [18].)

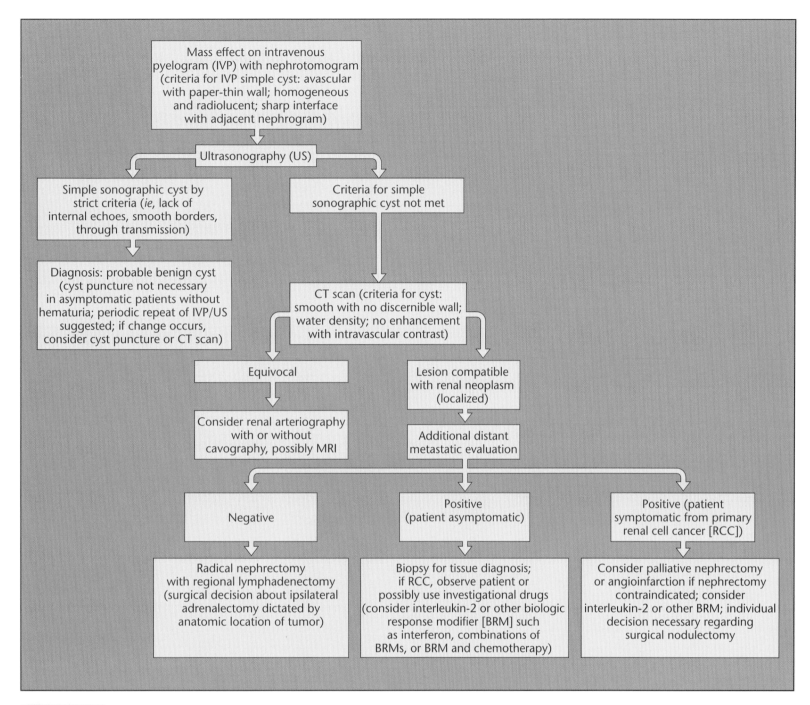

FIGURE 9-28.

Diagnostic evaluation of and therapeutic approach to primary renal cancer—an algorithm for diagnosis and management of a renal mass. The discovery of evidence during the history or physical examination that suggests a renal abnormality should be followed by either an intravenous pyelogram or an abdominal ultrasound. With increasing frequency, however, evidence of a space-occupying lesion in the kidney is found incidentally during radiographic testing for other unrelated conditions. Renal ultrasonography may help distinguish simple cysts from more complex abnormalities. A simple cyst is defined sonographically by the lack of internal echoes, the presence of smooth borders, and the transmission of the ultrasound wave. If these three features are present, the cyst is most likely benign. At one time, cyst puncture was used, but it seems to be unnecessary today in the asymptomatic patient without hematuria. Periodic repetition of the ultrasound is suggested for follow-up. If a change in the lesion occurs, cyst puncture, needle aspiration, or CT scanning should be considered to evaluate the lesion further.

If the sonographic criteria for a simple cyst are not met or the intravenous pyelogram suggests a solid or complex mass, a CT scan should be performed. If a renal neoplasm is demonstrated on CT scanning, renal vein or vena caval involvement should be assessed with CT scanning or magnetic resonance imaging. Although used frequently in the past, selective renal arteriography has assumed a more limited use, mainly in further evaluating the renal vasculature in patients who are to undergo partial nephrectomy (nephron-sparing surgery). CT scanning is also very helpful in determining the presence of lymphadenopathy.

The differential diagnosis of a renal mass detected on CT scanning includes primary renal cancers, metastatic lesions of the kidney, and benign lesions. The latter include angiomyolipomas (renal hamartomas), oncocytomas, and other rare or unusual growths.

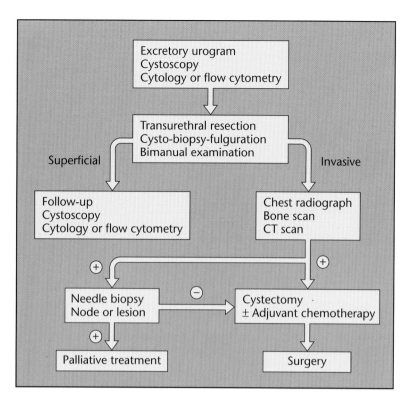

FIGURE 9-29.
Carcinoma of the bladder: clinical evaluation and treatment. This plan may be altered because of factors such as patient's age and general health. Most bladder tumors are transitional carcinomas and, less frequently, squamous cell and adenocarcinomas. Approximately 70% to 80% of these tumors are superficial (no muscle invasion), and local recurrences are fairly common; progressive muscle infiltrations occur only in approximately 20% of cases. Once infiltration occurs, the risk for regional and distant metastases is substantially increased. The disease is usually diagnosed in individuals between 60 and 70 years of age and affects men more frequently than women (3:1). CT—computed tomography. (*Adapted from* Kassabian and Graham [19].)

■ ENDOCRINE MALIGNANCIES

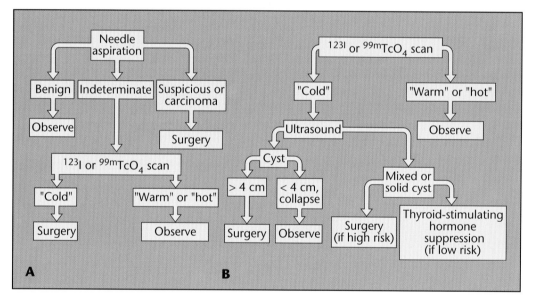

FIGURE 9-30.
Diagnostic approach to the patient with nodular thyroid disease. **A,** The general approach when an experienced cytopathologist is available. **B,** The general approach when a cytopathologist is not available. Solitary thyroid nodules are common in adults; however, 4% to 6% of these nodules are malignant. The approach to thyroid nodules requires prudent diagnostic considerations. There are two types of well-differentiated thyroid carcinomas: papillary and follicular. Papillary carcinoma is the most common type, comprising as many as 80% of all thyroid cancer. Distant metastases are rare with papillary carcinoma but are more frequent with follicular carcinoma. Anaplastic thyroid carcinoma is an aggressive malignancy usually occurring in older patients. (*Courtesy of* Steven D. Averbuch and Li-Teh Wu.)

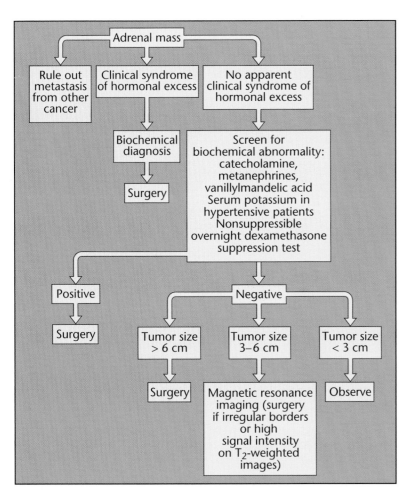

FIGURE 9-31.

Diagnostic approach to the patient with an adrenal mass. Biochemical assessments should be directed by the presenting syndrome in patients likely to have hormonal excess. For patients with a 3- to 6-cm mass, surgery is indicated if it is enlarging, has irregular borders, or has a high signal intensity (T$_2$-weighted) on magnetic resonance imaging. Adrenal carcinoma is a rare and aggressive cancer. Approximately 50% of patients manifest an endocrine hypersecretion syndrome such as Cushing's syndrome, virilization, feminization, or hyperaldosteronism. (*Courtesy of* Steven D. Averbuch and Li-Teh Wu.)

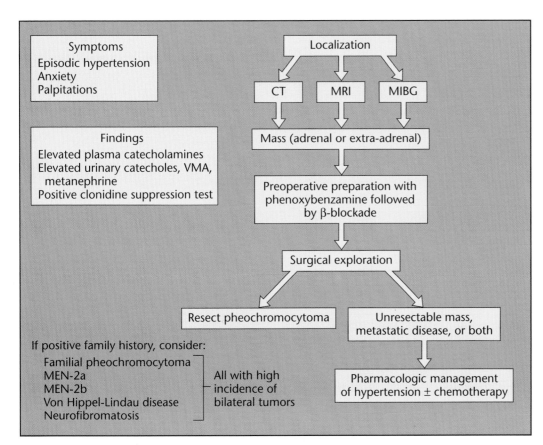

FIGURE 9-32.

Diagnosis and treatment of pheochromocytoma. Patients with pheochromocytoma present with sustained or intermittent hypertension with episodes of palpitations, headache, pallor, sweating, and anxiety from sudden release of catecholamines. Orthostatic hypertension is common. Overall, 13% of pheochromocytomas are malignant. Surgery is the only cure for this disease; however, prompt medical management is critical in preventing catastrophic hypertensive events before surgery or in the presence of unresectable functional tumor. CT—computed tomography; MEN-2a—multiple endocrine neoplasia-2a; MEN-2b—multiple endocrine neoplasmia-2b; MIBG—metaiodobenzyl-guanidine; MRI—magnetic resonance imaging; VMA—vanillymandelic acid. (*Adapted from* Macdonald *et al.* [20].)

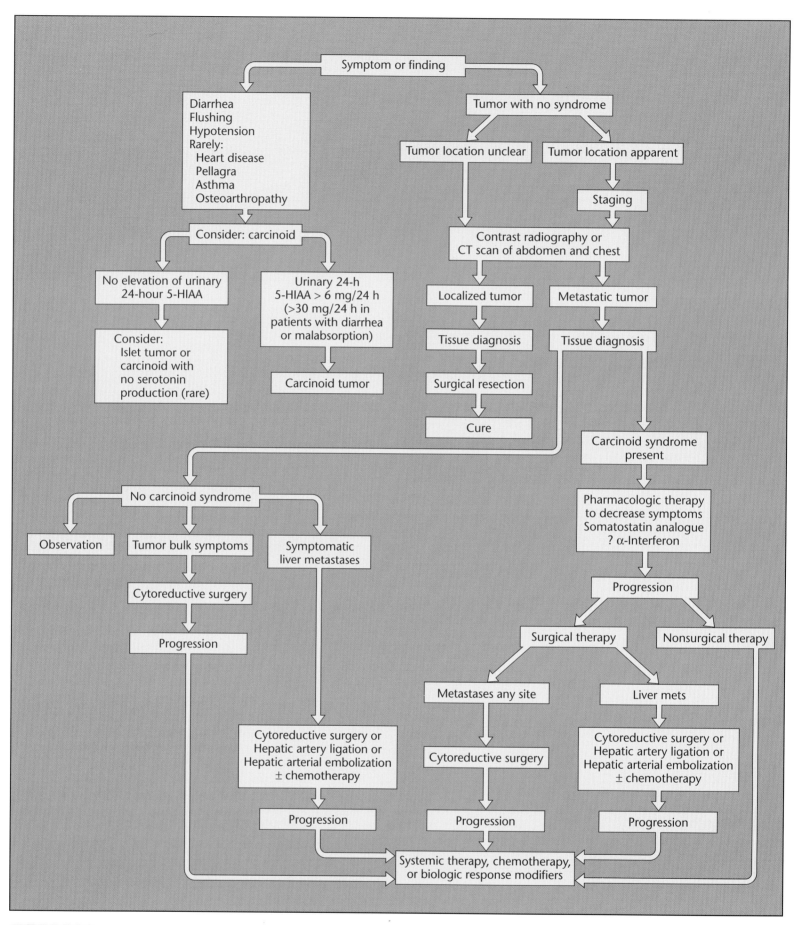

FIGURE 9-33.

Diagnosis and treatment of carcinoid tumors. Carcinoid tumors arise from enterochromaffin cells that produce serotonin; its precursor, 5-hydroxytryptophan (5-H1AA); and several peptide hormones. Most carcinoid tumors are found in the mid-gut (ie, intestine, appendix, right colon). These tumors are slow-growing and rarely metastasize when the primary lesion is less than 1 cm in size. In contrast, the incidence of metastasis increases significantly when the primary tumor is greater than 2 cm in size. When hormone products of carcinoid tumors reach the systemic circulation, usually in the presence of liver metastases, the carcinoid syndrome may occur. CT—computed tomography; mets—metastases. (*Adapted from* Macdonald *et al.* [20].)

■ SARCOMAS OF SOFT TISSUE AND BONE

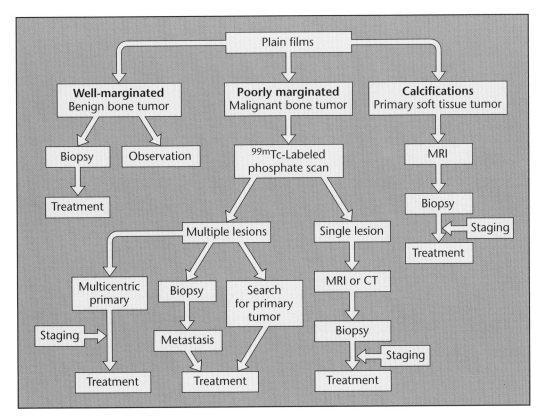

FIGURE 9-34.

Approach to musculoskeletal tumor evaluation. It is estimated that in 1998 there will be 8700 new cases of soft tissue sarcomas, with 4400 deaths; for bone tumors, it is estimated that approximately 2900 new cases will be diagnosed, with 1400 deaths occurring in 2001. Sarcomas can arise anywhere within the body, including connective tissue of visceral organs. Early diagnosis is difficult and requires a high index of suspicion. Biopsies of a suspicious mass must be planned with care so as not to jeopardize subsequent efforts to achieve local control if the mass proves to be malignant. CT—computed tomography; MRI—magnetic resonance imaging. (*Adapted from* Bridge *et al.* [21].)

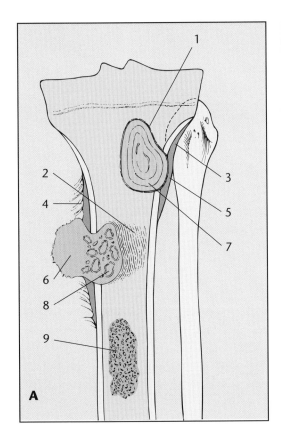

B. Benign versus Malignant Bone Lesions

Feature	Benign (Slow-growing Process)	Malignant (Aggressive Process)
Border	1. Sharply outlined, sclerotic (narrow zone of transition)	2. Poorly defined (wide zone of transition)
Periosteal reaction	3. Solid, uninterrupted	4. Interrupted (sunburst, Codman's triangle)
Soft-tissue extension or mass	5. Absent or contained by shell of periosteal new bone	6. Frank extension through destroyed periosteum
Type of bone destruction	7. Uniformly destroyed area with sharply defined border	8. Moth-eaten (likely malignant): destroyed areas with ragged borders
		9. Permeative (aggressive or malignant): ill-defined destruction spreading through marrow space

FIGURE 9-35.

Benign versus malignant bone lesions. The radiographic features illustrated (**A**) may help differentiate benign from malignant lesions (**B**). The numbers in *panel A* correspond with those in *panel B*. (*Adapted from* Skarin [22].)

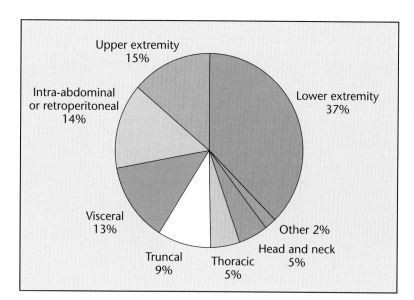

FIGURE 9-36.

Anatomic distribution of soft tissue sarcomas presenting to Memorial Sloan-Kettering Cancer Center (New York, New York) between 7/1/82 and 5/1/92 ($n = 1957$). It was estimated that there would be 6600 new cases of soft tissue sarcomas in 1997. (*Adapted from* Conlon and Brennan [23].)

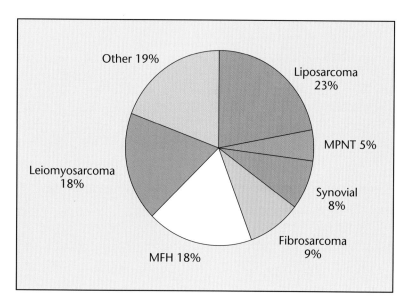

FIGURE 9-37.

Histopathology of soft tissue sarcomas for patients admitted between 7/1/82 and 5/1/92 ($n = 1957$). There are at least 30 different forms of soft tissue sarcomas. The histologic subclassification of sarcomas has been shown to differ from one medical center to another, even in the hands of pathologists familiar with this group of tumors. Clinical decisions regarding the treatment of soft tissue sarcomas place unique emphasis on the assessment of tumor grade rather than on histologic subclassification. High-grade tumors tend to metastasize early and are more likely to respond to chemotherapy. MFH—malignant fibrous histiocytoma; MPNT—malignant peripheral nerve tumor. (*Adapted from* Conlon and Brennan [23].)

Distribution and Differential Diagnosis of Tumors of the Central Nervous System

Intracranial Region	Adulthood Tumors	Childhood and Adolescent Tumors
Cerebral hemisphere	Astrocytoma	Astrocytoma
	Anaplastic astrocytoma	Anaplastic astrocytoma
	Glioblastoma	Ependymoma
	Meningioma	Oligodendroglioma
	Metastatic carcinoma	Embryonal tumor
	Oligodendroglioma	Ganglion cell tumor
	Ependymoma	
	Lymphoma	
	Sarcoma	
Lateral ventricle	Ependymoma	Ependymoma
	Meningioma	Choroid plexus papilloma
	Subependymoma	Subependymal giant cell astrocytoma
	Choroid plexus papilloma	
Third ventricle	Colloid cyst	Ependymoma
	Ependymoma	Choroid plexus papilloma
Peri-third ventricular region	Astrocytoma	Pilocytic astrocytoma
	Anaplastic astrocytoma	
	Glioblastoma	
	Oligodendroglioma	
	Ependymoma	
	Pilocytic astrocytoma	
Pineal region	Germ cell tumor	Germ cell tumor
	Pineal parenchymal tumor	Pineal parenchymal tumor
	Glioma	
Optic chiasm and nerve	Meningioma	Astrocytoma
	Astrocytoma	
Pituitary and sellar region	Pituitary adenoma	Craniopharyngioma
	Craniopharyngioma	Germ cell tumor
	Meningioma	Pituitary adenoma
	Germ cell tumor	
Corpus callosum	Astrocytoma	Astrocytoma
	Anaplastic astrocytoma	Anaplastic astrocytoma
	Glioblastoma	Oligodendroglioma
	Oligodendroglioma	Lipoma
	Lipoma	
Brain stem	Astrocytoma	Astrocytoma
	Anaplastic astrocytoma	Anaplastic astrocytoma
	Glioblastoma	Glioblastoma
Cerebellopontine angle	Acoustic neuroma	Ependymoma
	Meningioma	
	Epidermoid cyst	
	Choroid plexus papilloma	
Cerebellum	Hemangioblastoma	Medulloblastoma
	Metastatic carcinoma	Astrocytoma
	Astrocytoma	Dermoid cyst
	Medulloblastoma	
Fourth Ventricle	Ependymoma	Ependymoma
	Subependymoma	Choroid plexus papilloma
	Choroid plexus papilloma	
Region of foramen magnum	Meningioma	
	Schwannoma (neurilemoma)	

FIGURE 9-38.

Distribution and differential diagnosis of tumors of the central nervous system.
(*Adapted from* Skarin [24].)

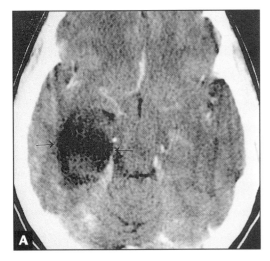

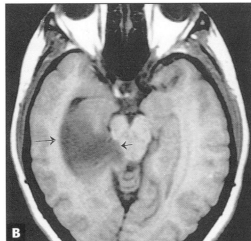

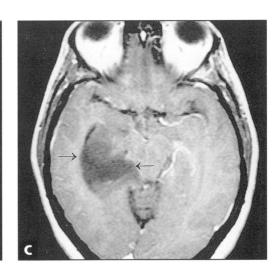

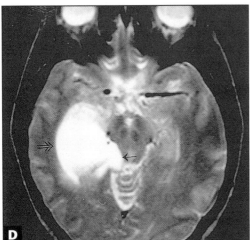

FIGURE 9-39.

Low-grade astrocytoma. **A,** A contrast-enhanced computed tomography (CT) scan of a low-grade astrocytoma shows a large, nonenhancing, low-attenuation right temporal lobe mass. **B,** Axial T$_1$-weighted magnetic resonance images before contrast. **C,** After contrast, no enhancement is seen (*arrows*). **D,** Axial T$_2$-weighted image shows lesion to have increased signal intensity (*open arrow*). A mass effect is seen posteriorly on the adjacent brain stem (*closed arrow*). CT scans usually are done with and without an iodinated contrast agent. The precontrast scan allows the abnormalities to be compared with brain density and areas of calcification and hemorrhage to be identified. The postcontrast scan demonstrates enhancement of the tumor in areas of blood–brain barrier disruption with magnetic resonance imaging T$_1$-weighted images with contrast help distinguish tumor from non-enhancing edema; T$_2$-weighted images effectively demonstrate edema and cerebrospinal fluid. (*Courtesy of* Richard M. Hellman.)

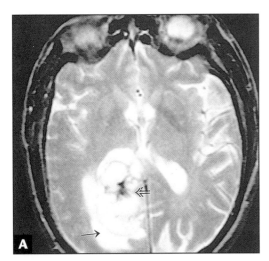

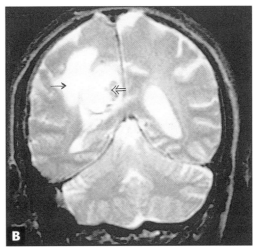

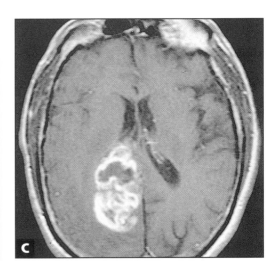

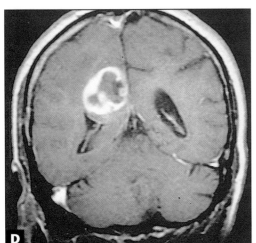

FIGURE 9-40.

Glioblastoma multiforme. An axial T$_2$-weighted magnetic resonance imaging scan (**A**) and a coronal T$_2$-weighted image (**B**) of a glioblastoma multiforme reveal a large, right-side heterogeneous mass involving the splenium of the corpus callosum (*open arrows*). The adjacent edema (*closed arrows*) is of increased signal intensity. After contrast, axial (**C**) and coronal (**D**) T$_1$-weighted images show this lesion to have typical peripheral, irregular enhancement. Glioblastoma multiforme is the most common glioma found in adults and has the most unfavorable prognosis. The tumors are usually solitary but occasionally are multifocal. (*Courtesy of* Richard M. Hellman.)

■ MELANOMA AND OTHER SKIN CANCERS

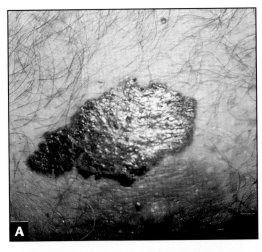

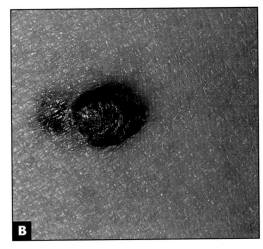

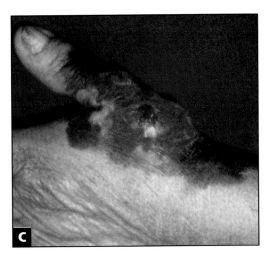

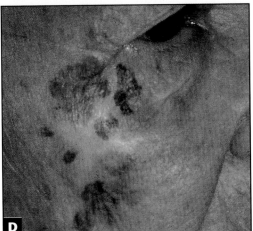

FIGURE 9-41.

Melanoma. Note the asymmetry, irregular border, variation in color, and diameter of 6 mm or more. **A,** Superficial spreading melanoma. **B,** Nodular melanoma. **C,** Acral lentiginous melanoma. **D,** Lentigo maligna melanoma. The diagnosis of melanoma begins with the clinical identification of a suspected tumor. The criteria for clinical diagnosis has been clustered into an "ABCD" mnemonic (Asymmetry in shape, Borders that are irregular in shape and indistinct, variable Colors or shades of a single color, and Diameter ≥ 6 mm). Most benign skin tumors are round or oval and have a uniform color pattern. (Panels A and C *courtesy of* Evan R. Farmer; panels B and D *courtesy of* SE Wolverton.)

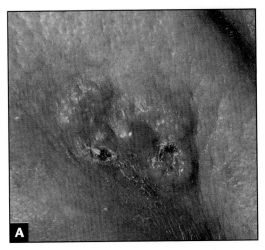

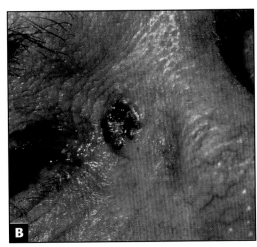

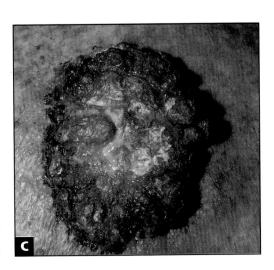

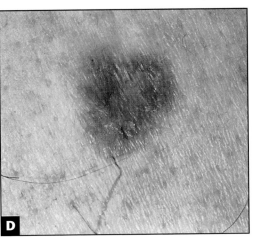

FIGURE 9-42.

Basal cell carcinoma. There are variations in appearance. **A,** Nodular basal cell carcinoma. Note the shiny waxy surface. **B,** Pigmented basal cell carcinoma. **C,** Sclerotic basal cell carcinoma. Note the white sclerotic areas in the center of the tumor. **D,** Superficial basal cell carcinoma. Note the thin plaquelike or dermatitislike appearance. Most basal cell carcinomas occur in people older than 40 years of age in the temperate and northern latitudes but can be seen in younger patients in the southern regions of the United States. The clinical criterion suggestive of a basal cell carcinoma is a smooth, shiny papule with overlying telangiectasia. There also may be ulceration or a history of bleeding with minor trauma. (Panels A and C *courtesy of* Evan R. Farmer; panels B and D *courtesy of* SE Wolverton.)

■ CANCERS OF UNKNOWN PRIMARY SITES

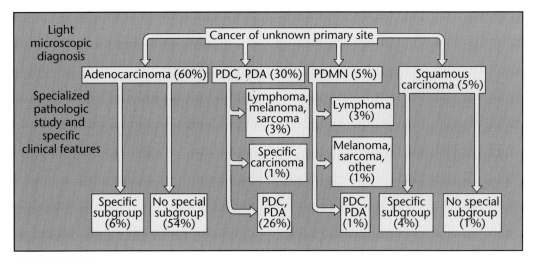

FIGURE 9-43.

Incidence of various histologic and clinical subgroups as defined by optimum pathologic and clinical evaluation. Most patients (approximately 60%) have well-differentiated adenocarci-

noma. The morphologic appearance of adenocarcinoma from various primary sites is similar, and routine light microscopic examination rarely provides specific clues regarding the primary sites. An additional 5% of patients have squamous carcinoma. In the remaining 35% of patients, less specific information regarding tumor lineage is provided by light microscopy. Identification of lineage is particularly important when the diagnosis is poorly differentiated neoplasm because these patients may have an unsuspected non-Hodgkin's lymphoma, which is potentially curable when treated. PDA—poorly differentiated adenocarcinoma; PDC—poorly differentiated carcinoma; PDMN—poorly differentiated malignant neoplasm. (*Courtesy of* Frank Anthony Greco and John D. Hainsworth.)

■ ONCOLOGIC EMERGENCIES

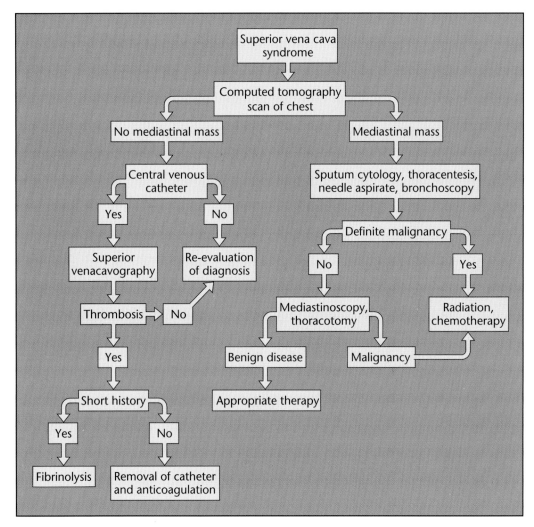

FIGURE 9-44.

Evaluation of the superior vena cava (SVC) syndrome. Because most of the lesions causing the syndrome are malignant, histologic diagnosis is necessary before instituting appropriate therapy; invasive diagnostic procedures, such as bronchoscopy, mediastinoscopy, and thoracotomy, can be performed with minimal additional risk in patients with SVC syndrome. The use of long-term central venous catheters has become common practice in patients with cancer and is another cause of the SVC syndrome. Patients with the syndrome usually have neck and facial swelling, dyspnea, and cough. Other symptoms include hoarseness, tongue swelling, nasal congestion, dysphagia, headaches, dizziness, syncope, lethargy, and pain. (*Courtesy of* Rasim Gucalp and Janice Dutcher.)

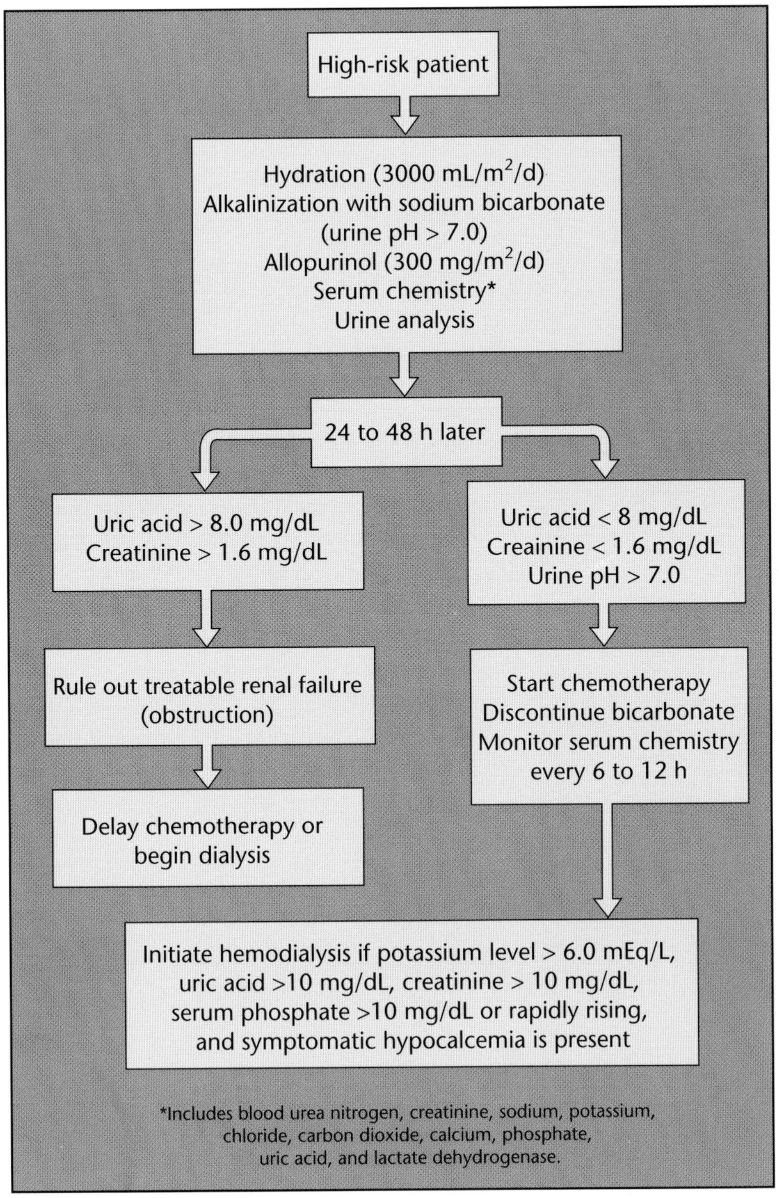
High-risk patient
Hydration (3000 mL/m²/d)
Alkalinization with sodium bicarbonate
(urine pH > 7.0)
Allopurinol (300 mg/m²/d)
Serum chemistry*
Urine analysis
24 to 48 h later
Uric acid > 8.0 mg/dL
Creatinine > 1.6 mg/dL
Uric acid < 8 mg/dL
Creainine < 1.6 mg/dL
Urine pH > 7.0
Rule out treatable renal failure
(obstruction)
Start chemotherapy
Discontinue bicarbonate
Monitor serum chemistry
every 6 to 12 h
Delay chemotherapy or
begin dialysis
Initiate hemodialysis if potassium level > 6.0 mEq/L,
uric acid >10 mg/dL, creatinine > 10 mg/dL,
serum phosphate >10 mg/dL or rapidly rising,
and symptomatic hypocalcemia is present
*Includes blood urea nitrogen, creatinine, sodium, potassium,
chloride, carbon dioxide, calcium, phosphate,
uric acid, and lactate dehydrogenase.

FIGURE 9-45.
Metabolic management of tumor lysis syndrome in patients at high risk. Acute tumor lysis syndrome is characterized by various combinations of hyperuricemia, hyperphosphatemia, hyperkalemia, lactic acidosis, and hypocalcemia caused by the massive destruction of many neoplastic cells. Frequently, acute renal failure develops, and combined with electrolyte abnormalities, may rapidly become life-threatening. Acute tumor lysis syndrome is most frequently associated with Burkitt's lymphoma, acute lymphoblastic leukemia, and other high-grade lymphomas, but it also may be seen with chronic leukemias and rarely with solid tumors including small cell lung cancer and breast cancer. Recognition of risk and prevention are the most important steps in managing this syndrome. Maintaining adequate hydration and urine flow is necessary to prevent renal failure, and metabolic derangements after chemotherapy-treatable causes of renal failure (*eg*, obstructive uropathy) should be managed before chemotherapy. Despite aggressive pretreatment management, the acute tumor lysis syndrome and oliguric or anuric renal failure may occur. Dialysis is often necessary. (*Adapted from* Cohen [25].)

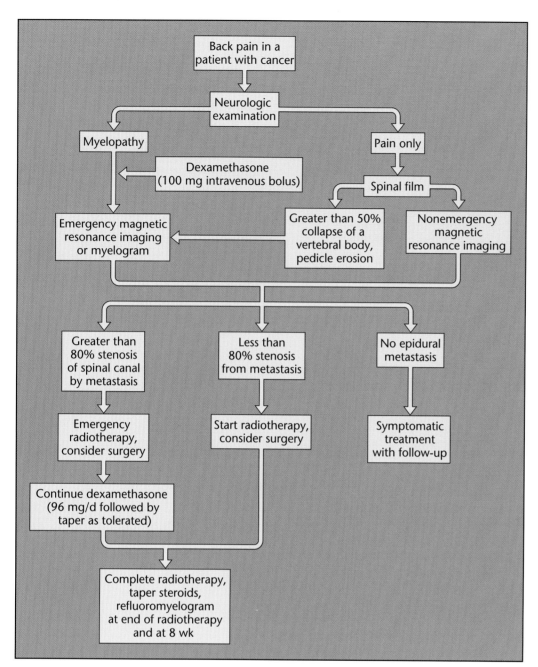

FIGURE 9-46.

Management of back pain in cancer patients. The most common initial symptom in patients with spinal cord compression is localized back pain and tenderness resulting from tumor involvement of the vertebrae. Pain may be present for days or months before other neurologic signs or symptoms appear. Local pain is exacerbated by movement, coughing, and sneezing. Worsening of pain by lying back differentiates cord compression from disk disease. Spinal cord compression is the third most common neurologic problem associated with cancer, occurring in 5% to 10% of patients. Metastatic tumor involving the vertebrae column occurs most commonly in patients with lung, breast, and prostate cancer. The thoracic spine is the most common site (70%) of metastatic vertebral involvement. Patients with known cancer who develop back pain should be evaluated for spinal cord compression. (*Adapted from* Henson and Posner [26].)

■ METASTATIC CANCER

Sites of Metastatic Involvement by Primary Tumor Type

	Site of Metastatic Involvement			
Primary Site	**Bone, %**	**Lung, %**	**Liver, %**	**Brain, %**
Lung	30–50	34	30–50	15–30
Breast	50–85	60	60	15–25
Thyroid	39	65	60	1
Pancreas	5–10	25–40	50–70	1–4
Liver	8	20	NA	0
Colorectal	5–10	25–40	71	1
Gastric	5–10	20–30	35–50	1–4
Renal	30–50	50–75	35–40	7–8
Ovary	2–6	10	10–15	1
Prostate	50–75	13–53	13	2

FIGURE 9-47.

Sites of metastatic involvement by primary tumor type. The lungs are a very common site for the development of metastases; however, the incidence of pulmonary involvement varies considerably with the underlying cancer diagnosis. The liver is the largest visceral organ in the human body and is a frequent site for metastatic cancer. Occasionally, hepatic metastases are the only clinically apparent metastatic site. Metastatic bone involvement is usually heralded by the onset of localized pain. Metastases to the brain occur in approximately 30% of all patients with cancer. NA—not applicable. (*Courtesy of* James L. Abbruzzese.)

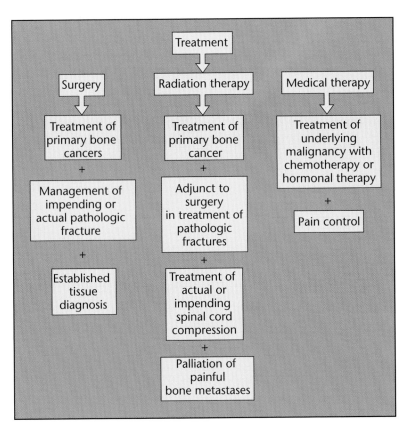

FIGURE 9-48.

Treatment approaches to the patient with bone metastases. Most patients with skeletal metastases are treated using a multimodality approach involving surgery, radiotherapy, chemotherapy, and hormonal manipulation. Surgical intervention is most commonly employed when a pending or actual pathologic fracture of a weight-bearing bone has been identified. Radiation therapy follows the surgical intervention or can be used as primary treatment for symptomatic bony metastases. Chemotherapy or hormonal therapy is usually given to treat the specific cancer systemically. (*Courtesy of* James L. Abbruzzese.)

■ MALIGNANT EFFUSIONS

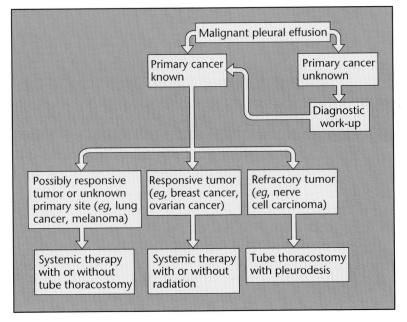

FIGURE 9-49.

Management of pleural effusions. Neoplasms are responsible for nearly 50% of pleural effusions. Breast cancer, lung cancer (primarily non–small cell), lymphoma, and ovarian cancer are the most common causes. Dyspnea, cough, weakness, and chest pain are the most common symptoms of large effusions. A diagnostic needle thoracentesis allows for evaluation of the appearance, protein content, lactic dehydrogenase level, bacterial content, and cytologic make-up of the specimen. Patients who have no symptoms from their malignant pleural effusion require no specific local therapy. Symptomatic malignant effusions are best managed by tube thoracostomy and closed drainage with subsequent chemical pleurodesis. Sclerosing agents include bleomycin, doxycycline, and talc slurry. The effusions in patients so treated are controlled in more than 50% of the time. (*Courtesy of* John Horton.)

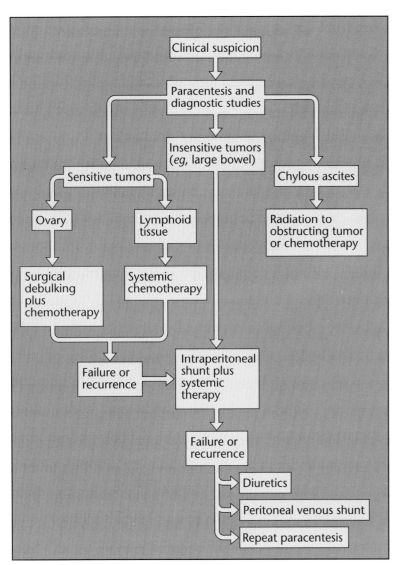

FIGURE 9-50.

Management of malignant ascites. Malignant ascites is most often caused by proteinaceous weeping from peritoneal tumor implants. Malignant ascites is a complication seen most often with carcinoma of the ovary but may occur with any intra-abdominal tumor or lymphoma. Most patients with a malignant ascites present with symptoms of abdominal distention and discomfort and weight gain. Management of the malignant ascites is determined by considering the pathogenesis of the ascites, the expected sensitivity of the tumor to local or systemic measures, and the patient's symptoms. For ovarian cancer, surgical debulking enhances the likelihood that systemic therapy would be used to control the remaining disease. (*Adapted from* Horton [27].)

■ CANCER PAIN

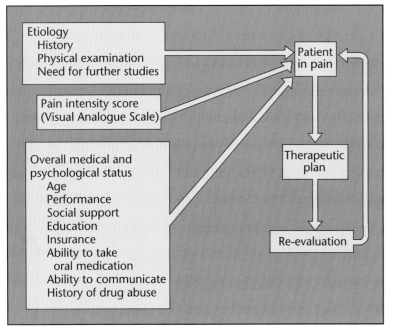

FIGURE 9-51.

Management of cancer pain. Pain is one of the most common and dreaded symptoms associated with cancer. Despite the importance of cancer pain and the excellent therapies available for it, cancer pain frequently is undertreated. Health care providers must rely heavily on patient reports of pain intensity because pain is an entirely subjective phenomenon. An accurate assessment of the etiology and intensity of cancer pain is critical to proper management. More than 80% of patients with cancer pain can be well-palliated with conventional oral medications. Opioids are the most effective analgesics, but many pharmacologic agents can be useful. (*Courtesy of* Stuart A. Grossman and Juraj Baumohl.)

■ PSYCHOLOGICAL ISSUES IN PATIENTS WITH CANCER

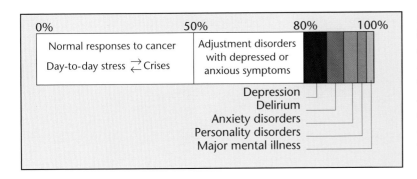

FIGURE 9-52.

Spectrum of psychiatric disorders in cancer. The best prevalence estimate available suggests that approximately 50% of cancer patients receiving active treatment suffer from some diagnosable mental disorder as defined by the current psychiatric nomenclature, the *Diagnostic and Statistical Manual of Mental Disorders, 4th Edition, Revised (DSM-IV)*. Differential diagnosis of psychological disorders is often complicated by the impact of the disease itself. Most people with psychological disorders can be treated effectively with medication, short-term psychotherapy, or both. (*Adapted from* Holland and Rowland [28].)

■ REFERENCES

1. Greenlee RT, Hill-Harmon MB, Murray T, Thun M: Cancer Statistics, 2001. CA Cancer J Clin 51:15–36, 2001.

2. Westin A, Harris CC: Chemical carcinogenesis. In *Cancer Medicine*, vol 1, edn 4. Edited by Holland JF, Bast RC Jr, Morton DL, *et al.* Baltimore: Williams & Wilkins; 1997:261–276.

3. Nesbitt JC, Lee JS, Komaki R, Roth JA: Cancer of the lung. In *Cancer Medicine*, vol 2, edn 4. Edited by Holland JF, Bast RC Jr, Morton DL, *et al.* Baltimore: Williams & Wilkins; 1997:1723–1803.

4. Mountain CF. Lung cancer staging classification. *Clin Chest Med* 1993, 14:43–53.

5. Skarin AT, ed: Tumors of the heart and mediastinum. In *Atlas of Diagnostic Oncology*. Philadelphia: JB Lippincott Co; 1991:2.35–2.42.

6. Skarin AT, ed: Breast cancer. In *Atlas of Diagnostic Oncology*. Philadelphia: JB Lippincott Co; 1991:6.2–6.31.

7. Donegan WL: Current concepts: evaluation of a palpable breast mass. *N Engl J Med* 1992, 327:937–942.

8. Beahrs OH, Henson DE, Hutter RV, Kennedy BJ, eds: Breast. In *Reference Manual for Staging of Cancer*, edn 4. Philadelphia: JB Lippincott; 1992:149–154.

9. Goldhirsch A, Glick JG, Gelber RD, Senn HJ: Meeting highlights: International Consensus Panel on Treatment of Primary Breast Cancer. J Natl Cancer Inst 1998, 90:1601.

10. Beart RW Jr: Colon and rectum. In *Clinical Oncology*. Edited by Abeloff MD, Armitage JO, Lichter AS, Niederhuber JE. New York: Churchill Livingstone; 1995:1267–1286.

11. Niederhuber JE. Tumors of the liver. In *American Cancer Society Textbook of Clinical Oncology*. Edited by Murphy GP, Lawrence W Jr, Lenhard RE Jr. Atlanta: American Cancer Society; 1995:269–280.

12. Helzlsouer KJ: Challenges of population screening. In *Early Detection of Cancer Molecular Markers*. Edited by Srivastciva S, Lippman SM, Hong WK, Mulshine J. Armonk: Futura Publishing Co; 1994.

13. Look KY: Epidemiology, etiology, and screening of ovarian cancer. In *Ovarian Cancer*. Edited by Rubin SC, Sutton GP. New York: McGraw-Hill; 1993:175–187.

14. Crawford RAF, Shepherd JH: Management of epithelial ovarian cancer. In *Gynecologic Oncology: Current Diagnosis and Treatment*. Edited by Shingleton HM, Fowler WC Jr, Jordan JA, Lawrence WD. Philadelphia: WB Saunders; 1996:203–214.

15. Herman ML, Grosen EA: Cervix. In *Cancer Treatment*, edn 4. Edited by Haskell CM. Philadelphia: WB Saunders Company; 1995:662–675.

16. Scher HI, Isaacs JT, Fuks Z, Walsh PC: Prostate. In *Clinical Oncology*. Edited by Abeloff MD, Armitage JO, Lichter AS, Niederhuber JE. New York: Churchill Livingstone; 1995:1439–1472.

17. Carter HB, Hamper UM, Sheth S, *et al.*: Longitudinal evaluation of prostate-specific antigen levels in men with and without prostate disease. *JAMA* 1992, 267:2215–2220.

18. Small EJ, Torti JM: Testes. In *Clinical Oncology*. Edited by Abeloff MD, Armitage JO, Lichter AS, Niederhuber JE. New York: Churchill Livingstone; 1995:1493–1526.

19. Kassabian VS, Graham SD Jr: Urologic and male genital cancer. In *American Cancer Society Textbook of Clinical Oncology*. Edited by Murphy GP, Lawrence W Jr, Lenhard RE Jr. Atlanta: American Cancer Society; 1995:311–329.

20. Macdonald J, Haller D, Weigel RJ: Endocrine system. In *Clinical Oncology*. Edited by Abeloff MD, Armitage JO, Lichter AS, Niederhuber JE. New York: Churchill Livingstone; 1995:1047–1081.

21. Bridge JA, Schwartz HS, Neff JR: Bone sarcomas. In *Clinical Oncology*. Edited by Abeloff MD, Armitage JO, Lichter AS, Niederhuber JE. New York: Churchill Livingstone; 1995:1715–1797.

22. Skarin AT, ed: Sarcomas of bone and soft tissue. In *Atlas of Diagnostic Oncology*. Philadelphia: JB Lippincott Co; 1991:8.2–8.42.

23. Conlon KC, Brennan MF. Soft tissue sarcomas. In *American Cancer Society Textbook of Clinical Oncology*. Edited by Murphy GP, Lawrence W Jr, Lenhard RE Jr. Atlanta: American Cancer Society; 1995:435–450.

24. Skarin AT, ed: Neoplasms of the central nervous system. In *Atlas of Diagnostic Oncology*. Philadelphia: JB Lippincott Co; 1991:10.2–10.43.

25. Cohen LF, Balow JE, Magrath IT, *et al.*: Acute tumor lysis syndrome: a review of 37 patients with Burkitt's lymphoma. *Am J Med* 1980, 68:486–491.

26. Henson JW, Posner JB: *Cancer Medicine* Philadelphia: Lea & Febiger; 1993.

27. Horton J: Malignant effusions. In *Comprehensive Textbook of Oncology*, edn 2. Edited by Moosa AR, Schimpff SS, Robson MC. Baltimore: Williams & Wilkins; 1991:1690–1696.

28. Holland JC, Rowland JH, eds: *Handbook of Psychooncology: Psychological Care of the Patient with Cancer*. New York: Oxford University Press; 1989.

Hematology

THOMAS P. DUFFY

Hematologic abnormalities cover a broad terrain of clinical and laboratory findings that may have their origin in primary hematologic disorders or constitute hematologic manifestations of systemic disease. A hematologic abnormality is frequently the window that opens access to a wide range of pathology and often serves as the fulcrum of the differential diagnosis surrounding a patient's illness. Many hematologic abnormalities are the signs of serious pathology involving other organ systems; conversely, malfunctioning of organ systems may occur secondary to primary hematologic disease. Iron deficiency anemia is a finding that creates a responsibility to identify the source of blood loss and may be the initial sign of an otherwise occult malignancy; migratory thrombophlebitis is a different presentation that may also have its cause in an underlying malignancy. Severe anemia may masquerade as angina pectoris or create a puzzling picture that is confused with cardiopulmonary disease. The canvas of hematologic disease is a very large one, and no aspect of the body's functioning escapes the potential impact of disorders in this system.

The prominence of hematologic abnormalities in medicine is complemented by the ease with which laboratory specimens can be obtained and studied for pathologic alterations. Staining techniques have been available in hematology for more than 100 years, linking laboratory and clinical diagnosis as the definition of hematologic disease. These original descriptive methods are now joined with the vast array of molecular analytic tools that serve both diagnostic and investigative roles. Sickle cell disease is the original molecular disease, a designation that was made possible by the linkage of the clinical problem of sickling with the new technology of hemoglobin electrophoresis. Genetic alterations as the cause of disease have their proof in chromosomal markers that accompany leukemias and lymphomas; these markers allow identification of individuals with subtle but life-threatening conditions such as hemochromatosis. This chapter encompasses a broad reach that extends from the patient to the standard hematology testing to the most modern molecular technology.

■ ANEMIAS

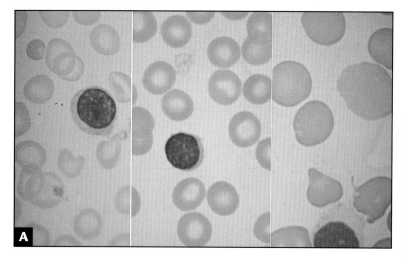

FIGURE 10-1.
Erythrocyte size. **A,** The three categories of microcytic (*left*), normocytic (*middle*), and macrocytic (*right*) anemia are generated by electronic counters, permitting assignment of the causes of anemias to a limited number of specific etiologies. A normocytic erythrocyte is approximately the diameter of the nucleus of a mature lymphocyte. Microcytic indices point to deficient or defective hemoglobin synthesis, most commonly attributable to iron deficiency. Marked macrocytosis (> 115 fl) is almost always secondary to vitamin B12 or folate deficiency. All anemias are initially normocytic until the abnormal cell population predominates [1]. **B,** Erythrocyte size (mean corpuscular volume) is an essential determinant in framing the differential diagnosis of anemia.

B. Differential Diagnosis of Anemia on the Basis of Erythrocyte Mean Corpuscular Volume

Mean Corpuscular Volume, *fl*	Diagnosis
< 80	Iron deficiency
	Anemia of chronic disease
	Thalassemia
	Sideroblastic anemia
80–90	Initial stage of all anemias
	Anemia of chronic disease
	Erythropoietin deficiency
	Hemolytic anemia
	Stem cell disorders
	Endocrine disorders
	Myelophthisic anemia
> 95	Dysproteinemias
	Megaloblastic anemia
	B12 or folate deficiency
	Myelodysplasia
	Purine or pyrimidine abnormalities
	Nonmegaloblastic
	Liver disease
	Hypothyroidism
	Reticulocytosis
	Cold agglutinins

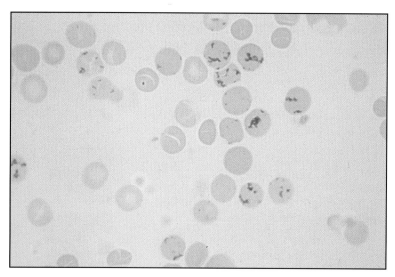

FIGURE 10-2.
Reticulocyte stain. Supravital staining of the peripheral blood allows quantitation of the reticulocyte count—young erythrocytes with residual polyribosomal material as the marker of their recent release from the marrow. A low reticulocyte count (< 2%) in the presence of anemia supports a defect in erythrocyte production, a hypoproliferative anemia; an elevated reticulocyte count (> 2%) accompanies blood loss or a hemolytic process, a hyperproliferative anemia. Because of their importance in determining the causes of anemia, reticulocyte counts and mean corpuscular volume are essential measurements in the approach to the patient with anemia.

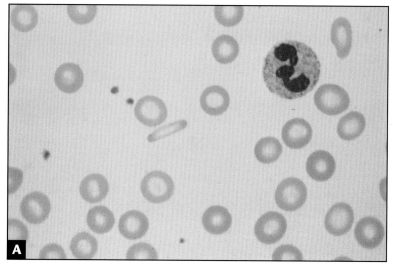

FIGURE 10-3.
Microcytic anemia (mean corpuscular volume < 80 fl). All microcytic anemias share deficient erythrocyte hemoglobin synthesis as their cause; the defective hemoglobin synthesis has its etiologies in absolute iron deficiency, defective iron delivery (anemia of chronic disease), or abnormalities in heme (sideroblastic) or globin chain (thalassemia) synthesis. Iron indices (serum iron and iron binding capacity, serum ferritin), marrow iron stores, and hemoglobin electrophoresis help differentiate between these separate causes of microcytic anemias. **A,** Iron-deficient erythrocytes with increased pallor (hypochromia) secondary to a decreased hemoglobin concentration.

(Continued)

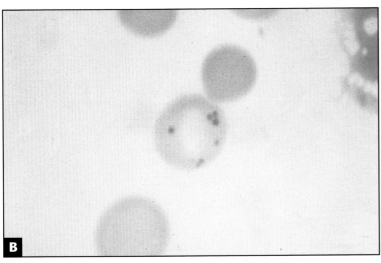

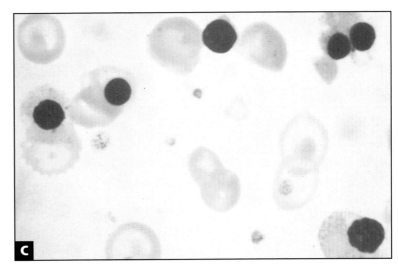

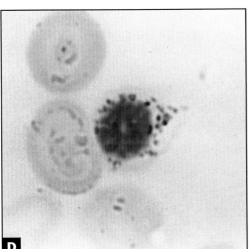

FIGURE 10-3. *(CONTINUED)*

B, Small siderotic (iron) granules in hypochromic erythrocytes, the clue to a sideroblastic marrow process. **C,** Target erythrocytes, which are characteristic of thalassemia.

Sideroblastic anemias [2] have characteristic perinuclear erythrocyte iron accumulation responsible for the "ringed" designation. The iron is deposited in erythrocyte mitochondria, the site of altered protoporphyrin and heme synthesis in sideroblastic anemia. **D,** Prussian blue staining of the marrow, which permits recognition of this iron-loading abnormality in erythrocyte precursors. The iron hang-up precludes normal heme production, resulting in a hypochromic cell in the face of excess iron. (*Courtesy of* Pharmacia & Upjohn Co, Kalamazoo, MI.)

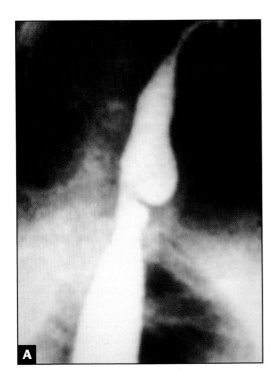

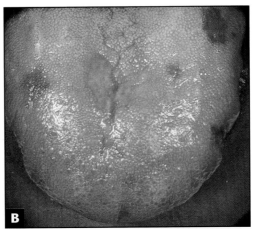

FIGURE 10-4.

The most common cause of a microcytic anemia is iron deficiency; it may rarely be associated with characteristic clinical findings of dysphagia secondary to Plummer-Vinson syndrome, or esophageal web formation; glossitis, or sore tongue; and koilonychia, or spooning of the nails. Pica, an abnormal appetite for unusual foods, is an association unique to iron deficiency [3]. **A,** A barium swallow demonstrating an esophageal web. **B,** A smooth tongue with loss of papillae occurring in iron deficiency. **C,** Loss of the normal concave nail shape constituting spooning of the nails.

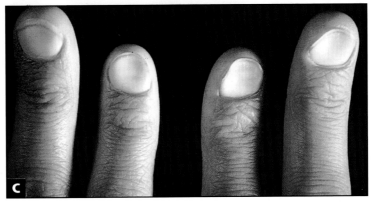

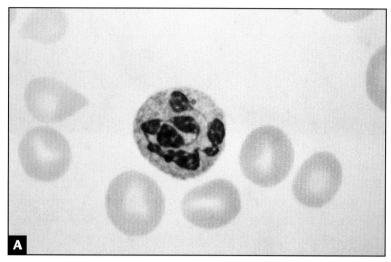

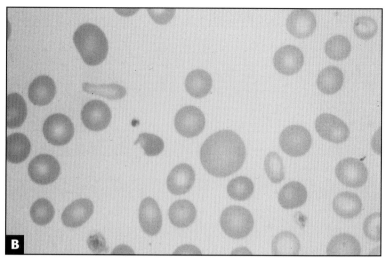

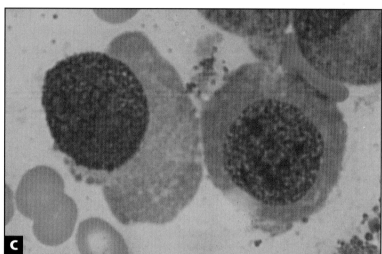

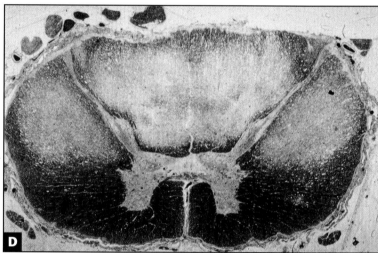

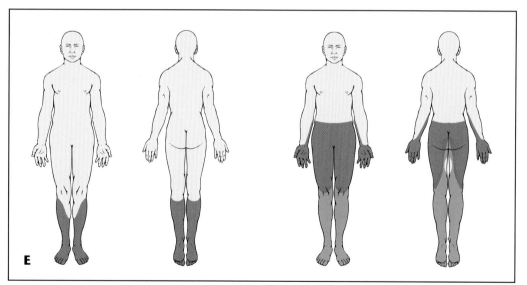

FIGURE 10-5.

Macrocytic anemias (mean corpuscular volume > 95 fl) [4]. The most common cause of macrocytosis is a megaloblastic process that has its origin in vitamin B12 or folate deficiency. Megaloblastic hematopoiesis is a morphologic diagnosis gleaned from examination of the blood and bone marrow. Its hallmark is nuclear-cytoplasmic dissociation with nuclear immaturity relative to cytoplasmic maturation; these cells undergo premature death or apoptosis within the marrow, resulting in markedly ineffective hematopoiesis. A, A polymorphonuclear cell demonstrating megaloblastic features of hypersegmentation. B, Macro-ovalocytes and macrocytes. C, Megaloblastic erythroid precursors with very immature "open-faced" nuclei. Other evidence of a megaloblastic process is hypersegmentation of polymorphonuclear cells (more than five or six lobes) and macro-ovalocytes on the peripheral blood smear.

The hematologic lesions caused by folate and vitamin B12 deficiency are morphologically indistinguishable, with both deficiencies affecting the synthesis of DNA. The development of a demyelinating lesion involving the dorsolateral columns of the spinal cord leading to a loss of vibratory and position sensation in the lower extremities is restricted to vitamin B12 deficiency and is not present in folate deficiency. D, Spinal cord cross-section with loss of myelin in the posterior lateral columns. E, Pattern (in black) of neurosensory loss in vitamin B12 deficiency.

Measurement of serum vitamin B12 and erythrocyte folate levels establishes the causes of these anemias. If vitamin B12 deficiency is identified, a Schilling test helps establish the cause of the deficiency. Pernicious anemia, an autoimmune disorder, is a frequent cause of vitamin B12 deficiency [5].

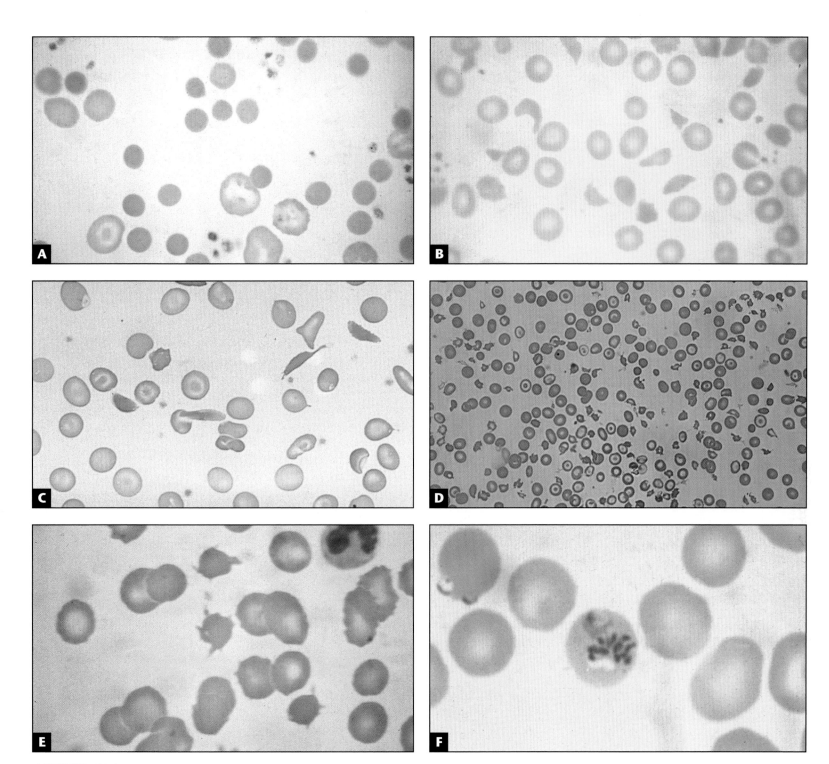

FIGURE 10-6.

Hemolytic anemia. All hemolytic anemias have alterations in erythrocyte morphology as the final common pathway determining their premature destruction; loss of the essential properties of plasticity and deformability secondary to membrane alterations or frank rupture of the membrane shortens their survival, which is normally 90 to 100 days. Examination of the peripheral smear is therefore the most critical source of information in pursuing the cause of hemolytic anemia. Spherocytosis may be a clue to inherited defects in the erythrocyte membrane or an acquired alteration secondary to immune sensitization. **A,** Spherocytes, small, dense erythrocytes that lack the central pallor of normal erythrocytes. **B,** Traumatic hemolysis is the accompaniment of a spectrum of disorders that ranges from the Waring Blender syndrome created by artificial heart valves to the microangiopathic lesions that may occur with malignant hypertension, disseminated intravascular coagulation, and thrombotic thrombocytopenic purpura. Schistocytes (sickle-like forms), helmet cells, and spherocytes are the morphologic evidence of traumatic hemolysis. **C,** Sickle forms, which

are usually present on the peripheral smear of patients with sickle cell anemia [6]. Hemoglobinopathies leave their characteristic imprints on erythrocyte morphology with the sickle forms of sickle hemoglobin, the crystals of hemoglobin C, and the target cells of thalassemia.

Hemolysis may result from progressive organ dysfunction of the liver and kidney and other systemic insults, such as infection. **D,** Acanthocytes with loss of erythrocyte symmetry and irregular membrane projections represent an erythrocyte membrane lipid abnormality present in advanced liver disease. **E,** Burr cells with multiple nipple-like foldings of the erythrocyte membrane. Burr cells are a feature of renal failure. A catastrophic hemolysis may complicate clostridial sepsis wherein a bacterial lecithinase leads to lysis of the erythrocyte membrane. **F,** Thick smear preparations allow a larger number of erythrocytes to be examined for intracellular parasites such as malaria, present here. The presence of parasites such as malaria or *Bartonella* in thick smears of the peripheral blood is the diagnostic method for these infections when hemolysis is a central feature of the pathophysiology of the disorder.

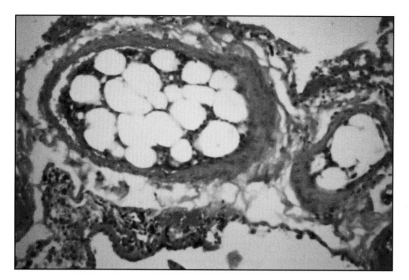

FIGURE 10-7.

Sickle cell anemia. Lung cross section demonstrating fat embolism from a patient with sickle cell anemia who died from the acute chest syndrome [7].

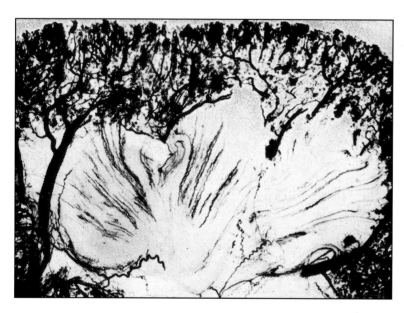

FIGURE 10-8.

Contrast injection of a kidney from a patient with sickle cell anemia. There has been thrombotic obliteration of the vasculature of the renal medulla, creating an anatomic/papillectomy with loss of the countercurrent mechanism and concentrating ability in that kidney. Renal failure in the patient with sickle cell anemia creates a double jeopardy by exaggerating the underlying hemolytic anemia with a superimposed hypoerythropoietin state [8].

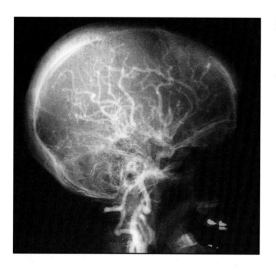

FIGURE 10-9.

Cerebral angiogram demonstrating the characteristic moya-moya lesions in a patient with sickle cell disease. A collateral circulation of delicate vessels form, at the base of the brain, giving rise to the "puff of smoke" sign of sickle cerebrovascular disease [9].

■ OTHER BLOOD DYSCRASIAS

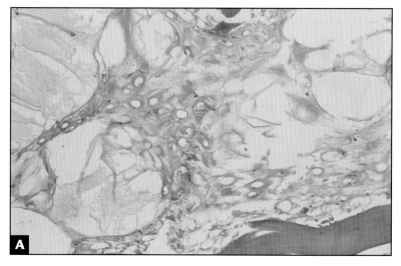

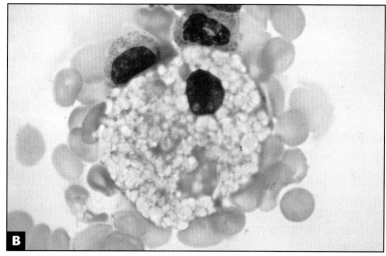

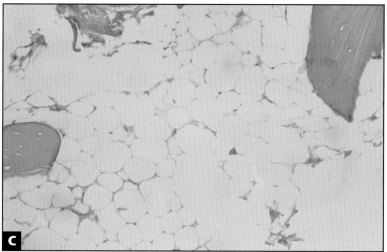

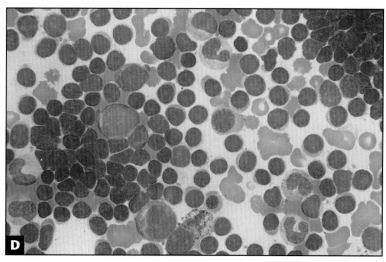

FIGURE 10-10.

Pancytopenia. Reduction in all three elements (*ie*, erythrocyte, leukocyte, platelet) in the peripheral blood defines the entity of pancytopenia. It may have its origin in hypersplenism or in any of the insults that affect the population of hematopoietic elements within the marrow [10]. These include famine, pestilence, warfare, and abnormal clones, and each have parallels in hematopoiesis. **A**, An eosinophilic mucopolysaccharide, which accumulates in the bone marrow of patients with anorexia nervosa. Other examples of famine are vitamin B12, folate, and protein-caloric malnutrition.

B, A histiocyte with "ingested" cells. Hemophagocytosis of marrow elements may occur with viral infections. Other examples of pestilence are mycobacterial and fungal infections. **C**, Bone marrow with total aplasia of hematopoietic elements. A biopsy is necessary to gauge the severity of marrow cellular depletion. Other examples of warfare are exposure to drugs, x-rays, and toxins. **D**, Marrow infiltration in chronic lymphocytic leukemia. Normal marrow stem cells may be replaced or inhibited by pathologic clones. Other examples of abnormal clones are lymphoma and immune disorders.

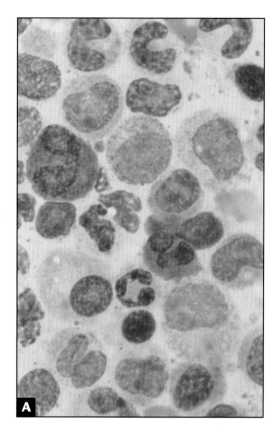

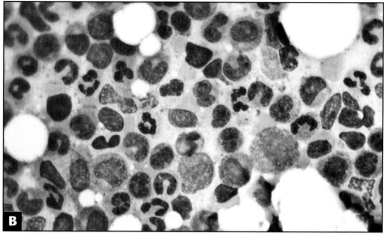

FIGURE 10-11.

Marrow aspirate with no erythroid precursors in pure erythrocyte aplasia [11]. Selective elimination of marrow erythrocyte elements may occur secondary to immune suppression in association with thymomas or lymphoproliferative disorders. A life-threatening erythrocyte aplasia may complicate chronic hemolytic anemias when parvovirus destroys the marrow erythroblast; a more chronic anemia may persist when this infection occurs in an immunosuppressed patient with AIDS [12]. High- (**A**) and low-power (**B**) views of erythrocyte aplasia with striking myeloid prominence.

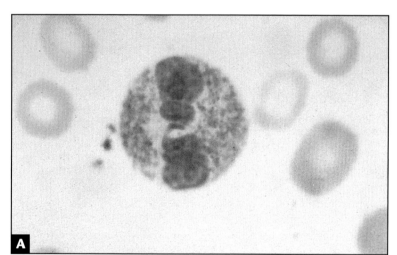

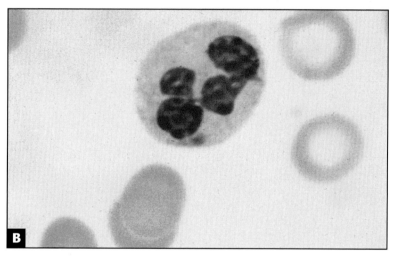

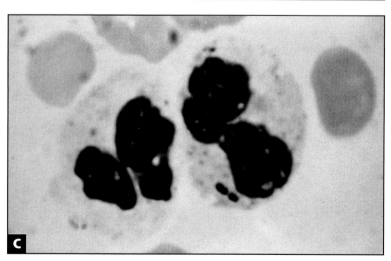

FIGURE 10-12.

The leukocyte in infection. Leukocytosis with a "shift-to-the left" composed of a predominance of polymorphonuclear cells and band forms is the hematologic evidence of a bacterial infection. Other leukocyte manifestations of such infections include toxic granulations, Döhle bodies, and vacuolization of leukocytes. **A,** Toxic "prominent" granulation of neutrophils during sepsis. **B,** Döhle bodies, blue-gray particles in the cytoplasm of neutrophils. **C,** A vacuolated polymorphonuclear cell with a prominent microorganism on Gram stain. In overwhelming sepsis with meningococcemia and pneumococcal infections, Gram stain of the peripheral blood may reveal circulating microorganisms in vacuolated leukocytes.

(Continued)

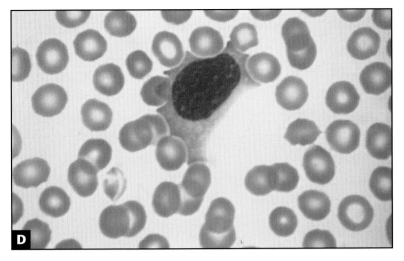

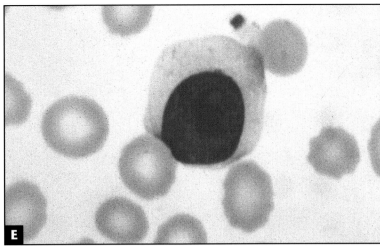

FIGURE 10-12. *(CONTINUED)*

Leukopenia with a relative lymphocytosis often accompanies viral infections and may support this diagnosis, especially when atypical lymphocytes are noted. Atypical lymphocytes are characterized by a large amount of cytoplasm that frequently is indented by surrounding erythrocytes. These "virocytes" represent activated T cells in infectious mononucleosis that have been mobilized to contain the viral-infected B cells. **D** and **E**, Atypical lymphocytes may vary in the degree of nuclear size relative to cell cytoplasm [13]. (Part C *courtesy of* Pharmacia & Upjohn Co, Kalamazoo, MI.)

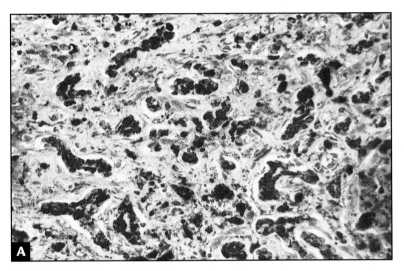

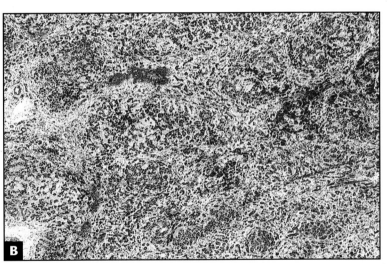

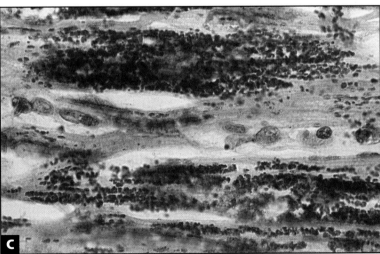

D. Diagnostic Tests for Hemochromatosis

Serum iron/transferrin saturation > 50% to 60%

Serum ferritin as a reflection of total body iron stores

Liver biopsy with quantitative iron determination and histochemistry

Identification of HFE, the genetic mutation present in more than 85% of patients with hemochromatosis

Examination of the bone marrow is of no value in the detection of iron overload

FIGURE 10-13.

Primary hemochromatosis. The accumulation of pathologic amounts of iron secondary to excessive gastrointestinal absorption in primary hemochromatosis may result in cirrhosis, diabetes, cardiomyopathy, arthropathy, and endocrine deficiency [14]. Recognition of this autosomal recessive disorder is necessary prior to the development of these complications in the "bronzed diabetic" (ie, a hyperpigmented diabetic patient with iron overload). This is now possible with the use of serum markers of iron stores, liver biopsy for iron quantification, and a newly available chromosomal marker (HFE). **A**, Prussian blue iron stain of a cirrhotic liver in hemochromatosis. **B**, Iron stain of pancreas. **C**, Iron stain of myocardium. **D**, Diagnostic tests for hemochromatosis.

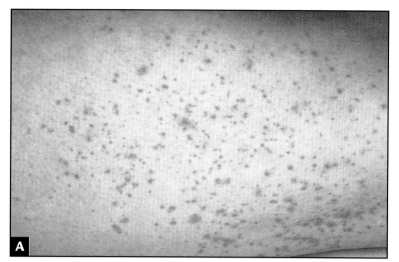

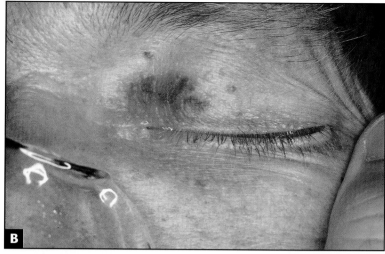

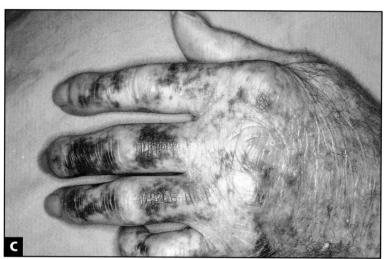

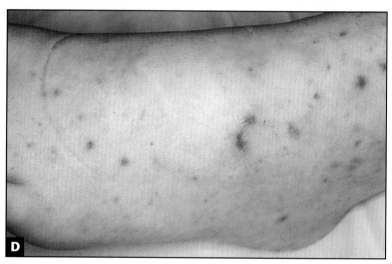

FIGURE 10-14.

Purpura. The morphologic appearance of purpuric skin lesions often contains the clues to the etiology of the condition. Soft tissue ecchymoses (black and blue spots) are characteristic of abnormalities in the soluble coagulation pathway (hemophilia, von Willebrand disease, excessive anticoagulation); petechial lesions are the imprint of platelet deficiency states resulting in minute defects in the endothelium with erythrocyte extravasation. **A,** Perifollicular hemorrhage, the hallmark of scurvy. Perifollicular petechial hemorrhage occurs with scurvy secondary to a vascular collagen deficiency created by vitamin C deficiency. **B,** Post-ptussive periorbital purpura are the four P's suggesting amyloidosis. Periorbital purpura is the hallmark of amyloidosis [15]. Palpable purpura connotes a vasculitis that often contains immunoglobulin deposition such a cryoglobulins. **C,** Purpura and gangrene of the extremities in purpura fulminans. Purpura fulminans, consisting of acral cyanosis, purpura, and gangrene, may arise when disseminated intravascular coagulation complicates meningococcal or pneumococcal sepsis [16]. **D,** Typical purpural skin rash in meningococcemia.

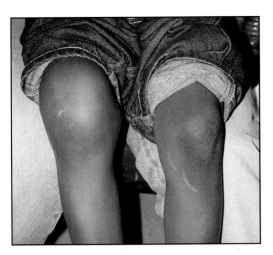

FIGURE 10-15.

Hemarthrosis in hemophilia. Painful bleeding into joints is characteristic of hemophilia A and B. Acute bleeding episodes are managed with aspiration and factor replacement therapy. Recurrent bleeding may result in a chronic arthropathy with marked restriction of joint mobility. More aggressive factor replacement and exercise regimens are lessening these limiting complications. Hemophilia disorders are seen as potential targets for successful treatment with gene therapy [17].

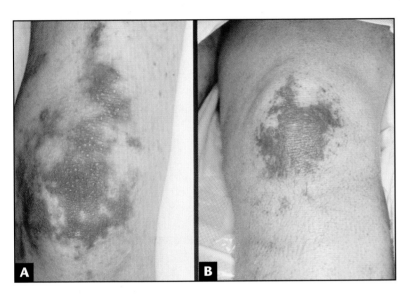

FIGURE 10-16.

Thrombotic microangiopathy. **A, B,** The irregular borders of the purpuric lesions indicate thrombosis of the vascular arcade in the subepidermal layers of the skin. This is characteristic of occlusions seen with anticardiolipid antibodies. Other dermal manifestations of the antiphospholipid syndrome include livedo reticularis, a mottled vascular pattern on the extremities. This livedo pattern may be associated with Sneddon's syndrome, a central nervous system thrombosis in an antiphospholipid constellation. Recurrent miscarriages are also characteristic of this acquired thrombophilic state.

Thrombosis of large vessels can also occur with antiphospholipid antibodies. One complication is phlegmasia cerulea dolens, a thrombosed, swollen, painful, cyanotic extremity. Similar thrombosis can occur with heparin-induced thrombosis-thrombocytopenia syndrome (HITTS). This thrombotic-thrombocytopenic state is life-threatening and necessitates switching to a nonheparin anticoagulant (hirudin) when thrombocytopenia occurs with heparin administration [18].

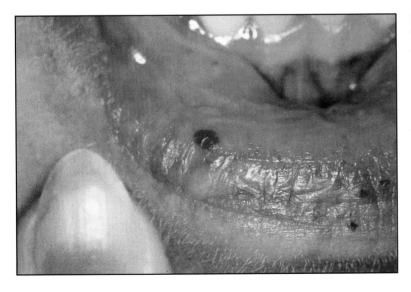

FIGURE 10-17.

Telangiectasias. Hereditary hemorrhagic telangiectasia is an autosomally dominant inherited disorder complicated by chronic bleeding secondary to fragile vascular telangiectasias (venous capillary dilations) in the nasal mucosa and gastrointestinal and genitourinary tracts. Life-threatening hemorrhage may occur secondary to the presence of pulmonary arteriovenous malformations; brain abscesses, strokes, and transient ischemia attack are also attributable to these vascular shunts. The diagnosis rests in the recognition of the blanching vascular lesions on the lips, buccal mucosa, and periungual areas [19].

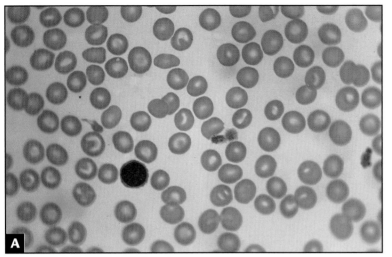

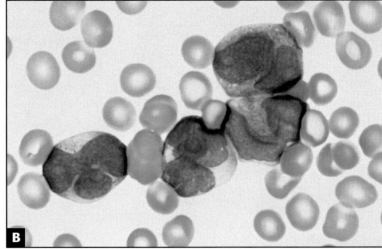

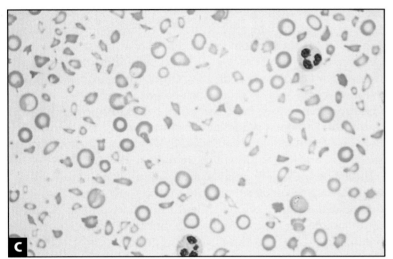

D. Differential Diagnosis of ITP, DIC, and TTP Using Erythrocyte Morphology and FSP Measurements

	Microangiopathic Erythrocyte	Fibrin-split Products
ITP	0	0
DIC	+	+++
TTP or HUS	+++	+

0—absent; +—present; +++—strongly present.

FIGURE 10-18.

Thrombocytopenia. The discovery of thrombocytopenia on electronic Coulter counting always requires confirmation of the platelet deficiency by examination of the peripheral smear; each platelet counted in any high-power field multiplied by 7000 approximates the peripheral platelet count. Agglutination of platelets, easily apparent on examination of the blood smear, may create a misleading "pseudo" thrombocytopenia.

Thrombocytopenia may result from a problem of inadequate production or accelerated destruction. Decreased production may occur with aplastic and hypoplastic anemias, absence of megakaryocytes, marrow replacement with leukemia and lymphoma, and the effect of toxins (such as alcohol) on platelet production. The three major causes of accelerated platelet destruction (in addition to hypersplenism) are immune thrombocytopenia (ITP), disseminated intravascular coagulation (DIC), and thrombolytic states such as thrombotic thrombocytopenic purpura (TTP) and hemolytic-uremic syndrome (HUS). These peripheral platelet consumptive states can be identified by using a simple combination of coagulation assays and an examination of the peripheral smear erythrocyte morphology. **A**, A peripheral blood smear with low to absent platelets and normal erythrocyte morphology, compatible with ITP. **B**, Promyelocytic leukemia, which is often accompanied by thrombocytopenia caused by DIC. **C**, Traumatic erythrocyte damage with thrombocytopenia, which is characteristic of TTP and HUS [20].

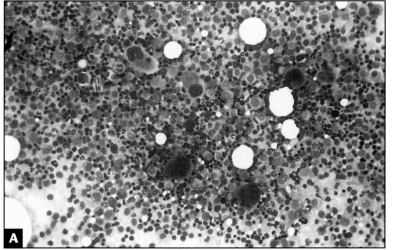 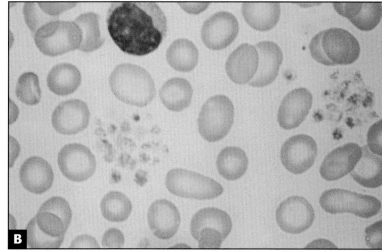

FIGURE 10-19.

Essential thrombocythemia. Essential thrombocythemia (thrombocytosis) is a clonal myeloproliferative disorder characterized by a sustained hyperproliferation of megakaryocytes and a markedly elevated peripheral platelet count [21]. Unlike another myeloproliferative disorder, chronic myelogenous leukemia, there is no defining chromosomal abnormality in essential thrombocythemia. Its diagnosis requires exclusion of secondary causes of thrombocytosis, such as bleeding, iron deficiency, malignancies, and so on. Helpful clues to its presence are megakaryocyte clustering within the marrow and marked variability in the size and shape of platelets on the peripheral smear. **A,** Bone marrow aspiration with megakaryocyte clustering in essential thrombocythemia. **B,** Excess platelets with clumping in essential thrombocythemia.

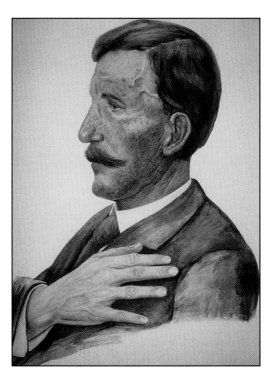

FIGURE 10-20.

Polycythemia vera. This portrait represents the patient in the original case history of polycythemia vera (PCV) (Osler Weber-Rendu disease) described by Sir William Osler in 1903. The ruddy, plethoric complexion with acral cyanosis and conjunctival injection are often joined by splenomegaly as the physical findings in this myeloproliferative disorder. Untreated PCV poses a special risk of thrombotic complications with hepatic and portal veins as frequent sites of involvement. Leukocytosis and thrombocytosis frequently accompany the elevation in hematocrit and red cell mass. Low to absent levels of serum erythropoietin are characteristic of this polycythemic state; this measurement helps to distinguish primary PCV from the many causes of secondary polycythemia (hypoxemia, erythropoietin-secreting tumors, etc.).

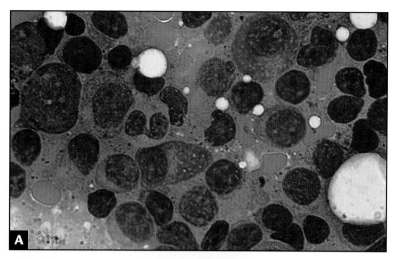

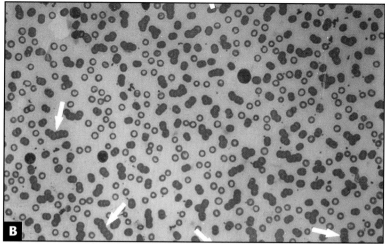

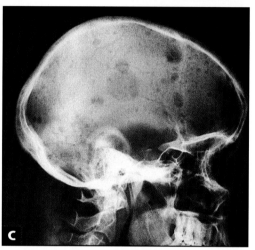

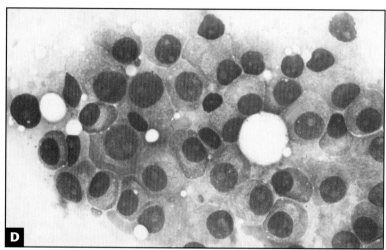

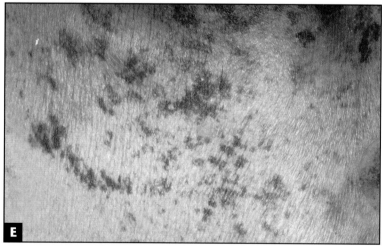

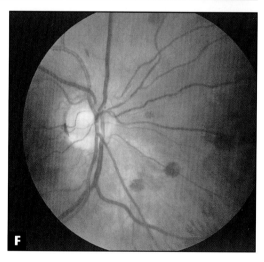

FIGURE 10-21.

Dysproteinemias. Multiple myeloma is a neoplastic proliferation of plasma cells associated with a monoclonal immunoglobulin spike in the serum or urine; the clinical presentation is most frequently with bone pain secondary to osteolytic bony lesions [22]. Renal failure secondary to any combination of hypercalcemia, dehydration, hyperuricemia, and light-chain deposition often occurs; amyloidosis may further complicate the clinical picture. The diagnosis is based on a constellation of findings that includes marrow plasmacytosis (A), a monoclonal protein spike, anemia, azotemia, hypercalcemia, and osteolytic lesions shown on bone radiographs. The erythrocyte sedimentation rate is usually greater than 100 mm/h in myeloma, an abnormality that is suggested by the presence of marked rouleauxing of erythrocytes on the peripheral smear. **B,** "Stacking" of erythrocytes with rouleaux formation in multiple myeloma. **C,** Osteolytic skull lesions in multiple myeloma. **D,** Lymphoplasmacytoid infiltration of bone marrow in

Waldenström's macroglobulinemia [23]. Macroglobulinemia of Waldenström has its origin in a lymphoplasmacytoid proliferation of marrow elements that synthesize IgM monoclonal proteins. Bony lesions and renal failure do not complicate this dysproteinemia. **E,** Purpuric lesions with dysproteinemia. Hyperviscosity with prominent central nervous system manifestations and bleeding problems are the most common clinical involvements in Waldenström's syndrome. **F,** Hemorrhagic lesions in retina in Waldenström's syndrome. Serum protein electrophoresis and marrow examination constitute the diagnostic approach to the condition. Funduscopic examination may reveal so-called "boxcars" or fundus paraproteinaceous where segmentation of blood flow within the vessels is often accompanied by hemorrhage. Measurement of serum viscosity allows recognition of the threat hyperviscosity presents and the need for intervention with plasmapheresis. (Part C *from* Hoffstrand *et al.* [24]; with permission.)

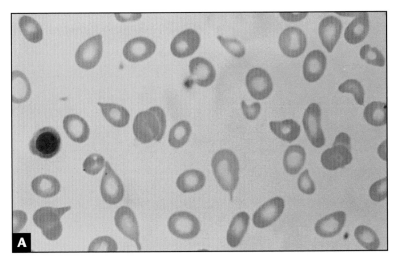

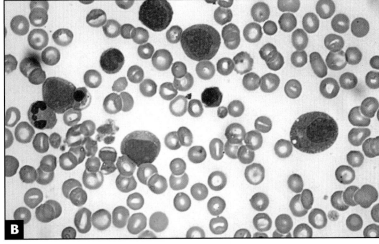

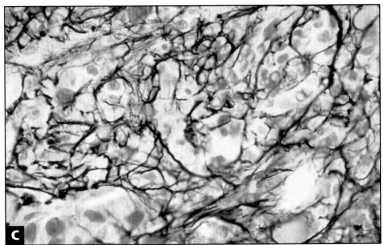

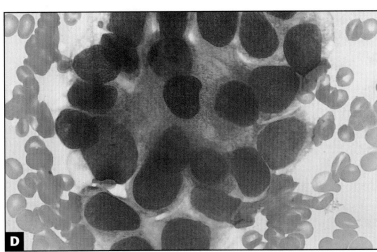

FIGURE 10-22.

Leukoerythroblastic anemia. **A,** Teardrop and nucleated erythrocytes in leukoerythroblastic anemia. A leukoerythroblastic blood picture is characterized by teardrop erythrocytes, leukocytosis with immature leukocyte forms, and large irregular platelet forms. Its importance is its mirroring of a significant pathologic marrow process that includes myelofibrosis and myelophthisic processes associated with malignancy

and granulomatous infections. **B,** Immature leukocytes, nucleated erythrocytes, and large platelet forms in a leukoerythroblastic blood picture. **C,** Dense reticulum in myelofibrosis. **D,** A cluster of metastatic tumor cells in the marrow. In a patient with a known malignancy, the presence of a leukoerythroblastic anemia is very supportive of marrow involvement with the malignancy.

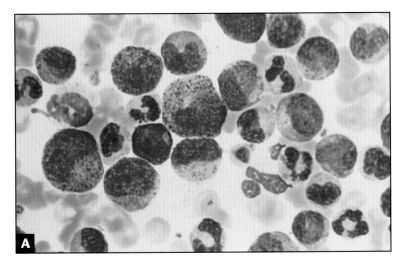

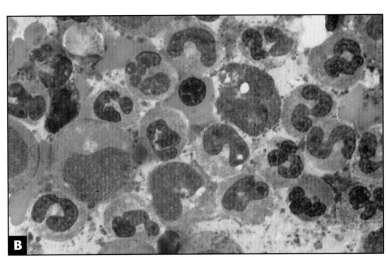

FIGURE 10-23.

Chronic myelogenous leukemia (CML) [25]. The marked increase in the granulocyte mass in CML has its origins and cause in a translocation between chromosomes 9 and 22, resulting in the production of a BCR-cABL chimeric gene product. There is an orderly maturation of myeloid

elements in the peripheral blood (**A**) and bone marrow (**B**) in CML, a characteristic that distinguishes this entity from acute leukemic processes.

(Continued)

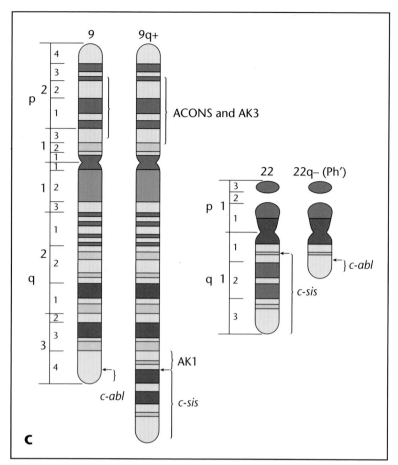

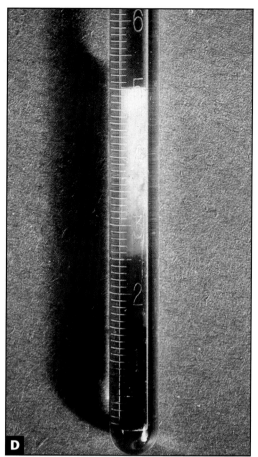

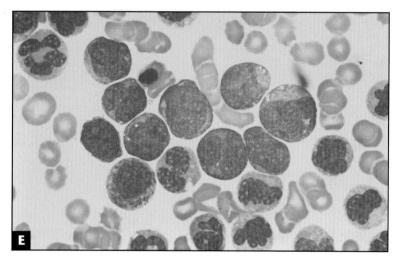

FIGURE 10-23. *(CONTINUED)*
The 9-22 translocation, the Philadelphia chromosome (**C**), is present in more than 85% of bone marrow from CML patients; a decreased to absent concentration of a neutrophil enzyme, alkaline phosphatase, is an additional marker of this myeloproliferative disorder. **D**, Dramatic increase in the leukocyte buffy coat in hyperleukocytotic leukemia. A major threat of CML is hyperviscosity secondary to the dramatic leukocytosis that may occur in this disorder. **E**, Blast transformation of CML. Transformation into acute leukemia is a part of the natural history of CML.

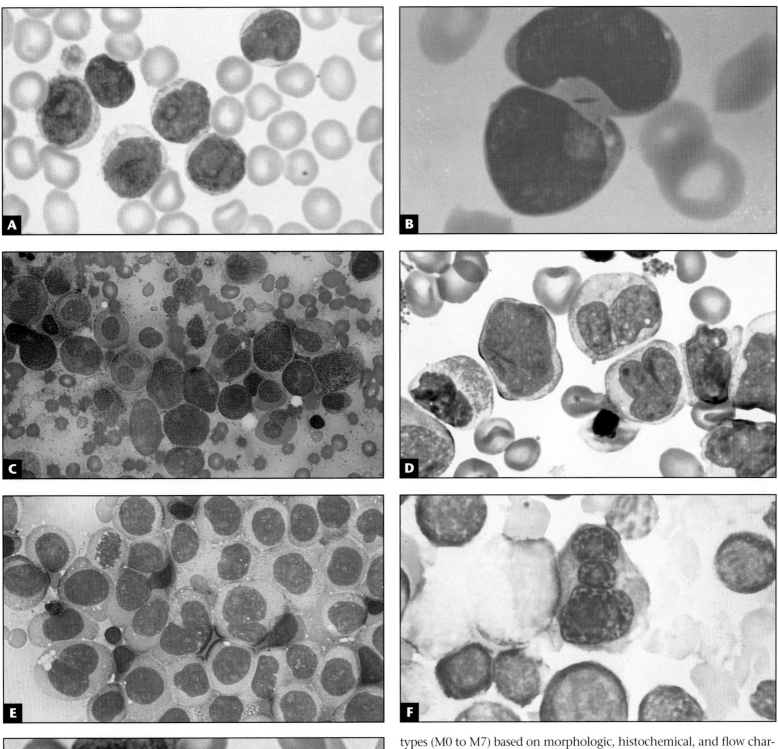

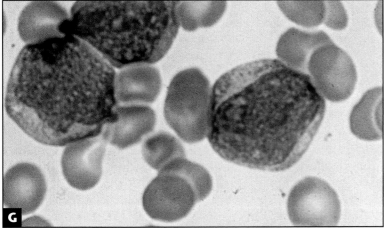

FIGURE 10-24.

Acute nonlymphocytic leukemia. The FAB (French-American-British) classification of acute nonlymphocytic leukemia recognizes eight sub-types (M0 to M7) based on morphologic, histochemical, and flow characteristics of the blast-cell population. Specific chromosomal markers also help assign leukemias to a specific subtype and serve to define prognostic categories on the basis of certain translocations. The diagnosis of leukemia requires that more than 30% of the marrow element be of leukemic origin. These leukemic cells represent an "arrested" stage in the differentiation sequence of developing marrow elements; the specific stage of the arrest determines the subtypes of leukemia. Although the term *leukemia* implies leukocytes, leukemic transformation may involve erythroid and megakaryocytic lines as well. Other marrow elements are inhibited in their development, leading to the anemia and thrombocytopenia that is part of the presentation of most leukemias. The M0 subtype (not shown) describes undifferentiated "stem" cell leukemia. **A**, M1, early acute myeloblastic leukemia. **B**, M2, acute myeloblastic leukemia with Auer rod. **C**, M3, acute promyelocytic leukemia. **D**, M4, acute myelomonocytic leukemia. **E**, M5, acute monocytic leukemia. **F**, M6, acute erythroleukemia. **G**, M7, acute megakaryoblastic leukemia [26].

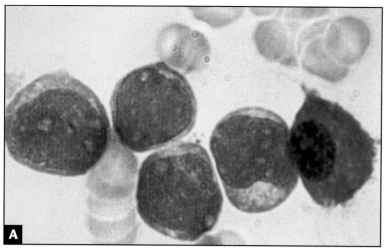

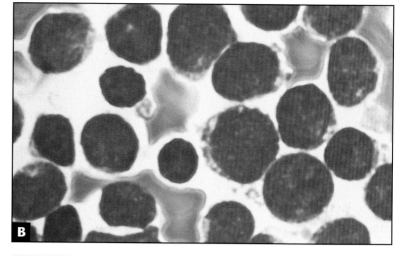

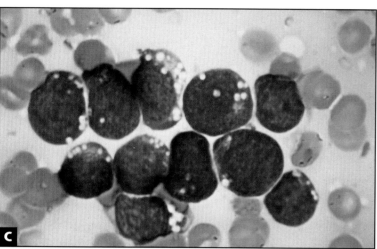

FIGURE 10-25.

Acute lymphocytic leukemia (ALL). There are three subtypes of ALL according to the FAB (French-American-British) classification. **A**, L1 is a CALLA (common ALL antigen) positive, non–B-, non–T-cell lymphocytic leukemia that is most common in childhood. **B**, L2 is composed of a more heterogeneous population of lymphoid cells that often includes the poor prognosis Philadelphia chromosome–positive ALL. **C**, L3 is an immunoblastic, Burkett's type of leukemia. ALL cells stain positive with periodic acid-Schiff, and flow cytometry permits subtyping of the leukemia [27].

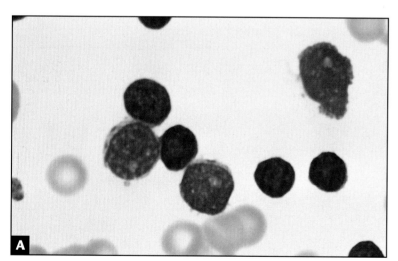

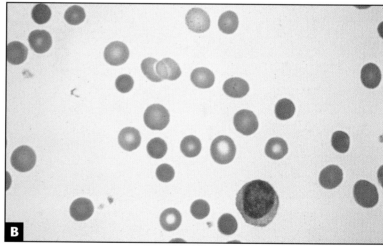

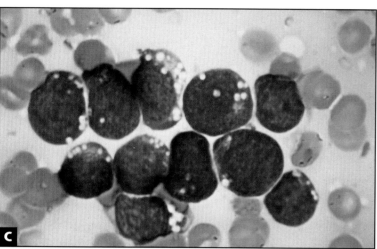

FIGURE 10-26.

Chronic lymphocytic leukemia (CLL). CLL (**A**) is an accumulation of immunologically incompetent cells; it is primarily a disease of the elderly and represents the most common leukemia worldwide [28]. It is associated with progressive lymphadenopathy and hepatosplenomegaly; acquired immunoglobulin deficiency gives rise to an increased risk of infection. A small percentage of CLL patients will develop autoimmune hemolytic anemia, immune thrombocytopenia, or both. CLL with spherocytic erythrocytes (**B**) may be evidence for an associated hemolytic anemia. Flow cytometry permits easy recognition of the characteristic monoclonal B-cell population in CLL. Other lymphatic leukemias need to be differentiated from CLL; these include hairy-cell leukemia (**C**), which has a characteristic cytoplasmic morphology,

(Continued)

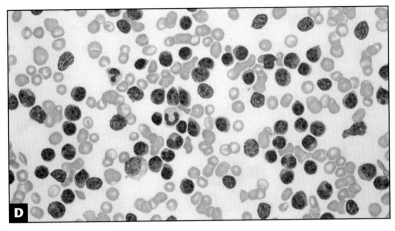

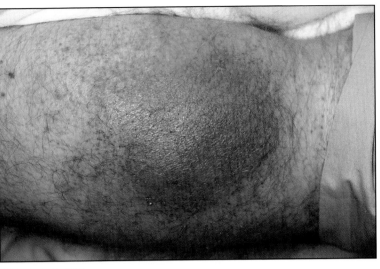

FIGURE 10-26. (CONTINUED)
and prolymphocytic leukemia (**D**), which has a less-differentiated population of lymphocytes and more prominent splenomegaly. (Part A *courtesy of* Pharmacia & Upjohn Co, Kalamazoo, MI.)

FIGURE 10-27.
Ichthyma gangrenosum. A classic skin lesion in the neutropenic patient following chemotherapy for leukemia is the exquisitely painful, erythematous lesion of ichthyma gangrenosum. Recognition of the clinical lesion and rapid initiation of antibiotics may be life-saving. Another devastating infectious complication in this patient population is Fournier's gangrene, a spreading bacterial infection of the perirectal-rectal-perineal fascial planes with severe local and systemic toxicity. Antibiotic therapy may be supplemented with white cell transfusions to control this frequently lethal infection.

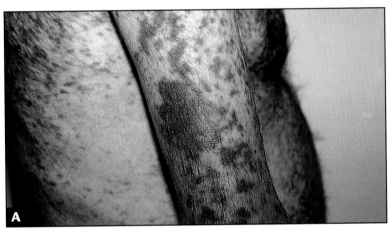

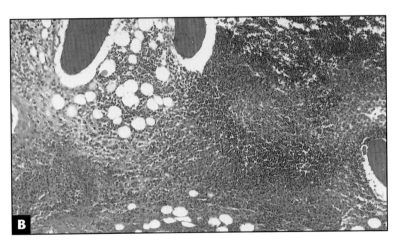

FIGURE 10-28.
Systemic mastocytosis. Systemic mast-cell disease is an abnormal accumulation of mast cells within the skin (urticaria pigmentosa) or other organs of the body, predominantly the spleen and bone marrow [29]. Its clinical manifestations are protean, attributable to the large number of active pharmacologic agents contained within the mast-cell granules. Diagnosis is possible by demonstrating mast cells in biopsies of the skin or bone marrow; elevated levels of serum tryptase are also helpful in arriving at this diagnosis. Gastrointestinal (*eg*, diarrhea, peptic ulcer disease), pulmonary (*eg*, bronchospasm, dyspnea), cardiovascular (*eg*, hypertension, syncope, angina), and dermatologic (*eg*, pruritus, urticaria) symptoms are common. **A**, Skin lesions of urticaria pigmentosa. **B**, Bone marrow infiltration with mast cells.

■ REFERENCES

1. Schnall S, Berliner N, Duffy TP, *et al.*: *Approach to the Adult and Child with Anemia.* In *Hematology: Principles and Practice* edn 3. Edited by Hoffman R. New York: Churchill Livingstone; 1999:367–382.

2. Andrews NC: Disorders of iron metabolism. *N Engl J Med* 1999, 341:1986–1995.

3. Federman DG, Kirsner RS, Federman GS: Pica: are you hungry for the facts? *Conn Med* 1997, 61:207–209.

4. Davenport J: Macrocytic anemia. *Am Fam Physician* 1996, 53:155–162.

5. Toh BH, van Driel IR, Gleeson PA: Pernicious anemia. *N Engl J Med* 1997, 337:1441–1448.

6. Bunn HF: Pathogenesis and treatment of sickle cell disease. *N Engl J Med* 1997, 337:762–769.

7. Vichinsky EP, Neumayr LD, Earles AN, *et al.*: Causes and outcomes of the acute chest syndrome in sickle cell disease. National Acute Chest Syndrome study group. *N Engl J Med* 2000, 342:1855–1865.

8. Ataga KI, Orringer EP: Renal abnormalities in sickle cell disease. *Am J Hematol* 2000, 63:205–211.

9. Powars DR, Conti PS, Wong WY, *et al.*: Cerebral vasculopathy in sickle cell anemia: diagnostic contribution of positron emission tomography. *Blood* 1999, 93(1):71–79.

10. Guinan EC: Clinical aspects of aplastic anemia. *Hematol Oncol Clin North Am* 1997, 11:1025–1044.

11. Erslev AJ, Soltan A: Pure red-cell aplasia: a review. *Blood Rev* 1996, 10:20–28.

12. Brown KE, Young NS: Parvovirus B19 in human disease. *Ann Rev Med* 1997, 48:59–67.

13. Seebach JD, Morant R, Ruegg R, *et al.*: The diagnostic value of the neutrophil left shift in predicting inflammatory and infectious disease. *Am J Clin Pathol* 1997, 107:582–591.

14. Barton JC, Edwards CQ. *Hemochromatosis.* Cambridge: Cambridge University Press; 2000.

15. Falk RH, Comenzo RL, Skinner M: Medical progress: the systemic amyloidoses. *N Engl J Med* 1997, 337:899–909.

16. Carpenter CT, Kaiser AB: Purpura fulminans in pneumococcal sepsis: case report and review. *Scand J Infect Dis* 1997, 29:479–483.

17. Mannucci PM, Tuddenham EG: The hemophilias—from royal genes to gene therapy. *N Engl J Med* 2001, 344(23):1773–1779.

18. Schaar CG, Ronday KH, Boets EP, *et al.*: Catastrophic manifestation of the antiphospholipid syndrome. *J Rheumatol* 1999, 26(10):2261–2264.

19. Guttmacher AE, Marchuk DA, White RI Jr: Hereditary hemorrhagic telangiectasia. *N Engl J Med* 1995, 333:918–924.

20. Anonymous: Diagnosis and treatment of idiopathic thrombocytopenic purpura: recommendations of the American Society of Hematology. The American Society of Hematology ITP Practice Guideline Panel. *Ann Intern Med* 1997, 126:319–326.

21. Murphy S, Peterson P, Iland H, Laszlo J: Experience of the Polycythemia Vera Study Group with essential thrombocythemia: a final report on diagnostic criteria, survival, and leukemic transition by treatment. *Semin Hematol* 1997, 34:29–39.

22. Larson RS, Sukpanichnant S, Greer JP, *et al.*: The spectrum of multiple myeloma: diagnostic and biological implications. *Hum Pathol* 1997, 28:1336–1347.

23. Andriko JA, Arguilera NS, Chu WS, *et al.*: Waldenstrom's macroglobulinemia: a clinicopathologic study of 22 cases. *Cancer* 1995, 80:1926–1935.

24. Hoffstrand AV, Pettit J: *Sandoz Slide Atlas of Clinical Hematology.* Philadelphia: Gower Medical Publishing; 1988.

25. Tefferi A, Litzow MR, Noel P, Dewald GW: Chronic granulocytic leukemia: recent information on pathogenesis, diagnosis, and disease monitoring. *Mayo Clin Proc* 1997, 72:445–452.

26. Taylor CG, Stasi R, Bastianelli C, *et al.*: Diagnosis and classification of the acute leukemias: recent advances and controversial issues. *Hematopathol Molec Hematol* 1996, 10:1–38.

27. Cortes JE, Kantarjian H, Freireich EJ: Acute lymphocytic leukemia: a comprehensive review with emphasis on biology and therapy. *Cancer Treat Res* 1996, 84:291–323.

28. Cheson BD, Bennett JM, Grever M, *et al.*: National Cancer Institute–sponsored Working Group guidelines for chronic lymphocytic leukemia: revised guidelines for diagnosis and treatment. *Blood* 1996, 87:4990–4997.

29. Longley J, Duffy TP, Kohn S: The mast cell and mast cell disease. *J Am Acad Dermatol* 1995, 32:545–561.

Gastroenterology

MARK FELDMAN

Internists frequently diagnose and treat adult patients with acute or chronic gastrointestinal disorders. This clinical spectrum ranges from managing acute diarrhea in adolescents to severe constipation in the elderly. More and more, general internists are also involved in screening (and preventing) digestive diseases, such as judicious use of fecal occult blood testing and flexible sigmoidoscopy to screen for colorectal cancer.

Disorders of the gastrointestinal (GI) tract, biliary tree, and pancreas are common in internal medicine practice. *Helicobacter pylori* gastritis is the most frequent bacterial infection of humans and is a risk factor for peptic ulcer disease and gastric malignancies [1]. Colorectal carcinoma is the second leading cause of cancer mortality in the United States, responsible for an estimated 56,500 deaths in 1998. Pancreatic cancer resulted in an additional 28,900 deaths [2]. Gallstone disease is also common in our society, as is an increasing reliance on laparoscopic cholecystectomy in symptomatic individuals. Inflammatory bowel diseases (ulcerative colitis, Crohn's disease) are also widespread in all segments of the population; their causes still elude us. Irritable bowel syndrome and other functional GI disorders, including functional abdominal pain syndrome, cause considerable morbidity and absenteeism and represent a sizable fraction of disorders seen by internists and gastroenterologists [3].

Striking advances in diagnostic and therapeutic GI endoscopy, GI radiology, or a combination of the two, such as endoscopic retrograde cholangiopancreatography, have occurred. Advances have also been made in the therapy of gastrointestinal disorders. Examples include cure of peptic ulcer disease by eradicating *Heliobacter pylori* with antimicrobial agents, healing of erosive esophagitis with proton pump inhibitor drugs, and use of anticytokines (anti-TNF compounds) in Crohn's disease [4]. Therapeutic endoscopic techniques have proliferated that reduce the need for surgical procedures. Endoscopic advances include placement of peroral endoscopic gastrostomy tubes for nutritional support; insertion of stents in the bile duct or esophagus to relieve malignant obstruction; removal of gallstones from the common bile duct; and the use of injection therapy, thermal coagulation, or laser therapy to treat bleeding ulcers and other lesions, including tumors.

This chapter of the second edition of *Atlas of Internal Medicine* is a collection of approximately 100 images that pictorially displays the diseases of the gastrointestinal tract, biliary tree, and pancreas in adults. The images selected were thought to be the most relevant to general internists in clinical practice or in training.

■ ESOPHAGEAL DISORDERS

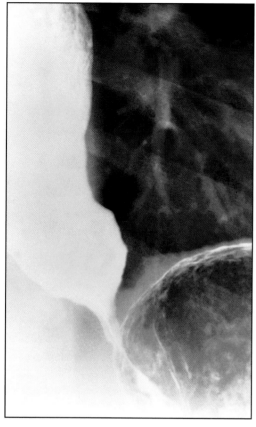

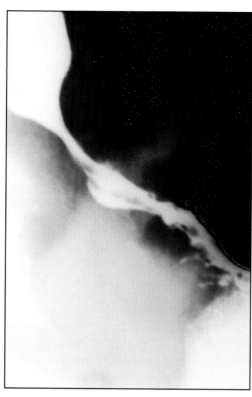

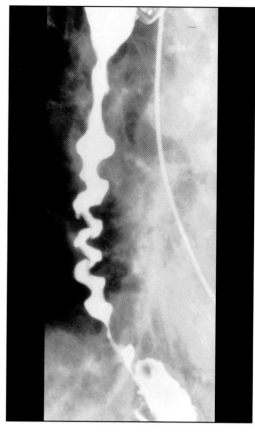

FIGURE 11-1.

Barium esophagogram and endoscopy are complementary to each other in the diagnosis of esophageal diseases. This figure represents the lower esophagus of a patient with dysphagia. Esophagogram showed a bird's beak appearance of the gastroesophageal junction and total aperistalsis of the esophageal body consistent with the diagnosis of achalasia. Therapeutic options include pneumatic dilation, laparoscopic or open myotomy, or endoscopic injection of botulinum toxin. (*Courtesy of* Wallace C. Wu.)

FIGURE 11-2.

Pseudoachalasia. When there is a short history of dysphagia and considerable weight loss and when a patient is age 60 or older, cancer may produce the image of achalasia, or pseudoachalasia. Pseudoachalasia is most commonly caused by esophageal gastric cancers, but pancreatic cancers and lymphoma also may cause it.

FIGURE 11-3.

Endoscopy is an excellent tool in the diagnosis of mucosal lesions. Unfortunately, it cannot differentiate between normal and abnormal peristalsis and hence is insensitive in the diagnosis of motility disorders of the esophagus. This figure depicts the esophagogram of a patient with dysphagia and chest pain. His endoscopy is completely normal. Esophagogram shows classic changes of diffuse esophageal spasm, with a "corkscrew" esophagus. Esophageal manometry confirms the diagnosis. (*Courtesy of* Wallace C. Wu.)

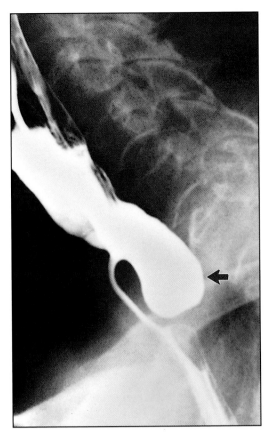

FIGURE 11-4.

Zenker's diverticulum. Radiograph of a 70-year-old patient with oropharyngeal dysphagia, coughing, choking spells, and recurrent pneumonia. Note the outpouching of the pharynx above the level of the cricopharyngeus (*arrow*). This outpouching is located in the posterior wall of the pharynx. Zenker's diverticulum is a true pulsion diverticulum and is the result of increased intrapharyngeal pressures during swallowing as a result of a noncompliant or nonrelaxing upper esophageal sphincter. There may be penetration of the barium into the laryngeal inlet and spilling into the tracheobronchial tree. The treatment of this condition in the setting of severe symptoms is usually cricopharyngeal myotomy, with or without a diverticulectomy or diverticulopexy. (*Courtesy of* Ravinder K. Mittal.)

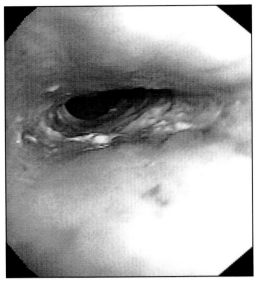

FIGURE 11-5.

Erosive esophagitis: endoscopic view. The hallmark of reflux esophagitis on endoscopy is the presence of one or more erosions within the distal esophagus [5]. Although the finding of such lesions is neither sensitive (being found in less than 50% of those whose heartburn is explored endoscopically) nor specific (because they can occur with other esophageal injuries), the diagnosis is established by the chronicity of symptoms coupled with the typical nature of the lesions in the absence of other definable causes (*eg*, infectious or pill-induced esophagitis). (*Courtesy of* Roy C. Orlando.)

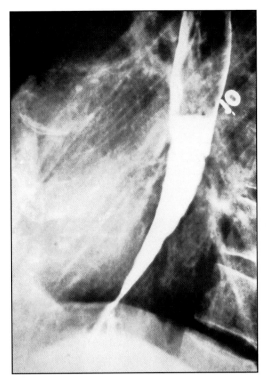

FIGURE 11-6.

Esophageal stricture. A barium esophagogram demonstrates the presence of a partially obstructing smooth-walled distal esophageal stricture secondary to reflux esophagitis. Patients with this complication may note amelioration of heartburn when a new symptom (*ie*, dysphagia for solid foods) becomes more pronounced. (*From* Orlando [6]; with permission.)

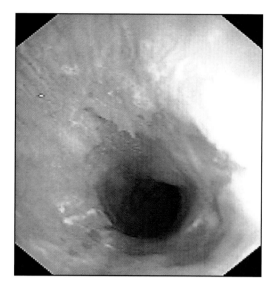

FIGURE 11-7.

Barrett's esophagus. The endoscopic appearance of a columnar-lined lower esophagus (*ie*, Barrett's) is shown for a patient with reflux esophagitis. The typical red coloration of the columnar epithelium distally is readily distinguished from the lighter pink or orange stratified squamous epithelium proximally. For a specific diagnosis, however, endoscopic biopsy is required for histologic confirmation of the specialized columnar epithelium lining the lower esophagus. Barrett's esophagus predisposes to esophageal adenocarcinoma, which occurs in approximately 5% to 10% of patients. (*Courtesy of* Roy C. Orlando.)

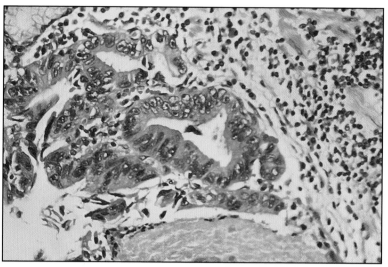

FIGURE 11-8.

Histology of Barrett's esophagus. Biopsies of the esophagus reveal glands consisting of specialized columnar epithelium rather than normal squamous epithelium (Barrett's metaplasia).

Proton Pump Inhibitors

Generic Name	Trade Name	GERD Dosage	Formulation
Omeprazole	Prilosec*	20 mg/d	Capsule
Lasoprazole	Prevacid†	30 mg/d	Capsule
Rabeprazole	Aciphex‡	20 mg/d	Tablet
Pantoprazole	Protonix§	40 mg/d	Tablet
Esomeprazole	Nexium*	20 mg/d	Capsule

*AstraZeneca, Wilmington, DE.
†TAP Pharmaceuticals, Lake Forest, IL.
‡Janssen Pharmaceutica, Titusville, NJ
§Wyeth-Ayerst, Philadelphia, PA.

FIGURE 11-9.

Proton pump inhibitors used in gastroesophageal reflux disease in the United States.

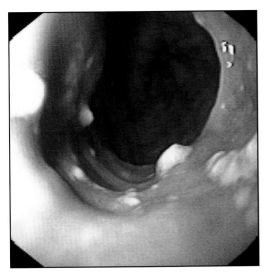

FIGURE 11-10.
Early findings of esophagitis caused by *Candida* with plaques not yet becoming confluent. As the infection worsens, there is associated hyperemia. The most common predisposing condition is HIV infection. (*Courtesy of* A. Tsuchida.)

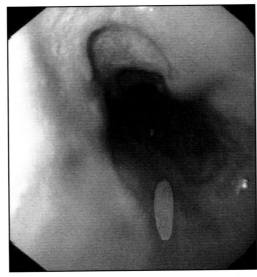

FIGURE 11-11.
The endoscopic characteristics of an esophageal ulcer caused by HIV are variable, ranging from small, superficial, shallow aphthous ulcers (0.5 to 1.0 cm) to, as shown here, large, deep ulcers with undermining borders (1 to 6 cm). To be considered as an ulcer caused by HIV other causes of esophageal ulceration must be excluded, such as *Candida*, cytomegalovirus, and herpes virus infections. This endoscopic photograph demonstrates a large 6-cm chronic ulcer with deep undermining edges and nodularity within the ulcer base. Idiopathic HIV-associated ulcers have been successfully treated with intravenous corticosteroid therapy. In one study, 23 of 24 patients (95.8%) improved. Relapses were common after discontinuation of therapy. To maintain remission, long-term therapy was required. These results must be tempered by the risk of additional long-term immunosuppressive therapy. (*Courtesy of* Matthew S.Z. Bachinski and Roy K.H. Wong.)

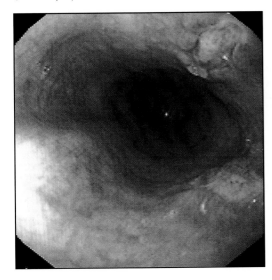

FIGURE 11-12.
Pill ulcers. A 25-year-old female developed dysphagia and odynophagia acutely. She had taken a dose of doxycycline for acne just before she went to bed the night before. Endoscopy showed two ulcers in the midesophagus, one at 1 o'clock and one at 4 o'clock. The history and endoscopic appearance are perfectly compatible with the diagnosis of esophagitis caused by medication in pill form. (*Courtesy of* Wallace C. Wu.)

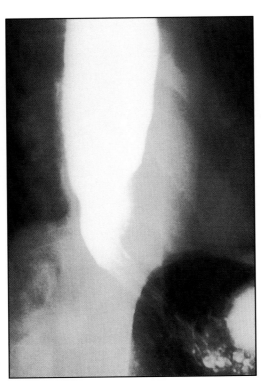

FIGURE 11-13.
Scleroderma. Dilated esophagus with absent motility in a patient with CREST syndrome. Reflux esophagitis and peptic strictures may also occur.

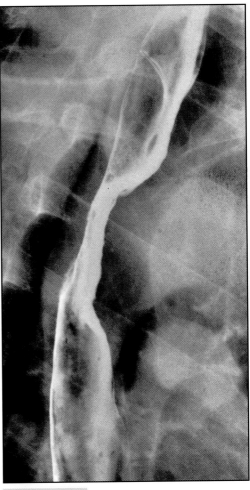

FIGURE 11-14.
Esophagogram from a patient who experienced progressive solid-food dysphagia for several months. He also experienced a 20-pound weight loss during that same period. Esophagogram showed a malignant neoplasm involving the esophagus, with luminal narrowing and mucosal irregularity. (*Courtesy of* Wallace C. Wu.)

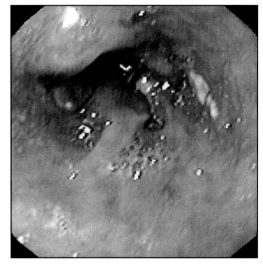

FIGURE 11-15.
Endoscopic view of the patient in Figure 11-14. Endoscopy confirmed the presence of an apparently malignant lesion in the esophagus. Biopsies showed a squamous cell carcinoma of the esophagus. (*Courtesy of* Wallace C. Wu.)

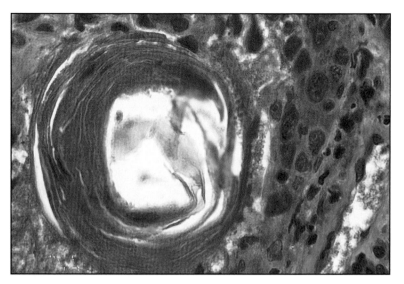

FIGURE 11-16.
Biopsies from the esophagus in Figures 11-14 and 11-15 showing squamous cell carcinoma. In the center is an esophageal "pearl," an accumulation of keratin protein.

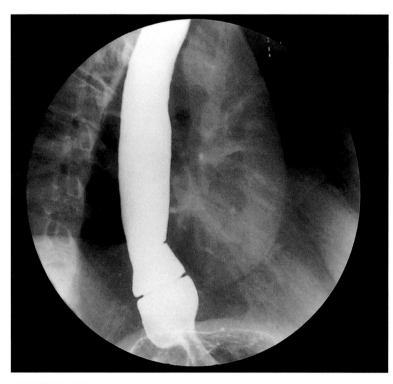

FIGURE 11-17.
Schatzki's ring on barium esophagram. Esophageal webs and rings are thin esophageal stenoses typically composed of only mucosa. Rings formed at the gastroesophageal junction, as described by Schatzki, are usually silent but become symptomatic when the internal diameter is less than 13 mm. (*From* McBride and Ergun [7]; with permission.)

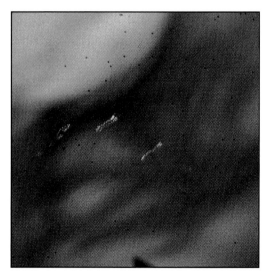

FIGURE 11-18.
Esophageal varices, as viewed by endoscopy. Enlarged, worm-like veins are visible. Varices usually indicate portal hypertension secondary to cirrhosis from hepatitis C, alcohol, or other causes of cirrhosis (*see* Chapter 12, *Hepatology*).

■ GASTRIC AND DUODENAL DISORDERS

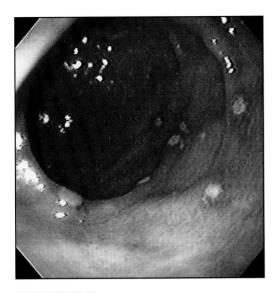

FIGURE 11-19.

Endoscopic erosive gastritis. The observations of multiple erosive and hemorrhagic lesions may be defined endoscopically as gastritis. This figure is an example of endoscopic erosive gastritis. Common settings that may lead to endoscopic gastritis include use of nonsteroidal anti-inflammatory drugs, alcohol abuse, and the physiologic stress associated with serious illnesses (stress gastritis). Other less common causes include ingestion of corrosives, chemotherapeutic agents, or irradiation. There may also be no known demonstrable associated factor present (idiopathic). The term gastritis may be a misnomer, as inflammation may be absent. Reactive gastropathy may be a more appropriate term. (*Courtesy of* W. Harford.)

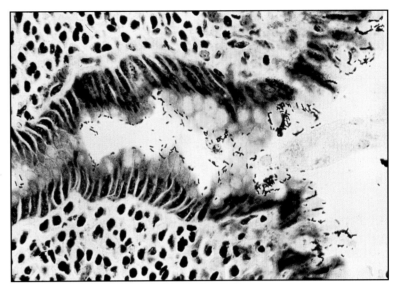

FIGURE 11-20.

Helicobacter pylori in gastric mucosa. As shown, at high-power magnification, *H. pylori* can be easily identified (Warthin-Starry silver stain). *H. pylori* can be almost as easily identified using the routine hematoxylin and eosin stain. Acute and chronic inflammation is present as well. (*From* Peterson *et al.* [8]; with permission.)

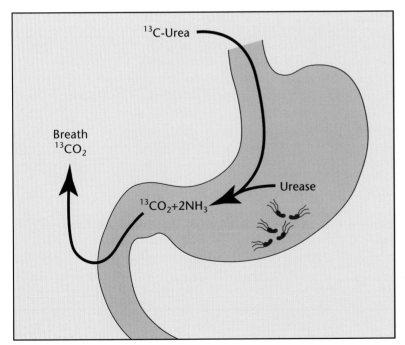

FIGURE 11-21.

^{13}C Urea breath tests. Diagnosis of *Helicobacter pylori* by the urea breath test is based on urease metabolism of ingested urea. Either ^{13}C– or ^{14}C–labeled urea is ingested. (The ^{13}C-labeled urea is a nonradioactive carbon isotope). If *H. pylori* is present, urea is metabolized to ammonia and carbon-labeled carbon dioxide. The labeled carbon dioxide is then excreted in breath as labeled carbon dioxide, which is then collected and quantified. (*Courtesy of* Byron Cryer and Edward Lee.)

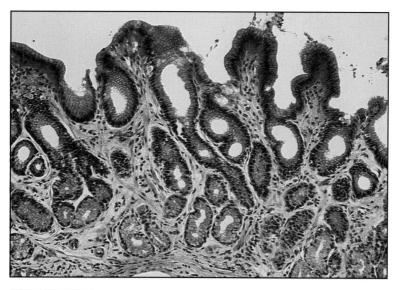
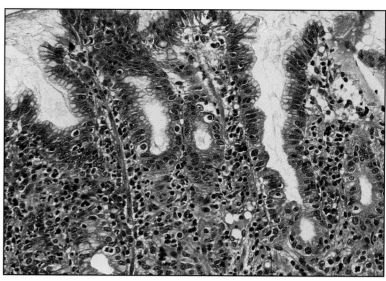

FIGURE 11-22.

A, Normal antral biopsy. **B,** Severe diffuse antral gastritis due to *Helicobacter pylori* infection. Most infected patients also have some inflammation in the gastric body as well.

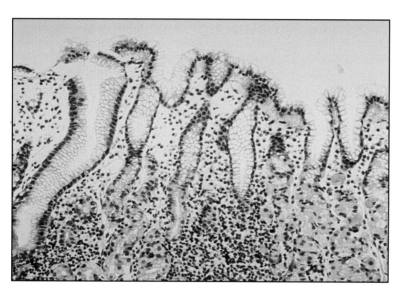

FIGURE 11-23.

Lymphoid follicle. *Helicobacter pylori* infection can be associated with mucosal lymphoid follicles as shown. *H. pylori* are visible within the base of gastric pits. Histologic identification of gastric lymphoid follicles, not normally observed in an uninfected stomach, strongly suggests a coexisting *H. pylori* infection, even if the organisms are not visualized in the same section as the lymphoid follicle.

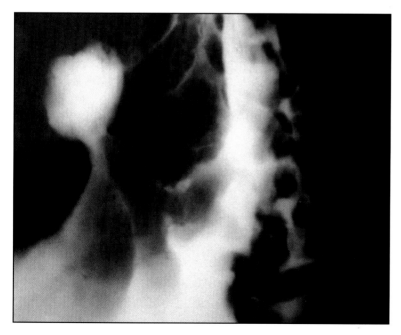

FIGURE 11-24.

Typical radiographic features of a benign gastric ulcer. A large well-circumscribed ulcer is seen on the angularis. Rugal folds can be seen radiating to the crater. Radiographic features suggestive of a benign ulcer include projection of the ulcer away from the lumen, absence of mass effect or mucosal nodularity, and rugal folds of normal appearance, which extend to the ulcer crater. The sensitivity of barium radiography for the diagnosis of gastric ulcer is approximately 65% to 90%; the sensitivity increases with the size of the lesion.

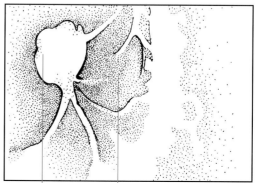

Ulcer crater   *Radiating folds*

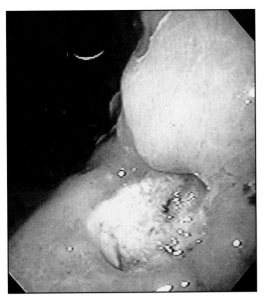

FIGURE 11-25.

The ulcer crater in Figure 11-24 as seen at endoscopy. The lesion is large and well circumscribed with a symmetrical appearance. Multiple biopsies did not demonstrate carcinoma, and the ulcer was demonstrated to heal on follow-up endoscopy. The most common risk factors are *H. pylori* infection and use of nonsteroidal anti-inflammatory drugs.

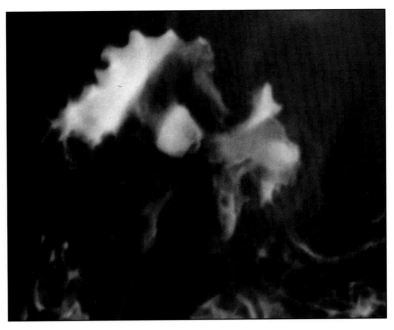

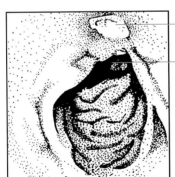

Ulcer crater

FIGURE 11-26.

Typical radiographic features of duodenal ulcer. This duodenal bulb ulcer is associated with marked edema, resulting in the appearance of radiating folds to the ulcer crater. The bulb is also distorted (scarred) secondary to previously existing ulceration. *Helicobacter pylori* is the most common risk factor for duodenal ulcers. (*Courtesy of* C. Mel Wilcox.)

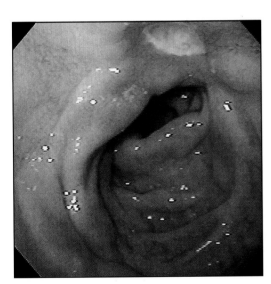

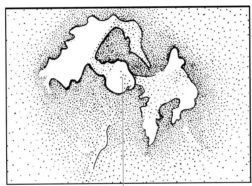

Ulcer crater

To second duodenum

FIGURE 11-27.

Duodenal ulcer at endoscopy. A well-circumscribed lesion as seen in a superior view. The remaining portion of the bulb is mildly edematous but without any associated subepithelial hemorrhage or erosions. (*Courtesy of* C. Mel Wilcox.)

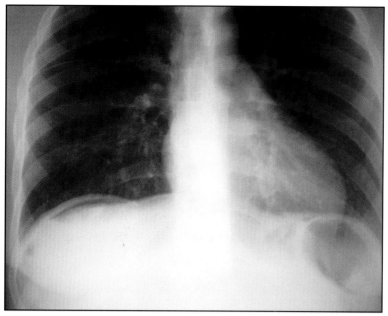

FIGURE 11-28.

Perforated peptic ulcer. A small amount of air is present under the right hemidiaphragm in a patient with acute severe abdominal pain. This patient had a perforated anterior duodenal bulbar ulcer. Recently, perforated ulcer has also been associated with cocaine use. (*Courtesy of* C. Mel Wilcox.)

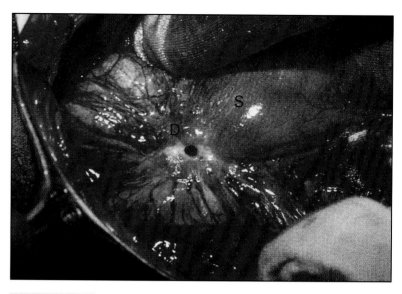

FIGURE 11-29.

Laparotomy view of perforated ulcer of duodenal bulb (D), with stomach(s) on the right. (*From* Molmenti [9]; with permission.)

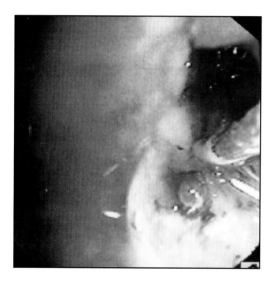

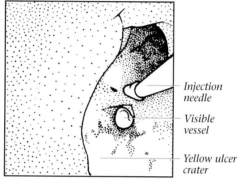

Injection needle

Visible vessel

Yellow ulcer crater

FIGURE 11-30.

Ulcer bleeding. Approximately 50% of patients with upper gastrointestinal hemorrhage have experienced bleeding from a peptic ulcer. Bleeding duodenal ulcers are somewhat more common than gastric ulcers. Endoscopic appearance of an ulcer, that is, the presence or absence of stigmata predicting recurrent bleeding, is of value in assessing prognosis. This visible vessel was seen in an ulcer in an edematous duodenal bulb (hence the close-up view). It is actively oozing. Endoscopic therapy is being applied using an injection catheter and needle. (*Courtesy of* Karl Fukunaga and Russell Yang.)

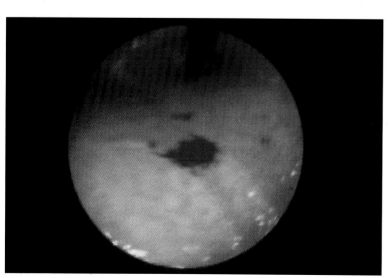

FIGURE 11-31.

Vascular ectasias of the stomach that may cause acute or chronic upper gastrointestinal bleeding (angiodysplasia). Note leaf-like pattern of lesion and a few smaller surrounding lesions. These are seen mostly in elderly patients.

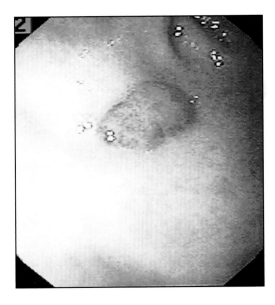

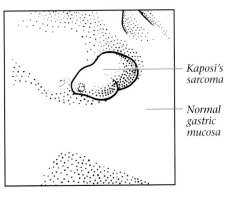

Kaposi's sarcoma

Normal gastric mucosa

FIGURE 11-32.

Gastric Kaposi's sarcoma. In the area of AIDS, a variety of bleeding gastrointestinal lesions have been noted. Kaposi's sarcoma is a spindle cell tumor that often has a submucosal location histologically; hence the yield of biopsy is low, 23%, despite a typical endoscopic appearance [10]. Although gastrointestinal Kaposi's sarcoma can occur in the absence of cutaneous lesions, increasing numbers of skin lesions predict a higher incidence of gastrointestinal lesions. The lesion is typically a well-circumscribed, submucosal, erythematous, or violaceous mass lesion. Bleeding gastrointestinal Kaposi's sarcoma lesions are a reflection of advanced immunosuppression and poor long-term survival. Some authors have, however, reported good acute control of active bleeding with endoscopic sclerotherapy [11]. (*Courtesy of* Karl Fukanaga and Russell Yang.)

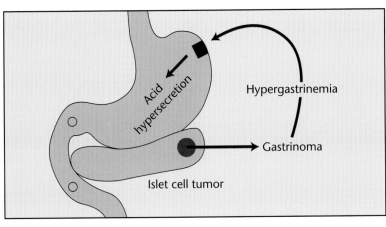

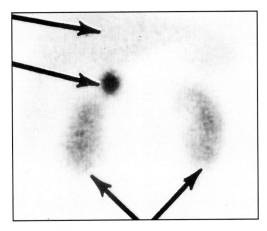

FIGURE 11-33.

Features of the Zollinger-Ellison syndrome. Gastrinomas are typically located in the pancreas, as shown here, or the duodenum. Ulcers (*circles*) occur typically in the duodenal bulb or more distally in the small bowel.

FIGURE 11-34.

Somatostatin receptor scintigraphy (SRS) localization of a gastrinoma in the pancreatic head area in a patient with ulcer disease due to Zollinger-Ellison syndrome (ZES). This figure shows the localization of a gastrinoma (*lower arrow at left*) in a patient with ZES using SRS with [^{111}In-DTPA-Dphe^1]-octreotide. As this figure shows, [^{111}In-DTPA-Dphe^1]-octreotide is primarily excreted by the kidneys (*arrows at bottom*); however, a small amount also is taken up by the liver (*upper arrow at left*). Recent data suggest SRS will be particularly helpful in diagnosis of gastrinomas [12–15]. Nearly 100% of gastrinomas are reported to possess increased numbers of somatostatin receptors [16]. Another advantage of SRS is its ability of also frequently detecting previously unrecognized distal metastases [14]. The false-positive rate, whether SRS will detect small duodenal gastrinomas, and whether it is more sensitive than angiography remain unclear [12,17]. (*Courtesy of* Robert T. Jensen.)

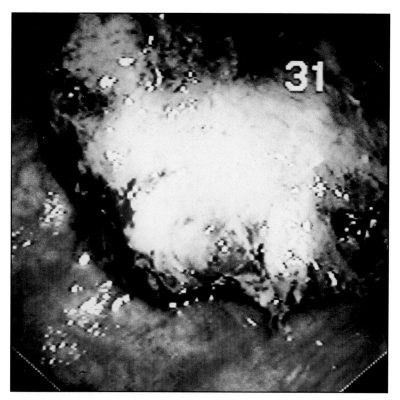

FIGURE 11-35.

Gastric carcinoma. The most common type of all malignant gastric neoplasms is the gastric adenocarcinoma. The average 5-year survival rate for patients with gastric adenocarcinoma is 15%. Treatment includes local resection for patients with "early gastric cancer," extensive resection and lymph node dissection for patients with advanced gastric cancer, and possibly the addition of chemotherapeutic modalities for those patients in whom there is evidence of widespread metastatic disease. The possible role of adjuvant, neoadjuvant, hormonal, or radiographic therapy in the treatment of patients with advanced gastric cancer remains uncertain. Certain groups of patients are at significantly higher risk than others, including postpartial gastrectomy patients; patients with pernicious anemia; patients of lower socioeconomic status; patients infected with *Helicobacter pylori*; and patients whose diet includes intake of large amounts of salted fish, starches, pickled vegetables, meat, smoked foods, nitrates, and nitrites. Even for such patients, routine endoscopic screening is not warranted. When a person from such a high-risk group develops symptoms, however, the patient should have upper gastrointestinal endoscopy. The possible endoscopic features seen can include such an ulcerated mass as shown in this figure. (*Courtesy of* Daniel C. DeMarco.)

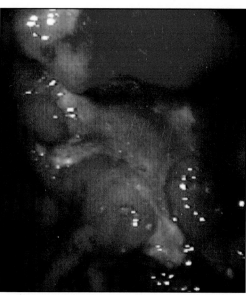

FIGURE 11-36.

Gastric lymphoma. Gastric lymphoma represents less than 5% of the gastric malignant neoplasms seen. The stomach remains the most common site of involvement for extranodal non-Hodgkin's lymphoma. Using only endoscopy and radiographic barium studies, lymphoma may be difficult to differentiate from gastric adenocarcinoma. Biopsies also are not particularly helpful in making the diagnosis. The 5-year survival rate for patients who have gastric lymphoma is approximately 50% when all combinations of patients and therapeutic modalities are considered. This endoscopic view reveals thickened folds. The differential diagnosis of thickened gastric folds includes many entities such as Zollinger-Ellison syndrome, Ménétrier's disease, varices, lues, idiopathic hypertrophic gastrophy, eosinophilic gastritis, pseudolymphoma, and lymphoma. (*Courtesy of* Daniel C. DeMarco.)

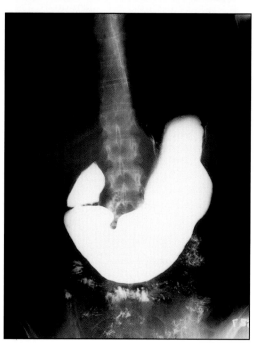

FIGURE 11-37.

Gastric motility. Gastric motility problems are not uncommon and often present with nausea and vomiting. The most common underlying etiology is diabetes mellitus. This barium radiograph shows virtually no gastric emptying of barium after more than an hour in a diabetic patient with gastroparesis.

■ SMALL INTESTINAL DISORDERS

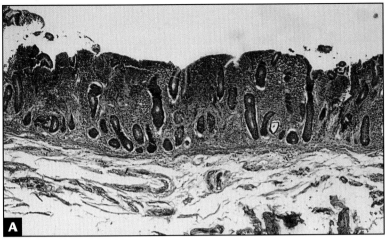

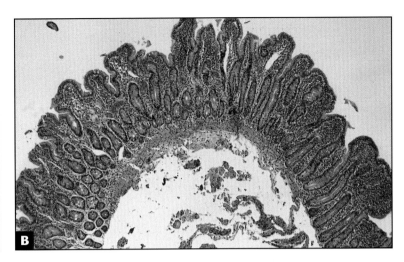

FIGURE 11-38.

Sprue. Jejunal mucosal biopsy from a patient with celiac sprue before (**A**) and 3 months after (**B**) treatment with a gluten-free diet. Celiac sprue is characterized by small intestinal mucosal damage and nutrient malabsorption in susceptible persons after ingesting gluten, the water-insoluble protein component of certain grains. *Panel A* illustrates the flat mucosal surface, absence of villi, hyperplastic crypts, and increased lamina propria cellularity that are characteristic of the disease. After 3 months of treatment (*panel B*) the mucosa is markedly improved and recognizable villi are present. The villi are short, however, and crypt hyperplasia and lamina propria hypercellularity persist.

The severity of malabsorption and clinical symptoms can vary markedly in patients with celiac sprue and are directly correlated with the length of the intestinal lesion. Usually, the proximal intestine is most involved, and disease severity decreases distally along the length of small bowel. Patients with severe disease have flatulence, progressive weight loss, and multiple nutrient deficiencies. The diarrhea is often voluminous and may float on water because of increased air and fat content. However, some patients have increased fecal mass without loose stools and complain of constipation. Removal of dietary gluten, present in wheat, rye, barely, oats, food additives, emulsifiers, and stabilizers, is essential for successful management. Patients who do not respond to a strict gluten-free diet may have refractory sprue or lymphoma. Diagnosis of celiac sprue is now facilitated by noninvasive serologic tests (see Figure 11-39). (*Courtesy of* Samuel Klein.)

Sensitivity and Specificity for IgA Anti-endomysial Antibody in Celiac Sprue	
Sensitivity	
Adults	68%–100%
Children	85%–100%
Specificity	99.7%–100%

FIGURE 11-39.

Sensitivity and specificity for IgA anti-endomysial antibody in celiac sprue. The endomysium is a part of the lining of smooth muscle bundles. The target for this antibody appears to be tissue transglutaminase [18,19].

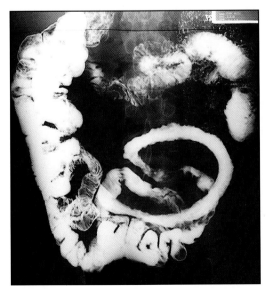

FIGURE 11-40.

Radiographic appearance of Crohn's disease of the terminal ileum. Nodularity, ulceration, narrowing, and irregularity of the lumen, characteristically affecting the terminal ileum, may result from transmural inflammation and lymphoid proliferation. Separation of involved loops of intestine from adjacent segments of bowel reflects luminal narrowing, thickening of bowel wall, and mesenteric hypertrophy. (*Courtesy of* Ellen J. Scherl and David B. Sachar.)

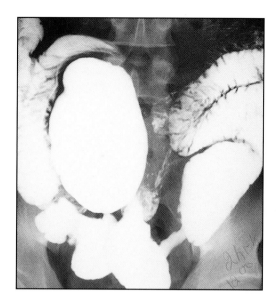

FIGURE 11-41.

When multiple strictures due to Crohn's disease produce multiple areas of massively dilated proximal bowel over periods of many years, huge sacs, or "saddlebags," may develop. This saccular pattern is often accompanied by clinical sequelae of malnutrition due to impaired intake, bacterial overgrowth, and malabsorption. (*Courtesy of* Ellen J. Scherl and David B. Sachar.)

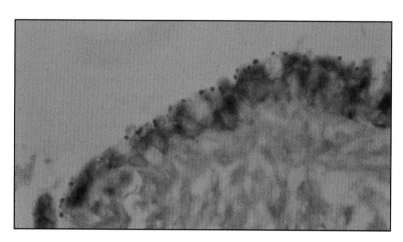

FIGURE 11-42.

Photomicrograph of intestinal biopsy—cryptosporidiosis. A small intestinal biopsy from a patient with AIDS reveals cryptosporidia adherent to the surface of the enterocytes. The organism does not invade and is confined to the surface of the epithelial cell [20]. A similar appearance can be seen in the colon. (*From* Banwell and Lake [20]; *courtesy of* R.L. Owen.)

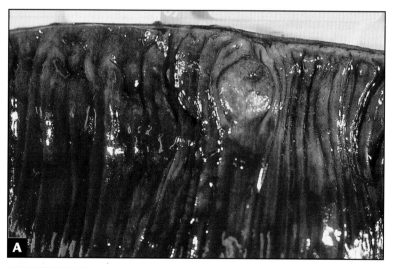

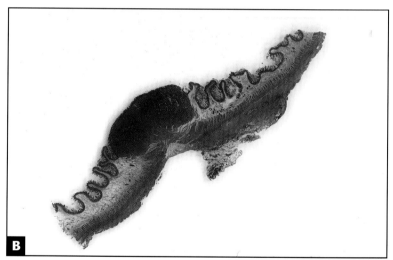

FIGURE 11-43.

Carcinoid. **A,** This surgical resection specimen shows a well-circumscribed intraluminal mass with apparently normal overlying mucosa and a central umbilication. On cut section, the tumor showed a pale-yellow meaty appearance, suggestive of a carcinoid; the muscular layer and serosa has undergone retractile changes that resulted in the formation of a knuckle of bowel, also suggestive of a carcinoid. **B,** The histology shows normal mucosa overlying the submucosal tumor, which consists of a monotonous array of bland tumor cells, which are characteristic of carcinoid. (*Courtesy of* Gordon D. Luk, Herbert J. Smith, and Edward L. Lee.)

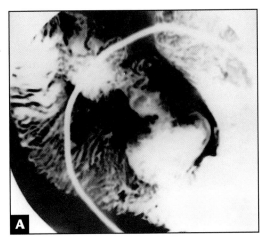

A

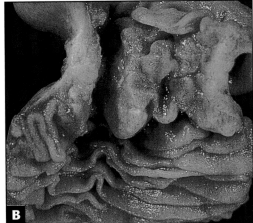

B

FIGURE 11-44.

Small bowel adenocarcinoma. Although many duodenal and proximal jejunal tumors may be seen by endoscopy or enteroscopy, most are beyond the reach of even the longest instruments. Such tumors require either conventional small-bowel follow-through radiograms or enteroclysis for their detection. **A,** In this patient who presented with weight loss and vomiting, the annular napkin-ringlike lesion was seen to best advantage at enteroclysis. **B,** The marked narrowing of the lumen by the circumferentially growing adenocarcinoma was seen in the resection specimen. (*Courtesy of* Gordon D. Luk, Herbert J. Smith, and Edward L. Lee.)

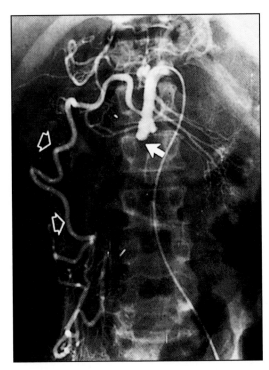

FIGURE 11-45.
Embolic occlusion of the superior mesenteric artery (SMA). The usual origin of a

mesenteric arterial embolus is a thrombus from the left atrium or ventricle. Predisposing conditions include atrial fibrillation, rheumatic heart disease, prosthetic heart valves, myocardial infarction, ventricular aneurysms, and invasive angiographic procedures. The clinician should be alert to the possibility of embolism to a major mesenteric artery when severe periumbilical abdominal pain, vomiting, diarrhea, and leukocytosis arise acutely in the appropriate clinical setting. Emboli to the SMA most often lodge in the middle colic branch, but can affect any of its four branches. Emboli tend to lodge within 3 to 8 cm of the origin of the SMA, usually where the vessel narrows. This angiogram reveals occlusion of the SMA by a thrombus. The *solid arrow* points to complete occlusion distal to the origin of the middle colic artery. The *open arrows* reveal some collateral flow through the middle colic–right colic anastomosis [21]. (*From* Rogers *et al.* [21]; *courtesy of* Stanley Baum.)

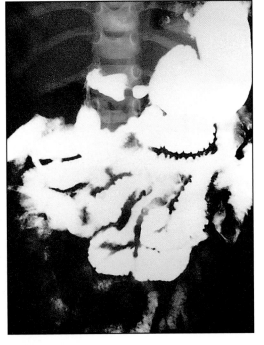

FIGURE 11-46.

Henoch-Schönlein purpura. Henoch-Schönlein purpura, a small-vessel vasculitis, frequently involves the gastrointestinal tract. It is characterized by nonthrombocytopenic purpura, renal involvement, and colicky abdominal pain (with or without bloody diarrhea). This disease is most often seen in children between the ages of 4 and 7 years old. Pain may be related to intramural hemorrhage, secondary to the vasculitis. Pain, nausea, and vomiting may also develop if hematoma formation or resultant edema causes intussusception. This upper gastrointestinal series was taken of a 2-year-old child who presented with anemia, abdominal pain, and gastrointestinal bleeding. It reveals narrowing and ulceration of the jejunum and ileum (*arrows*), which are most commonly involved, and thickened (spiculated) small bowel folds. This appearance can mimic Crohn's disease or lymphoma [22]. (*Courtesy of* Robert Feltman.)

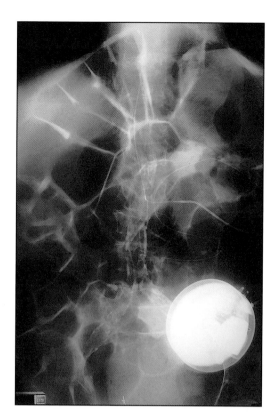

FIGURE 11-47.

Acute intestinal pseudoobstruction or ileus. Although ileus is an expected consequence of abdominal and other surgical procedures, it may also occur in other nonsurgical situations, such as in patients with pneumonia, pancreatitis, cholecystitis, myocardial infarction, and a variety of neurologic conditions. Occasionally, ileus may occur without an obvious cause (idiopathic ileus). This figure illustrates marked dilatation of small and large intestine, a finding consistent with ileus, in a patient with multiple sclerosis. Note patient also had an implanted pump (*see* lower right of photograph) to deliver the muscle relaxant baclofen. (*Courtesy of* Eamonn MM Quigley.)

■ ANAL, RECTAL, AND COLONIC DISORDERS

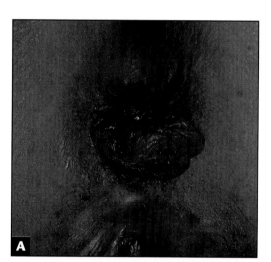

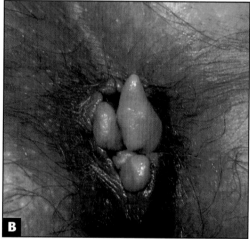

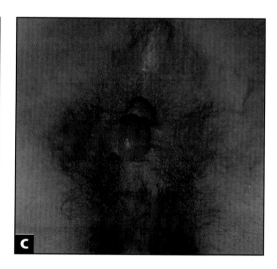

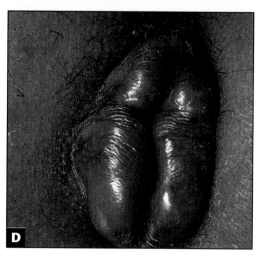

FIGURE 11-48.

External or perianal skin tags are soft, fleshy folds of fibrous connective tissue. They are often the sequelae after the clot from a thrombosed external hemorrhoid has resolved. External hemorrhoids arise from the inferior hemorrhoidal plexus and are located below the dentate line; they are covered by squamous epithelium. External hemorrhoids are usually asymptomatic unless thrombosis occurs. Internal hemorrhoids are submucosal vascular cushions arising from above the dentate line and are covered by rectal mucosa. Internal and external hemorrhoids may coexist as a mixed hemorrhoid. **A,** An external or perianal skin tag. Skin tags may interfere with adequate anal hygiene and may worsen anal irritation or pruritus. Surgical excision is rarely necessary. **B,** Prominent fibroepithelial anal canal tags. **C,** An acutely thrombosed external hemorrhoid. A thrombosed external hemorrhoid may be quite painful, and bleeding may occur if the overlying skin ulcerates and the hematoma is expressed. Most respond to conservative management, but if acute and painful, local incision and clot evacuation afford immediate relief. **D,** Acutely prolapsed large, bilateral external and internal (mixed) hemorrhoids. (*Courtesy of* R. Burney.)

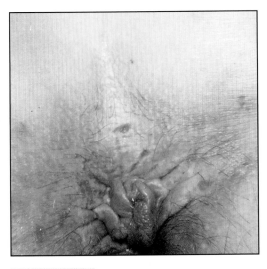

FIGURE 11-49.

Pruritus ani. This is characterized by intense perianal itching and burning discomfort. Causes include local irritants or sensitivities, benign and malignant dermatoses, infections, and anorectal diseases that lead to fecal contamination or leakage. This excoriated perianal skin was a result of idiopathic pruritus ani. (*Courtesy of* R. Burney.)

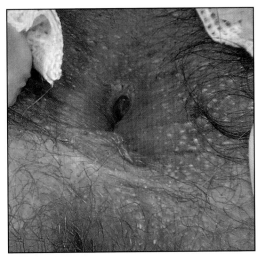

FIGURE 11-50.

Typical fissure in ano located in the posterior midline. An anal fissure is a painful, linear defect in the anal canal oriented perpendicularly to the dentate line. It is usually caused by a tearing that occurred during passage of a stool. The vast majority are located in the posterior midline; the remainder are anteriorly placed. A fissure located laterally should arouse suspicion of an underlying condition such as inflammatory bowel disease. An anal fissure is best identified by gentle but forceful lateral traction of the buttocks (after topical application of an anesthetic if necessary). Most acute anal fissures will heal with conservative medical management and time. Persistent acute fissures and many chronic fissures require definitive surgery, usually a lateral internal sphincterotomy to reduce resting sphincter tone. Application of topical nitroglycerine ointment or injection of botulinum toxin into the internal anal sphincter has been reported to heal chronic fissures. (*Courtesy of* Jeffery L. Barnett.)

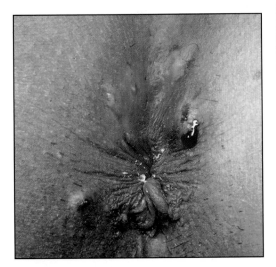

FIGURE 11-51.

Multiple perianal fistula sites from fistula in ano. Fistula is a chronic manifestation of suppurative anorectal infection, while abscess is an acute manifestation. Fistulous disease and abscess are caused by infection of the anal glands, secondary to ductal obstruction caused by fecal material or anal trauma. The primary fistulous orifice is found at the level of the dentate line and the secondary opening at the anal verge or elsewhere in the perineum. Fistula in ano usually causes discharge with occasional discomfort; abscess typically presents as pain and swelling. (*Courtesy of* R. Burney.)

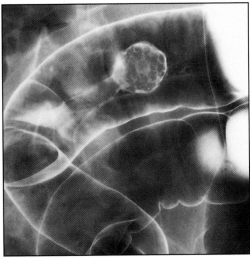

FIGURE 11-52.

A pedunculated sigmoid polyp. Most bleeding from colorectal polyps is occult or mild and intermittent. Rarely polyps may cause significant lower gastrointestinal hemorrhage. Left-sided and rectal neoplasms are more likely to cause gross bleeding than right-sided lesions. Diagnosis is made by endoscopy or barium enema. Treatment for bleeding polyps is usually by colonoscopic removal or surgery. (*Courtesy of* J. Lappas.)

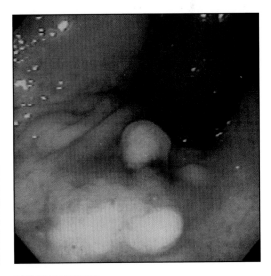

FIGURE 11-53.

Flexible sigmoidoscopic view of the distal rectum upon retroflexion of the sigmoidoscope, which demonstrates several small polyps. Periodic flexible sigmoidoscopy (every 5 years) and polypectomy reduces cancer incidence and mortality caused by cancer within the reach of the endoscope by approximately 70%. (*Courtesy of* Robert S. Bresalier.)

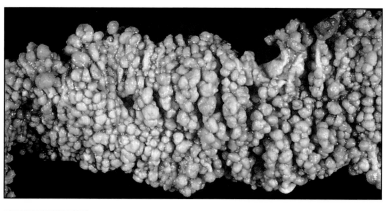

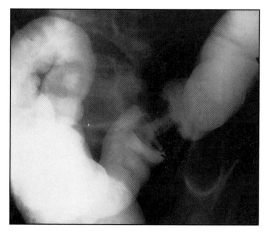

FIGURE 11-54.

Familial adenomatous polyposis. A portion of a colectomy specimen that shows complete carpeting of the mucosal surface by adenomatous polyps. In general, colons containing more than 100 adenomatous polyps are thought to have this autosomal dominant condition. The genetic defect appears to be caused by mutations or deletions in the *APC* gene located on the long arm of chromosome 5. (*Courtesy of* Ellen J. Scherl and Joel K. Greenson.)

FIGURE 11-55.

Colon cancer. Barium enema demonstrating an annular constricting lesion in the sigmoid colon. (*Courtesy of* Robert S. Bresalier.)

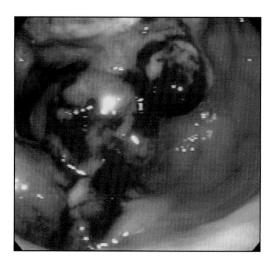

FIGURE 11-56.

Colonoscopic view of bleeding colon cancer. Colorectal cancers may present with gross bleeding (hematochezia) or result in the presence of occult blood in the stool. (*Courtesy of* Robert K. Bresalier.)

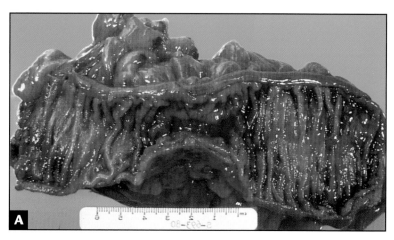

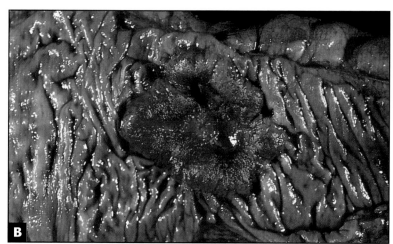

FIGURE 11-57.

Colon cancer. A, Gross surgical specimen of annular constricting or napkin-ring carcinoma of the colon. B, Colonic resection specimen shows an erythematous-raised tumor with a central umbilication. (*Courtesy of* Joel K. Greenson.)

American Cancer Society Recommendations For Early Colorectal Cancer Detection

Beginning at age 50, both men and women should follow one of these screening options:

- Yearly fecal occult blood test plus a flexible sigmoidoscopy every 5 years
- Colonoscopy every 10 years
- Double contrast barium enema every 5–10 years

Screening should be done earlier and more often if any of the following colorectal cancer risk factors are present:

- A strong family history of colorectal cancer or polyps (cancer or polyps in a first-degree relative younger than 60 or in two or more first-degree relatives of any age)
- Families with hereditary colorectal cancer syndromes (familial adenomatous polyposis and hereditary non-polyposis colon cancer)
- A personal history of colorectal cancer or adenomatous polyps
- A personal history of chronic inflammatory bowel disease

FIGURE 11-58.

Current American Cancer Society guidelines for screening average-risk patients for colorectal cancer. Beginning at age 50, both men and women should follow one of the three screening options listed, combined with a digital rectal exam at the time screening is done [23].

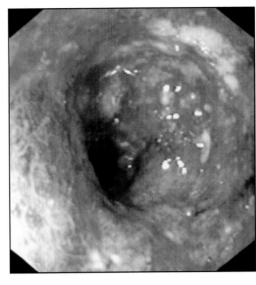

FIGURE 11-59.

Endoscopic features of active ulcerative colitis. Findings include diffusely erythematous, edematous, and granular mucosa with areas of submucosal hemorrhage and, when severe, frank mucopurulent exudate. Inflammation invariably begins in the rectum and extends proximally for varying extents. The chronicity of the process is suggested by the loss of colonic haustrations; otherwise, the endoscopic picture is nonspecific and could be consistent with acute infectious colitis, chronic ulcerative or Crohn's colitis, or any number of other specific causes of colitis. This example shows moderately severe ulcerative colitis with irregular, inflamed, ulcerated mucosa and a patchy exudate. (*Courtesy of* Lawrence S. Friedman, Fiona Graeme-Cook, and Robert H. Schapiro.)

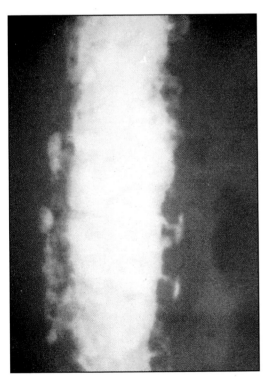

FIGURE 11-60.

Radiographic appearance of severe ulcerative colitis. This single-contrast barium enema demonstrates the typical ragged and ulcerative appearance of the mucosa in active ulcerative colitis. Characteristic collar-button or undermining ulcers are seen. In general, barium enema and colonoscopy should be avoided in fulminant ulcerative colitis because of the possibility of precipitating toxic megacolon. (*Courtesy of* Lawrence S. Friedman, Fiona Graeme-Cook, and Robert H. Schapiro.)

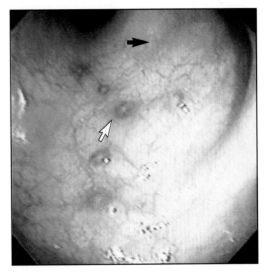

FIGURE 11-61.

Crohn's colitis—aphthous ulceration. Aphthous ulcers are tiny, pinpoint lesions with exudate (*open arrow*) surrounded by an erythematous margin. Microscopically, these are tiny foci of mucosal ulceration often overlying enlarged lymphoid follicles. Normal mucosa (*closed arrow*) is seen adjacent to the inflamed mucosa.

Aphthous ulcers may be the earliest recognizable lesion of Crohn's disease, but infiltration by lymphocytes, polymorphonuclear cells, and plasma cells probably precedes the development of the aphthous ulcer [24]. Aphthous ulcers can occur anywhere from the mouth to the anal area. These lesions may also be seen by air-contrast barium enema. (*Courtesy of* Anupama Chawla and Frederic Daum.)

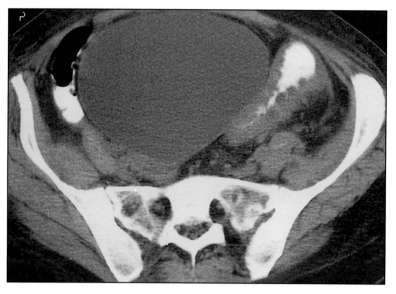

FIGURE 11-62.
Radiologic findings in Crohn's disease. Computed tomographic scan showing marked thickening of the colonic wall (to the left of the urinary bladder) typical of Crohn's disease. Computed tomographic scanning is also useful for detecting Crohn's abscesses and fistulas. (*Courtesy of* G. J. Whitman.)

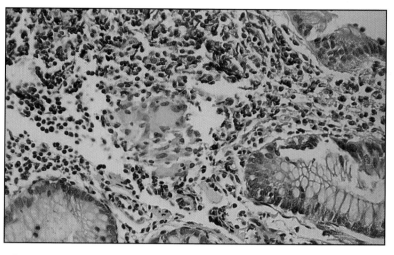

FIGURE 11-63.
Microscopic specimen from a patient with Crohn's colitis. The specimen has diffuse inflammation of the mucosa and submucosa with a small granuloma in the center. (*Courtesy of* Lawrence S. Friedman, Fiona Graeme-Cook, and Robert H. Schapiro.)

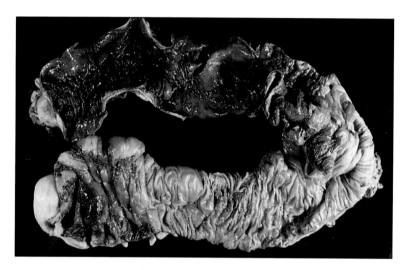

FIGURE 11-64.
Ischemic colitis. A colectomy specimen that shows a well-demarcated darkened area of hemorrhagic necrosis. The sharp border and diffuse involvement of the affected segment are characteristic of ischemic disease. (*Courtesy of* Joel K. Greenson.)

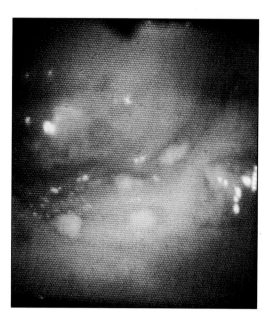

FIGURE 11-65.
Endoscopic appearance of pseudomembranous colitis. Pseudomembranous colitis characteristically results from the use of antibiotics and is caused by the toxin produced by *Clostridium difficile*. The characteristic appearance is yellow-white pseudomembranes. Pseudomembranous colitis also occurs with ischemia and in patients infected with *Escherichia coli* 0157:H7. (*Courtesy of* Lawrence S. Friedman, Fiona Graeme-Cook, and Robert H. Schapiro.)

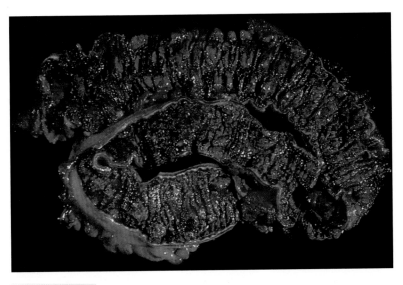

FIGURE 11-66.
A severe case of enterohemorrhagic *Escherichia coli* infection (serotype O157:H7) that required colectomy. The appearance of infection caused by enterohemorrhagic *E. coli* can mimic that of ischemic colitis or pseudomembranous colitis. On gross pathology, diffuse inflammation of the colonic mucosa is not confined to the distribution of a major mesenteric vessel. There are large areas of pseudomembrane formation and marked edema. Ingestion of rare meat, particularly hamburger, is a risk factor. (*Courtesy of* Lawrence S. Friedman, Fiona Graeme-Cook, and Robert H. Schapiro.)

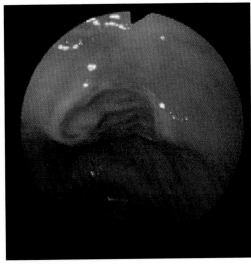

FIGURE 11-67.
Cytomegalovirus colitis. Cytomegalovirus may cause colitis, particularly in immunosuppressed hosts such as patients with AIDS or transplant recipients. Endoscopic findings may include diffuse colitis as well as solitary ulcers of the colon. As shown here, the half-moon shaped ulcer may be large with raised edges, but the surrounding mucosa is normal. (*Courtesy of* Lawrence S. Friedman, Fiona Graeme-Cook, and Robert H. Schapiro.)

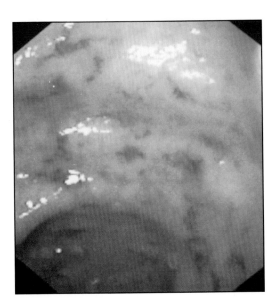

FIGURE 11-68.
Radiation colitis. Radiation colitis is seen most commonly as a complication of pelvic irradiation for malignancy. The endoscopic appearance may be indistinguishable from that of ulcerative colitis, but common characteristic mucosal telangiectatic lesions are seen. Luminal narrowing is frequent, and solitary ulcers may occur. (*Courtesy of* Lawrence S. Friedman, Fiona Graeme-Cook, and Robert H. Schapiro.)

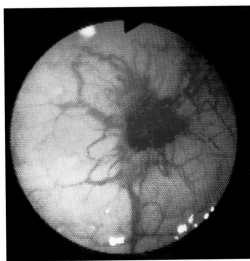

FIGURE 11-69.
Colonic angiodysplasia. Lesions appear flat or slightly raised, red, and 2 to 10 mm in diameter. They may be round, stellate, or fernlike [25]. There may be a prominent feeding vessel or a pale mucosal halo. Lesions may be missed if the patient is anemic or volume depleted. Most patients are elderly. Many lesions may mimic angiodysplasia, including lesions of hereditary hemorrhagic telangiectasia, ischemia, radiation colitis, and suction artifacts. (*Courtesy of* Christopher S. Cutler and Douglas K. Rex.)

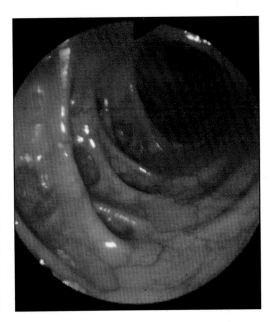

FIGURE 11-70.
Diverticulosis. Numerous diverticula with fold thickening in the sigmoid colon. Knowledge of the existence of diverticula is important in evaluating patients with left lower quadrant pain. (*Courtesy of* Timothy T. Nostrant.)

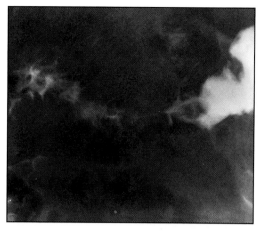

FIGURE 11-71.

This barium enema demonstrates a classic case of acute sigmoid diverticulitis. Note the long segment of colon involved in the inflammatory process and the luminal narrowing secondary to the inflammation. Endoscopic examination would reveal intense spasm and edema at the rectosigmoid junction. (*Courtesy of* David A. Rothenberger, Carlos Belmonte-Montes, J. Javier Perez-Ramirez.)

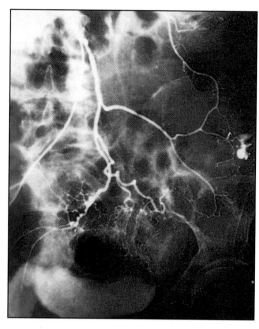

FIGURE 11-72.

Radiograph of a patient with an actively bleeding diverticula of the descending colon. Selective mesenteric angiography is effective in the diagnosis of active diverticular bleeding. Extravasation of contrast into a diverticula shown here at 3 o'clock is the diagnostic radiographic finding. Angiographic infusion of vasopressors may halt diverticular bleeding in 80% to 90% of patients [26]. Fifteen percent to 25% of these patients rebleed and eventually require surgery. Angiographic embolization may also be used, but below the ligament of Treitz, there is a 30% incidence of bowel ischemia or infarction. (*From* Dietzen *et al.* [27]; with permission.)

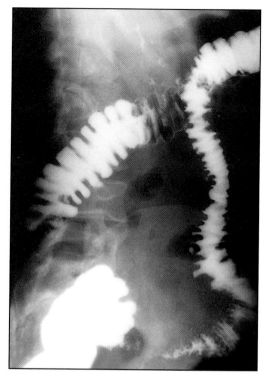

FIGURE 11-73.

Barium enema in a patient with irritable bowel syndrome (IBS). The extreme hypercontractility of the left and sigmoid colon is indicative of excessive segmenting motor activity. Several studies report a high frequency of hysteria, somatization disorder, depression, and anxiety in patients with irritable bowel syndrome. Many patients with IBS, however, have completely normal barium enemas. Functional (nonulcer) dyspepsia and other functional gastrointestinal disorders may be present. (*Courtesy of* Arnold Wald.)

Rome Criteria for Diagnosis of Functional Abdominal Pain Syndrome

Continuous or nearly continuous abdominal pain

No or only occasional relationship of pain with physiologic events (*eg*, eating, defecation, menses)

Some loss of daily functioning

The pain is not feigned (*eg*, malingering)

Insufficient criteria for other functional gastrointestinal disorders that would explain the abdominal pain

FIGURE 11-74.

Rome criteria for diagnosis of functional abdominal pain syndrome in patients presenting with chronic unexplained abdominal pain. Symptoms must be present for at least six months. (*Adapted from* Drossman *et al.* [3].)

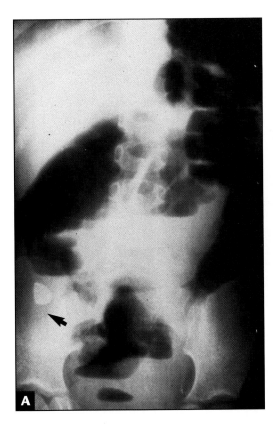

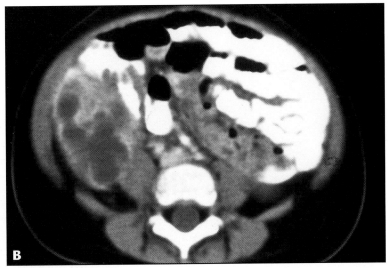

FIGURE 11-75.
Acute appendicitis. **A,** Abdominal radiograph showing appendicolith
(*arrow*) and local ileus in lower abdomen. This finding is specific but
uncommon (insensitive). Computed tomography (CT) scan with
oral and intravenous contrast agents is the most sensitive and specific test, although patients with classic presentation can be taken
straight to laparoscopic appendectomy for diagnosis and treatment.
B, CT scan showing localized appendiceal abscess in right lower
abdomen (*arrow*). (*Courtesy of* M. Siegel.)

■ GALLBLADDER AND BILIARY DISORDERS

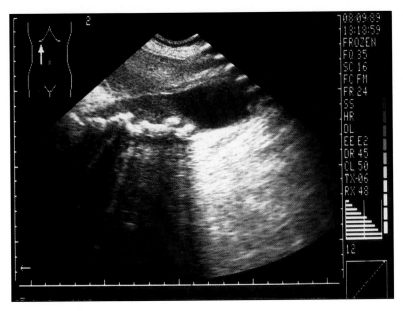

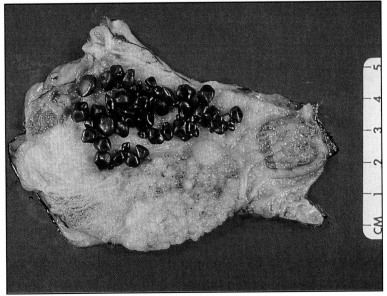

FIGURE 11-76.
Ultrasound scan (sagittal view) demonstrating sludge and multiple
stones in the gallbladder with shadowing behind the stones. There
is also generalized thickening of the gallbladder wall suggestive of
acute cholecystitis. Ultrasound is the most cost-effective test for
detecting stones in the gall bladder in patients with a history compatible with biliary tract disease. (*Courtesy of* Nahid E. Eshagi.)

FIGURE 11-77.
Cholesterol stones with a thin surface layer of black pigment, along
with an adenocarcinoma in the neck of the gallbladder (*extreme
right*). Gallstones increase the risk of gallbladder cancer. (*Courtesy of*
Johnson L. Thistle.)

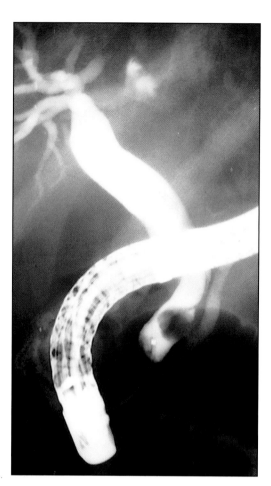

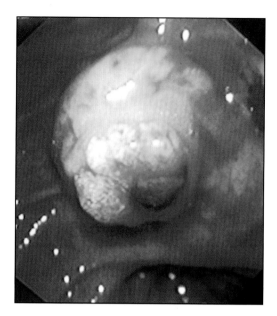

FIGURE 11-78.
Common bile duct stones. Endoscopic retrograde cholangiopancreatography is the most accurate invasive diagnostic modality and can clearly demonstrate intraluminal filling defects as well as proximal ductal dilatation, as shown here. Endoscopic ductal clearance rates are usually 95%. Endoscopic ductal clearance has a published mortality rate ranging from 0% to 3% and a recurrence rate of less than 5%. (*Courtesy of* Alfred D. Roston and David L. Carr-Locke.)

FIGURE 11-79.
Endoscopy in acute cholangitis. Stone disease remains the most common cause of cholangitis in most large series in the United States. Choledocholithiasis occurs in 8% to 15% of patients undergoing cholecystectomy; the incidence in patients older than 60 years of age is even higher, estimated at 15% to 60% in some series [28]. At endoscopy, the obstructing stone is often seen bulging from the papillary orifice, as in this figure. A recent randomized, controlled trial supports early endoscopic examination and intervention in cases of suspected stone-related acute cholangitis [29]. (*Courtesy of* Wendy Z. Davis and M. Stanley Branch.)

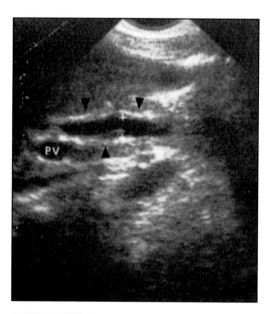

FIGURE 11-80.
AIDS cholangiopathy. Biliary tract disease is being reported with increasing frequency in the AIDS population. Abdominal pain and laboratory evidence of cholestasis are common clinical features that may prompt further investigation. Both ultrasound and computed tomography may demonstrate cholangiographic abnormalities. This ultrasound depicts dilation (13 mm) and thickening (*arrowheads*) of the common bile duct in a case of cholangitis associated with cryptosporidiosis. PV—portal vein. (*From* Teixidor *et al.* [30]; with permission.)

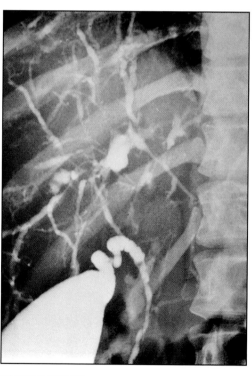

FIGURE 11-81.
Classic cholangiographic appearance of sclerosing cholangitis. Multifocal strictures and intervening cholangiectatic ductal segments are seen. There is a strong association with male gender and with inflammatory bowel diseases such as ulcerative colitis and Crohn's disease. (*Courtesy of* Keith D. Lindor.)

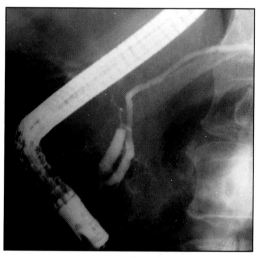

FIGURE 11-82.
This endoscopic retrograde cholangiopancreatography (ERCP) shows a patent pancreatic duct and, just above it, an occluded common bile duct in a patient with a distal cholangiocarcinoma. In patients with distal bile duct obstruction, the additional information provided by the pancreatogram may give useful diagnostic information. Thus, ERCP is the diagnostic test of choice when a distal lesion is suspected. (*Courtesy of* Henry A. Pitt.)

■ PANCREATIC DISORDERS

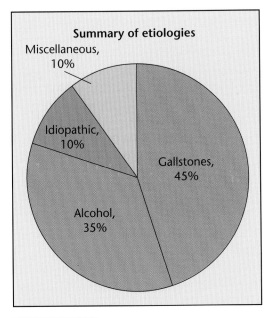

FIGURE 11-83.

Summary of the main etiologies for acute pancreatitis. A compilation of many studies from around the world reveals that gallstones account for 45% of cases, alcoholism for 35% of cases, miscellaneous causes for 10% of cases, and idiopathic for 10% of cases. (*Courtesy of* William M. Steinberg.)

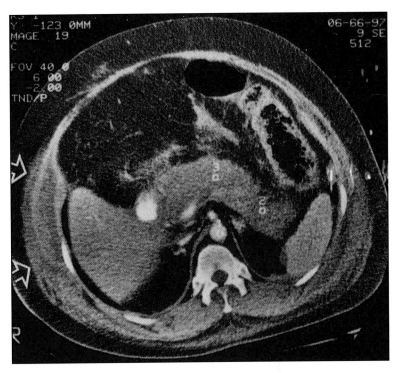

FIGURE 11-84.

Bolus contrast computed tomography (CT) in severe acute pancreatitis. Impairment of the pancreatic microcirculation leading to tissue ischemia may be an important factor in determining the extent of injury and necrosis of the pancreas and the ultimate severity of the disease process. A clinical correlate of this tissue ischemia may be failure of the pancreas to enhance its density on CT after intravenous injection of a bolus of radio contrast agent in patients with more severe acute pancreatitis. This CT scan shows poor perfusion of the pancreas. The presence of poor perfusion on CT scan has about a 90% predictive value of predicting necrosis at surgery; however, only about 60% of patients with necrosis on CT scan have a severe course clinically [31,32]. (*Courtesy of* William M. Steinberg.)

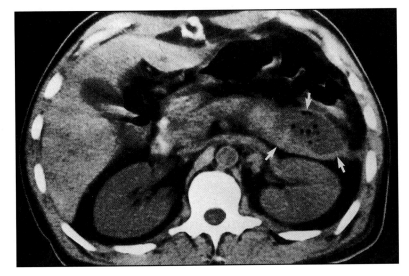

FIGURE 11-85.

A computed tomography (CT) scan of the pancreas indicating gas bubbles within the tail of the pancreas. This suggests pancreatic abscess secondary to gas-producing organisms; however, sterile necrosis with microcommunication with the gut can lead to this CT finding. Only with a fine-needle aspirate with gram stain and culture can one diagnose an abscess with assurance. (*From* Freeny *et al.* [33]; with permission.)

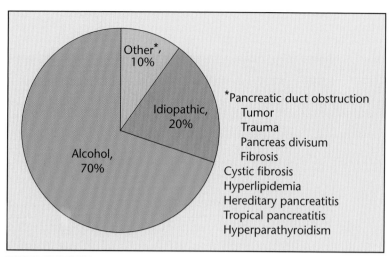

FIGURE 11-86.

Suummary of the main etiologies for chronic pancreatitis. Chronic pancreatitis may also be classified by its presumed cause. Chronic alcoholism accounts for approximately 70% of all cases of chronic pancreatitis. Prolonged and substantial abuse is generally required to produce chronic pancreatitis, and most (but not all) patients who present with an episode of acute pancreatitis caused by alcohol consumption already have chronic pancreatic damage. Chronic obstruction of the pancreatic duct may also produce chronic pancreatitis, such as that caused by tumors, trauma, pseudocysts, inflammation and fibrosis (such as after a severe episode of acute

pancreatitis), pancreas divisum (with associated minor papilla stenosis), and even after prolonged endoscopic stenting of the pancreatic duct. After traumatic injury to the pancreatic duct (such as after a motor vehicle accident or a stab wound), chronic pancreatitis may develop within a few months. Pancreas divisum commonly occurs as a normal variant (in 5%–10% of the population), and most patients remain asymptomatic. This variant occurs after nonfusion of the two pancreatic buds during development, so that most pancreatic secretion in the dorsal segment drains through the minor papilla rather than the major papilla. A small subset of patients have both pancreas divisum and obstruction at the minor papilla, which may produce both acute relapsing pancreatitis or, more rarely, chronic obstructive pancreatitis. Cystic fibrosis is an important cause of chronic pancreatitis in children, although with improved pulmonary care these patients may live to adulthood. Hyperlipidemia, particularly when the serum triglycerides are above 1000 mg/dL, may produce both acute and chronic pancreatitis. Pancreatitis may be hereditary, due to a mutation in the gene for trypsinogen, which increases its activity [34]. Tropical chronic pancreatitis, probably caused by malnutrition and toxic products in the diet, is rare in the United States. Hyperparathyroidism and other hypercalcemic conditions may cause chronic pancreatitis. Despite careful evaluation, about 20% of patients (in some studies as high as 30%) have no specific identifiable etiology, and are thus classified as having idiopathic chronic pancreatitis. (*Courtesy of* Chris E. Forsmark and Phillip P. Toskes.)

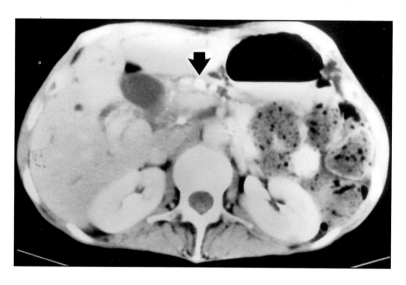

FIGURE 11-87.

Pathophysiology of chronic pancreatitis. The specific mechanism by which alcohol produces chronic pancreatitis is unknown, but it does appear to require substantial alcohol ingestion over at least 6 to 12 years. Various physiologic abnormalities have been documented in both animal models and in humans, including a direct toxic effect of pancreatic acinar cells, stimulation of pancreatic secretion, interference with normal intracellular protein trafficking, and the promotion of the formation of protein plugs within the ductal system. These plugs often become calcified, producing pancreatic ductal stones. Whether these stones contribute to the pathogenesis of alcoholic chronic pancreatitis by obstructing the pancreatic ducts is unknown. They may merely be a marker of alcoholic chronic pancreatitis rather than its cause. Multiple calcified stones within the pancreatic duct on a computed tomography scan (*arrow*). (*Courtesy of* Chris E. Forsmark and Phillip P. Toskes.)

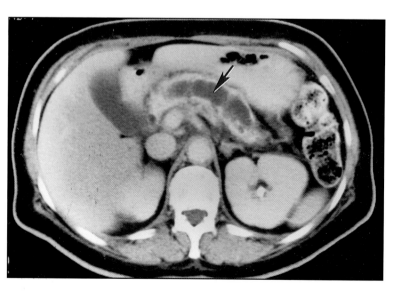

FIGURE 11-88.

Computed tomography (CT) in chronic pancreatitis. Findings on CT that suggest chronic pancreatitis include diffuse calcification, ductal dilation, gland atrophy, irregular contour, and associated pseudocysts. CT is less accurate than endoscopic retrograde pancreatography for the diagnosis of chronic pancreatitis, although spiral CT technology allows improved resolution of small structures, such as the pancreatic duct, and appears more accurate than earlier scanning methods. A markedly dilated pancreatic duct (*arrow*) with atrophy of the pancreas is seen in this figure.

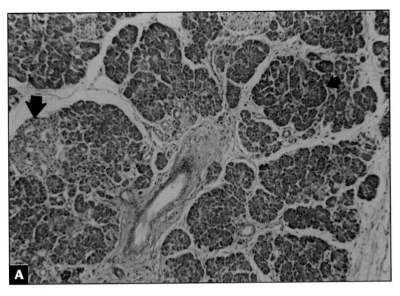

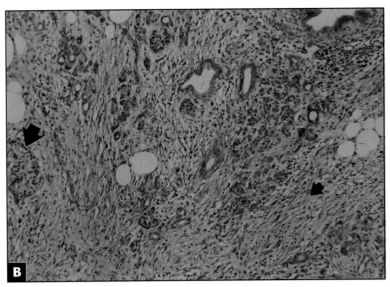

FIGURE 11-89.

Histology of chronic pancreatitis. Regardless of the specific cause of chronic pancreatitis, the histologic result is similar. Pancreatic inflammation, together with progressive fibrosis, leads to destruction of the acinar cells either focally or diffusely, producing exocrine insufficiency and steatorrhea. Intraductal concretions and stones may form, which may block the flow of pancreatic secretions and augment the damage. Inflammation involving pancreatic nerves is also commonly found. The endocrine tissue (the islets of Langerhans) is typically spared until late in the disease process, making diabetes mellitus a late complication. **A,** Normal pancreatic tissue is demonstrated with a normal acinar architecture (*small arrow*) and islets of Langerhans (*large arrow*). **B,** Changes of chronic pancreatitis include destruction of acinar tissue with replacement by fibrosis (small arrow), but the islets remain intact (large arrow). (*Courtesy of* Chris E. Forsmark and Phillip P. Toskes.)

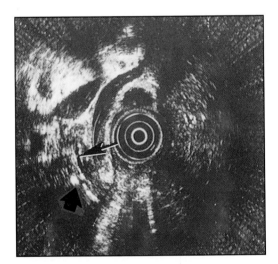

FIGURE 11-90.

Transabdominal ultrasonography in chronic pancreatitis. Ultrasound is an inexpensive, noninvasive diagnostic test that does not submit the patient to ionizing radiation. It is limited by its poor sensitivity (60% to 70%) and inability to image the pancreas in the presence of overlying intestinal gas. Endoscopic ultrasonography is used to evaluate chronic pancreatitis. Shown here is an endosonographic image of the body of the pancreas with a visible pancreatic duct (*thin arrow*) and calcifications within the gland (*thick arrow*). The circular target structure in the center is the instrument.

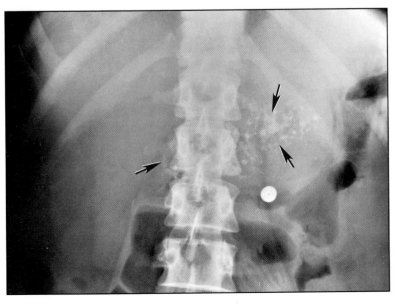

FIGURE 11-91.

Plain abdominal radiograph in chronic pancreatitis. The finding of diffuse pancreatic calcification is a specific marker of chronic pancreatitis, but it is only seen in far-advanced disease. Focal calcification is not diagnostic of chronic pancreatitis, and may be seen in a number of other diseases. Although patients with alcoholic chronic pancreatitis will commonly develop diffuse calcifications (70% of patients after 15 years of observation), patients with idiopathic pancreatitis do so only rarely (20% to 40% after 15 years of follow-up). The low sensitivity of plain radiographs limits their use as a diagnostic tool. This figure demonstrates diffuse pancreatic calcification (*arrows*). (*Courtesy of* Chris E. Forsmark and Phillip P. Toskes.)

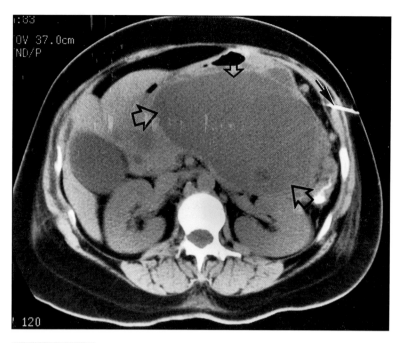

FIGURE 11-92.

Pseudocysts in chronic pancreatitis. A large pseudocyst (*open arrows*), which is being percutaneously drained (*closed arrow*). Pseudocysts that develop in chronic pancreatitis are most commonly caused by duct obstruction, with the formation of a "retention" cyst in the upstream duct or side branch. Unlike the pseudocysts associated with acute pancreatitis, these pseudocysts do not contain activated enzymes and are usually not a reflection of a necrotizing inflammatory process. These pseudocysts are less likely to produce complications than those associated with acute necrotizing pancreatitis, but they are paradoxically also less likely to resolve. Many of these pseudocysts remain asymptomatic, but they may be complicated by infection, rupture or leak, bleeding, or obstruction of a neighboring hollow viscus (*eg*, duodenum, bile duct, colon, or ureter, among others). Pseudocysts may also worsen chronic pain or even initiate a wasting syndrome.

Recent clinical experience suggests that in patients with pseudocysts smaller than 6 cm, if there is a mature pseudocyst wall on radiographic imaging that does not resemble a cystic neoplasm, minimal symptoms, and no evidence of active alcohol abuse, the risk of complications is extremely small (10%). These patients may be safely observed with little risk of serious complication [34,35]. Even larger asymptomatic pseudocysts can be considered for expectant management in this group of patients. Symptomatic pseudocysts or those producing complications require therapy.

Surgical decompression remains the standard criterion for symptomatic pseudocysts with low mortality and little recurrence. Surgical therapy also allows the differentiation of true pseudocysts from cystic pancreatic neoplasms. Percutaneous drainage of symptomatic pseudocysts is usually successful in the short-term, but pseudocyst recurrence is common (although the recurrent pseudocyst may remain asymptomatic!). Percutaneous drainage seems to be particularly effective for infected pseudocysts; however, it is usually ineffective for other complications, such as bleeding, rupture, or leak. Bleeding is a rare event, but carries substantial mortality, often because the bleeding source is a medium-sized artery that has formed a pseudoaneurysm. (*Courtesy of* Chris E. Forsmark and Phillip P. Toskes.)

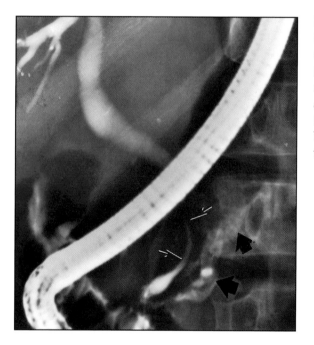

FIGURE 11-93.

Common bile duct stricture in chronic pancreatitis. Common bile duct stricture may develop as a consequence of compression by an adjacent pseudocyst or by progressive fibrosis of the head of the pancreas. This figure demonstrates an endoscopic retrograde cholangiopancreatography with changes of chronic pancreatitis (*thick arrows*) and a coexistent smooth stricture of the intrapancreatic common bile duct (*thin arrow*). Symptomatic obstruction of the bile duct usually requires surgical biliary bypass, sometimes in conjunction with a Peustow procedure (pancreatico-jejunostomy). (*Courtesy of* Chris E. Forsmark and Phillip P. Toskes.)

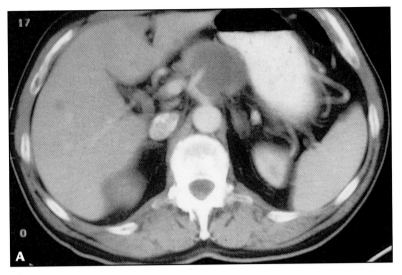

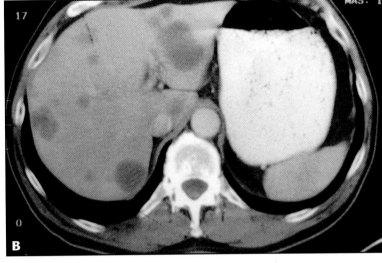

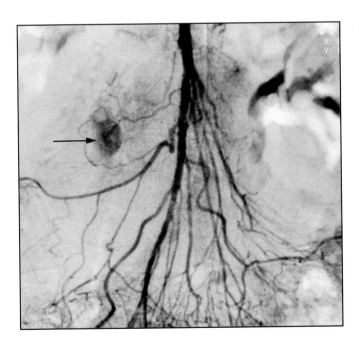

Mass in the head of the pancreas

Superior mesenteric artery

FIGURE 11-94.

Pancreatic cancer. **A,** Computed tomography (CT) scan demonstrates encasement of the superior mesenteric artery by a cancerous mass in the head of the pancreas. **B,** CT scan of the liver in the same patient showing the presence of multiple liver metastases. This patient's tumors would not be resectable because of involvement of a major vascular structure and the presence of metastatic disease. (*Courtesy of* Mark T. Toyama, Amy H. Kusske, and Howard A. Reber.)

FIGURE 11-95.

Pancreatic islet cell tumor. A 75-year-old woman who was admitted to the hospital for the evaluation of syncope and mental status changes was noted to have inappropriately elevated levels of plasma insulin. An Indium (In)-111 pentetreotide planar anterior view and SPECT images of the upper abdomen were normal. Computed tomography image of the upper abdomen did not reveal any abnormality involving the pancreas. Angiography seen here demonstrated a hypervascular focus (*arrow*) in the head of the pancreas. The lesion was enucleated at surgery and proved to be a 1.3 cm insulinoma by immunohistology.

Approximately 50% of patients with insulinoma will have normal results with In-111 pentetreotide scintigraphy. These insulinomas may express a subtype of somatostatin receptor that does not concentrate the radiopharmaceutical adequately for imaging purposes. It is also possible that some insulinomas may have either no receptors or may have an inadequate number of receptors to allow for their detection by scintigraphy. (*Courtesy of* Rodney V. Pozderac and Thomas M. O'Dorisio.)

■ ACKNOWLEDGMENT

Many physicians contributed to the images in this chapter, which is divided into several sections (Roy Orlando, Esophageal Disorders; Mark Feldman, Gastric and Duodenal Disorders; Lawrence Schiller, Small Intestinal Disorders; Richard Boland, Anal, Rectal, and Colonic Disorders; Nick LaRusso, Gallbladder and Biliary Disorders; and Phillip Toskes, Pancreatic Disorders). I am very grateful for their efforts.

■ REFERENCES

1. Spechler SJ, Fischbach L, Feldman M Clinical aspects of genetic variability in Helicobacter pylori. *JAMA* 2000, 283:1264–1266.

2. Landis SH, Murray T, Bolden S, Wingo PA: Cancer statistics, 1998. *CA Cancer J Clin* 1998, 48(1):6–29.

3. Drossman DA, Corazziari E, Talley NJ, *et al.*: *Rome II. The Functional Gastrointestinal Disorders. Diagnosis, Pathophysiology and Treatment: A Multinational Consensus.* 2nd ed. McLean, VA: Degnon Associates; 2000: 1–764.

4. Targan SR, Hanauer SB, van Deventer SJH, *et al.*: A short-term study of chimeric monoclonal antibody cA2 to tumor necrosis factor α for Crohn's disease. *N Engl J Med* 1997, 337:1029–1035.

5. Weinstein WM, Goboch ER, Bowes KL: The normal human esophageal mucosa: a histologic reappraisal. *Gastroenterology* 1975, 68:40.

6. Orlando RC: Reflux esophagitis. In *Textbook of Gastroenterology.* Edited by Yamada T, Alpers DH, Owyang C, *et al.* Philadelphia: JB Lippincott; 1991:1123–1147.

7. McBride MA, Ergun GA: Role of upper endoscopy in the management of esophageal strictures. *Gastrointestin Endoc Clin North Am* 1994, 4:595–621.

8. Peterson WL, Lee E, Feldman M: Relationship between *Campylocater pylori* and gastritis in healthy humans after administration of placebo or indomethacin. *Gastroenterology* 1988, 95:1185–1197.

9. Molmenti EP: Perforated duodenal ulcer. *N Engl J Med* 1997, 336:1499.

10. Friedman S, Wright T, Altman D: Gastrointestinal Kaposi's sarcoma in patients with acquired immunodeficiency syndrome: endoscopic and autopsy findings. *Gastroenterol* 1985, 89:751–755.

11. Lew E, Dieterich D: Severe hemorrhage caused by gastrointestinal Kaposi's syndrome in patients with the acquired immunodeficiency syndrome. *Am J Gastroenterol* 1992, 87:1471–1474.

12. Orbuch M, Doppman JL, Strader DB, *et al.*: Imaging for pancreatic endocrine tumor localization: recent advances. In *Endocrine Tumors of the Pancreas: Recent Advances in Research and Management.* Edited by Mignon M, Jensen RT. Basel: Karger; 1995:268–281.

13. Kwekkeboom DJ, Krenning EP, Oei HY, *et al.*: Use of radiolabeled somatostatin to localize islet cell tumors. In *Endocrine Tumors of the Pancreas: Recent Advances in Research and Management.* Edited by Mignon M, Jensen RT. Basel: Karger; 1995:298–308.

14. Lamberts SW, Bakker WH, Reubi JC, Krenning EP: Somatostatin-receptor imging in the localization of endocrine tumours. *N Engl J Med* 1990, 323:1246–1249.

15. Lamberts SWJ, Chayvialle JA, Krenning EP: The visualization of gastro-enteropancreatic endocrine tumors. *Digestion* 1993, 54(suppl 1):92–97.

16. Krenning EP, Kwekkeboom DJ, Bakker WH, *et al.*: Somatostatin receptor scintigraphy with [^{111}In-DTPA-D-Phe^1]-[^{123}I-Tyr^3]-octreotide: the Rotterdam experience with more than 1000 patients. *Eur J Nucl Med* 1993, 20:716–731.

17. Nakamura Y, Larsson C, Julier C, *et al.*: Localization of the genetic defect in multiple endocrine neoplasia type I within a small region of chromosome 11. *Am J Hum Genet* 1989, 44:751–755.

18. Sulkanen S, Halttunen T, Laurila K, *et al.*: Tissue transglutaminase autoantibody enzyme-linked immunosorbent assay in detecting celiac disease. *Gastroenterol* 1998, 115:1322–1328.

19. Sollid LM, Scott H: New tool to predict celiac disease on its way to the clinics. *Gastroenterol* 1998, 115:1584–1586.

20. Banwell JG, Lake AM: *Undergraduate Teaching Project. Unit 17. Gut Immunology and Ecology.* Bethesda, MD: American Gastroenterological Association.

21. Rogers AI, David S: Intestinal blood flow and diseases of vascular impairment. In *Bockus Gasroenterology*, vol 2, edn 5. Edited by Haubarich WS, Fenton S. Philadelphia: WB Saunders; 1995:1212–1234.

22. Harris MT, Lewis BS: Systemic diseases affecting the mesenteric circulation. *Surg Clin North Am* 1992, 72:245–259.

23. American Cancer Society. Colon and Rectum Cancer. Available at: http://www.cancer.org/ . Accessed June 18, 2001.

24. Dourmashkin RR, Davies H, Wells C, *et al.*: Epithelial patchy necrosis in Crohn's disease. *Hum Pathol* 1983, 14:643–648.

25. Deal SE, Zfass AM, Duckworth PF, *et al.*: Arteriovenous malformation (AVMs). Are they concealed by meperidine ? [abstract] *Am J Gastroenterol* 1991, 86:1351.

26. Reinus JF, Brandt LJ: Vascular ectasies and diverticulosis. Common causes of lower intestinal bleeding. *Gastroenterol Clin North Am* 1994, 23:1–20.

27. Dietzen CD, Pemberton JH: Diverticulitis. In *Atlas of Gastroenterology* Edited by Yamada T. Philadelphia: JB Lippincott; 1992:279–285.

28. NIH Consensus Conference Statement. *Am J Surg* 1993, 165:387–548.

29. Lai ECS, Mok FPT, Tan ES, *et al.*: Endoscopic biliary drainage for severe acute cholangitis. *N Engl J Med* 1992, 326:1582–1586.

30. Teixidor HS, Godwin TA, Ramirez EA: Cryptosporidiosis of the biliary tract in AIDS. *Radiology* 1991, 180:51–56.

31. Bradley EL, Murphy F, *et al.*: Prediction of pancreatic necrosis by dynamic pancreatography. *Ann Surg* 1990, 210:495–504.

32. London NJM, Lesse T, *et al.*: Rapid bolus contrast enhanced dynamic computed tomography in acute pancreatitis: a prospective study. *Br J Surg* 1991, 78:1452–1456.

33. Freeny PC, Lawson TL: *Radiology of the Pancreas.* New York: Springer-Verlag; 1982:334.

34. Vitas GJ, Sarr MG: Selected management of pancreatic pseudocysts: operative versus expectant management. *Surgery* 1992, 111:123–130.

35. Yeo CJ, Bastidas JA, Lynch-Nyhan A, *et al.*: The natural history of pancreatic pseudocysts documented by computed tomography. *Surg Gynecol Obstet* 1990, 170:411–417.

Hepatology

WILLIS C. MADDREY

Interest in the liver and its diseases has never been greater. Much of what is new, exciting, and of interest to clinicians is presented here in the form of tables and photomicrographs in this chapter of the second edition of the Atlas of Internal Medicine. Considerable attention is directed towards what is known about acute and chronic viral hepatitis.

The remarkable advances in the identification of viruses that cause hepatitis have led to considerable emphasis on these important diseases which affect millions of people around the world. In a span of 40 years, the viruses that cause hepatitis A through E have been identified and excellent diagnostic tests developed. The epidemiology and natural histories of the liver diseases caused by these viruses have been investigated. The development and deployment of effective vaccines to prevent hepatitis A and hepatitis B represent milestones in improvement in public health. Hepatitis B and hepatitis C are the leading causes of chronic hepatitis, cirrhosis, and eventually hepatocellular carcinoma. Hepatitis D has been identified as a virus that is present only in association with hepatitis B. Chronic hepatitis C and the liver diseases that develop in patients who are persistently infected with this virus have been shown to represent the most important liver-related health problems in the United States. Of great importance are the observations regarding routes of transmission, extrahepatic manifestations, and the accelerating effect on progression of disease in patients who also use alcohol.

There have been important advances in the understanding of the pathogenesis of autoimmune hepatitis, and autoimmune responses to drugs and hepatitis viruses have been identified and are described in figures in this chapter.

Much has been learned about cholestatic disorders. Primary biliary cirrhosis (chronic non-suppurative cholangitis) is being identified much earlier in its natural history because of increased awareness and the expanded use of antimitochondrial antibodies. The association of sclerosing cholangitis and inflammatory bowel disease are now well known, and, with the use of endoscopic retrograde cholangiography, this disorder can be readily recognized.

There is increasing interest in the spectrum of drug-induced liver injuries. Therapeutic drugs cause a broad array of liver disorders ranging from minimal elevations in biochemical tests to acute hepatitis, acute liver failure, chronic hepatitis, chronic cholestatic liver diseases even with the vanishing bile duct syndrome, cirrhosis, and a variety of vascular disorders and tumors.

This chapter features several illustrations that outline many processes within the liver including the pathway of bilirubin excretion, the natural histories of the liver diseases caused by the various hepatitis viruses, the association of chronic hepatitis B and C with cancer, and the pathogenesis of alcohol-induced liver injury. Advances in imaging techniques allow visualization of the liver, bile duct, and intra-abdominal vasculature with increasing precision. There are illustrations outlining the major complications of cirrhosis including the development of esophagogastric varices, ascites, spontaneous bacterial peritonitis, and hepatic encephalopathy.

Liver transplantation has now been established as a clinically useful procedure. Broader application of liver transplantation to include patients with alcohol-induced liver disease, cirrhosis-induced chronic hepatitis B, and even hepatocellular carcinoma has increased the demand for liver transplantation. The marked disparity between the number of organs available for transplantation and the growing need for donor organs have led to new innovations in transplantation include living-related donor procedures and the splitting of livers to provide an organ for two individuals.

Many of the advances in therapy of patients with liver disease are noted within this chapter. Interferon/ribavirin combination therapy has become the standard of care for hepatitis C, and both lamivudine and interferon therapy have proven successful in patients with chronic hepatitis B. There are more effective approaches to preventing recurrence of esophagogastric variceal hemorrhage and spontaneous bacterial peritonitis.

Progress in understanding the liver and its diseases coupled with increasingly effective therapies provide much more extensive information which will be useful to clinicians.

■ JAUNDICE

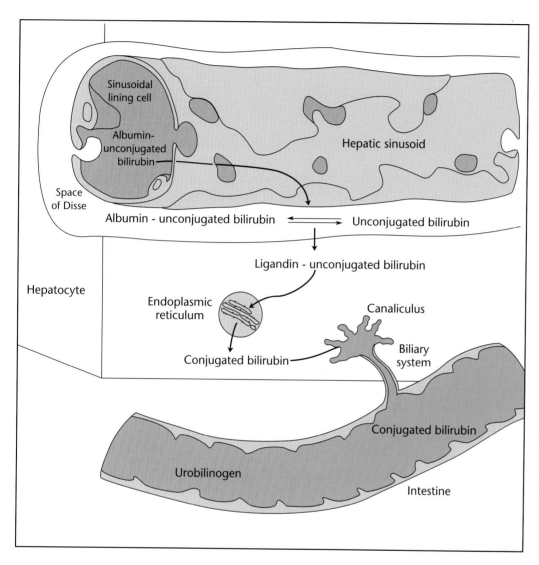

FIGURE 12-1.

Pathway of bilirubin excretion. Because of its poor solubility in physiologic aqueous solution, unconjugated bilirubin circulates in the blood as a noncovalent complex with albumin. The pores in the hepatic sinusoids are sufficiently large so that the bilirubin-albumin complex readily diffuses to the plasma membrane of the hepatocyte as blood flows through the liver. It is there unconjugated bilirubin dissociates from albumin and enters the cytosol. This dissociation occurs by facilitated transport. Within the hepatocyte cytosol, unconjugated bilirubin is bound to the protein ligandin (glutathione-S-transferase). The bilirubin molecule is subsequently conjugated with one or two molecules of glucuronic acid by the enzyme uridine diphosphate-glucuronyl transferase, which is located in the interior of the endoplasmic reticulum, and conjugated bilirubin is excreted across the canalicular membrane into bile. Conjugated bilirubin remains largely intact during passage through the biliary tract and the small intestine, but it is degraded by colonic bacteria to a series of tetrapyrroles that are collectively termed urobilinogen. These compounds partially account for the color of stool. A portion of urobilinogen is absorbed and excreted in bile; less than 2% is excreted in urine under normal circumstances. (*Adapted from* Bloomer [1].)

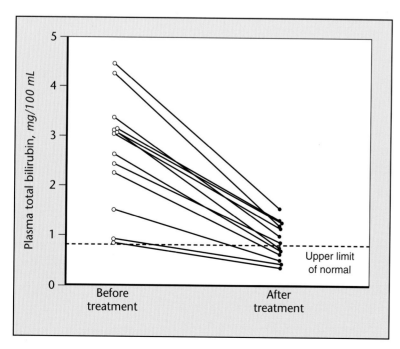

FIGURE 12-2.

Effect of phenobarbital administration on plasma bilirubin in Gilbert's syndrome. In this study, 13 patients with Gilbert's syndrome were given 180 mg/d of phenobarbital for 2 weeks. In each case, the plasma bilirubin level fell significantly. This reduction was evident as early as 2 to 3 days after treatment was begun; this lowering was maintained as long as the medication was continued. Reduction in the plasma bilirubin level was associated with, and was thought to be the result of, an increase in hepatic bilirubin UDP-glucuronyl transferase activity. (*Adapted from* Black and Sherlock [2].)

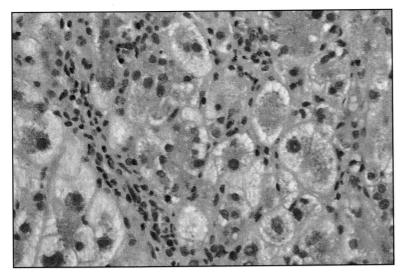

FIGURE 12-3.

Liver biopsy in fatty liver of pregnancy. Acute fatty liver of pregnancy is a rare disorder of the third trimester in which the hepatocytes become infiltrated with microvesicular fat in a pattern similar to that seen in Reye's syndrome. The incidence is estimated at 1/13,000 deliveries and is more common in primigravidas. The cause is unknown but may be an abnormality in lipid metabolism or mitochondrial function. Liver histology reveals microvesicular fat in a centrilobular distribution. The fat is primarily in the form of triglycerides and free fatty acids. Patients present with nausea, malaise, fatigue, and mild abdominal distress. Jaundice follows several weeks later. Renal dysfunction is a frequent complication. Prognosis is poor with maternal and fetal mortality rates at about 50%. Most authorities recommend prompt delivery of the infant once this entity is recognized because survival rates of both infant and mother are improved.

■ HEPATITIS

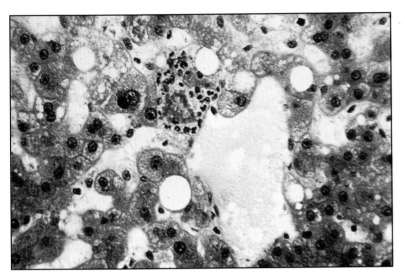

FIGURE 12-4.

Liver biopsy in alcoholic hepatitis. Alcoholic hepatitis is a common cause of jaundice in adults. Even if the patient denies alcohol consumption, one is suspicious of alcoholism if liver chemistries' results reveal moderate elevations of the transaminases with an aspartate aminotransferase that is two or more times greater than the alanine aminotransferase. Coupled with an elevated γ-glutamyl transpeptidase level and an elevated erythrocyte mean corpuscular volume, alcohol is the probable cause. If the diagnosis remains in doubt, liver biopsy may be indicated. Alcoholic hepatitis has a characteristic, although not pathognomonic, appearance. Marked fatty infiltration is usually present. Ballooning degeneration of hepatocytes is seen with Mallory hyalin often present in a centrilobular location. Mallory hyalin appears to be composed of intermediate filaments of the microtubular apparatus. Polymorphonuclear cell infiltration often occurs in association with Mallory hyalin. Finally, fibrosis may be present.

■ ACUTE VIRAL HEPATITIS

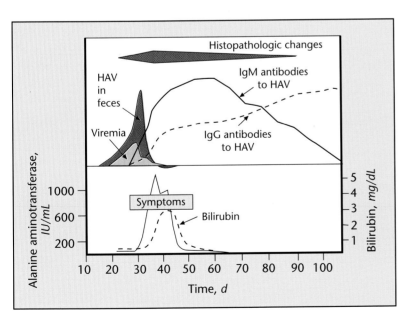

FIGURE 12-5.

Hepatitis A virus (HAV) serologic events. Fecal shedding of HAV is first seen during the latter half of the incubation period, before the development of histopathologic changes in the liver, and reaches a peak with the onset of symptoms and elevation of the alanine aminotransferase levels. Viral shedding declines rapidly thereafter and is often absent within a week after the onset of symptoms. Viremia is usually short-lived. Immunoglobulin M (IgM) antibodies to HAV appear concomitant with the onset of symptoms, reach peak levels within several weeks, and may disappear at 3 to 6 months. In contrast, immunoglobulin G (IgG) antibodies to HAV, the neutralizing, protective antibody, reach peak levels during the convalescent phase and decline slowly over many decades. (*Adapted from* Brown *et al.* [3].)

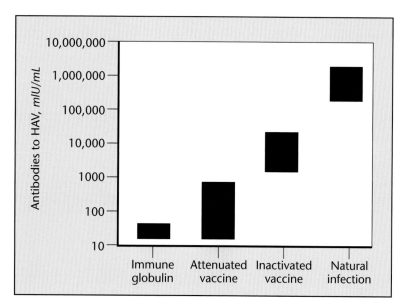

FIGURE 12-6.

Serum levels of antibodies against hepatitis A virus (HAV). Although the absolute level of antibodies to HAV necessary for protection from infection is not established, it seems probable that levels in excess of 10 to 20 mIU/mL, a range of values seen after injection of immune globulin, are protective. As shown here, antibodies to HAV levels reach very high levels following natural infection. Levels after administration of inactivated HAV vaccines are lower, but exceed by several fold those reported to be induced by attenuated vaccine preparations. It is presumed that the higher the level of antibodies to HAV, the longer the duration of protection will be. (*Adapted from* Lemon and Stapleton [4].)

Immunoprophylaxis of Hepatitis A: Immune Globulin vs Inactivated HAV Vaccine

Feature	Immune Globulin	Inactivated HAV Vaccine
Derived from blood	Yes	No
Acquisition of anti-HAV	Passive	Active
Prefered injection site	Deltoid	Deltoid
Peak anti-HAV level	Low	High, approaching level in natural infection
Pre-exposure efficacy	Yes	Yes
Duration of protection	2–3 months	>10 to 30 years
Postexposure efficacy	Yes, if given within 2 weeks of exposure	Possibly, but limited data
Combined use	May be given at separate deltoid sites for rapid induction of immunity	

FIGURE 12-7

Immune globulin, used for passive immunoprophylaxis of hepatitis A virus (HAV) infection for nearly 50 years, is a relatively inexpensive blood product that provides good pre-exposure protection and some postexposure protective efficacy if give early after exposure [5]. Unfortunately, peak antibodies to HAV (anti-HAV) levels are low and the passively acquired antibodies disappear and protection wanes after a few months. In contrast, the more costly two-dose inactivated HAV vaccine induces anti-HAV production, which may reach levels similar to those seen after natural infection. Pre-exposure protective efficacy is excellent [6] and, based on anti-HAV levels, it is likely that protection may last for years. Whether the inactivated HAV vaccine is effective in postexposure settings requires further study.

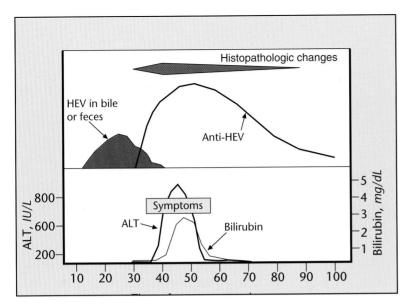

FIGURE 12-8.

Serologic events in hepatitis E virus (HEV) infection. Although information on the subject is very limited, the incubation period of HEV is, as shown here, approximately 40 days. HEV particles may appear in bile and then feces during the second half of the incubation period. Fecal HEV shedding may peak before the onset of jaundice or during the first week after the onset of jaundice. HEV disappears rapidly; it has not been identified in stool samples obtained 8 to 15 days after the onset of jaundice. Antibodies to HEV (Anti-HEV) have been found in sera taken during the acute phase. Although levels of Anti-HEV appear to decline during the late convalescent phase, the duration of detectable Anti-HEV remains uncertain. ALT—alanine aminotransferase. (*Adapted from* Brown *et al.* [3].)

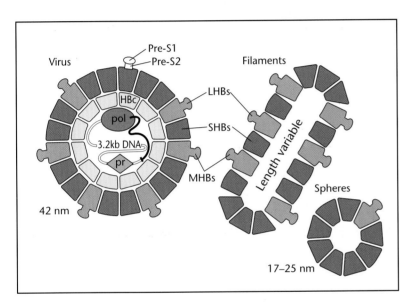

FIGURE 12-9.

Hepatitis B virus (HBV) particles. This schematic diagram shows the 42-nm HBV particle, tubular filaments, and spherical particles composed of the HBV envelope proteins, which also appear in the circulation of HBV–infected individuals. The envelope of intact HBV contains the so-called small (SHBs), middle-sized (MHBs), and large (LHBs) envelope proteins (hepatitis B surface antigen [HBsAg]). Although the filaments contain similar proportions of these proteins, the spheres contain less of the large protein. The small protein of HBsAg is specified by the S gene, the middle protein by *S* and *Pre-S2*, and the large protein by *S*, *Pre-S1*, and *Pre-S2*. The *S*, *Pre-2*, and *Pre-S1* domains are shown on the LHBs of the HBV particle. The 3.2-kb DNA, HBV DNA polymerase (pol), and a primase protein (pr) are shown within the capsid (HBc). (*Adapted from* Gerlich [7].)

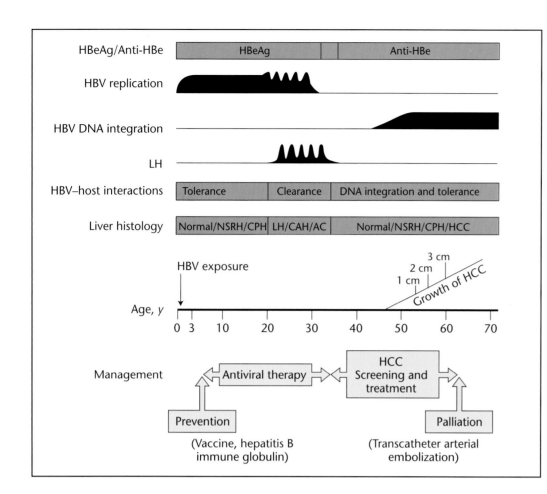

FIGURE 12-10.

Natural history of hepatitis B virus (HBV) infection. The natural history of HBV infection in individuals who acquire infection early in life, in the absence of immunoprophylaxis, is depicted in this schematic. During the early period after HBV acquisition, replication is high, hepatitis B e antigen (HBeAg) is present, and liver histology may be normal or show mild chronic hepatitis. Antiviral therapy at this point may alter the natural history of the disease. In its absence, over a period of time, HBV replication may diminish, HBeAg may disappear, and hepatic inflammation may increase. Eventually, HBV DNA genomic or subgenomic integration into the host hepatocyte may occur. Over many years, especially in patients who develop cirrhosis, hepatocellular carcinoma (HCC) may develop. AC—active cirrhosis; Anti-HBe—antibodies to HBeAg; CAH—chronic active hepatitis; CPH—chronic persistent hepatitis; LH—lobular hepatitis; NSRH—nonspecific reactive hepatitis. (*Adapted from* Chen [8].)

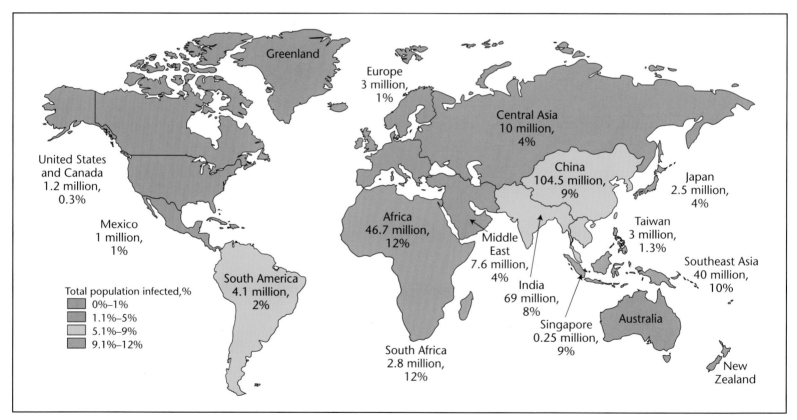

FIGURE 12-11.

Hepatitis B virus (HBV) worldwide. Chronic HBV infection is believed to affect close to 300 million people throughout the world. The prevalence of the hepatitis B surface antigen carrier state varies widely from area to area and even within the same country. Nonetheless, very high carrier rates have been identified in sub-Saharan Africa, in Southeast Asia, and in China. In addition to persistent infection, a very large proportion of the population of these regions has been exposed to HBV and infected by this virus. However, in contrast to the carriers, these individuals have successfully cleared the virus and resolved the infection. (*Adapted from* Hamilton and Gross [9].)

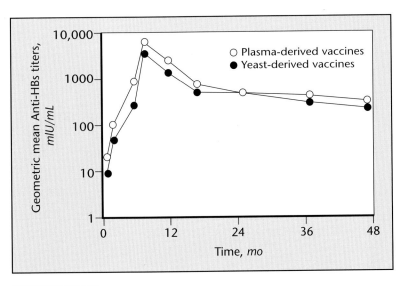

FIGURE 12-12.

Hepatitis B virus (HBV) vaccine–induced antibodies to hepatitis B surface antigen (anti-HBs). HBV vaccines were originally produced by hepatitis B surface antigen (HBsAg)–positive plasma treated with chemicals (urea, pepsin, formaldehyde) to inactivate residual HBV. In contrast, the recombinant vaccines have been produced through genetic engineering: the S open reading frame of HBV DNA is incorporated into the DNA of a yeast cell. The cell then produces HBsAg which is used as the immunogen in the vaccine. In the results of the study illustrated here, peak levels of anti-HBs produced after the conventional 0, 1, 6-month vaccination schedule were shown to be comparable for both plasma- and yeast-derived vaccines, and anti-HBs persisted equally in recipients on follow-up through 48 months. (*Adapted from* Scheiermann *et al.* [10].)

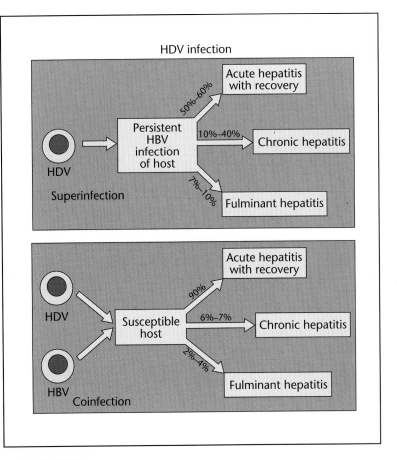

FIGURE 12-13.

Sequelae of hepatitis D virus (HDV). In general, the sequelae of HDV infection are more serious when superinfection of the host with persistent hepatitis B virus (HBV) infection occurs. As shown in the *upper panel*, superinfection is associated with a risk of chronic hepatitis in 10% to 40% of patients; fulminant disease is seen in 7% to 10%. In contrast, as shown in the *lower panel*, HDV and HBV coinfections are less often associated with grave outcomes. Only 6% to 7% coinfections lead to chronic hepatitis and only 2% to 4% end with fulminant hepatitis. (*Adapted from* Conjeevaram and Di Bisceglie [11].)

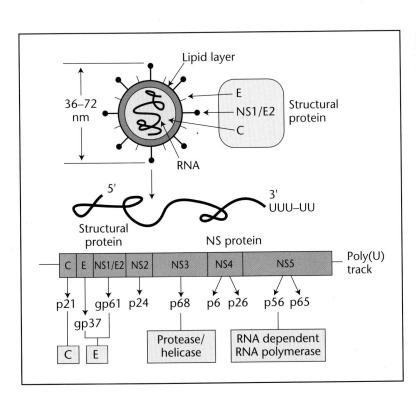

FIGURE 12-14.

Hepatitis C virus (HCV) particles and genome. This schematic diagram indicates that HCV is a positive sense, single-stranded RNA virus, with an estimated diameter of 36 to 72 nm. HCV is believed to represent a distinct genus in the *Flaviviridae* family. A viral envelope comprising a lipid layer and envelope proteins, surrounds a core (capsid) structure enclosing the viral nucleic acid. HCV RNA is 9.4 kb in length and consists of a 5'-nontranslated region, followed by core (C), envelope (E), and nonstructural (NS) protein encoding regions. The latter is followed by a short 3'-noncoding region with a poly(U) track at its end. Glycosylated (gp) and nonglycosylated (p) putative protein products of the structural and NS regions are shown. The NS protein products include a serine proteinase, helicase, and an RNA–dependent RNA polymerase. (*Adapted from* Esumi and Shikata [12].)

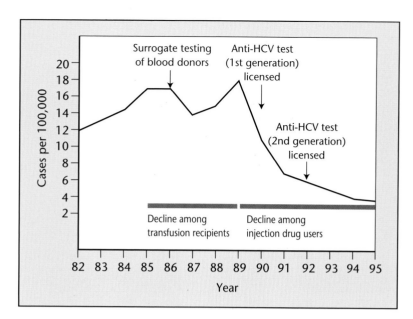

FIGURE 12-15.

Estimated incidence of acute hepatitis C virus (HCV) in the United States. The Centers for Disease Control and Prevention have estimated the incidence of acute viral hepatitis caused by HCV between 1982 and 1995. Based on data from their four-sentinel county study, and allowing for adjustments for underreporting, this figure suggests a dramatic decline in incidence after 1989. This decline is believed to reflect a decrease in HCV infection among injection drug users and in transfusion-associated HCV infection. While as many as 150,000 HCV infections may have occurred annually during the late 1980s, by the late 1990s this figure fell to less than 30,000 annually. Nonetheless, because of the high frequency of progression to chronicity, there may be as many as 2.7 million currently infected individuals in the United States. (*Adapted from* Alter and Moyer [13].)

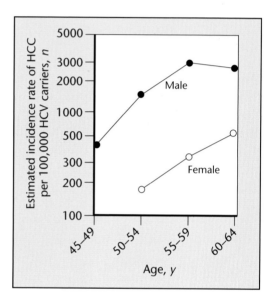

FIGURE 12-16.

Incidence of hepatocellular carcinoma (HCC) in hepatitis C virus (HCV) carriers. Osaka, Japan has been recognized as one of the highest risk regions for HCV–related HCC in the world. Based on second-generation assays for antibodies to HCV (anti-HCV), the prevalence of HCV RNA among volunteer blood donors in Osaka, the frequency of anti-HCV among cases of HCC, and data from the Osaka Cancer Registry, estimates of the probability of developing HCC were drawn for HCV carriers and plotted by 5-year age groups for both males and females. The estimated HCC incidence was higher in males than females and peaked for males at ages 55 to 59, whereas no peak could be identified in females. The cumulative risk of developing HCC in 50-year-old male HCV carriers was 28% within the following 15 years; for female HCV carriers the risk was 6%. This gender difference remains poorly understood. (*Adapted from* Tanaka *et al.* [14].)

■ AUTOIMMUNE HEPATITIS

Autoimmune hepatitis

Definite diagnosis	Probable diagnosis
Piecemeal necrosis +/- Lobular hepatitis +/- Bridging necrosis	Piecemeal necrosis +/- Lobular hepatitis +/- Bridging necrosis
No biliary lesions	No biliary lesions
AST/ALT elevation	AST/ALT elevation
Normal serum α_1 antitrypsin, copper, ceruloplasmin	Abnormal copper and ceruloplasmin if Wilson's disease excluded
Gamma globulin or IgG >1.5 x normal	Any gamma globulin or IgG elevation
ANA, SMA, or LKM1 > 1:80	ANA, SMA, or LKM1 ≥ 1:40 Other autoantibodies Anti-HCV positive/RIBA negative
IgM Anti-HAV, HBsAg, IgM Anti-HBc, Anti-HCV negative	
No active cytomegalovirus, Epstein-Barr virus	Alcohol (< 50 g/d)
No blood/drug exposures	Previous blood/drug exposure

FIGURE 12-17.

Diagnostic criteria for autoimmune hepatitis. The International Autoimmune Hepatitis Group met for the first time in Brighton, England, in June 1992. This panel formulated the criteria for a definite and probable diagnosis of autoimmune hepatitis [15]. The 6-month criterion of disease activity to establish chronicity was waived. Levels of significant hypergammaglobulinemia and auto-antibody titer were described, and elimination factors were strictly defined [15]. Lobular hepatitis was accepted within the spectrum of the disease. Laboratory and histologic features of cholestasis precluded the definite diagnosis as did markers of true viral infection [15]. The criteria recognized the possibility of an acute, even fulminant, onset of the disease and permitted the diagnosis even in those patients without conventional immunoserologic markers [15]. ALT—alanine aminotransferase; ANA—antinuclear antibodies; Anti-HAV—antibodies to hepatitis A virus; Anti-HBc—antibodies to hepatitis B core antigen; Anti-HCV—antibodies to hepatitis C virus; AST—aspartate aminotransferase; HBsAg—hepatitis B surface antigen; IgG—immunoglobin G; IgM—immunoglobin M; LKM1—liver-kidney microsome type 1; RIBA—recombinant immunoblot assay; SMA—smooth muscle antibodies. (*Courtesy of* Albert J. Czaja.)

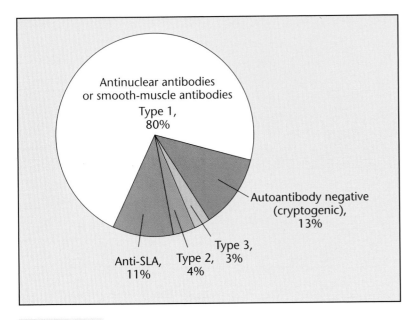

FIGURE 12-18.

Frequency of the different subtypes of autoimmune hepatitis in adults in the United States. Type 1 autoimmune hepatitis is the most common subtype [16,17]. Types 2 and 3 autoimmune hepatitis are very uncommon in American adults [18,19]. Autoantibody-negative autoimmune hepatitis (cryptogenic chronic hepatitis) is the second most common diagnosis. These patients may have escaped detection by conventional immunoserologic assays. Assessment for antibodies to soluble liver antigen (anti-SLA) and antibodies to liver–pancreas may allow reclassification of these patients as autoimmune hepatitis in 18% and 33% of patients, respectively [20,21]. Unfortunately, 11% of patients with type 1 autoimmune hepatitis have anti-SLA, and it is uncertain that these autoantibodies define a distinct subpopulation of patients [19].

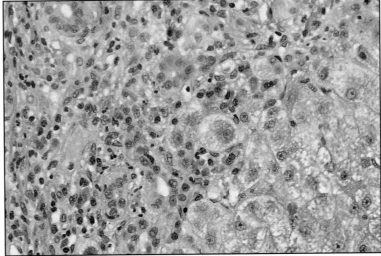

FIGURE 12-19.

Histologic findings of plasma cell infiltration of the portal tracts in type 1 autoimmune hepatitis (hematoxylin and eosin; original magnification, x400). Moderate-to-severe plasma cell infiltration of the portal tracts is found in 66% of tissue specimens [21]. Assessments using monoclonal antibodies have indicated that the major component of the inflammatory cell infiltrate in the portal tracts is the T lymphocyte [22]. Nevertheless, the recognition of plasma cells has diagnostic value [21]. In portal and periportal regions, the helper/inducer cells (CD4) are more numerous than the suppressor/cytotoxic T cells (CD8) [23]. In the lobule and in areas of piecemeal necrosis, the reverse is true [23].

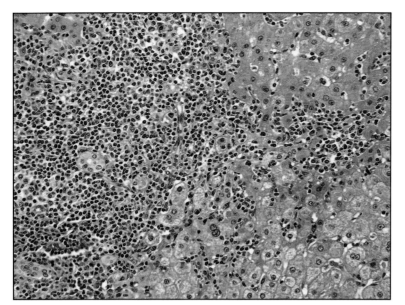

FIGURE 12-20.
Histologic findings in chronic hepatitis C that resemble those in type 1 autoimmune hepatitis (hematoxylin and eosin; original magnification, x100). Moderate interface hepatitis and portal plasma cell infiltration can occur in patients with true hepatitis C (hepatitis C virus [HCV] infection) [21,24]. In such instances, steatosis and portal lymphoid aggregates are absent and the findings suggest an autoimmune hepatitis. These patients may have autoimmune hepatitis with coexistent background HCV infection (overlap syndrome) or chronic hepatitis C with associated autoimmunity. Autoantibodies and hypergammaglobulinemia may also be present [24].

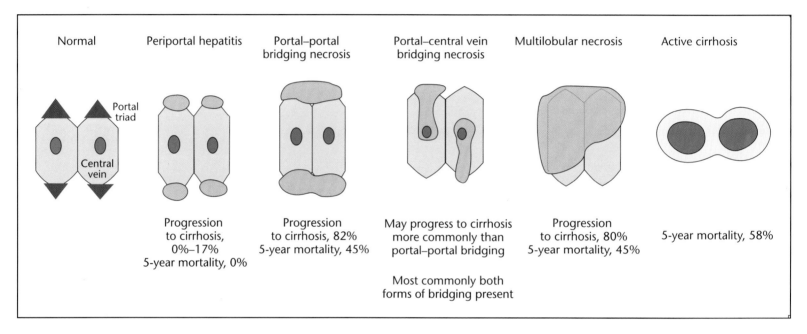

FIGURE 12-21.
Prognoses of initial histologic patterns in untreated type 1 autoimmune hepatitis. The severity and aggressiveness of the inflammatory process can be estimated by the histologic pattern at presentation [25,26]. The type and degree of hepatic inflammation can be assessed by needle biopsy with 90% accuracy [25]. Sampling variation and intraobserver interpretive error limit the ability of needle biopsy to evaluate cirrhosis [25]. Portal–portal and portal–central bridging necrosis are frequently mixed findings or are difficult to distinguish. Periportal hepatitis, which is the hallmark lesion of autoimmune hepatitis, typically has a benign prognosis and does not require therapy per se [17,25]. Transitions can occur between the various histologic patterns spontaneously or during therapy [17,25].

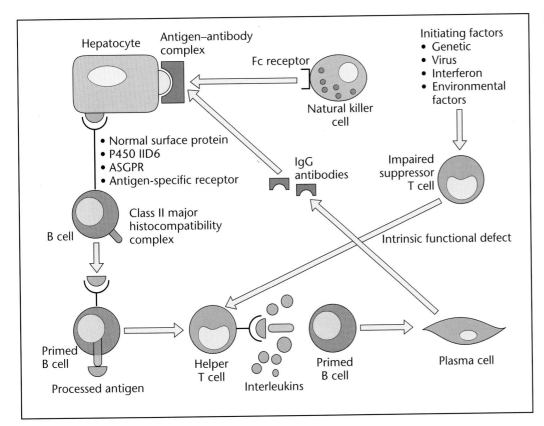

FIGURE 12-22.

Pathogenic hypothesis based on antibody-dependent, cell-mediated cytotoxicity. The principal defect is impairment of suppressor T-cell function [25–27]. Immunoglobulin G (IgG) production by plasma cells is inadequately modulated and antibodies complex with normal proteins on the hepatocyte surface [28]. Candidate target antigens are asialoglycoprotein receptor (ASGPR) and P450 IID6 (CYP2D6). The antigen–antibody complex is the target for natural killer cells that have Fc receptors. The natural killer cells do not require prior sensitization to a specific antigen, but the antibody complex does provide some antigen specificity [28]. Causes for suppressor cell dysfunction are unknown, but initiating factors may include genetic predisposition, viral infection, exogenous or endogenous interferon, and environmental factors [28]. Corticosteroids improve nonantigen–specific suppressor T-cell dysfunction. Antigen-specific suppressor T-cell dysfunction is not affected by corticosteroid treatment and may perpetuate the disease. Unfortunately, this type of defect has not been consistently demonstrated in autoimmune hepatitis. (*Adapted from* Czaja [28].)

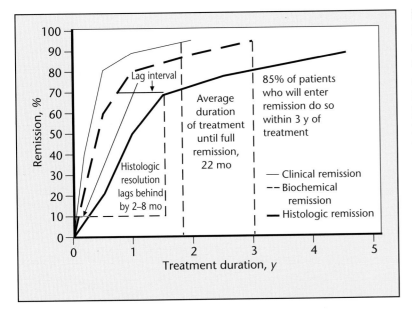

FIGURE 12-23.

Probabilities of clinical, biochemical, and histologic remission during corticosteroid therapy. Most patients (85%) who enter remission during therapy do so within 3 years [25]. The average duration of treatment to achieve remission is 22 months [17,25,29]. Because histologic remission lags behind clinical and biochemical remission by 3 to 6 months, treatment should be continued for at least this long following laboratory resolution. A liver biopsy assessment is useful to establish a confident treatment endpoint [30].

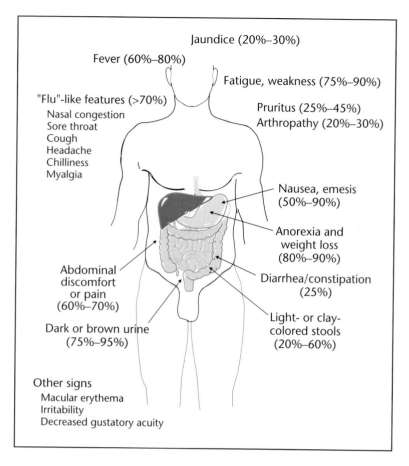

Jaundice (20%–30%)

Fever (60%–80%)

Fatigue, weakness (75%–90%)

"Flu"-like features (>70%)
Nasal congestion
Sore throat
Cough
Headache
Chilliness
Myalgia

Pruritus (25%–45%)
Arthropathy (20%–30%)

Nausea, emesis
(50%–90%)

Anorexia and
weight loss
(80%–90%)

Abdominal
discomfort
or pain
(60%–70%)

Diarrhea/constipation
(25%)

Dark or brown urine
(75%–95%)

Light- or clay-
colored stools
(20%–60%)

Other signs
Macular erythema
Irritability
Decreased gustatory acuity

FIGURE 12-24.

Constellation of symptoms reported by patients with acute hepatitis B. Most patients experiencing an acute HBV infection will have a non-icteric or asymptomatic illness [31]. The frequency of recognized acute hepatitis B is correlated to age at the time of infection. Adults are more likely to manifest evidence of illness, whereas infants and children rarely do. Patients who do not have icterus in the presence or absence of symptoms are at higher risk for developing chronic disease [32]. Although only a quarter of patients will become clinically jaundiced [33], a larger proportion will report evidence consistent with a cholestatic process by describing changes in color of urine and stool. Most symptoms experienced by patients are protean and frequently attributed to a nonspecific "viral" syndrome.

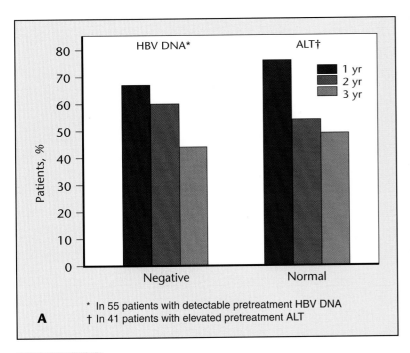

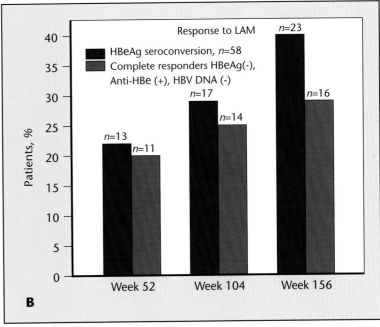

FIGURE 12-25.

Complete response to treatment with lamivudine (LAM) is defined as a loss of serum HBV DNA and seroconversion to an HBeAg negative, anti-HBe positive status in patients initially HBeAg positive. In Phase I/II studies, short term LAM therapy led to significant decreases in serum HBV DNA with return to pretreatment levels after discontinuation of drug [34]. Dosing studies and clinical trials with extended treatment periods suggested that LAM was effective in suppressing, but perhaps not in preventing viral replication [34–37]. Additional clinical trials assessing drug efficacy and safety for periods of up to 3 years demonstrated increased HBeAg seroconversion with increasing duration of LAM treatment [35,37–40]. Furthermore, when patients with HBeAg-negative/HBV DNA positive chronic hepatitis B and, liver transplant recipients with recurrent HBV disease were treated for 1 year with LAM, response rates were nearly equal or superior to that seen in non transplant patients with wild type chronic hepatitis B [41–43]. Leung *et al.* [40] reported on 58 Chinese patients participating in a Phase 3 multicenter trial who received LAM 100 mg daily for 3 years.

A, Of the 55 patients who had detectable serum HBV DNA at entry, 24 (44%) remained HBV DNA negative after 3 years of continuous treatment. Of the 41 (71%) patients with elevated ALT values at entry, 20 (49%) had normal ALT values at the end of 3 years. **B**, At the conclusion of the 3-year treatment, 23 of 58 (40%) patients had undergone HBeAg seroconversion and 16 of 55 (29%) were complete responders. Significant improvement in hepatic histologic scores paralleled the virologic response in from 52%-67% of patients receiving LAM for 1 year and in 57% of patients treated for 3 years [35,37,39,41–44]. The durability of the HBeAg seroconversion in LAM responsive patients has yet to be determined. One study reported that 32 (91%) of 35 complete responders to LAM remained HBeAg negative after short-term follow up (median 6 months) [45]. More recently only 6 (17%) of 35 patients, HBeAg negative pretreatment, who were HBV DNA negative following 52 weeks of LAM therapy, maintained a complete response when examined 6 months after discontinuing LAM [46].

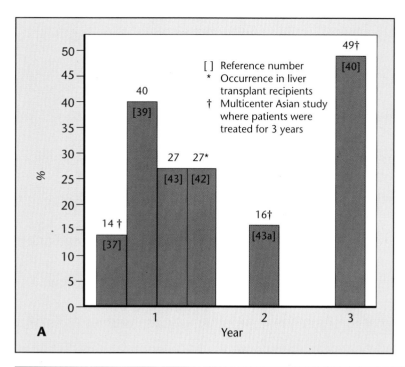

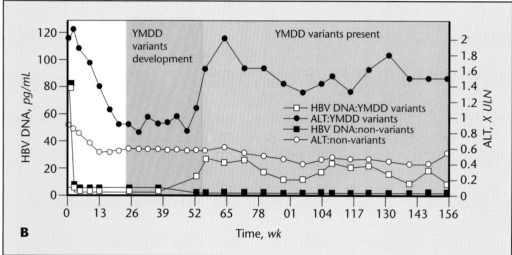

FIGURE 12-26.

YMDD variants of HBV. HBV replicates DNA via reverse transcription of an RNA intermediate. The half-life of HBV infected cells is in excess of 100 days [47] and as long-term administration of LAM is necessary to suppress HBV replication, the stage is set for emergence of resistant strains. HBV resistance to LAM is a consequence of mutations in the YMDD motif of the HBV polymerase gene (substitutions for methionine by valine or isoleucine at position 552 and a leucine to methionine substitution at position 528) and results in a defective HBV

reverse transcriptase. LAM resistance increases with time usually beginning after 6 months of treatment [48]. **A,** The rate of appearance for YMDD mutations and viral breakthrough is a function of the duration of LAM therapy. Studies denoted by + represent sequential serum analyses for YMDD variants in a large population of Asians treated for up to 3 years. The frequency of YMDD tripled in patients treated for 3 years as opposed to those receiving LAM for 2 years. **B,** The clinical implications of viral breakthrough with YMDD variants are problematic. YMDD variants can be detected in serum by PCR months before HBV DNA breakthrough but is not present in pretreatment serum [49]. Moreover, when treatment with LAM is discontinued there is a re-takeover by wild type HBV within 3 to 4 months which may be accompanied by clinical relapse [49]. Patients with the YMDD variant who are continued on LAM therapy remain capable of HBeAg seroconversion, demonstrate histologic improvements, and maintain median ALT as well as HBV DNA levels below the values observed just prior to initiation of LAM therapy [40,50]. The likelihood that patients treated with LAM harbor YMDD variants is 99% when they are HBeAg positive following 24 weeks of LAM treatment with ALT levels greater than 1.3 times upper limits of normal and serum HBV DNA levels greater than 20 pg/mL (using solution hybridization methodology) [50]. LAM has been used in combination with interferon as well as with nucleoside analogues. Logic would suggest that several modalities of treatment in combination, with each possessing a different mechanism(s) of anti HBV activity, would be more likely to succeed in eradicating the virus. Unfortunately, clinical observations have not as yet proven that combination LAM and interferon or LAM with other nucleoside analogues provide benefit beyond that seen with LAM alone [51,52].

Lamivudine versus Interferon: Similarities and Contrasts

Characteristics	Lamivudine	IFN
Chemical classification	Pyrimidine nucleoside and cytidine analogue metabolized intracellularly to lamivudine triphosphate	Glycoproteins
Mechanism of action	Inhibits HBV DNA replication	Inhibits HBV DNA replication
Administration	Oral dose of 100 mg daily for 1 year	Enhances cell-mediated immunity
Frequency of response (loss of HBeAg, HBV DNA, development of anti Hbe)	Equivalent	Subcutaneous or intramuscular injections for 4–6 months
Histologic improvement with treatment	Proven	Equivalent
Safety issues	Minimal/none	Proven
	Well tolerated	Significant
Factors associated with decreased treatment response	HBV variants (?)	Normal aminotransferases
		HIV co-infection/immune suppressed
		Decompensated cirrhosis
		HBV "mutants"

FIGURE 12-27.

Lamivudine, the negative enantiomer of 2' 3'-dideoxy3'-thiacytidine is the first of the nucleoside analogues approved by the United States Food and Drug Administration (December 1998) for the initial treatment of chronic hepatitis B. Indeed, lamivudine not only represents an alternative form of therapy to IFN, it may well supplant it. Although the specific mechanism for lamivudine (and other nucleoside analogues) action is not clear, it is a potent inhibitor of HBV replication by suppressing HBV DNA polymerase. While viral replication may be terminated and the number of infected hepatocytes decreased, intracellular covalent circular-core DNA persists and with cessation of treatment, promotes recurrent viral replication [53]. Lamivudine possesses many attractive features including ease of administration, treatment results and safety issues to promote its use as initial therapy.

■ HEPATITIS C

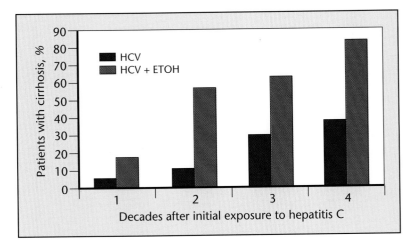

FIGURE 12-28.

Impact of alcohol consumption on disease progression. Mild alcohol consumption in patients with hepatitis C has been associated with an increased risk of developing cirrhosis. The rate of the development of cirrhosis is accelerated in hepatitis C patients who drink alcohol when compared with those hepatitis C patients who avoid alcohol [54].

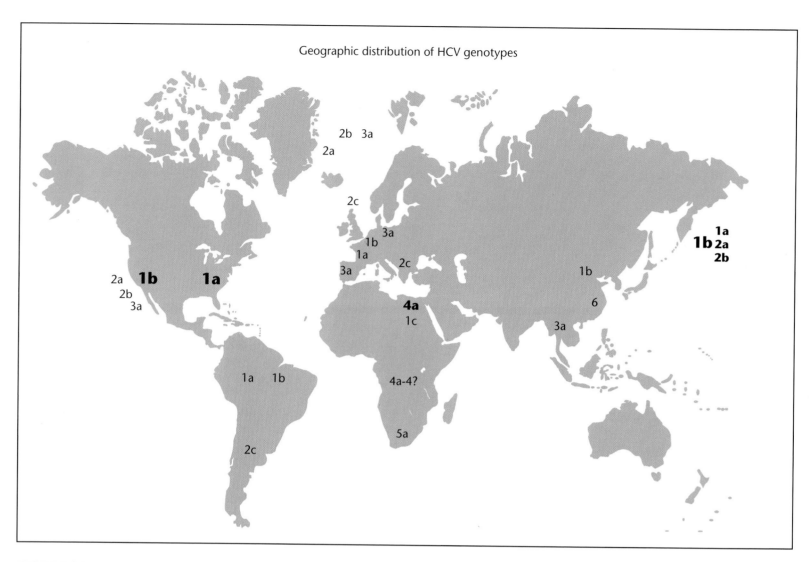

Geographic distribution of HCV genotypes

FIGURE 12-29.

Geographic distribution of hepatitis C virus (HCV) genotypes. There are six major genotypes. The most common genotype seen in the United States and Canada is type 1. Type 1b is associated with a more aggressive clinical course and appears to be more resistant to interferon therapy [55–57]. Several studies have associated genotype 1b with a higher risk for the development of

hepatocellular carcinoma type 2 is commonly seen in Japan and Europe and appears to respond better to both interferon monotherapy and combination interferon/ribavirin therapy. Genotype appears to have a role in determining the duration of treatment in native patients receiving combination interferon/ribavirin therapy. (*Courtesy of* M. Urdea.)

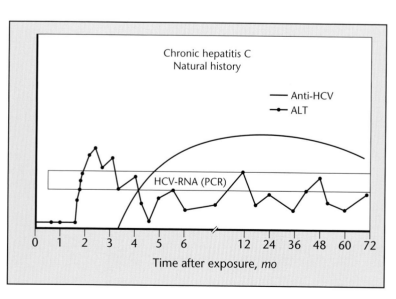

Chronic hepatitis C
Natural history

— Anti-HCV
— ALT

HCV-RNA (PCR)

Time after exposure, *mo*

FIGURE 12-30.

Serologic sequence in chronic hepatitis C virus (HCV). HCV-RNA appears approximately 2 to 4 weeks after exposure. Symptoms and jaundice may appear 6 to 24 weeks after exposure. Antibody to HCV (Anti-HCV) appears 12 to 14 weeks after exposure and its presence is lifelong. Anti-HCV does not denote chronicity or active infection. HCV-RNA denotes active disease. Nevertheless, most patients do not present during the acute phase of the illness but instead are diagnosed years later with chronic HCV [58,59]. ALT—alanine aminotransferase; PCR—polymerase chain reaction. (*Adapted from* Hoofnagle [60].)

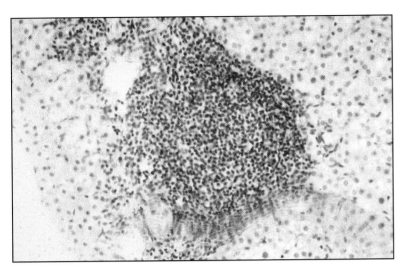

FIGURE 12-31.
Although the histologic features of chronic hepatitis C are not diagnostic, there are certain characteristic findings that are frequently found. Lymphoid follicular-like aggregates in the portal areas, fatty infiltration, bile ductular changes, and sinusoidal inflammation are common. Furthermore, there may be secondary iron deposition, evidence of coinfection with hepatitis B, or alcoholic liver injury in these patients. This figure illustrates one lymphoid follicular-like infiltrate.

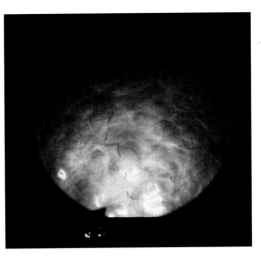

FIGURE 12-32.
Laparoscopic view of a patient with chronic active hepatitis and early cirrhosis [61,62]. Percutaneous liver biopsy with or without ultrasonic guidance is a standard diagnostic approach for establishing the presence of chronic hepatitis. Laparoscopic liver biopsy, which is used in several large referral centers, has the advantage of minimizing the sample error by facilitating gross inspection of the liver and thus ensuring an adequate biopsy sample size.

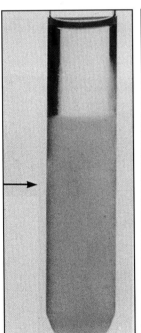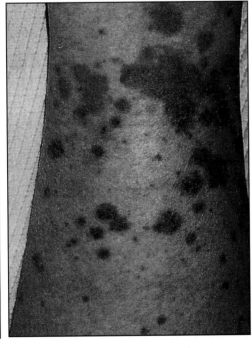

FIGURE 12-33.
Vasculitis and cryoglobulinemia related to hepatitis C virus. Mixed essential cryoglobulinemia has been associated with many chronic liver diseases. However, there appears to be high prevalence of cryoglobulinemia in patients with hepatitis C. The figure on the **right** depicts an area of palpable purpura approximately 2 by 3 cm on the medial aspect of the lower extremity of a patient with hepatitis C (*arrow*). The photograph on the **left** shows uncentrifuged serum after 48 hours at 4° C with the arrow indicating cryoprecipitate [63–65].

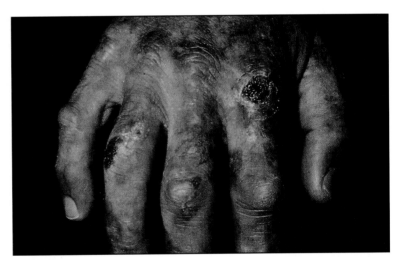

FIGURE 12-34.
Porphyria cutanea tarda. Fifty percent to 70% of cases of porphyria cutanea tarda (PCT) in the United States are positive for antibodies to hepatitis C virus. Hepatitis C is known to trigger the development of PCT. The exact mechanism of hepatitis C-induced PCT is unknown. Several proposed mechanisms include decreased intracellular glutathione concentration, decreased uroporphyrinogen carboxylase activity, elevated hepatocellular iron, and damaged hepatocyte production of an uroporphyrinogen decarboxylase inhibitor. All PCT patients should be tested for the presence of hepatitis C [66–69].

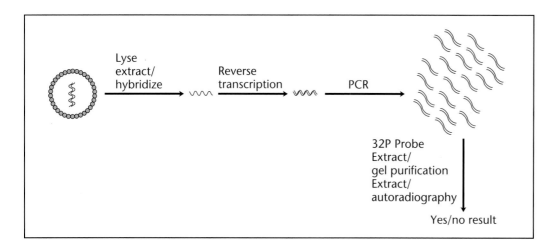

FIGURE 12-35.
Polymerase chain reaction (PCR) is an amplification technique used to detect hepatitis C virus (HCV)-RNA in both the serum and the liver. PCR is difficult to perform and contamination may occur leading to false-positive results. False-negative results may occur if there are important mismatches between the primers used in the PCR assay and the nucleotide sequences of the HCV genotype under study. Both qualitative and quantative PCR assays are readily available [70,71]. (*Adapted from* Chiron Corp., Emeryville, CA.)

■ DRUGS AND THE LIVER

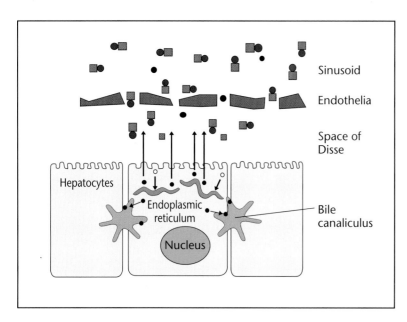

FIGURE 12-36.
Entry of drugs into the hepatocyte. Most drugs are fat soluble or lipophilic to a variable extent. Fat solubility is important because in order to reach the systemic circulation, an orally administered drug must generally diffuse across the lipid membrane of the enterocyte. A drug with little or no lipophilic property is poorly absorbed and is excreted in the stool. In contrast, a drug that is absorbed is then bound to protein, usually albumin, and distributes itself to various tissues, including fat. Unless rendered more polar or water soluble, such drugs tend to accumulate in the body over a prolonged period and may affect cellular processes. Whether given orally or parenterally, drugs eventually pass through the liver. The degree of hepatic drug extraction depends on hepatic blood flow and the activity of the drug-metabolizing enzymes. In the hepatic sinusoids the drugs (*open circles*) bound to protein (*open squares*) pass through openings (fenestrae) in the endothelium and gain access to the space of Disse, from which they enter the hepatocytes, where enzymes convert them into more polar compounds (*solid circles*). Some of these water-soluble molecules pass back to the sinusoids, whereas others enter the biliary canaliculi. (*Adapted from* Watkins [72].)

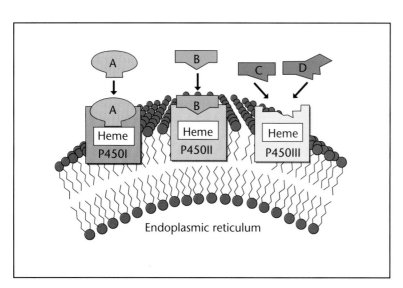

FIGURE 12-37.
Catalytic specificity of P450s. Each human P450 isoenzyme appears to be expressed by a particular gene. The *P450* genes, however, are distributed among different chromosomes. One P450 isoenzyme may be involved in the metabolism of one or more drugs, and a single drug may be acted upon by multiple enzymes. Many drugs, however, are largely metabolized by a single form of P450. These findings may be explained by the observation that relative binding affinities for specific drugs vary among the different P450s. Drugs must bind to the P450 at the substrate binding site, which is located close to the enzyme's heme prosthetic group. The binding affinity between certain drugs and P450 may vary so that a single P450 may be largely responsible for the metabolism of some drugs. Drug A and drug B are metabolized individually by P450I and P450II, respectively. These drugs will not bind with the other P450s, but each P450 can metabolize more than one drug as shown by the ability of a single P450III to bind drugs C and D. (*Adapted from* Watkins [72].)

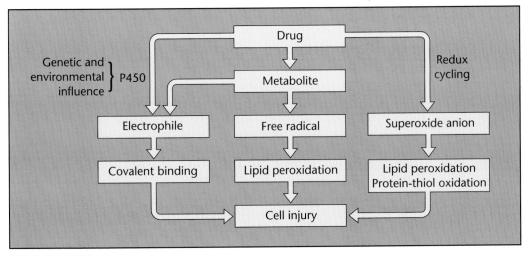

FIGURE 12-38.

Mechanisms of drug-induced hepatic necrosis. Because compounds that are known to be direct toxins are not used as pharmacologic agents in clinical practice, the hepatotoxicity associated with drugs is generally idiosyncratic and unpredictable rather than intrinsic and predictable. Moreover, because it is idiosyncratic in nature, the drug-induced hepatotoxicity seen in clinical practice cannot be entirely eliminated based on the results of previous animal studies alone. Idiosyncratic drug toxicity may result from a metabolic derangement that leads to the production of toxic reactive metabolites. It may also result from hypersensitivity (allergy). Some hypersensitivity results from migration of a toxic derivative (such as haptene) to the surface plasma membrane where it may evoke an immune response. Hepatocellular injury is usually not caused by the drug itself, but by its metabolic products [73]. The drug-metabolizing enzymes (P450 system), under genetic and environmental influences, cause the generation of electrophilic substances, which seek and accept electrons from other compounds, thereby forming covalent bonds. Electrophiles may form bonds with thiol (sulfur-containing groups), as is seen in acetaminophen toxicity, or with amino groups, as evident in halothane toxicity. Covalent binding of potent alkylating, arylating, or acylating agents to hepatic molecules adversely affects normal cell function and cell necrosis ensues. This condition becomes especially true when levels of intracellular protective substances like glutathione, which are capable of preferentially combining with toxic metabolites, are depleted. Cell necrosis/apoptosis can also result from the generation of free radicals (metabolites with unpaired electrons) in the course of oxidative drug metabolism. These free radicals can bind both to proteins and unsaturated fatty acids of the cell membranes, resulting in lipid peroxidation, membrane damage, and disruption of membrane and mitochondrial functions. The effect of lipid peroxidation may be mediated via the release of various cytokines (*ie*, tumor necrosis factor). An example of free radical–mediated injury is carbon tetrachloride hepatoxicity. Lipid peroxidation can also result from the generation of superoxide anion through redox cycling. Necrosis may be greatest in the centrilobular zone where the sinusoidal oxygen tension is lowest and where the concentration of P450 enzymes tends to be highest.

Arrayed against these mechanisms of liver injury are protective compounds. Foremost is glutathione. Some electrophiles preferentially attack the thiol of glutathione, a reaction that is catalyzed by the glutathione S-transferase. Another defense mechanism is mediated by scavengers that interfere with the free radical chain reaction of lipid peroxidation. The leading free radical scavenger against lipid peroxidation is tocopherol, but such endogenous substances as uric acid, bilirubin, ascorbic acid, and vitamin A may be important also.

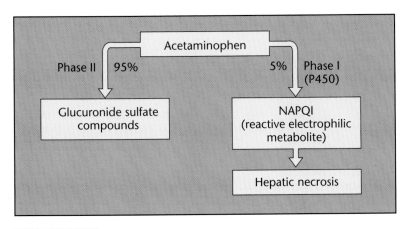

FIGURE 12-39.

Mechanisms of acetaminophen toxicity [74]. The major bulk of acetaminophen is metabolized by phase II reaction (95% or more), mainly through glucuronidation and sulfation, whereas only 5% or less undergo oxidation that results in the formation of a reactive electrophilic metabolite, N-acetyl-P-benzoquinoneimine (NAPQI). NAPQI preferentially binds to glutathionine (GSH), and when cytosolic (and especially mitochondrial) GSH concentration falls, NAPQI toxicity ensues. Mitochondrial function is impaired. The isoenzyme (P450IIE$_1$) that catalyzes the oxidation of acetaminophen also metabolizes ethanol, so that chronic ethanol ingestion induces this enzyme and increases the proportion of acetaminophen that undergoes oxidative degradation. Thus, in such patients the concomitant ingestion of acetaminophen, even in ordinary therapeutic doses (3 to 4 g/day), may result in serious hepatotoxicity. Depletion of GSH by starvation, alcohol ingestion, or other drugs are important contributory factors in acetaminophen toxicity. Therapy is aimed at increasing GSH synthesis by providing N-acetylcysteine. Because isoniazid also induces P450IIE, patients taking both this antituberculosis agent and acetaminophen are also at risk for possible acetaminophen hepatotoxicity.

■ ACUTE LIVER FAILURE

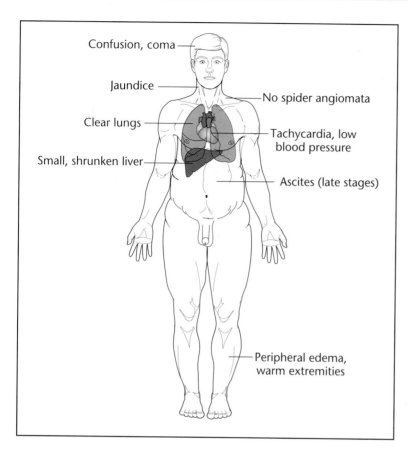

Confusion, coma

Jaundice

Clear lungs

Small, shrunken liver

No spider angiomata

Tachycardia, low
blood pressure

Ascites (late stages)

Peripheral edema,
warm extremities

FIGURE 12-40.
Basic physical findings in acute liver failure. Typical features observed in the patient with acute liver failure include confusion, agitation, or even hallucination. Mental status often deteriorates to coma soon after presentation, making history-taking impossible. Most patients will be icteric, although some barely so, and spider angiomata as seen in cirrhotic patients should be absent. Tachycardia, tachypnea, and relative hypotension are common. Asterixis, so commonly observed in chronic hepatic encephalopathy, is rarely seen. *Fetor hepaticus*, a sweet odor caused by mercaptans excreted in the breath, is often observed. Percussion over the rib cage to detect hepatic dullness reveals that the liver span is considerably decreased, and there may be no dullness appreciated, as evidence of the loss of hepatic mass. At autopsy, the normal liver mass of approximately 1600 g may be reduced to as little as 600 g. Edema is not observed initially but may develop in the hospital. Although the extremities are often cold, after resuscitation "warm shock" is the rule.

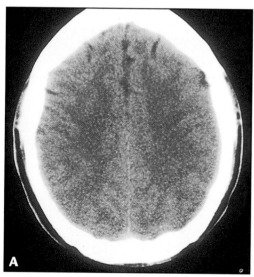

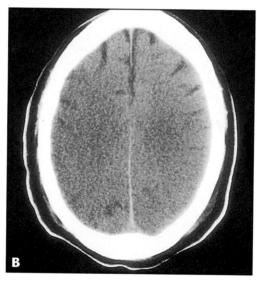

FIGURE 12-41.
Cerebral edema on computerized tomographic (CT) scanning in a patient with acute liver failure. **A**, CT of a normal brain showing clear demarcation between gray and white matter.

B, A similar section showing obliteration of gray and white matter demarcation caused by increased cerebral water. Obliteration of brain sulci is also seen but is a less consistent finding. Evidence of edema using CT is a late and inconstant finding in cerebral edema patients and thus is not a reliable guide to therapy. The presence of edema has two possible adverse effects. First, it decreases cerebral blood flow and may result in brain anoxia. The cerebral perfusion pressure (systemic blood pressure minus intracerebral pressure) should be maintained above 40 mm Hg to preserve adequate brain oxygenation. Second, herniation of the brain stem through the falx cerebri caused by cerebral edema is uniformly fatal. Erratic changes in blood pressure, temperature, or breathing pattern imply impending herniation.

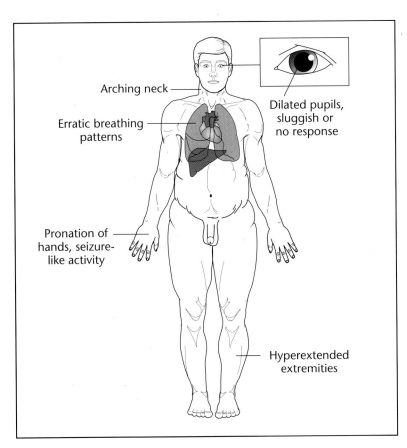

FIGURE 12-42.

Physical findings in patients with advanced hepatic encephalopathy and cerebral edema. Typically, patients will experience a brief period of agitation before the development of coma. Hepatic coma is usually graded as I through IV—grade I is signified by altered personality and subtle changes in cognition; grade II typically demonstrates confusion, slurred speech, and possibly asterixis, but the patient remains able to follow commands; grade III is characterized by deepening coma responsive to strong stimuli with some purposeful movements; grade IV patients are totally unresponsive. Hyperventilation is universal in all stages of hepatic coma. In grade IV coma, decerebrate posturing, changes in breathing patterns, seizures, and pupillary abnormalities all occur in the presence of cerebral edema. These signs, alone or in association with systemic hypertension, warrant immediate intervention with mannitol and pursuit of transplantation, if available. Corticosteroids, hyperventilation, and use of phenobarbital, although recommended for head trauma patients to decrease cerebral edema, are of little benefit in acute liver failure. Diuretics have been used in addition to mannitol but are of uncertain value.

Labels in figure:
- Arching neck
- Dilated pupils, sluggish or no response
- Erratic breathing patterns
- Pronation of hands, seizure-like activity
- Hyperextended extremities

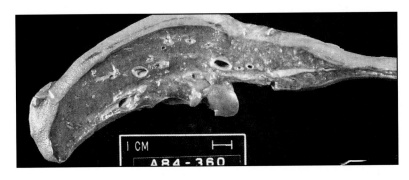

FIGURE 12-43.

Massive liver necrosis secondary to halothane anesthesia. This 55-year-old woman died 35 days after halothane anesthesia for a cholecystectomy. Twenty years prior, she had undergone a hysterectomy with halothane. The patient became ill 2 weeks after her surgery and became comatose 2 weeks later, never regaining consciousness. The liver was small and shrunken, with a wrinkled capsule, and weighed only 680 g (normal liver weight 1400–1600 g). This finding was formerly referred to as *acute yellow atrophy*.

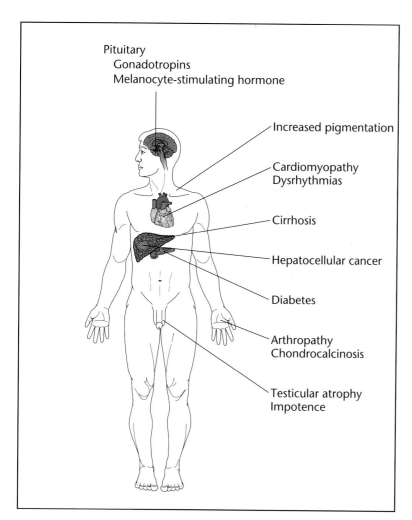

Pituitary
Gonadotropins
Melanocyte-stimulating hormone

Increased pigmentation

Cardiomyopathy
Dysrhythmias

Cirrhosis

Hepatocellular cancer

Diabetes

Arthropathy
Chondrocalcinosis

Testicular atrophy
Impotence

FIGURE 12-44.

Clinical manifestations of hereditary hemochromatosis. The clinical manifestations of hereditary hemochromatosis are protean. The most common abnormalities are found in the liver, and the development of hepatocellular carcinoma is 200 times more common in patients with untreated hemochromatosis than in the general population. In the 1990s, it is distinctly unusual to identify someone with the original triad of pigmentation, cirrhosis, and diabetes. With the advent of screening iron studies on routine chemistry panels, hemochromatosis is now often identified in asymptomatic individuals. (*Courtesy of* Bruce R. Bacon.)

■ HEMOCHROMATOSIS AND WILSON'S DISEASE

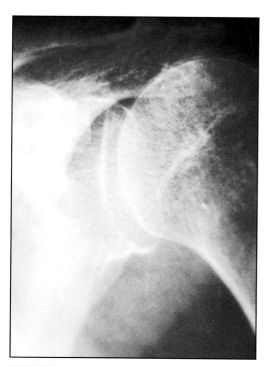

FIGURE 12-45.

Shoulder radiograph. The other arthritic changes seen in hereditary hemochromatosis are the development of chondrocalcinosis or pseudogout. This condition is depicted in this radiograph from a patient with hemochromatosis.

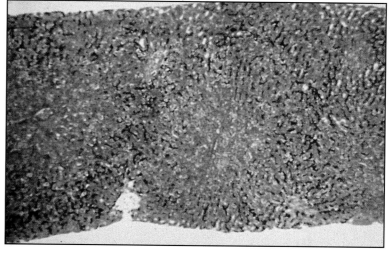

FIGURE 12-46.

A liver biopsy specimen shown at low power. The liver biopsy procedure has been essential to establish the diagnosis of hemochromatosis. Histochemical staining with Perls' Prussian blue reagent stains storage iron blue against the counterstain which is red. Shown here is a liver biopsy specimen from a 34-year-old man with newly diagnosed hereditary hemochromatosis (HH). At low power, the iron deposition is seen predominantly in a periportal distribution. With the availability of genetic testing, the need for liver biopsy to diagnose HH has decreased. Recent studies have shown that patients who are C282Y homozygotes (with abnormal blood studies of HH), who are less than 40 years old (with normal liver enzymes), may not need to have a liver biopsy performed since fibrosis/cirrhosis will not be present [75].

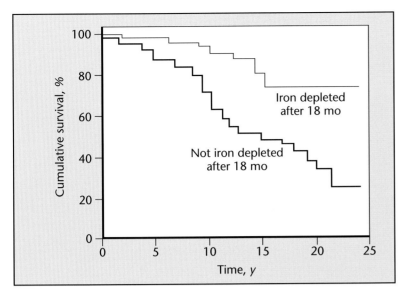

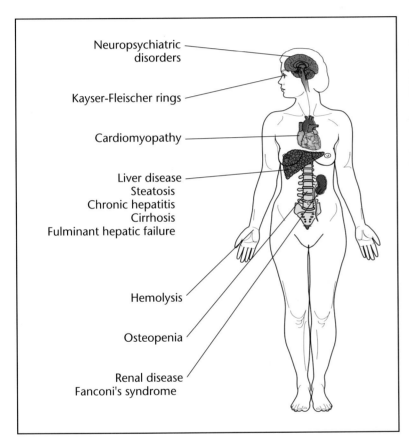

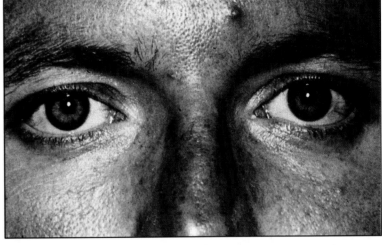

FIGURE 12-47.

Survival in hereditary hemochromatosis versus iron removal. When the total amount of excess iron could be removed within 18 months (indicating less severe iron overload), the survival was equivalent to the control population. However, when the iron burden was such that the excess iron could not be removed within 18 months of phlebotomy therapy, survival was decreased. These heavily iron-loaded patients also presented with cirrhosis and diabetes. (*Adapted from* Niederau *et al.* [76].)

FIGURE 12-49.

Kayser-Fleischer rings. This young man has classical Kayser-Fleischer rings, identified as the golden-brown pigment deposits in Descemet's membrane in the periphery of the iris. These rings can be seen with the naked eye, but occasionally, a slit-lamp examination is necessary to identify them. Another unusual ophthalmologic manifestation of Wilson's disease is sunflower cataracts.

FIGURE 12-48.

Clinical manifestations of Wilson's disease. There are numerous clinical manifestations of Wilson's disease including the presence of Kayser-Fleischer rings. Many psychiatric symptoms and disorders are typical of Wilson's disease. Rarely, cardiomyopathy ensues. All patients with Wilson's disease have hepatic involvement that can range from fairly mild steatosis to the insidious development of cirrhosis or the often fatal fulminant hepatic failure. The renal disease that occurs in Wilson's disease is comparable with that seen in Fanconi's syndrome. Hemolysis is caused by copper toxicity; many patients have significant osteopenia [77–79].

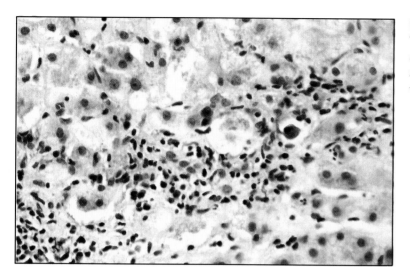

FIGURE 12-50.
This figure shows chronic active hepatitis with piecemeal necrosis and parenchymal inflammation. Some studies have suggested that as many as 25% of young individuals with nonviral chronic hepatitis have Wilson's disease.

Pathogenetic Mechanisms

Genetic factors
HLA Associations A3 (B7, B14)
Gene location, chromosome 6; frequency 5%
Autosomal recessive
HFE mutation analysis for C282Y, H63D
Pathophysiology
HFE binds to transferrin receptor (TfR) and participates in regulation of iron absorption
2—4 mg/d; 100 mg/y
Clinical evidence of toxicity at >20 g total body iron stores

FIGURE 12-51.
Pathogenetic mechanisms. The genetic factors in hereditary hemochromatosis indicate that it is an autosomal recessive disorder with the gene located on the short arm of chromosome 6. The gene frequency is 5% with the prevalence of homozygosity being approximately one in 250 with a heterozygote frequency of approximately one in 10 individuals. The disease is seen predominantly in white patients of Northern European descent. Approximately 85% to 90% of typical hemochromatosis patients are homozygous for C282Y. The inherited disorder results in an inappropriate gastrointestinal absorption of iron, and instead of the usual 1 to 2 mg/d, patients with hemochromatosis absorb 2 to 4 mg/d.

HFE Mutations in Hereditary Hemochromatosis

Genotype	Patients, *n*	Patients, %
	980	100
C282Y/C282Y	843	86
C282Y/H63D*	33	3.3
C282Y/Wild type	13	1.3
H63D/H63D	8	0.8
-H63D/Wild type	26	2.6
Wild type/Wild type	57	5.8

*Compound heterozygote.

FIGURE 12-52.
HFE mutations in hereditary hemochromatosis. Numerous studies have been performed worldwide where *HFE* genotyping was performed on a series of patients with typical hemochromatosis. In nine series, totaling 980 patients, 86% were homozygous for C282Y.

FIGURE 12-53.
After therapy is initiated for the proband, it should be remembered that hemochromatosis is an inherited disease and screening should be performed on all first-degree relatives. Screening studies should include measuring serum iron, transferrin saturation, and ferritin levels. If any of these are abnormal, a liver biopsy should be performed for histochemical staining and biochemical iron determination. HLA studies are only useful to evaluate siblings of an affected proband or when performing pedigree analysis. HLA studies should not be used in individual patients.

Characteristic Laboratory Features of Wilson's Disease

	Normal	Wilson's Disease
Serum copper, *μg/dL*	80–140	<80
Urine copper, *μg/24 h*	<40	>100
Serum cerulospasm, *mg/dL*	20–40	<20
Hepatic copper concentration, *μg/g dry weight*	15–50	250–3000

FIGURE 12-54.
Characteristic laboratory features of Wilson's disease. Serum copper levels are typically depressed, but this feature is not a highly sensitive and specific laboratory finding. Twenty-four–hour urine copper excretion is the best confirmatory test, along with hepatic copper concentration as determined by liver biopsy. Serum ceruloplasmin levels are depressed in the majority of patients with Wilson's disease but can be depressed in severe malabsorption and malnutrition.

■ ALCOHOL-INDUCED LIVER DISEASE

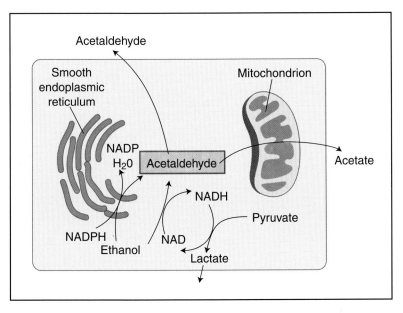

FIGURE 12-55.
Metabolism of alcohol. Once alcohol is absorbed from the gastrointestinal tract, over 90% is oxidized in the liver. The amount of alcohol available for hepatic oxidation is affected by factors such as gastric oxidation, rate of gastric emptying, volume of distribution, and hepatic extraction from portal blood. There are three major hepatic oxidation pathways. Most oxidation proceeds through the cytosolic alcohol dehydrogenase pathway and the microsomal enzyme oxidizing system (MEOS) located in the endoplasmic reticulum. Chronic alcohol consumption results in increased MEOS activity. The catalase pathway, located in peroxisomes, is a minor pathway. All three pathways result in the production of acetaldehyde. Usually, this highly toxic metabolite is rapidly metabolized to acetate by mitochondrial aldehyde dehydrogenase. Chronic alcohol consumption reduces the activity of this enzyme resulting in increased levels of acetaldehyde [80].

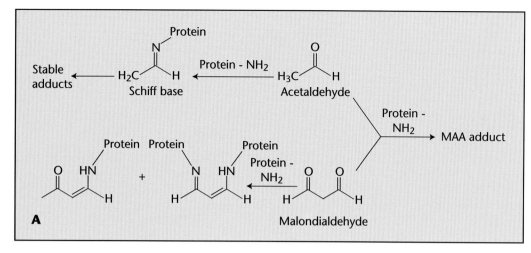

FIGURE 12-56.

Alcohol and fibrogenesis. **A,** Acetaldehyde and the lipid peroxidation-derived aldehyde malondialdehyde react together with proteins in a synergistic manner to form distinct hybrid adducts (MAA-adducts). These play a role in modulation of hepatic inflammatory response by recruiting leukocytes to hepatocytes. In turn, these recruited leukocytes, through cytokine release, may further exacerbate the fibrogenic and inflammatory responses of stellate cell as well as have a direct cytotoxic effect on hepatocytes, resulting in the release of more MAA-adducts. **B,** A continuous self-perpetuating cycle is established that leads to more severe fibrosis and cirrhosis [81].

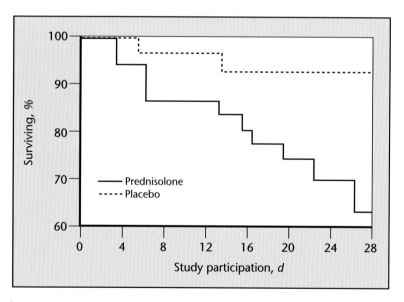

FIGURE 12-57.

Corticosteroids. Corticosteroids (Methylprednisolone 32 mg/d or Prednisolone 40 mg/d, for 28 days) have been shown to significantly improve short-term survival and markers of hepatic dysfunction in a subgroup of patients with severe alcoholic hepatitis [82,83]. The subgroup characteristics include presence of hepatic encephalopathy or a Maddrey index > 32, and absence of renal failure, active infection, or active gastrointestinal bleeding. The putative mechanisms include deactivation of the enhanced immune response to release of neoantigens and inhibition of cytokine production.

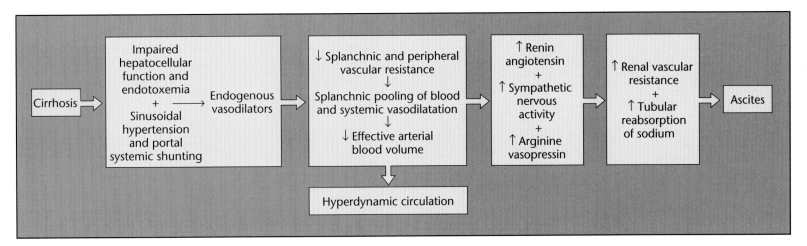

FIGURE 12-58.

One of several theories proposed to explain the pathogenesis of renal sodium and water retention in cirrhosis is the *Peripheral Arterial Vasodilatation Hypothesis*. Profound hemodynamic changes complicate the clinical course of chronic liver disease. There is opening of arteriovenous shunts and splanchnic and peripheral arteriolar vasodilatation. This results in a fall in arterial blood pressure and systemic vascular resistance, leading to a reduction in the effective arterial blood volume and a hyperdynamic circulation.

This in turn activates neurohumoral pressor systems, promoting renal sodium and water retention in an attempt to restore the effective arterial blood volume and maintain blood pressure. When increased renal sodium reabsorption cannot compensate for the arterial vasodilatation, arterial underfilling occurs. Then the cascade of further activation of various neurohumoral pressor systems begins, leading to increased renal sodium retention and ultimately, ascites formation.

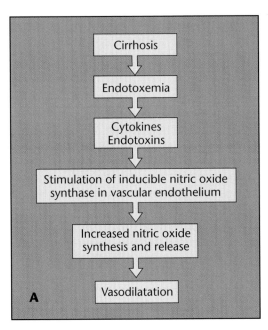

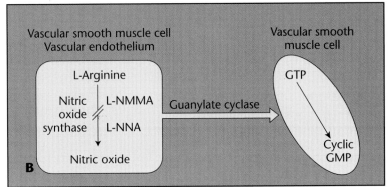

FIGURE 12-59.

A, The most recently proposed vasodilator is nitric oxide or endothelial-derived relaxing factor. It has been suggested that chronic endotoxemia associated with cirrhosis may stimulate synthesis and release of nitric oxide through increased cytokine expression, although several growth factors are also known to stimulate the production of nitric oxide synthase, the enzyme responsible for nitric oxide synthesis. It is likely that shear stress on the endothelium secondary to portal hypertension is the more important factor in the production of nitric oxide. **B,** Nitric oxide released from the endothelium stimulates the enzyme guanylate cyclase in the myocytes, leading to the production of cyclic guanosine monophosphate in the vascular smooth muscle cell. This results in smooth muscle cell relaxation and vasodilatation. Nitric oxide also mediates the vasodilatory effects of acetylcholine and bradykinin. However, recent studies in animal models examining the role of nitric oxide as a vasodilator have yielded conflicting results. Therefore, the role of nitric oxide remains controversial. GMP—guanosine monophosphate; GTP—guanosine triphosphate; L-NMMA—N^G-monomethyl-L-arginine; L-NNA—N^G-nitro-L-arginine. (*Adapted from* Stark and Szurszewski [84].)

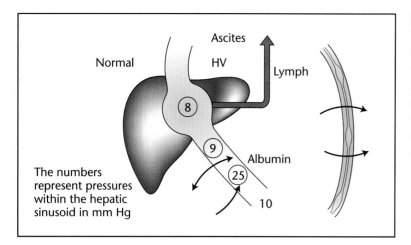

FIGURE 12-60.
The hepatic sinusoidal bed is normally a low pressure venous bed resulting from high presinusoidal resistance in the hepatic arterioles. Sinusoidal hydrostatic pressure is therefore very low. There is minimal pressure gradient from the portal venous end to the hepatic venous end of the sinusoidal bed. Interstitial fluid that escapes from the sinusoids into the hepatic parenchyma is drained away by hepatic lymphatics; very little fluid escapes through the liver capsule into the peritoneal cavity. HV—hepatic vein.

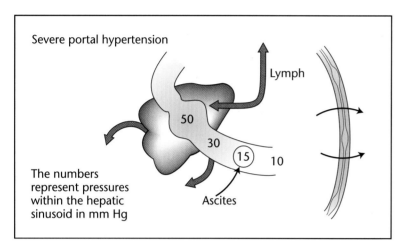

FIGURE 12-61.
When cirrhosis develops, there is a hepatic venous outflow block, leading to sinusoidal portal hypertension. Sinusoidal hydrostatic pressure increases markedly, which favors transudation of fluid into the interstitial space. There remains no oncotic pressure gradient across the sinusoids caused by free passage of albumin through the sinusoidal fenestrae. Regional hepatic lymphatics become tortuous and dilated and increase their drainage capacity as much as 20-fold. Fluid begins to escape through the liver capsule into the peritoneal cavity as ascites. Once sequestered within the peritoneal cavity, ascitic fluid can be reabsorbed by the peritoneal lymphatics at a maximal rate of 900 mL/d. The ascites can also be drained by the subdiaphragmatic peritoneum. When hepatic lymph production exceeds the drainage capacities of the hepatic and peritoneal lymphatics, ascites will accumulate.

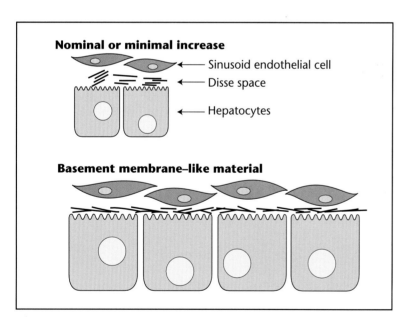

FIGURE 12-62.
In the later stage of cirrhosis the fenestration is lost, and a basement membranelike material that *capillarises* the sinusoid is laid down. This membrane reduces the sinusoidal permeability; an oncotic pressure gradient develops between the hepatic interstitial space and the sinusoidal lumen. In patients with alcoholic cirrhosis, there is a deposition of immunoglobulin A underneath the sinusoidal endothelium, further reducing the sinusoidal permeability. This acts to counterbalance the hydrostatic pressure gradient, thereby decreasing hepatic lymph production. When there is an accumulation of ascitic fluid in the peritoneal cavity, the resultant rise in intra-abdominal pressure is transmitted back to the hepatic parenchyma. This leads to a rise in interstitial pressure, counteracting further fluid loss. At this stage of cirrhosis, however, these compensatory mechanisms are no longer adequate to eliminate ascites. (*Adapted from* Orrego *et al.* [85].)

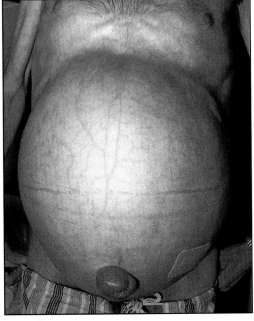

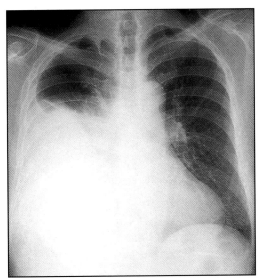

FIGURE 12-64.
Pleural effusion is present in about 6% of patients with ascites and more often it is on the right side. This is the result of a defect in the diaphragm that allows the ascitic fluid to pass up into the pleural cavity. In contrast, a left-sided pleural effusion in an ascitic patient may indicate pulmonary pathology. Occasionally, a pleural effusion can be seen (in the absence of ascites), caused by the negative intrathoracic pressure drawing the ascitic fluid through the diaphragmatic defect and into the pleural cavity. Thoracentesis is followed by rapid refilling of the pleural cavity because of the negative intrathoracic pressure. Control of the pleural effusion can only be achieved with the control of ascites.

FIGURE 12-63.
Increased intra-abdominal pressure favors development of hernias in the umbilicus and inguinal regions and through abdominal incisions. Pressure from the ascites-filled hernial sacs may cause considerable discomfort.

■ PORTAL HYPERTENSION

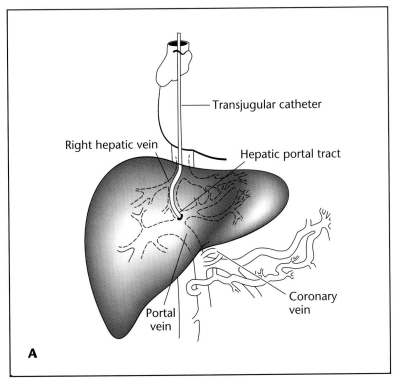

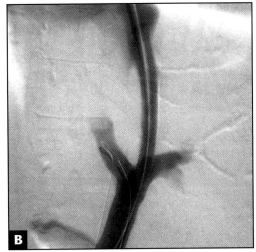

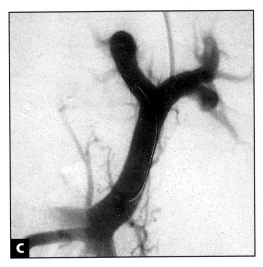

FIGURE 12-65.
A, The right hepatic vein is cannulated using the transjugular approach. Under fluoroscopic guidance, a needle is then passed through the cannula to puncture the liver, aiming at a main branch of the portal vein. Once the needle is in the portal vein, the cannula is advanced over the needle. **B,** Results of a portal venogram confirm that the portal vein has been entered. The cannula is then replaced with an angioplasty balloon. The intrahepatic tract is dilated. **C,** The angioplasty catheter is then replaced with the stent, which is then deployed in the intrahepatic tract. A repeat venogram confirms the patency of the shunt.

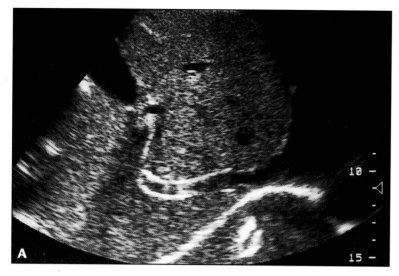

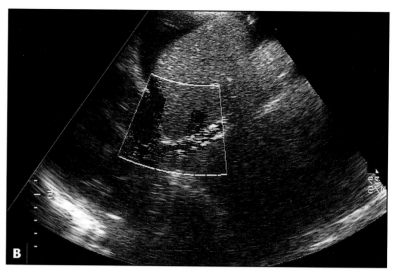

FIGURE 12-66.

Subsequent assessment of shunt patency can be performed using Doppler ultrasound. **A,** The metal shunt appears as a bright echogenic object on ultrasound. **B,** Doppler measurement of shunt flow velocity greater than 100 cm/s confirms shunt patency. Shunt obstruction can be managed by balloon dilatation of the shunt. If this is not successful, a new shunt can be inserted parallel to the original shunt. It is recommended that shunt patency assessment be performed immediately after insertion, at 1 month, and thereafter every 3 months.

■ SPONTANEOUS BACTERIAL PERITONITIS

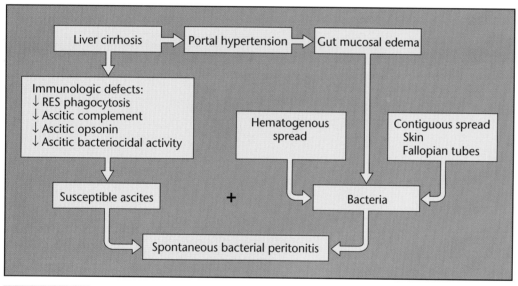

FIGURE 12-67.

Recent publications suggest that spontaneous bacterial peritonitis is the result of translocation of bacteria across the gastrointestinal epithelium into the lymphatics and then into the peritoneal cavity with seeding of susceptible ascites. Intestinal hypomotility appears to favor bacterial overgrowth and bacterial translocation [86]. Decompensated and especially jaundiced cirrhotic patients have impaired reticuloendothelial function with reduced phagocytic activity, low ascitic fluid protein concentration, and low ascitic opsonin activity, all of which predispose the patient to spontaneous infection within the ascites. RES—reticuloendothelial system.

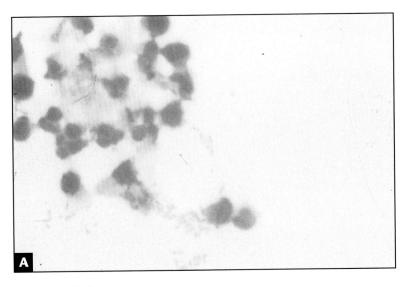

FIGURE 12-68.

A, Gram stains of ascitic fluid are only positive in 10% to 50% of infected patients. **B**, Cultures may take up to 48 hours to become positive. The percentage of possibility is maximized by injection of 10 mL of ascitic fluid directly into blood culture bottles at the bedside.

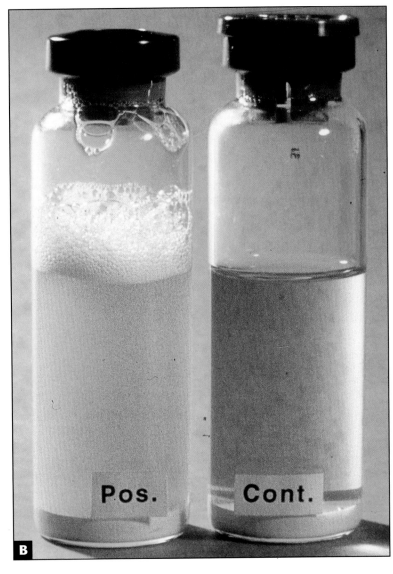

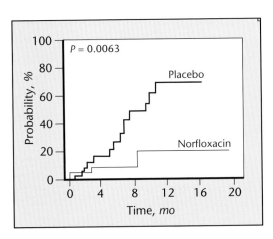

FIGURE 12-69.

Various therapeutic modalities have been tried to reduce the risk of recurrence. Diuretic therapy has been shown to increase ascitic protein content and opsonin activity but not to influence outcome. Selective intestinal decontamination to eliminate aerobic gram-negative bacilli with oral nonabsorbable antibiotics has proved to be effective in reducing the recurrence of spontaneous bacterial peritonitis. Norfloxacin (400 mg/d) has been shown to be significantly better than placebo to reduce the incidence of recurrence of spontaneous bacterial peritonitis. It is the drug of choice because it has the advantages of rarely causing bacterial resistance and of having a low incidence of side effects when administered long term. (*Adapted from* Gines *et al.* [87].)

■ BLEEDING VARICES AND HEPATIC ENCEPHALOPATHY

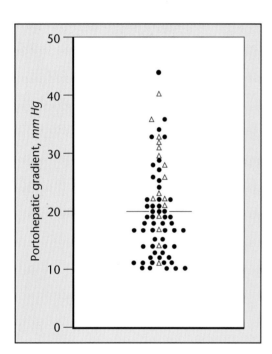

FIGURE 12-70.

Active hemorrhage from an esophageal varix. Pressure within esophageal varices averages almost 30 mm Hg in cirrhotic patients. Coughing, straining, defecation, or lifting may increase variceal pressure to arterial pressure levels. Indeed, bleeding at such high pressures may give rise to arterial jets, as shown in this remarkable endoscopic photograph. Needless to say, large volumes of blood can quickly be lost from such lesions. (*Courtesy of* N. Currey.)

FIGURE 12-71.

Portal venous pressure in patients who bled from esophageal varices. The hepatic vein pressure gradient (HVPG), *ie*, the wedged or occluded hepatic venous pressure minus the free hepatic venous pressure, is the *corrected* portal venous pressure. Patients who bled from esophageal varices invariably have a HVPG greater than 12 mm Hg. The pressure tends to be highest at the moment of hemorrhage and to decrease thereafter. This decrement is expected in alcoholic cirrhosis, in which hepatic fatty deposition and inflammation decrease during abstinence after admission to the hospital. Indeed, the HVPG was significantly lower among the 56 patients who survived more than 2 weeks after variceal hemorrhage (mean 26 mm Hg; *closed circles*) than in the 16 patients who died within the first 2 weeks (mean 20 mm Hg; *open triangles*) [88]. The failure to establish a relationship between the height of the HVPG and the risks of variceal hemorrhage and death could represent in part, at best, an artifact of retrospective analysis [89], *ie*, patients with the higher portal venous pressure levels may die before they survive long enough to have their portal venous pressure measured. (*Adapted from* Vinel *et al.* [88].)

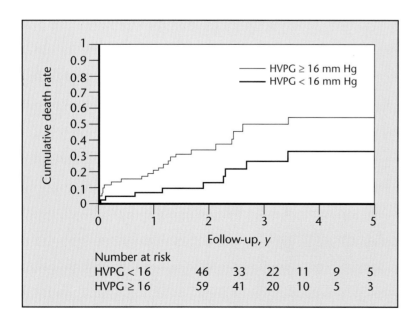

FIGURE 12-72.

Cumulative death rate in relation to free hepatic venous pressure gradient (HVPG). Ideally, a single, accurate prognostic portal venous pressure measurement is all that is needed to make pertinent clinical decisions in patients after hemorrhage from varices. The HVPG appeared to be such an indicator of survival in a heterogenous group of 105 alcoholic and nonalcoholic cirrhotic patients when measured after stabilization within 11 days of variceal bleeding. Patch *et al.* [90] found that the cumulative mortality rate was significantly higher in patients whose HVPG was ≥ 16 mm Hg than in those whose HVPG was < 16 mm Hg. These data confirm the belief that the portal pressure level probably peaks at the time of hemorrhage and decreases thereafter.

Furthermore, those patients whose HVPG decreased by > 15% had a better prognosis than those whose pressure gradient decreased to a lesser degree. The reduction in pressure is multifactorial and is induced by the mobilization of fat and a decrease in inflammation in the liver. Although such indices, when based on heterogenous factors may not be invariably correct, this indicator is compatible with previous studies of portal venous pressure [90].

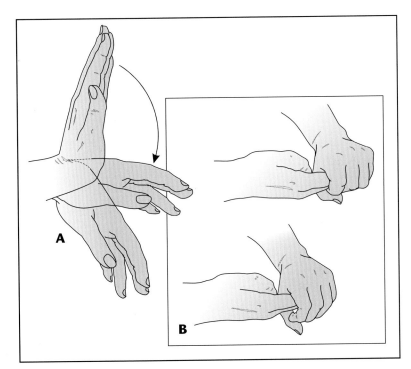

FIGURE 12-73.

Assessing asterixis: two techniques. Asterixis is a nonspecific neurologic sign that appears to result, at least in part, from dysfunction of the descending reticular system [91]. It may be seen in almost all types of metabolic encephalopathy of both hepatic and nonhepatic origin. **A**, It is defined as a defect of movement that is characterized by an inability to sustain a fixed posture such as holding one's hand in a dorsiflexed position at the wrist. Within 30 seconds, repetitive, irregular, involuntary movements of the hand occur. They appear to be flapping motions, hence its colloquial name *the flapping tremor*. Both the active and opposing muscles are activated. When asterixis is present, transient interruptions in electrical current, which last from 50 to 100 msec, occur. When the current is cut off, the hand falls forward by force of gravity; when the current returns, the position is resumed. Similar abnormalities can be induced in experimental animals by infusion of ammonium salts [92]. **B**, It can be tested for by having the patient squeeze two of the examiner's fingers. When asterixis is present, intermittent relaxation of the squeezing fingers can be felt by the examiner, whose fingers are being squeezed within 30 seconds. (**A**, *adapted from* Leavitt and Tyler [91]; **B**, *adapted from* Conn and Lieberthal [92].)

■ VASCULAR DISEASES, ABSCESSES, AND CYSTS

ISCHEMIC HEPATITIS

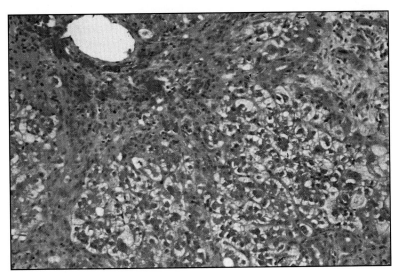

FIGURE 12-74.

Ischemic hepatitis. Transient decreases in arterial flow to the liver may result in ischemic necrosis of the centrilobular perivenular zone of the liver (zone 3). In some patients, even a brief episode of hypotension is sufficient to cause ischemic injury. Patients with severe left or right heart failure are at highest risk. Ischemia may also occur during or following cardiac bypass. Prognosis in these patients is poor because of the underlying cardiopulmonary disease and not from the liver injury itself [93]. Apoptosis appears to be a response to acute ischemia, while atrophy and nodular hyperplasia occur when the ischemia becomes chronic [94].

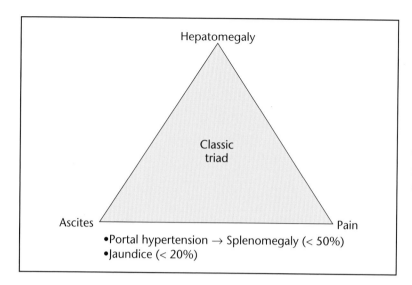

FIGURE 12-75.
Clinical manifestations of Budd-Chiari syndrome. The classic triad of abdominal pain, hepatomegaly, and ascites is present in the majority of patients with Budd-Chiari syndrome. Of these, pain is the least constant finding. Jaundice is rare, occurring in less than 20% of patients, and is an ominous sign. Splenomegaly is found in almost 50%. In some instances, splenomegaly is a consequence of an underlying hematologic disorder, such as polycythemia rubra vera, whereas in others it results from portal hypertension. The remaining clinical signs are those associated with portal hypertension per se.

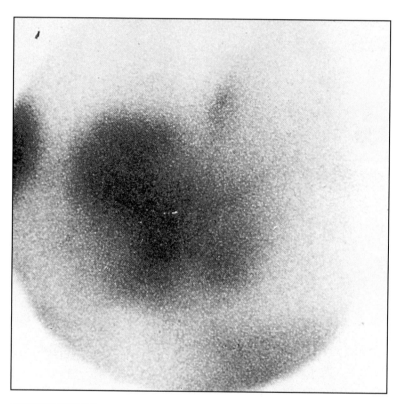

FIGURE 12-76.
Use of liver scintiscan for diagnosis of Budd-Chiari syndrome. [99]Technetium liver spleen scans often provide clues for making a positive diagnosis of Budd-Chiari syndrome. There is usually decreased uptake of tracer in the right and left lobes of the liver, corresponding to occlusion of the right, middle, and left hepatic veins. By contrast, the caudate lobe, which has a separate venous drainage, is often hypertrophied and has increased tracer uptake.

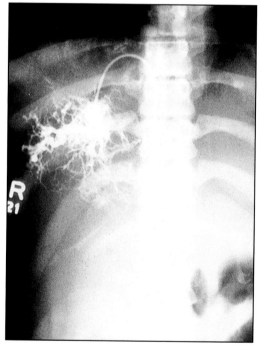

FIGURE 12-77.
The spider web pattern illustrates collateral flow from the small hepatic veins directly into the systemic circulation. Although seen infrequently, the spider web pattern of hepatic venography is almost definitely diagnostic of Budd-Chiari syndrome. This pattern is speculated to result from the formation of collateral anastomoses between the small hepatic veins and the systemic circulation, which occurs when the obstruction to venous outflow has existed for a prolonged period. (Courtesy of K. R. Reddy.)

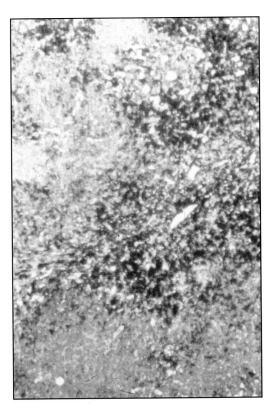

FIGURE 12-78.

Liver biopsy is often needed to establish duration of Budd-Chiari syndrome and to exclude the existence of cirrhosis before making decisions about therapy. Acute obstruction of the hepatic veins leads to severe sinusoidal dilatation often associated with congestion and necrosis of hepatocytes in zone 3. These hepatocytes are replaced by erythrocytes within the space of Disse. The periportal zone is affected much less than the centrilobular perivenular zone.

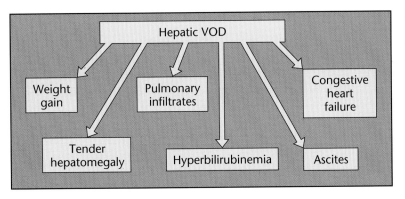

FIGURE 12-79.

Clinical manifestations of hepatic veno-occlusive disease (VOD). The syndrome of VOD involves multiple organs including the liver. Typically, patients experience rapid weight gain, tender hepatomegaly, and early development of ascites. Pulmonary infiltrates and clinical signs of congestive heart failure are observed in the most severe cases; severe jaundice is a poor prognostic sign. Transjugular intrahepatic portosystemic shunts have been used with limited success [95].

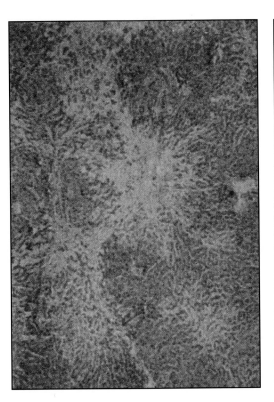 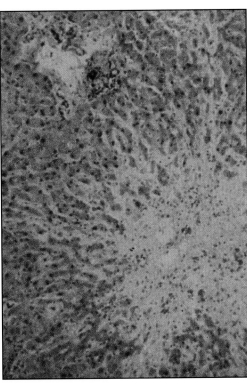

FIGURE 12-80.

Histologic manifestations of hepatic veno-occlusive disease. In the early stages, endotheliitis associated with proliferative changes is present. Progressively, there is more fibrotic reaction in the endothelial space, eventually leading to obliteration of the terminal hepatic venules. The portal areas are spared. Sinusoids are dilated; often atrophy of hepatocytes in the surrounding perivenular zone exists [96]. (*Courtesy of* K. R. Reddy.)

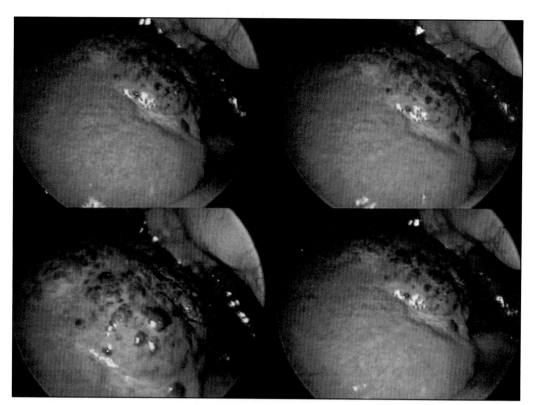

FIGURE 12-81.

Hepatic cavernous hemangioma. This tumor is the most common benign mesenchymal tumor, found in 3% to 5% of all autopsies. Hemangiomas are usually single and small, but multiple hemangiomas occur in about 10% of cases [97]. They are usually millimetric, but may reach up to 20 cm in size. In very rare cases, over a period of time, hemangiomas may increase in size [98]. The majority of patients are asymptomatic and have normal liver chemistries. Large lesions (larger than 4 cm) may cause symptoms such as a sensation of a mass and abdominal pain. (*Courtesy of* K. R. Reddy.)

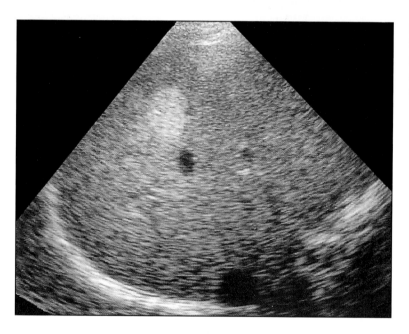

FIGURE 12-82.

Ultrasound in the diagnosis of hepatic hemangiomas. On imaging with ultrasound, hemangiomas appear as single echogenic lesions with well-defined borders. Posterior acoustic enhancement is characteristic.

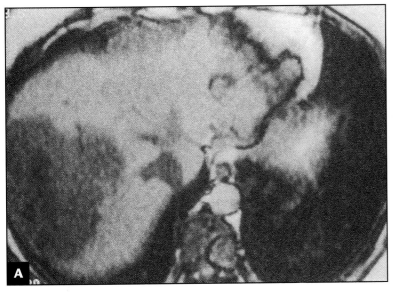

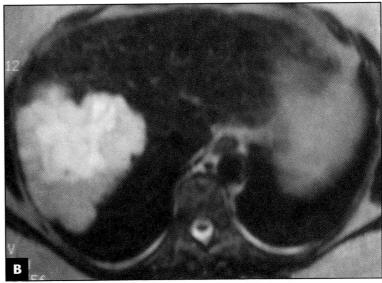

FIGURE 12-83.

Magnetic resonance imaging is very useful in characterizing hemangiomas, especially those measuring less than 5 cm. On magnetic resonance imaging, hemangiomas appear as well-circumscribed homogeneous lesions with low signal intensity in T_1-weighted images (**A**) and a characteristic high intensity in T_2-weighted images (**B**), which distinguishes them from other neoplasms [99].

HEPATIC CYSTS

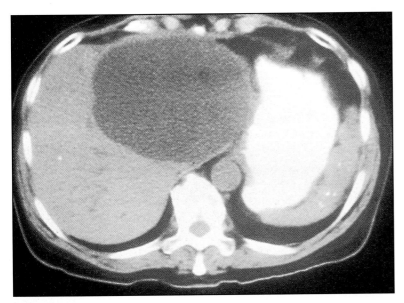

FIGURE 12-84.

Simple hepatic cyst. Simple hepatic cysts are the most common cystic lesions of the liver. They are usually small and asymptomatic, whereas large cysts may produce symptoms. Intrahepatic cysts are seen on CT scans as a low-attenuation space-filling lesion. The attenuation coefficient is usually similar to water and always lower than blood. They do not fill with administration of IV contrast dye. Large cysts may be excised surgically although percutaneous ultrasound-guided drainage followed by tetracycline chloride infusion has been used with success [100].

AMEBIC ABSCESSES

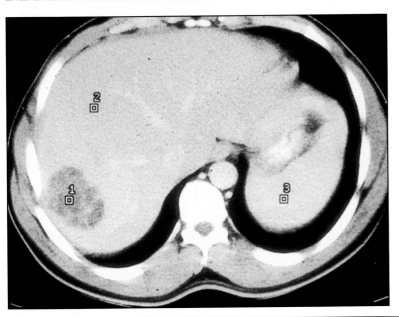

FIGURE 12-85.

Amebic abscesses are the most common type of liver abscesses worldwide. They are more frequently localized in the right lobe superoanteriorly, near the diaphragm. They are usually single, but may also be multiple and involve both lobes. Computed tomographic scan is very sensitive in the detection of amebic abscesses. It is also very useful in detecting extrahepatic involvement such as in the pleural space or lung. Amebic abscesses appear as a hypodense round or oval lesions with irregular borders. Abscesses can virtually always be treated medically with metronidazole or chloroquine. Indications for percutaneous drainage include superinfection by bacteria and impending pleural or pericardial involvement [101]. Both ultrasound and computed tomographic scan may be used when drainage is indicated and as follow-up after institution of medical therapy.

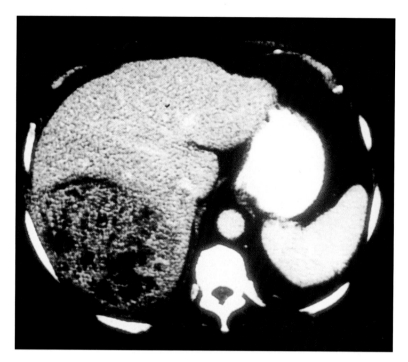

FIGURE 12-86.

Computed tomographic scan is highly sensitive in the localization of pyogenic liver abscesses. These lesions are hypodense areas that may sometimes show an air-fluid level indicating a gas-producing organism. Both computed tomography and ultrasound may be used in the aspiration of pyogenic abscesses, which can be done for both diagnostic and therapeutic purposes. It appears that catheter drainage may be more effective than needle aspiration [102].

■ TUMORS OF THE LIVER

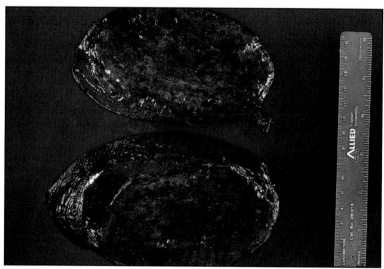

FIGURE 12-87.

Cut surface of a large hepatocellular adenoma. Hepatocellular adenoma is a benign neoplastic condition of hepatocytes. Although relatively rare, its incidence seems to have increased over the past few decades since the introduction and widespread use of oral contraceptives (incidence 3 to 4/100,000 long-term oral contraceptive users) [103]. It has also been associated with the use of anabolic steroids and is a complication of some types of glycogen storage disease. This tumor occurs almost exclusively in adult women. Most female patients with adenoma have a history of oral contraceptive use, either current or remote. The duration of oral contraceptive use in such patients is variable and may even have been as short as 1 to 2 years. The most common presenting symptom is right upper quadrant abdominal pain or discomfort. The most feared complication of hepatocellular adenoma is free intra-abdominal rupture related to hemorrhage and necrosis within the tumor. This complication may be life threatening and requires urgent resuscitation and surgery. Liver biopsy is almost always required for confirmation of the diagnosis of adenoma. If this diagnosis is suspected in advance, biopsy may be best done at the time of surgical resection.

The histologic appearance of hepatocellular adenoma is of benign-looking hepatocytes often arranged in cords. Evidence of bile production may be noted. Surgical resection is usually recommended because of the risks of rupture. Possible exceptions to this recommendation are very small adenomata or in those where the patient is not fit for surgery. Shrinkage of these tumors has been noted in some cases with discontinuation of oral contraceptive use; although this maneuver may be attempted in some cases, it should not replace the need for resection in most instances. (*Courtesy of* E. Brunt.)

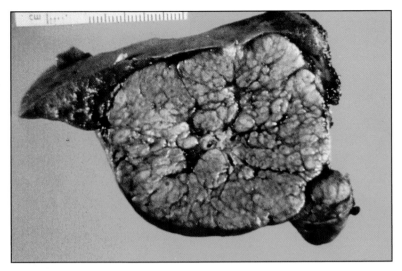

FIGURE 12-88.

A heterogenous group of lesions occurring in the liver may give a neoplastic appearance. Some of them may also cause diagnostic confusion with cirrhosis. This figure shows the cut surface of a focal nodular hyperplasia (FNH), approximately 5 to 6 cm in diameter. Note the cirrhosis-like appearance (pseudocirrhosis) around a central area of fibrous tissue. This lesion represents a focal benign proliferation of hepatocytes occurring around an abnormal artery within the liver [104]. These lesions rarely cause symptoms and are most often found incidentally at the time of abdominal surgery (often at cholecystectomy). They are usually smaller than 5 cm in diameter. The cut surface typically shows a central stellate scar that contains the abnormal artery within it. As with hepatocellular adenoma, features of bile production and cholestasis may be seen both macroscopically and microscopically. The presence of central scar tissue may sometimes give the appearance of cirrhosis with regenerating nodules surrounded by fibrosis. This lesion is localized, however, rather than being throughout the liver and no bile ducts are seen within the lesions, whereas they would be present in most cases of cirrhosis. Interpretation of needle biopsy specimens obtained from FNH may be particularly difficult. Usually no treatment is required because these lesions rarely cause symptoms and are not prone to rupture or malignant transformation. In fact, they are very often removed at the time of excision biopsy. The differential diagnosis includes nodular regenerative hyperplasia, which is a diffuse nodular condition of the liver with no significant fibrosis and partial nodular transformation, a rare nodular condition usually confined to the hilar area of the liver.

Lesion		Size	Single/ Multiple	Common Underlying Causes	Comment
Nodular regenerative hyperplasia		Usually <1 cm	Multiple	Immunologic disorders (*eg*, rheumatoid arthritis) Myeloproliferative disorders	Pathogenesis related to portal venopathy and decreased blood flow; usually presents with portal hypertension
Focal nodular hyperplasia		Usually <5 cm	Single	None recognized	Often an incidental finding
Hepatocellular adenoma		May be very large	Usually single; occasionally multiple	Estrogen use	Requires resection because of risk of rupture or hemorrhage
Hepatocellular carcinoma		May be very large	Often multiple	Cirrhosis Chronic viral hepatitis	Probably arises from within dysplastic nodules
Partial nodular transformation		1–5 cm	Multiple but localized to perihilar area	None recognized	Rare entity; presents with portal hypertension

FIGURE 12-89.

Nodular diseases of the liver.

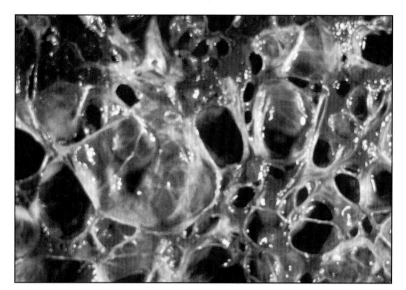

FIGURE 12-90.

Macroscopic appearance of polycystic disease of the liver. Note the presence of innumerable cysts, some filled with clear fluid. Small amounts of normal hepatic parenchyma are noted between cysts. Adult polycystic disease is an autosomally dominant inherited disease associated with multiple cysts within the liver, pancreas, and spleen. Hepatic cysts are sometimes associated with abdominal discomfort. Rarely, they may be complicated by infection [105]. Hepatocellular function is rarely compromised. No specific treatment is available. Liver transplantation has occasionally been performed for polycystic disease because of the patient's intolerable abdominal discomfort.

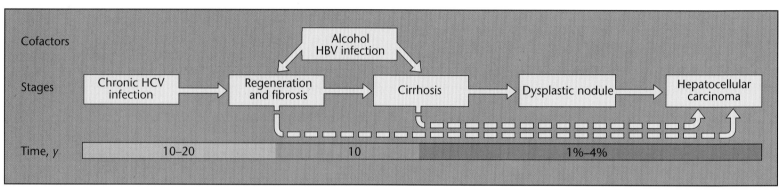

FIGURE 12-91.

Pathogenesis of hepatitis C virus (HCV)-related hepatocellular carcinoma (HCC). This figure illustrates the stepwise progression in liver disease associated with the chronic HCV infection leading to the development of HCC. *Dashed lines* show possible or unusual pathways. HBV—hepatitis B virus.

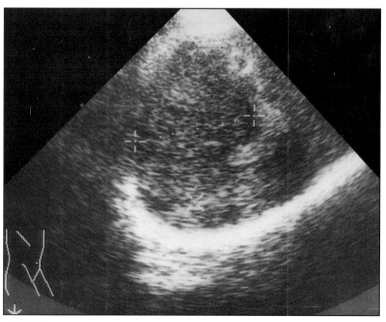

FIGURE 12-92.

Ultrasound examination of the liver showing a 5 x 10 cm hypoechoic mass (between markers). Ultrasound is one of the most sensitive methods for detecting tumors within the liver and is also relatively inexpensive and noninvasive [106]. Hepatocellular carcinoma often has echogenicity different from that in the remainder of the liver. Thus, small tumors are often hyperechoic with a thin hypoechoic rim. With time, and as the tumor grows, the whole tumor often becomes hypoechoic, and finally, when the tumor is large, it often has mixed echogenicity.

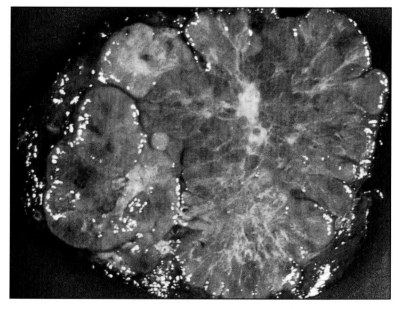

FIGURE 12-93.

Characteristic fibrotic lamellae coursing throughout a fibrolamellar hepatocellular carcinoma (HCC). This tumor is a variant with distinct morphologic features and is also associated with a better prognosis than other forms of HCC [107]. Thus, the surrounding nontumorous liver is usually not cirrhotic. (*Courtesy of* Z. Goodman.)

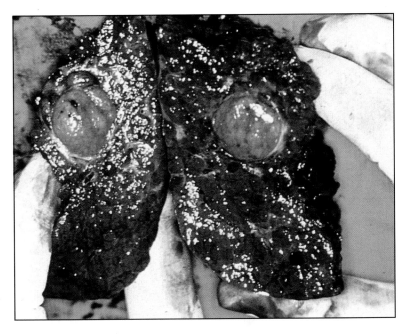

FIGURE 12-94.

Resected specimen of cirrhotic liver with a small (2.5 cm diameter) hepatocellular carcinoma (HCC). Therapy of HCC is difficult and the prognosis is poor. The best chance of cure or long-term

survival appears to be with resection. Because of the associated cirrhosis, extensive resection is usually not possible and the usual operation is a "segmentectomy" or enucleation of the tumor. Even so, a high rate of tumor recurrence exists within the first few years after surgery. Liver transplantation appears to be a suitable modality of therapy for HCC less than 5 cm in diameter with no evidence of extrahepatic spread [128]. Again, there is a high rate of recurrence (although less than resection) and attempts to prevent this complication have used adjuvant chemotherapy before and after transplantation. The value of this approach is currently being evaluated.

Other approaches that may be used for small tumors include ablation by injection with absolute alcohol or cryoablation. For large unresectable tumors, chemoembolization has been used in an attempt to shrink the tumor. The rationale for this approach is based on the fact that, whereas the liver as a whole has a dual blood supply (from the hepatic artery and portal vein), HCC derives its supply exclusively from the hepatic artery. Thus, when this blood supply is cut off, tumor necrosis and shrinking can be seen. The use of systemic chemotherapy and external radiation appear to be of little benefit in HCC. Chemotherapy directed to the tumor by intra-arterial infusion of targeting with Lipiodol (Therapex, Montreal, Quebec, Canada) may be more helpful. (*From* Di Bisceglie [109]; with permission.)

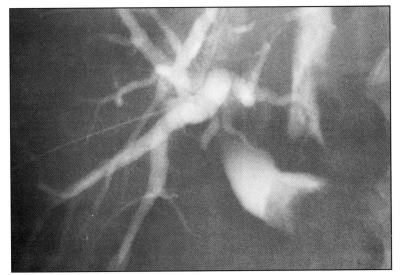

FIGURE 12-95.

Endoscopic retrograde cholangiopancreatography (ERCP) scan from a patient with long-standing primary sclerosing cholangitis (PSC) and cholangiocarcinoma. Note the convex upwards obstruction at the lower end of the common bile duct and the changes of PSC in the peripheral branches of the biliary tree. Such tumors may be very difficult to detect. Their presence may be signaled by sudden worsening in jaundice in a patient with PSC or may be found incidentally at the time of diagnostic ERCP or liver transplantation for PSC.

■ LIVER TRANSPLANTATION

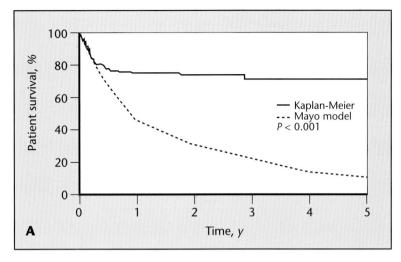

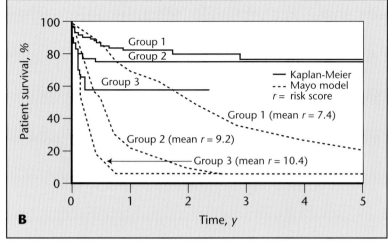

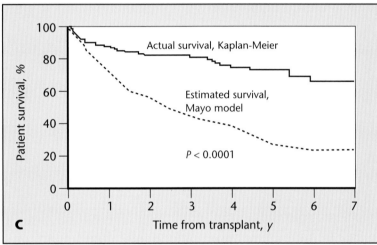

FIGURE 12-96.

A–C, To optimize the timing of transplantation, a clear understanding of the natural history of the disease is needed. The use of standard listing criteria has largely supplanted the ability to time transplantation for the individual patient. For primary biliary cirrhosis (PBC) and primary sclerosing cholangitis (PSC), the Mayo models make it possible to calculate the probability of survival at differing time points based on certain clinical features. However, the Mayo models appear to be no better than the Childs-Pugh score for evaluating cholestatic liver disease. Nonetheless, Wiesner *et al.* [110] performed Kaplan-Meier analyses of survival with and without transplantation in 161 patients with PBC (*panel A*) and 216 patients with PSC (*panel C*) who underwent orthotopic liver transplantation (OLT) at the Mayo Clinic. Overall, long-term survival improved for both diseases with transplantation. In addition, patients in the low and moderate risk groups (groups 1 and 2 in *panel B*) derived the largest survival benefit. This fact provides evidence that performing transplantation earlier in the disease has a more profound impact on long-term patient survival. In addition, Wiesner *et al.* [110] showed that OLT in low and moderate risk patients was less costly. These data were recently confirmed by a study from the National Institute of Diabetes and Digestive and Kidney Diseases Liver Transplantation Database. In this study, the factor that contributed the greatest variance in the cost of OLT was the degree of liver dysfunction as indicated by the Childs-Pugh score [111]. Increased use of live donors could allow more accurate timing of OLT and also may lower the costs associated with OLT. (**A** and **B**, *adapted from* Markus *et al.* [112]; **C**, *adapted from* Wiesner *et al.* [110].)

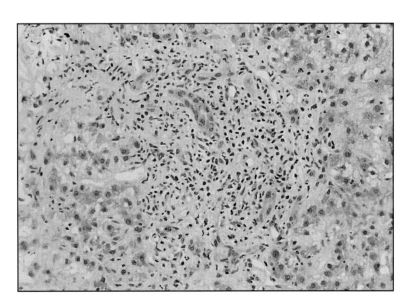

FIGURE 12-97.

One of the most difficult postorthotopic liver transplantation (post-OLT) problems is to differentiate between acute cellular rejection and post-OLT hepatitis C on liver biopsy. This figure shows a post-OLT biopsy from a patient transplanted for hepatitis C virus (HCV) cirrhosis. The patient developed a histologic picture of both acute cellular rejection and recurrent hepatitis C after transplantation. Her liver dysfunction progressed despite intensive treatment of the rejection and resulted in graft loss. In this histologic section, the prominent bile duct damage and mixed cell (*ie*, eosinophils) infiltrate suggest rejection, whereas the piecemeal necrosis and acidophil bodies suggest hepatitis C. None of these findings taken alone is specific for either diagnosis. All patients with pre-OLT HCV infection will be HCV-RNA positive post-OLT [115]. However, not all HCV-RNA–positive patients will have histologic hepatitis. In the past, if rejection and hepatitis coexisted on biopsy, many thought it was reasonable, in difficult to distinguish cases, to treat the rejection. However, a number of studies have suggested that one of the most important predictors of outcome in this patient population is the number of treated rejection episodes. Thus, treating a mild component of rejection in this group may not benefit the patient.

■ REFERENCES

1. Bloomer JR: Jaundice—why it happens—what to do. *Med Times* 1979, 107:43–52.

2. Black M, Sherlock S: Treatment of Gilbert's syndrome with phenobarbitone. *Lancet* 1970, 1:1359–1362.

3. Brown EA, Ticehurst J, Lemon SM: Immunopathogenesis of hepatitis A and E virus infections. In *Immunology of Liver Disease.* Edited by Thomas HC, Waters J. Dordrecht: Kluwer Academic Publishers; 1994:11–37.

4. Lemon SM, Stapleton JT: Prevention. In *Viral Hepatitis.* Edited by Zuckerman AJ, Thomas HC. Edinburgh: Churchill Livingstone; 1993:61–79.

5. Winokur PL, Stapleton JT: Immunoglobulin prophylaxis for hepatitis A. *Clin Infect Dis* 1992, 14:580–586.

6. Innis BL, Snitbhan R, Kunasol P, *et al.*: Protection against hepatitis A by an inactivated vaccine. *JAMA* 1994, 271:1328–1334.

7. Gerlich W: Structure and molecular virology. In *Viral Hepatitis.* Edited by Zuckerman AJ, Thomas HC. Edinburgh: Churchill Livingstone; 1993:83–113.

8. Chen D-S: Natural history of chronic hepatitis B virus infection: New light on an old story. *J Gastroenterol Hepatol* 1993, 8:470–475.

9. Hamilton J, Gross N: The huge bounty on a global killer. *Business Week* April 4, 1994:92–94.

10. Scheiermann N, Gesemann M, Maurer C, *et al.*: Persistence of antibodies after immunization with a recombinant yeast-derived hepatitis B vaccine following two different schedules. *Vaccine* 1990, 8(suppl):S44.

11. Conjeevaram HS, Di Bisceglie AM: Natural history. In *Viral Hepatitis.* Edited by Zuckerman AJ, Thomas HC. New York: Churchill Livingstone, 1993:341–349.

12. Esumi M, Shikata T: Hepatitis C virus and liver disease. *Pathology International* 1994, 44:85–95.

13. Alter MJ, Moyer LA: The importance of preventing hepatitis C virus infection among injection drug users in the United States. *J Acquir Immune Defic Syndr Hum Retrovirol* 1998, 18(suppl 1):S6–S10.

14. Tanaka H, Hiyama T, Tsukuma H, *et al.*: Cumulative risk of hepatocellular carcinoma in hepatitis C virus carriers: Statistical estimations from cross-sectional data. *Jpn J Cancer Res* 1994, 85:485–490.

15. Johnson PJ, McFarlane IG, Alvarez F, *et al.*: Meeting report. International autoimmune hepatitis group. *Hepatology* 1993, 18:998–1005.

16. Czaja AJ: Chronic active hepatitis: The challenge of a new nomenclature. *Ann Intern Med* 1993, 119:510–517.

17. Czaja AJ: Autoimmune hepatitis: Current therapeutic concepts. *Clin Immunother* 1994, 1:413–429.

18. Czaja AJ, Manns MP, Homburger HA: Frequency and significance of antibodies to liver–kidney microsome type 1 in adults with chronic active hepatitis. *Gastroenterology* 1992, 103:1290–1295.

19. Czaja AJ, Carpenter HA, Manns MP: Antibodies to soluble liver antigen, P450IID6, and mitochondrial complexes in chronic hepatitis. *Gastroenterology* 1993, 105:1522–1528.

20. Stechemesser E, Klein R, Berg PA: Characterization and clinical relevance of liver–pancreas antibodies in autoimmune hepatitis. *Hepatology* 1993, 18:1–9.

21. Czaja AJ, Carpenter HA: Sensitivity, specificity and predictability of biopsy interpretations in chronic hepatitis. *Gastroenterology* 1993, 105:1824–1832.

22. Frazer IH, Mackay IR, Bell J, Becker G: The cellular infiltrate in the liver in auto-immune chronic active hepatitis: Analysis with monoclonal antibodies. *Liver* 1985, 5:162–172.

23. Hashimoto E, Lindor KD, Homburger HA, *et al.*: Immunohistochemical characterization of hepatic lymphocytes in primary biliary cirrhosis in comparison with primary sclerosing cholangitis and autoimmune chronic active hepatitis. *Mayo Clin Proc* 1993, 68:1049–1055.

24. Czaja AJ, Carpenter HA: Histological findings in chronic hepatitis C with autoimmune features. *Hepatology* 1997, 26:459–466.

25. Czaja AJ: Diagnosis, prognosis, and treatment of classical autoimmune chronic active hepatitis. In *Autoimmune Liver Diseases.* Edited by Krawitt EL, Wiesner RH. New York: Raven Press; 1991:143–166.

26. Czaja AJ, Rakela J, Ludwig J: Features reflective of early prognosis in corticosteroid-treated severe autoimmune chronic active hepatitis. *Gastroenterology* 1988, 95:448–453.

27. Krawitt EL, Kilby AE, Albertini RJ, *et al.*: An immunogenetic study of suppressor cell activity in autoimmune chronic active hepatitis. *Clin Immunol Immunopathol* 1988, 46:249–257.

28. Czaja AJ: Autoimmune hepatitis; evolving concepts and treatment strategies. *Dig Dis Sci* 1995, 40:435–456.

29. Czaja AJ, Davis GL, Ludwig J, *et al.*: Autoimmune features as determinants of prognosis in steroid-treated chronic active hepatitis of uncertain etiology. *Gastroenterology* 1983, 85:713–717.

30. Czaja AJ, Davis GL, Ludwig J, Taswell HF: Complete resolution of inflammatory activity following corticosteroid treatment of HBsAg-negative chronic active hepatitis. *Hepatology* 1984, 4:622–627.

31. Koff RS: Viral hepatitis. In *Diseases of the Liver.* Edited by Schiff L, Schiff ER. Philadelphia: JB Lippincott Company, 1993: 492–577.

32. Seeff LB, Koff RS: Evolving concepts of the clinical and serologic consequences of hepatitis B infection. *Semin Liver Dis* 1986, 6:11–22.

33. Hoofnagle JH, Schafer DF: Serologic markers of hepatitis B virus infection. *Semin Liver Dis* 1986, 6:1–10.

34. Dienstag JL, Perrillo RP, Schiff ER, *et al.*: A preliminary trial of lamivudine for chronic hepatitis B infection. *N Engl J Med* 1995, 333:1657–1661.

35. Lai CL, Chien RN, Leung NWY, *et al.*: A one-year trial of lamivudine for chronic hepatitis B. Asia Hepatitis Lamivudine Study Group. *N Engl J Med* 1998, 339:61–68.

36. Nevens F, Main J, Honkoop P, *et al.*: Lamivudine therapy for chronic hepatitis B: a six-month randomized dose-ranging study. *Gastroenterology* 1997, 113:1258–1263.

37. Honkoop P, DeMan RA, Zondervan PE, *et al.*: Histological improvement in patients with chronic hepatitis B virus infection treated with lamivudine. *Liver* 1997, 17:103–106.

38. Liaw YF, Lai CL, Leung NWY, *et al.*: Two-year lamivudine therapy in chronic hepatitis B infection. Results of a placebo controlled multicenter study in Asia. *Gastroenterol* 1998, 114:A1289.

39. Dienstag J, Schiff E, Wright T, *et al.*: Lamivudine treatment for one year in previously untreated U.S. hepatitis B patients: histologic improvement and hepatitis BE-antigen (HBeAg) seroconversion. *Gastroenterology* 1998, 114:A1235.

40. Leung NWY, Lai CL, Chang TT, *et al.*: Three-year lamivudine therapy in chronic HBV. *J Hepatol* 1999, 30:59S.

41. Ben-Ari Z, Zemel R, Kazetsker A, *et al.*: Efficacy of lamivudine in patients with hepatitis B virus precore mutant infection before and after liver transplantation. *Am J Gastro* 1999, 94:663–667.

42. Perrillo R, Rakela J, Dienstag J, *et al.*: Multicenter study of lamivudine therapy for hepatitis B after liver transplantation. *Hepatology* 1999, 29:1581–1586.

43. Tassopoulos NC, Volpes R, Pastore G, *et al.*: Efficacy of lamivudine in patients with hepatitis Be antigen-negative/hepatitis B virus DNA-positive (precore mutant) chronic hepatitis B. *Hepatology* 1999, 29:889–896.

44. Leung N, Wu PC, Tsang S, *et al.*: Continued histological improvement in Chinese patients with chronic hepatitis B with 2 years lamivudine. *Hepatology* 1998, 29:489A.

45. Schiff E, Cianciara J, Kowdley K, *et al.*: Durability of HBeAg seroconversion after lamivudine monotherapy in controlled phase II and III trials. *Hepatology* 1998, 28:163A.

46. Tassopoulos NC, Volpes R, Pastore G, *et al.*: Post lamivudine treatment follow up of patients with HBeAg negative chronic hepatitis B. *J Hepatol* 1999, 30:117A.

47. Zeuzen S, deMan RA, Honkoop P, *et al.*: Dynamics of hepatitis B virus infection in vivo. *J Hepatol* 1997, 27:431–436.

48. Bartholomew MM, Jansen RW, Jeffers LJ, *et al.*: Hepatitis B virus resistance to lamivudine given for recurrent infection after orthotopic liver transplantation. *Lancet* 1997, 349:2–22.

49. Chayama K, Suzuki Y, Kobayashi M, *et al.*: Emergence and takeover of YMDD motif mutant hepatitis B virus during long-term lamivudine therapy and re-takeover by wild type after cessation of therapy. *Hepatology* 1998, 27:1711–1716.

50. Atkins M, Hunt CM, Brown N, *et al.*: Clinical significance of YMDD mutant hepatitis B virus (HBV) in a large cohort of lamivudine-treated hepatitis B patients. *Hepatology* 1998, 28:319A.

51. Heathcote J, Schalin SW, Cianciara J, *et al.*: Lamivudine and intron A combination treatment in patients with chronic hepatitis B infection. *J Hepatol* 1998, 29:43A.

52. Schiff E, Karayalcin S, Grimm I, *et al.*: A placebo controlled study of lamivudine and interferon alpha 2b in patients with chronic hepatitis B who previously failed interferon therapy. *Hepatology* 1998, 28:388A.

53. Shaw T, Locarnini SA: Preclinical aspects of lamivudine and famciclovir against hepatitis B virus. *J Viral Hepatitis* 1999, 6:89–106.

54. Wiley TE, McCarthy M, Breidi L, *et al.*: Impact of alcohol on the histological and clinical progression of hepatitis C infection. *Hepatology* 1998, 28:805–809.

55. Kanazawa Y, Hayashi N, Mita E, *et al.*: Influence of viral quasispecies on effectiveness of interferon therapy in chronic hepatitis C patients. *Hepatology* 1994, 20:1121–1130.

56. McOmish F, Yap PL, Dow BC, *et al.*: Geographic distribution of hepatitis C virus genotypes in blood donors: an international collaborative study. *J Clin Microbiol* 1994, 32:884–892.

57. Simmonds D, Alberti A, Alter HJ, *et al.*: A proposed system for the nomenclature of hepatitis C viral genotypes. *Hepatology* 1994,

58. Alter HJ, Purcell RH, Shih JW, *et al.*: Detection of antibody to hepatitis C virus in prospectively followed transfusion recipients with acute and chronic non A, non B hepatitis. *N Engl J Med* 1989, 321:1494–1500.

59. Tremolada F, Casarin C, Tragger A, *et al.*: Antibody to hepatitis C virus in post-transfusion hepatitis. *Ann Intern Med* 1991, 114:277–281.

60. Hoofnagle J: Chronic hepatitis. In *Liver Biopsy Interpretation for the 1990s. AASLD Postgraduate Course Syllabus 1991*. Edited by Hoofnagle JH, Goodman Z. Thorofare: Slack Inc; 1991:124.

61. Vargas C, Bernstein DE, Reddy KR, *et al.*: Diagnostic laparoscopy: a 5-year experience in a hepatology training program. *Am J Gastroenterol* 1995, 90:1258–1262.

62. Soloway RD, Baggenstoss AH, Schoenfield LJ, *et al.*: Observer error and sampling variability testing in evaluation of hepatitis. *Am J Dig Dis* 1971, 16:1082–1086.

63. Ferri C, Greco F, Longombardo G, *et al.*: Cryoglobulinemia in chronic liver disease: role of hepatitis C virus and liver damage. *Gastroenterology* 1994, 106:1291–1300.

64. Lunel F, Musset L, Cacoub P, *et al.*: Cryoglobulinemia in chronic liver diseases: role of hepatitis C virus and liver damage. *Gastroenterology* 1994, 106:1291–1300.

65. Shakil AO, DiBisceglie AM: Images in clinical medicine: vasculitis and cryoglobulinemia related to hepatitis C. *N Engl J Med* 1994, 331:1624.

66. DeCastro M, Sanchez J, Herrera JF, *et al.*: Hepatitis C virus antibodies and liver disease in patients with porphyria cutanea tarda. *Hepatology* 1993, 17:551–557.

67. Bonkovsky HL, Poh-Fitzpatrick M, Pimstone N, *et al.*: Porphyria cutanea tarda, hepatitis C, and HFE gene mutations in North America. *Hepatology* 1998, 27:1661–1669.

68. English JC, Peake MK, Becker LE: Hepatitis C and porphyria cutanea tarda. *Cutis* 1996, 57:404–408.

69. Lim HW, Harris HR, Fotiades J: Hepatitis C virus infection in patients with porphyria cutanea tarda in New York. *Arch Dermatol* 1995, 131:849.

70. Okamoto H, Sugiyama Y, Okada S, *et al.*: Typing hepatitis C virus by PCR with type specific primer: applications to clinical surveys and tracing infectious sources. *J Gen Virol* 1992, 73:673–679.

71. Zaaijer HL, Cuypers HTM, Reesink HW, *et al.*: Reliability of polymerase chain reaction for detection of hepatitis C virus. *Lancet* 1993, 341:722–724.

72. Watkins PB: Role of cytochrome P450 in drug metabolism and hepatotoxicity. *Semin Liver Dis* 1990, 10:235–250.

73. Kaplowitz N: Drug metabolism and hepatotoxicity. In *Liver and Biliary Diseases*. Edited by Kaplowitz N. Baltimore: Williams & Wilkins; 1992:82–97.

74. Nelson SD: Molecular mechanisms of the hepatoxicity caused by acetaminophen. *Semin Liver Dis* 1990, 10:267–278.

75. Bacon BR, Olynyk JK, Brunt EM, *et al.*: Hemochromatosis genotype: diagnostic implications in patients with hereditary hemochromatosis and in patients with liver disease. *Ann Intern Med* 1999, 130:953–962.

76. Niederau C, Fischer R, Sonnenberg A, *et al.*: Survival and causes if death in cirrhotic and noncirrhotic patients with primary hemochromatosis. *N Engl J Med* 1985, 313:1256–1262.

77. Scheinberg IH, Sternlieb I: Wilson's disease. In *Major Problems in Internal Medicine Series*. Edited by Smith LH. Philadelphia: WB Saunders; 1984.

78. Sternlieb I: Perspectives on Wilson's disease. *Hepatology* 1990, 12:1234–1239.

79. Stremmel W, Meyerow KW, Niederau C, *et al.*: Wilson's disease: Clinical presentation, treatment, and survival. *Ann Intern Med* 1991, 115:720–726.

80. Lieber CS: Alcohol and the liver: 1994 update. *Gastroenterology* 1994, 106:1085–1105.

81. Tuma DJ, Thiele GM, Xu D, *et al.*: Acetaldehyde and malondialdehyde react together to generate distinct protein adducts in the liver during long-term ethanol administration. *Hepatology* 1996, 23:872–880.

82. Lapuerta P, Rajan S, Bonacini M: Neural networks as predictors of outcomes in alcoholic patients with severe liver disease. *Hepatology* 1997, 25:302–306.

83. Carithers RL, Herlong HR, Diehl AM, *et al.*: Methylprednisolone therapy in patients with severe alcoholic hepatitis. *Ann Intern Med* 1989, 110:685–692.

84. Stark ME, Szurszewski JH: Role of nitric oxide in gastrointestinal and hepatic function and disease. *Gastroenterology* 1992, 103:1928–1949.

85. Orrego H, Medline A, Blendis LM, *et al.*: Collagenisation of the Disse space in alcoholic liver disease. *Gut* 1979, 20:673–679.

86. Perez-Paramo M, Muñoz J, Freile I, *et al.*: Propranolol accelerates intestinal transit time and decreases bacterial translocation in cirrhotic rats with ascites [abstract]. *Hepatology* 1998, 28:510A.

87. Gines P, Rimola A, Planas R, *et al.*: Norfloxacin prevents spontaneous bacterial peritonitis recurrence in cirrhosis: results of a double-blind placebo controlled trial. *Hepatology* 1990, 12:716–724.

88. Vinel JP, Cassigneul J, Levade M, *et al.*: Assessment of short-term prognosis after variceal bleeding in patients with alcoholic cirrhosis by early measurement of portohepatic gradient. *Hepatology* 1986, 6:116–117.

89. Conn HO: The varix-volcano connection. *Gastroenterology* 1980, 79:1333–1337.

90. Patch D, Armonis A, Sabin C, *et al.*: Single portal pressure measurement predicts survival in cirrhotic patients with recent bleeding. *Gut* 1999, 44:264–269.

91. Leavitt S, Tyler HR: Studies in asterixis. *Arch Neurol* 1964, 10:360–368.

92. Conn HO, Lieberthal MM: *The Hepatic Coma Syndromes and Lactulose*. Baltimore: Williams & Wilkins; 1978:49.

93. Fuchs S, Bogomolski-Yahalom V, Paltiel O, *et al.*: Ischemic hepatitis: clinical and laboratory observations of 34 patients. *J Clin Gastroenterol* 1998, 26:183–186.

94. Shimamamtsu K, Wanless IR: Role of ischemia in causing apoptosis, atrophy and nodular hyperplasia in human liver. *Hepatology* 1997, 26:343–350.

95. Fried MW, Connaghan DG, Sharma S, *et al.*: Transjugular intrahepatic portosystemic shunt for the management of severe venoocclusive disease following bone marrow transplantation. *Hepatology* 1996, 24:588–591.

96. Shulman HM, Fischer LB, Schoch HG, *et al.*: Veno-oclusive disease of the liver after marrow transplantation: histological correlates of clinical signs and symptoms. *Hepatology* 1994, 19:1171–1181.

97. Ishak KG: Mesenchymal tumors of the liver. In *Hepatocellular Carcinoma*. Edited by Okuda K, Peters RL. New York: John Wiley and Sons; 1976:242.

98. Ngheim HV, Bogost GA, Ryan JA, *et al.*: Cavernous hemangiomas of the liver: enlargement over time. *Am J Roentgenol* 1997, 169:919.

99. Outwater EK, Ito K, Siegelman E, *et al.*: Rapidly enhancing hepatic hemangiomas at MRI: distinction from malignancies with T2-weighted images. *J Magn Reson Imaging* 1997, 7:1033–1039.

100. Lopes HM, Portela FA, de Silva Pontes JM, *et al.*: Treatment of benign hepatic cysts by instillation of tetracycline hydrochloride. *Hepatogastroenterology* 1998, 45:496–499.

101. Ralls PW, Barnes PF, Johnson MB, *et al.*: Medical treatment of hepatic amebic abscess: rare need for percutaneous drainage. *Radiology* 1987, 165:805–807.

102. Rajak CL, Gupta S, Jain S, *et al.*: Percutaneous treatment of liver abscesses: neeedle aspiration versus catheter drainage. *Am J Roentgenol* 1998, 170:1035–1039.

103. Kerlin P, Davis GL, McGill DB, *et al.*: Hepatic adenoma and focal nodular hyperplasia: Clinical, pathologic, and radiologic features. *Gastroenterology* 1983, 84:994–1002.

104. Stromeyer FW, Ishak KG: Nodular transformation (nodular "regenerative" hyperplasia) of the liver. *Hum Pathol* 1981, 12:60–71.

105. Telenti A, Torres VE, Gross JB, *et al.*: Hepatic cyst infection in autosomal dominant polycystic kidney disease. *Mayo Clin Proc* 1990, 65:933–942.

106. Kobayashi K, Sugimoto T, Makino H, *et al.*: Screening methods for early detection of hepatocellular carcinoma. Hepatology 1985, 5:1100–1105.

107. Craig JR, Peters RL, Edmundson HA, Omata M: Fibrolamellar carcinoma of the liver. A tumor of adolescents and young adults with distinctive clinicopathologic features. *Cancer* 1980, 46:372–379.

108. Mazzaferro V, Regalia E, Doci R, *et al.*: Liver transplantation of small hepatocellular carcinoma in patients with cirrhosis. *N Engl J Med* 1996, 334:693–699.

109. Di Bisceglie AM: Tumors of the liver. In *Current Practice of Medicine*. Edited by Bone R. Philadelphia: Current Medicine; in press.

110. Wiesner RH, Porayko MK, Dickson ER, *et al.*: Selection timing of liver transplantation in primary biliary cirrhosis and primary sclerosing cholangitis. *Hepatology* 1992, 16:1290–1299.

111. Showstack J, Katz PP Lake JR, *et al.*: The association of patient and clinical characteristics with resource use for liver transplantation. *JAMA* 1999, 281:1381–1386.

112. Markus BH, Dickson ER, Grambsch PM, *et al.*: Efficiency of liver transplantation in patients with primary biliary cirrhosis. *N Engl J Med* 1989, 320:1709–1713.

113. Everhart JE, Wei Y, Eng H, *et al.*: Recurrent and new hepatitis C virus infection after liver transplantation. *Hepatology* 1999, 29:1220–1226.

Nephrology

WILLIAM M. BENNETT

Nephrology is a broad-based discipline interrelating with many fields of internal medicine. Nephrologic disorders including fluid and electrolyte and acid-base problems overlap with other diseases, many of which a busy clinician encounters frequently in practice. For example, hypertension is very common in patients with kidney disease and, conversely, is also a major cause of kidney disease. Diabetes affects the kidney, while the kidney affects the diabetic state in many ways.

The images collected in this chapter of the second edition of the *Atlas of Internal Medicine* are designed to illustrate key points in the evaluation, diagnosis, and management of these disorders. Primary care physicians will find a practical approach to many common disorders having important nephrologic aspects. This chapter will attempt to span the breadth of nephrology by providing color photographs, photomicrographs, tables, and algorithms for approaching patients with kidney and electrolyte disorders. While the selected material cannot be comprehensive, the compilation is a reasonable and representative sample of the field of nephrology.

■ EVALUATION OF PATIENTS WITH NEPHROLOGIC PROBLEMS

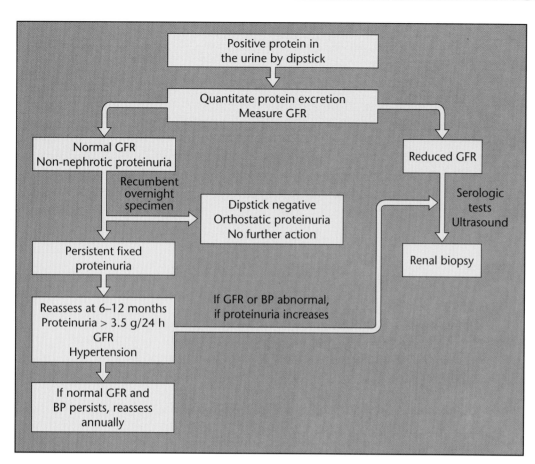

FIGURE 13-1.
Evaluation of patients with isolated asymptomatic urinary sediment abnormalities. Renal disorders are often detected by routine urinalysis. A standard dipstick test may be positive for urinary protein or blood; microscopic examination of the urine may then detect the presence or absence of casts or abnormal cells in the urine. Discovery of such abnormalities often leads to a specific renal diagnosis.

The characteristic abnormality in glomerular disease is excessive excretion of protein in the urine (>150 mg/24 h). If a patient presents with a full-blown nephrotic syndrome consisting of edema, proteinuria >3.5 g/24 hr, hypoalbuminemia, and hypercholesterolemia, a significant glomerular disorder is likely. BP—blood pressure; GFR—glomerular filtration rate. (*Adapted from* Johnson and Feehally [1].)

Common Glomerular Diseases Presenting as Nephrotic Syndrome in Adults

Disease	Associations	Serologic Tests for Diagnosis
Minimal change disease	Allergy, atopy, NSAIDs, Hodgkin's disease	None
Focal segmental glomerulosclerosis	Blacks	—
	HIV infection	HIV antibody
	Heroin	—
Membranous nephropathy	Drugs: gold, penicillamine, NSAIDs	—
	Infections: hepatitis B, C; malaria	Hepatitis B surface antigen, anti-HCV antibody
	Lupus nephritis	Anti-DNA antibody
	Malignancy: breast, lung, gastrointestinal tract	—
Membranoproliferative glomerulonephritis (Type I)	C4 nephritic factor	C3 ↓, C4 ↓
Membranoproliferative glomerulonephritis (Type II)	C3 nephritic factor	C3 ↓, C4 normal
Cryoglobulinemic MPGN	Hepatitis C	Anti-HCV antibody, rheumatoid factor
Amyloid		C3 ↓, C4 ↓, CH_{50} ↓
	Myeloma	Serun protein electrophoresis, urine immunoelectrophoresis
	Rheumatoid arthritis, bronchiectasis, Crohn's disease (and other chronic inflammatory conditions), familial Mediterranean fever	—
Diabetic nephropathy	Other diabetic microangiopathy	None

FIGURE 13-2.
Common glomerular diseases presenting as nephrotic syndrome in adults. If proteinuria is present with hematuria the likelihood of a glomerular disorder is increased; a biopsy should be done even if the urinary protein is between 500 mg–1 g/24 h. (*Adapted from* Johnson and Feehally [1].)

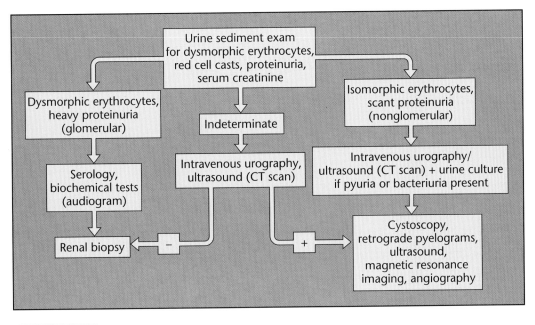

FIGURE 13-3.

Approach to the evaluation of hematuria. The evaluation of hematuria depends on clues provided by the history and physical examination. Hematuria, or abnormal urinary excretion of erythrocytes, can be classified as glomerular or nonglomerular based on findings in urinalysis, and this categorization directs further evaluation. Other formed elements, such as casts, may also be helpful.

Patients are classified into three groups based on findings in urine sediment examination: 1) glomerular: microcytic, poorly hemoglobinized, and dysmorphic erythrocytes predominate and red cell casts may also be found; 2) nonglomerular: normocytic, well-hemoglobinized isomorphic erythrocytes predominate; and 3) indeterminate: no clear predominance of isomorphic or dysmorphic erythrocytes. Glomerular hematuria directs evaluation to renal parenchymal causes (eg, glomerulonephritis). Nonglomerular hematuria directs attention to urinary tract abnormalities (eg, stones, tumors), renal neoplasia, or polycystic kidney disease. (*Courtesy of* Richard J. Glassock.)

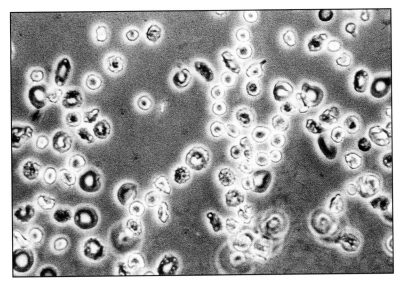

FIGURE 13-4.

Glomerular hematuria. Phase-contrast microscopy of a urinary sediment from a patient with acute glomerulonephritis. Note the small size of many erythrocytes, the distorted shape, and the loss of hemoglobin in many cells (ghost cells). (*Courtesy of* Ken Fairley.)

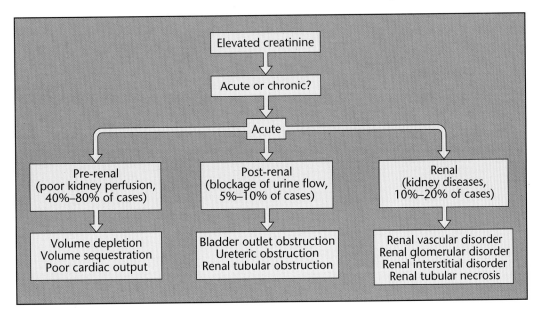

FIGURE 13-5.

General approach to diagnosis of acute renal failure (ARF). ARF is common among hospitalized patients. It can be divided into pre-renal, post-renal, or renal causes. Correct diagnosis relies on a careful history, physical examination, urinalysis, and biochemical measurement in urine. Occasionally, renal biopsy is required for correct diagnosis. (*Courtesy of* Heather T. Sponsel and Robert J. Anderson.)

■ HYPERTENSION

The Etiology of Hypertension

Essential (primary)

Secondary

  Unilateral/bilateral renal arterial stenosis

  Renal parenchymal disease (glomerulonephritis)

  Endocrine (primary hyperaldosteronism, Cushing's syndrome,
    adrenogenital syndrome, birth control pills, licorice ingestion)

  Pheochromocytoma

  Coarctation of the aorta

  Lead poisoning

  Porphyria (acute, intermittent)

  Brain tumors, subarachnoid bleed

  Acute bulbar poliomyelitis

  Renin secreting tumors

  Partial renal infarction (emboli/thrombosis)

  Liddle's syndrome

FIGURE 13-6.

Etiology of hypertension.

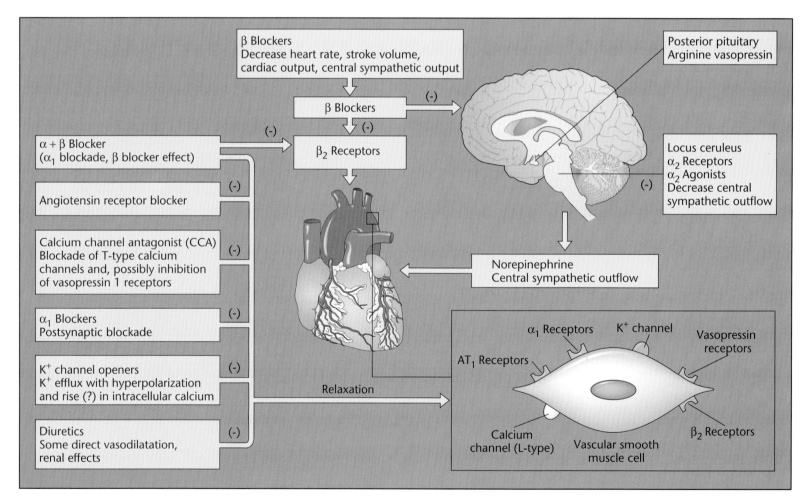

FIGURE 13-7.

Pharmacologic mechanisms and sites of action of different classes of antihypertensive drugs. Many agents can effectively lower blood pressure by working at multiple sites throughout the body. Inhibition is indicated by a minus sign. AT_1—angiotensin. (*Adapted from* Johnson and Feehally [1].)

Treatment of Hypertensive Emergency and Hypertensive Urgency

Drugs	Mechanism	Dose	Onset of Action	Side Effects
Hypertensive emergency				
Vasodilators				
Sodium nitroprusside	↑ cyclic GMP; blocks cell Ca^{2+}	0.25–10 µg/kg/min	Immediate	Nausea, severe hypertension, thiocyanate toxicity (check levels every 48 h especially in renal failure)
Nitroglycerine	↑ nitrate receptors	5–100 µg/min	2–5 min	Headache, vomiting, methemoglobinemia, tachyphylaxis
Hydralazine	Opens K$^+$ channels	10–50 mg q 4–6 h (IM, IV)	15–30 min	Hypotension, reflex sympathetic stimulation, exacerbates angina, myocardial infarction
Diazoxide	Direct acting	50–150 mg q 5 min or 15–30 mg/min	2–4 min	Nausea, flushing, reflex sympathetic stimulation, exacerbates angina, myocardial infarction
Fenoldopam	Dopamine DA$_1$ receptor agonist	0.1–0.3 µg/kg/min	< 5 min	Tachycardia, headache, nausea, flushing
Nicardipine	Calcium channel blocker	5–15 mg q 1 h (IV)	1–5 min	Hypotension, tachycardia, nausea, vomiting, phlebitis
Enalaprilat	ACE inhibitor	0.625–1.25 mg q 6 h	15–30 min	Severe hypotension, delayed excretion in renal failure
Adrenergic blockers				
Labetalol	α, β blocker	20–80 mg IV bolus q 10 min or 0.5–2.0 mg/min infusion	5–10 min	Nausea, hypotension, asthma, CHF, formication
Hypertensive urgency				
Captopril	ACE inhibitor	25 mg q 1–2 h	15–30 min	Angioedema, acute renal failure
Clonidine	Central α$_2$-adrenoceptor agonist	0.1–0.2 mg q 1–2 h	30–60 min	Hypotension, sedation, dry mouth
Labetalol	α, β blocker	200–400 mg q 2–3 h	30–120 min	Heart block, bronchoconstriction, orthostatic hypotension

FIGURE 13-8.

Treatment of hypertensive emergencies and urgencies. *Hypertensive emergency* is a rare situation with diastolic blood pressure > 130 mm Hg and symptomatic evidence of encephalopathy or angina. Diastolic blood pressure of 110 mm Hg or more with either mild or no acute end-organ damage and no clinical symptoms is defined as *hypertensive urgency*. (*Adapted from* Johnson and Feehally [1].)

Criteria for Initial Drug Therapy

Reduce peripheral vascular resistance
No sodium retention
No compromise in regional blood flow
No stimulation of the renin-angiotensin-aldosterone system
Favorable profile with concomitant diseases
Once a day dosing
Favorable adverse effect profile
Cost-effective (low direct and indirect cost)

FIGURE 13-9.

Selection of initial drug therapy. The Sixth Report of the Joint National Committee on Prevention, Detection, Evaluation, and Treatment of High Blood Pressure (JNC VI) recommends that either a diuretic or a β-blocker be chosen as initial drug therapy, based on numerous randomized controlled trials that show reduction in morbidity and mortality with these agents [2]. Not all authorities agree with this recommendation.

In selecting an initial drug therapy to treat a hypertensive patient, several criteria should be met. The drug should decrease peripheral resistance, the pathophysiologic hallmark of all hypertensive diseases. It should not produce sodium retention with attendant pseudotolerance. The drug should neither stimulate nor suppress the heart, nor should it compromise regional blood flow to target organs such as the heart, brain, or the kidney. It should not stimulate the renin-angiotensin-aldosterone axis. Drug selection should consider concomitant diseases such as arteriosclerotic cardiovascular and peripheral vascular disease, chronic obstructive pulmonary disease, diabetes mellitus, hypertensive cardiovascular disease, congestive heart failure, and hyperlipidemia. Drug dosing should be infrequent. The drug's side effect profile, including its effect on physical state, emotional well-being, sexual and social function, and cognitive activity, should be favorable. Drug costs, both direct and indirect, should be reasonable. It is readily apparent that no current class of antihypertensive drug fulfills all these criteria [3,4].

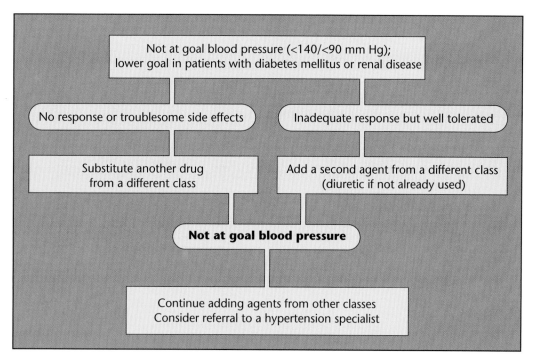

FIGURE 13-10.

Options for subsequent antihypertensive therapy. The majority of patients with mild to moderate hypertension can be controlled with one drug. If, after a 1- to 3-month interval, the response to the initial choice of therapy is inadequate, however, three options for subsequent antihypertensive drug therapy may be considered: 1) increase the dose of the initial drug; 2) discontinue the initial drug and substitute a drug from another class; or 3) add a drug from another class (combination therapy). Recommendations from the Sixth Report of the Joint National Committee on Detection, Evaluation, and Treatment of High Blood Pressure (JNC VI) are provided [2].

Causes of Resistant Hypertension

Patient's failure to adhere to drug therapy
Physician's failure to diagnose a secondary cause of hypertension
  Renal parenchymal hypertension
  Renovascular hypertension
  Mineralocorticoid excess state (*eg*, primary aldosteronism)
  Pheochromocytoma
  Drug-induced hypertension (*eg*, sympathomimetic, cyclosporine)
  Illicit substances (*eg*, cocaine, anabolic steroids)
  Glucocorticoid excess state (*eg*, Cushing's syndrome)
  Coarctation of the aorta
  Hormonal disturbances (*eg*, thyroid, parathyroid, growth
    hormone, serotonin)
  Neurologic syndromes (*eg*, Guillain-Barré syndrome,
    porphyria, sleep apnea)
Physician's failure to recognize an adverse drug-drug interaction
  See *Physician's Desk Reference*
Physician's failure to recognize the development of secondary
  drug resistance
  Sodium retention with pseudotolerance, secondary to diuretic
    resistance or excess sodium intake
  Increased heart rate, cardiac output secondary to drug-induced
    reflex tachycardia
  Increased peripheral vascular resistance secondary to drug-
    induced stimulation of the renin-angiotensin system

Causes of Endocrine Hypertension

Pituitary	Thyroid
Cushing's disease	Hypothyroidism
Acromegaly	Hyperthyroidism
Adrenal cortex	Renin-secreting tumors
Primary aldosteronism	Others
Pseudoaldosteronism	Hyperparathyroidism?
Cushing's syndrome	Endothelioma
Adrenal medulla	
Pheochromocytoma	

FIGURE 13-12.

Causes of endocrine hypertension. (*Adapted from* Johnson and Feehally [1].)

FIGURE 13-11.

Resistant hypertension. Causes of failure to achieve or sustain control of blood pressure with drug therapy are listed [3,4].

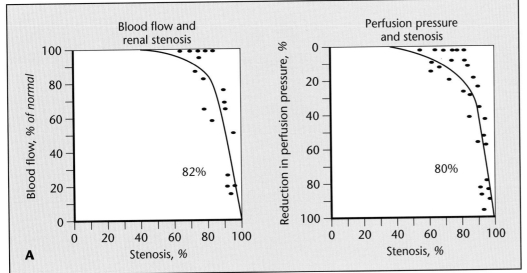

A

B

FIGURE 13-13.
Hemodynamic effects of stenotic lesions.
A, B, Obstruction to renal blood flow by
either atherosclerotic disease or fibromuscular hyperplasia is a common form of secondary hypertension. Changes in blood flow
and arterial pressure across arterial lesions
that have been carefully quantitated show
very little change until the cross-sectional
area of the vessel goes above 80%. Anatomic
lesions of less significance seldom cause
decreases in renal blood flow or perfusion
pressure. (*Adapted from* Johnson and
Feehally [1].)

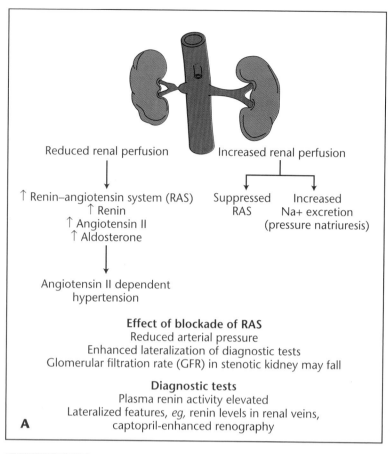

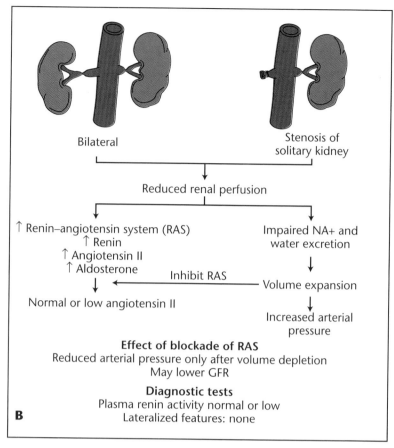

A *(left panel)*

Reduced renal perfusion   Increased renal perfusion

↑ Renin–angiotensin system (RAS)   Suppressed   Increased
↑ Renin   RAS   Na+ excretion
↑ Angiotensin II   (pressure natriuresis)
↑ Aldosterone

Angiotensin II dependent
hypertension

Effect of blockade of RAS
Reduced arterial pressure
Enhanced lateralization of diagnostic tests
Glomerular filtration rate (GFR) in stenotic kidney may fall

Diagnostic tests
Plasma renin activity elevated
Lateralized features, *eg,* renin levels in renal veins,
captopril-enhanced renography

B *(right panel)*

Bilateral   Stenosis of
solitary kidney

Reduced renal perfusion

↑ Renin–angiotensin system (RAS)   Impaired NA+ and
↑ Renin   water excretion
↑ Angiotensin II
↑ Aldosterone   Inhibit RAS   Volume expansion

Normal or low angiotensin II   Increased arterial
pressure

Effect of blockade of RAS
Reduced arterial pressure only after volume depletion
May lower GFR

Diagnostic tests
Plasma renin activity normal or low
Lateralized features: none

FIGURE 13-14.

Pathogenesis of renovascular hypertension in **A**, one-kidney versus **B**, two-kidney model. When critical levels of renal artery stenosis occur, a sequence of events activating the renin-angiotensin system leads to elevation of arterial pressure and retention of sodium by the stenotic kidney. If this stenosis is unilateral, the kidney with reduced perfusion stimulates the renin-angiotensin system resulting in the laboratory and clinical features of angiotensin-dependent hypertension. When there is stenosis to the entire renal mass, as with a solitary functioning kidney or a patient with bilateral renal artery stenosis, reduced perfusion pressure to the stenotic kidneys occurs in the absence of a normal kidney to excrete sodium. This leads to volume retention with suppressed or relatively suppressed parameters of the renin-angiotensin system. (*Adapted from* Johnson and Feehally [1].)

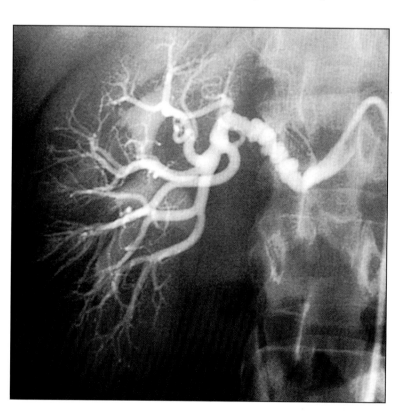

FIGURE 13-15.

Arteriogram in unilateral renovascular hypertension due to fibro-muscular hyperplasia. A selective renal arteriogram in a young woman with unilateral renovascular hypertension due to fibromus-cular hyperplasia: Note the irregular bead-like lesions along the renal artery. This is a common cause of renovascular hypertension in young women. (*From* Hallet [5]; with permission.)

■ FLUID, ELECTROLYTE, AND ACID-BASE DISORDERS

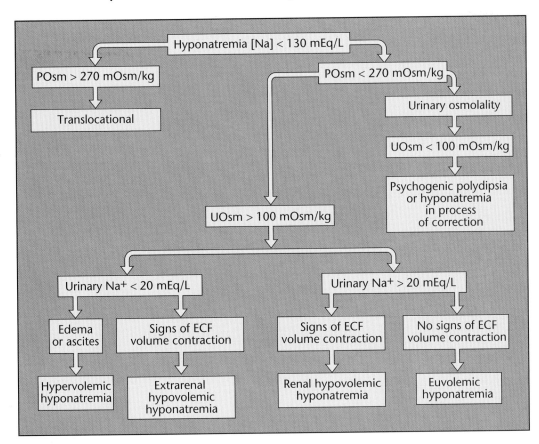

FIGURE 13-16.

Algorithm for evaluating a patient with hyponatremia (plasma sodium [P_{Na^+}] <130 mEq/L). A normal plasma osmolality (POsm) in the face of reduced [P_{Na^+}] suggests "pseudohyponatremia" due to abnormally high serum lipids (triglycerides) or protein. A high POsm suggests "translocational hyponatremia" due to osmotic redistribution of intracellular H_2O into the extracellular fluid (ECF) because of an osmotically active agent added to plasma (mannitol, glucose). An inappropriately high UOsm (>100 mOsm/Kg H_2O) and high urinary Na^+ excretion suggest euvolemic hyponatremia, commonly due to the syndrome of inappropriate antidiuretic hormone release. (*Courtesy of* Fariba Zarinetchi and Tomas Berl.)

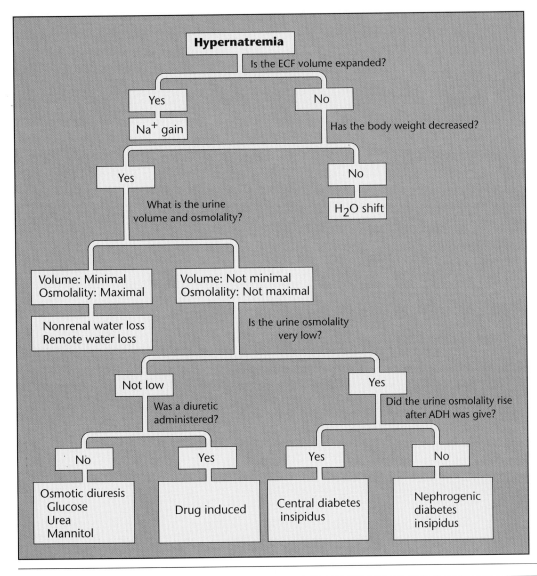

FIGURE 13-17.

Evaluation of hypernatremia. An algorithm for evaluation of hypernatremia (> 50 mEq/L). Note the critical step of extracellular fluid (ECF) volume status in evaluation. Loss of total body water rather than gain of sodium is the most common underlying mechanism. Water loss may occur through skin, lungs, gastrointestinal tract, or kidneys. ADH—antidiuretic hormone. (*Adapted from* Halperin and Goldstein [6].)

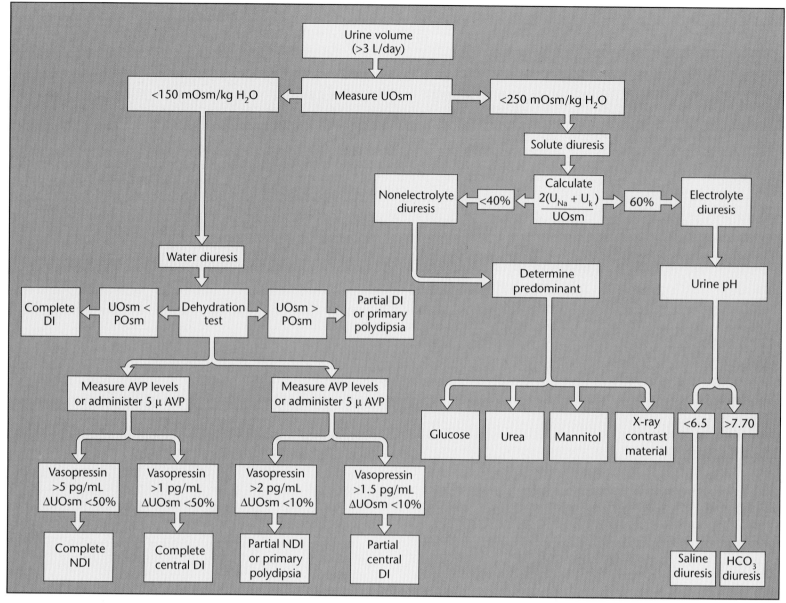

FIGURE 13-18.

Approach to polyuria. Polyuria (urine volumes consistently exceeding 3 L/d or 2.1 mL/min) can result from inadequate urinary concentrating power (diabetes insipidus, pituitary or nephrogenic), excessive H_2O intake, or excessive urinary excretion of osmotically active solutes (electrolyte or nonelectrolyte). Continued H_2O losses in the absence of appropriate H_2O intake (thirst-mediated) can lead to hypernatremia [7]. AVP—arginine vasopressin; DI—diabetes insipidus; NDI—nephrogenic diabetes insipidus; POsm—plasma osmolality; U_K—urinary potassium; U_{Na}—urine sodium concentration; UOsm—urine osmolality. (*Adapted from* Gonzalez and Suki [8].)

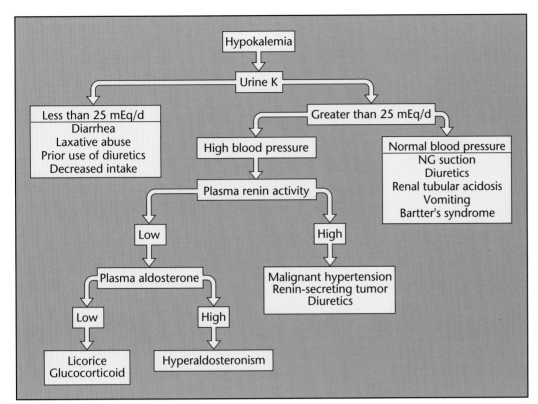

FIGURE 13-19.

Approach to a patient with hypokalemia ([K$^+$] < 3.5 mEq/L). Note the central role of measurement of urine potassium excretion in diagnosis. The potassium concentration in extracellular fluid is regulated by insulin, glucagon, aldosterone, the adrenergic system (α and β), blood pH, plasma osmolality, and renal function. Disorders of plasma potassium concentration need to be evaluated by taking these factors into account. NG—nasogastric. (*Courtesy of* Mohamed Medhat Salem and Daniel C. Battle.)

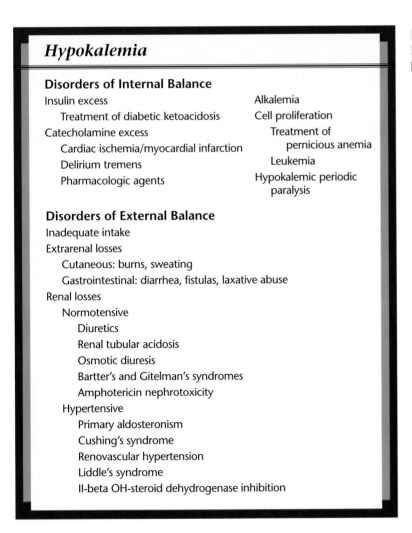

FIGURE 13-20.

Hypokalemia due to disorders of internal and external potassium balance.

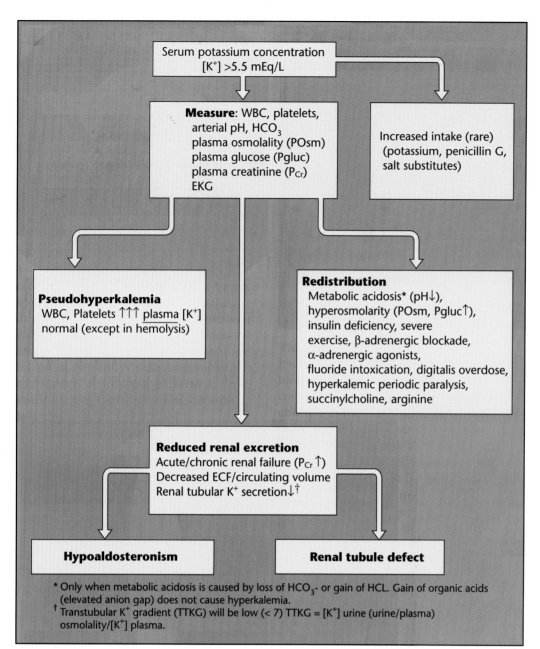

FIGURE 13-21.

The approach to the patient with hyperkalemia. Note the need to distinguish between cellular translocation and reduced renal potassium excretion. ECF—extracellular fluid; WBC—white blood cell count.

The flowchart contents:

Serum potassium concentration [K⁺] >5.5 mEq/L

Measure: WBC, platelets, arterial pH, HCO₃ plasma osmolality (POsm) plasma glucose (Pgluc) plasma creatinine (PCr) EKG

Increased intake (rare) (potassium, penicillin G, salt substitutes)

Pseudohyperkalemia
WBC, Platelets ↑↑↑ plasma [K⁺] normal (except in hemolysis)

Redistribution
Metabolic acidosis* (pH↓), hyperosmolarity (POsm, Pgluc↑), insulin deficiency, severe exercise, β-adrenergic blockade, α-adrenergic agonists, fluoride intoxication, digitalis overdose, hyperkalemic periodic paralysis, succinylcholine, arginine

Reduced renal excretion
Acute/chronic renal failure (PCr ↑)
Decreased ECF/circulating volume
Renal tubular K⁺ secretion↓†

Hypoaldosteronism

Renal tubule defect

* Only when metabolic acidosis is caused by loss of HCO₃- or gain of HCL. Gain of organic acids (elevated anion gap) does not cause hyperkalemia.
† Transtubular K⁺ gradient (TTKG) will be low (< 7) TTKG = [K⁺] urine (urine/plasma) osmolality/[K⁺] plasma.

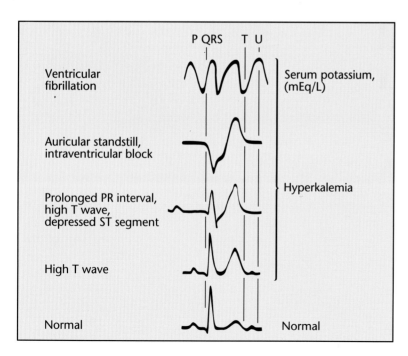

FIGURE 13-22.

Electrocardiographic changes in hyperkalemia. Note the progressive loss of P waves, "peaking" of T waves (tall, narrow based), and eventual development of a "sine wave." (*Courtesy of* Mohamed Medhat Salem and Daniel C. Battle.)

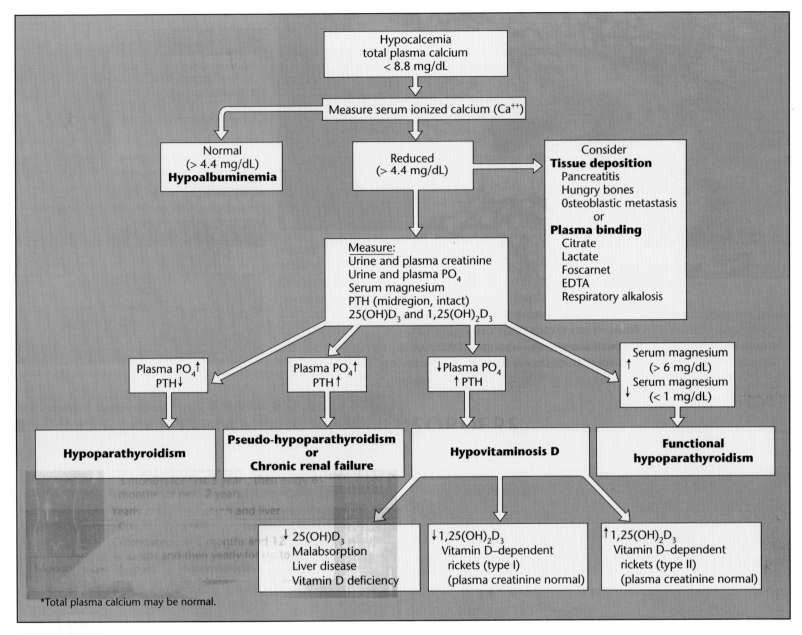

FIGURE 13-23.

Evaluation of hypocalcemia (serum total calcium < 8.8 mg/dL or < 4.4 mEq/L; serum ionized calcium < 4.4 mg/dL or < 2.2 mEq/L). Note the central role of measurement of ionized calcium, serum phosphate, vitamin D, and parathyroid hormone (PTH) (intact, mid-region) levels.

Disturbances in plasma calcium concentration arise from perturbations in calcium absorption from gastrointestinal tract, reabsorption or uptake of calcium from bone, or alteration of renal excretion of calcium or phosphate. Marked fluctuation of calcium concentration from normal can have significant effects on the heart, skeletal muscle, and nervous system. EDTA—ethylenediaminetetraacetic acid.

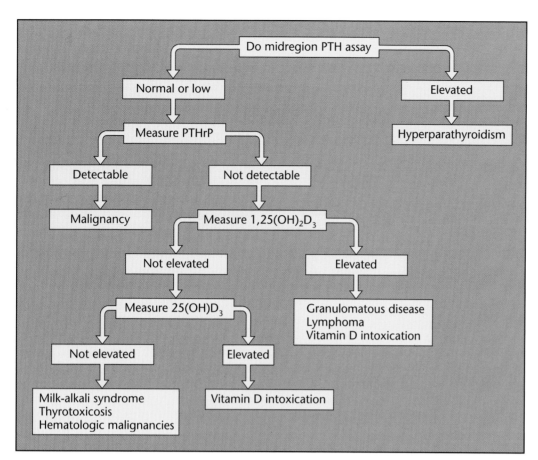

FIGURE 13-24.

An algorithm for the evaluation of patients with hypercalcemia, in the absence of renal failure (serum total calcium > 10.5 mg/dL or > 5.2 mEq/L; serum ionized calcium > 5.2 mg/dL or > 2.6 mEq/L). Note that measurement of a mid-region (intact) parathyroid hormone level (PTH) is the initial test of choice (PTHrP — PTH-related protein). The separation of true hyperparathyroidism from hypercalcemia of malignancy is particularly important. Urine calcium excretion will be elevated in hyperparathyroidism due to a parathyroid adenoma but will be reduced in familial hypocalciuric hypercalcemia, despite elevated PTH levels in both conditions. (*Courtesy of* Zalman S. Agus.)

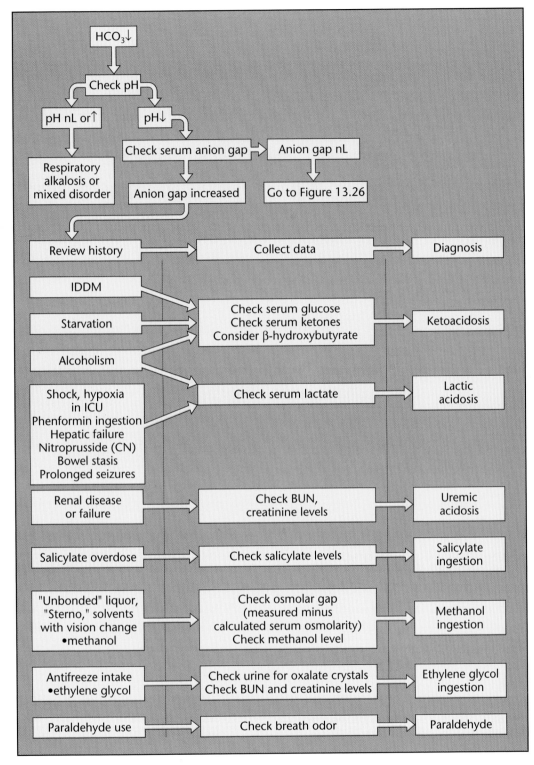

FIGURE 13-25.

Evaluation of the patient with acidemia (arterial pH < 7.40), reduced plasma HCO_3^- concentration < 23 mEq/L, and elevated anion gap (> 14 mEq/L), presumed to have a form of metabolic acidosis (osmolar gap = measured plasma osmolality 2 (2 [Na^+] + [blood urea nitrogen] 2.8 + [glucose]/18. Normal values do not usually exceed 9 MOsm/kg H_2O). Note that a few carefully selected tests (plasma glucose, plasma ketones, serum creatinine, urinalysis, and calculation of the osmolar gap) provide critical clues to the origin of metabolic acidosis with elevated anion gap. BUN—blood urea nitrogen; IDDM—insulin-dependent diabetes mellitus; ICU—intensive care unit. (*Courtesy of* Melvin E. Laski and Neil A. Kurtzman.)

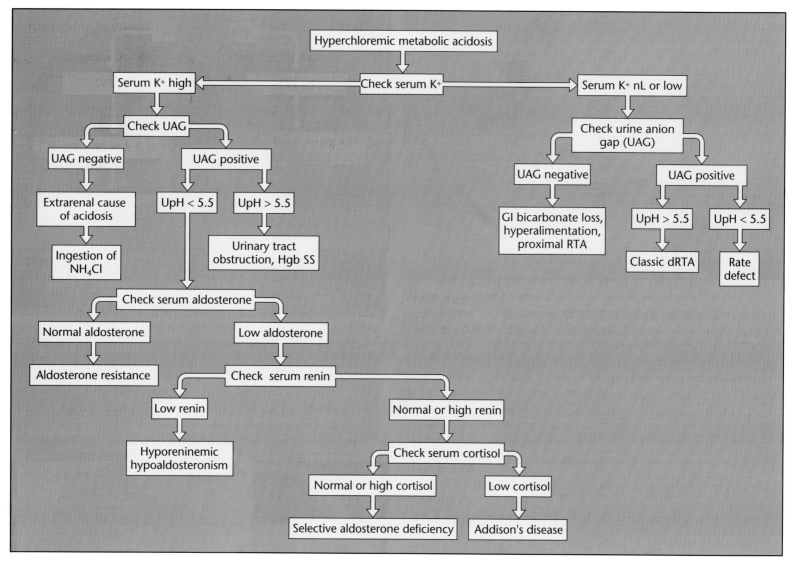

FIGURE 13-26.

Evaluation of the patient with acidemia (arterial pH < 7.40), reduced plasma HCO_3^- concentration (< 23 mEq/L) and a normal anion gap (6–14 mEq/L) (hyperchloremic metabolic acidosis). Urine anion gap (UAG) = (urine [Na^+] + urine [K^+] - urine [Cl^-] + urine [HCO_3^-]; urinary [HCO_3^-] can be presumed to be negligible if urine pH > 6.0). Normally, UAG is negative (urine [Cl^-] exceeds sum of urine ([Na^+] + [K^+]) because of NH_4^+ excretion. The UAG becomes increasingly negative with gastrointestinal losses of HCO_3^- or in proximal forms of renal tubular acidosis (renal HCO_3^- wastage). The UAG becomes positive in classical distal renal tubular acidosis (dRTA), in aldosterone deficiency, or in other distal tubule abnormalities (*eg*, urinary tract obstruction). GI—gastrointestinal; Hgb ss—hemoglobin ss; RTA—renal tubular acidosis; UpH—urine pH. (*Courtesy of* Melvin E. Laski and Neil A. Kurtzman.)

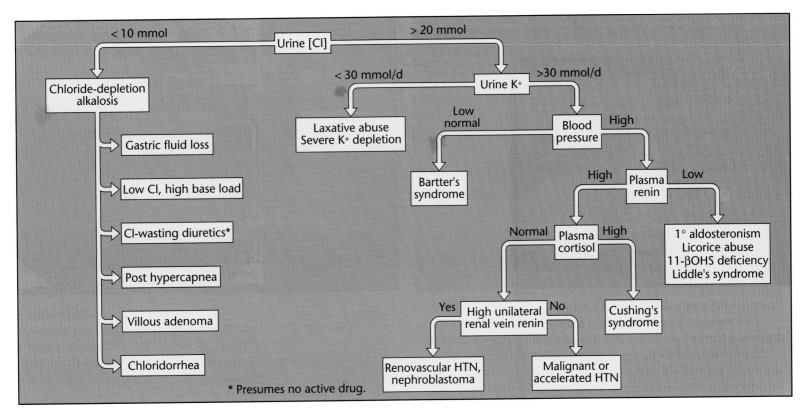

FIGURE 13-27.

Evaluation of the patient with alkalemia (arterial pH > 7.40) and elevated plasma bicarbonate (> 28 mEq/L) (metabolic alkalosis). The measurement of urinary [Cl⁻] provides a critical differentiation step.

The measurement of urinary [Cl⁻] should be done in the absence of diuretic use for 24 to 48 hours. HTN—hypertension; OHS—hydroxylase. (*Courtesy of* John H. Galla and Robert G. Luke.)

Diagnosis and Treatment of Metabolic Alkalosis

Differential Diagnosis

Saline Responsive

Contraction alkalosis

Renal alkalosis

   Diuretics

   Post-hypercapnia

   Poorly reabsorbed anion (CBCN, PCN, SO_4^{2-}, PO_4^{3-})

Gastrointestinal alkalosis

   Gastric alkalosis

   Chloride diarrhea

Exogenous alkali

   $NaHCO_3$

   Salts (sodium lactate, sodium citrate)

   Antacids

Saline Unresponsive

Renal alkalosis

   Normotensive

      Bartter's syndrome

      Severe K⁺ depletion

      Refeeding alkalosis

      Hypercalcemia/hypoparathyroidism

   Hypertensive

      Endogenous steroids

         Primary aldosteronism

         Hyperreninism

         Adrenal 11 or 17 hydroxylase deficiency

         Liddle's syndrome

      Exogenous substances

         Licorice

         Carbenoxolone

Treatment

ECF Contracted

   Adequate renal function

      Potassium

      Re-expand, NaCl

   Renal failure

      Need to re-expand

      Dialysis

ECF Expanded

   Adequate renal function

      Acetazolamide

      Acidifying agent

         Oral $CaCl_2$

         Titrated amino acids (peripheral IV)

         HCl—central IV

         NH_4Cl

   Renal failure

      Hemofiltration

      Dialysis

FIGURE 13-28.

Differential diagnosis and treatment of metabolic alkalosis. Metabolic alkalosis is common in hospitalized patients. Alkalosis is a risk factor for adverse cardiac events due to hypokalemia, hypocalcemia, and hypomagnesemia. Cardiac arrhythmias and respiratory depression are common.

Causes of Magnesium Deficiency and Hypomagnesemia

Redistribution
    Acute pancreatitis
    Catecholamine excess states (ETOH)
    Insulin administration
    Hungry bone syndrome
    Acute respiratory alkalosis
    Excessive lactation and sweating
Reduced intake
    Starvation
Reduced absorption
    Specific magnesium malabsorption
    Generalized malabsorption syndrome
    Extensive bowel resections
    Chronic diarrhea, laxative abuse

FIGURE 13-29.
Magnesium deficiency and hypomagnesemia. Magnesium is the fourth most abundant cation and the second most abundant intracellular cation in the body. It is important for muscle contraction as well as central and peripheral nervous system function. Gastrointestinal absorption of magnesium varies with diet; with a normal dietary magnesium intake, approximately 30% to 40% is absorbed. The percentage absorbed can vary inversely, with the dietary intake ranging from 80% in low magnesium states to 25% with high magnesium intake.

Redistribution from extracellular to intracellular fluids as well as reduced intake and reduced absorption may cause reduction of extracellular magnesium absorption. Magnesium may be lost through the kidney secondary to renal causes, *eg*, primarily tubular disorders or extrarenal factors that increase magnesuria.

Clinical Consequences of Hypermagnesemia

Mg^{++} level > 4 mEq/L
    Inhibition of neuromuscular transmission, deep tendon reflexes are abolished
    Inhibition of cardiac electrical conduction
Mg^{++} level > 7 mEq/L
    Lethargy
Mg^{++} level > 10 mEq/L
    Paralysis of voluntary muscles and respiratory failure
Mg^{++} level 5–10 mEq/L
    Hypotension and prolongation of the PR and QT intervals as well as QRS duration
Mg^{++} level > 15 mEq/L
    Complete heart block or asystole

FIGURE 13-30.
Clinical consequences of hypermagnesemia. Hypermagnesemia and magnesium toxicity are rare. They usually are associated with decreases in glomerular filtration rates plus either exogenous (laxatives and antacids, high-dose vitamin D analogs, parenteral management of toxemia in pregnancy) or endogenous (diabetic ketoacidosis, severe burns) loads.

■ OBSTRUCTIVE UROPATHY

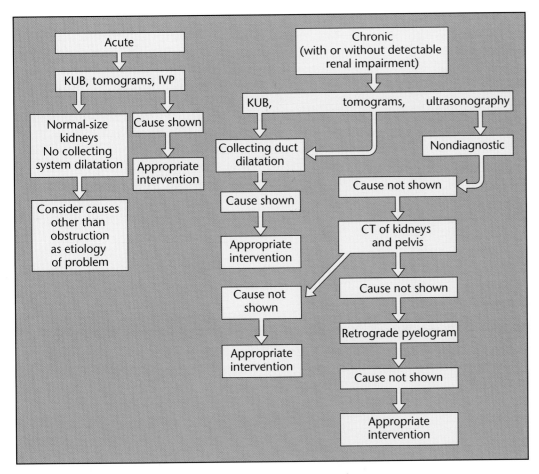

FIGURE 13-31.
Evaluation of patients suspected of ureteric obstruction. Obstruction of urinary flow can arise anywhere along the urinary tract, but it most commonly occurs in the proximal urethra (prostate), distal ureters (stones, cervical cancer), or in the renal pelvocalyceal system. The site of obstruction can usually be determined noninvasively (ultrasound, pyelography, computed tomography scan). Tumors, nephroliths, and extrinsic compression are among the most frequently observed causes. IVP—intravenous pyelography; KUB—supine plain films of the abdomen to image the kidneys and urinary bladder (without contrast media). (*Adapted from* Klahr and Bander [9].)

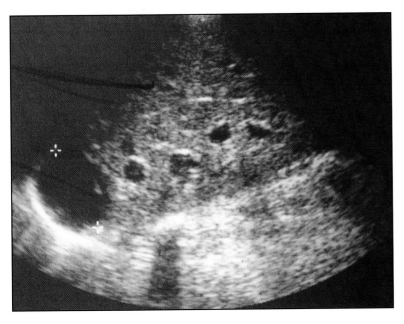

FIGURE 13-32.
Ultrasound of hydronephrosis due to urethral obstruction. An ultrasonographic image of bilateral hydronephrosis in a patient with proximal urethral obstruction due to prostate enlargement. The obstruction is "decompensated" due to loss of competence of the cysto-ureteric junction with resultant dilatation of the upper urinary system. (*From* Klahr and Harris [7]; with permission; *courtesy of* Bruce L. McClennan and the Mallinckrodt Institute of Radiology.)

■ NEPHROLITHIASIS

Epidemiology and Risks of Nephrolithiasis

Incidence: 0.1%–0.3%
Prevalence: 1%–5%
    Males, 1%–10%
    Females, 0.8%–5%
Hospitalization: 1/1000 per year
Age: 18–45 years
Composition
    Calcareous: calcium oxalate, calcium phosphate
    Noncalcareous: uric acid, struvite, cystine
Risks
    White male, 20%
    White female, 5%–10%
    Black male, 6%
    Black female, 2%

FIGURE 13-33.
Epidemiology and risks for nephrolithiasis. Genetic factors associated with nephrolith formation are mutations in gene *CLCN5* (Dent's disease) and gene *AGXT*. Fluid intake and sodium, protein, and calcium consumption as well as medullary sponge kidney, crystal-cell interaction, and nanobacter infection are other factors.

Primary hypercalciuria, an important factor in nephrolith formation, is defined as urinary calcium excretion > 0.1 mmol/L/kg/day. Secondary causes of hypercalciuria are hypercalcemia, hyperparathyroidism, granulomatous diseases, vitamin D intoxication, glucocorticoid excess, thyrotoxicosis, and immobilization.

Evaluation and Laboratory Assessment of Patients with Nephrolithiasis

Evaluation of Patients with Chronic Nephrolithiasis
History
    Previous results of nephrolith analysis
    Family history
    Nephrolith formation history
    Previous urologic intervention
    Medication
        Acetazolamide (calcium/phosphorus crystallization)
        Salicylic acid (increases urate and oxalate)
        Drugs that precipitate in the urine (acyclovir, indinavir, methyldopa,
            triamterene)
    Related medical illnesses
        Malabsorptive conditions that lead to enteric hyperoxaluria
        Chrohn's disease (calcium/oxalate nephrolith)
        Ileocecal resection (calcium/oxalate nephrolith)
        Jejunoileal bypass (calcium/oxalate nephrolith)
        Colectomy (uric acid nephrolith)
    Other diseases
        Sarcoidosis
        Hyperparathyroidism
        Renal tubular acidosis
        Skeletal disease
        Recurrent UTIs
        Neoplasm
Physical examination
Blood pressure
Evidence of bone loss via height and kyphosis
Evidence of subcutaneous calcification

Laboratory Assessment

Patient with Single Nephrolith
Urinalysis
Spot urine for cystine
    Serum
    Calcium
    Phosphorus
    Parathyroid hormone (if calcium and potassium abnormal)
    Uric acid
    Electrolytes
    Creatinine
Patient with Multiple or Complex Nephroliths
Repeat workup as for single stone former
Two consecutive 24-hour urine collections
    Volume
    Calcium
    Phosphate
    Sodium
    Uric acid
    Oxalate
    Citrate
    Creatinine
    pH
    Cystine (dependent on clinical situation)
    Magnesium (dependent on clinical situation)

FIGURE 13-34.
Evaluation and assessment of patients with nephrolithiasis. Dietary modifications and conservative therapy are suggested for various types of nephroliths. Although drug therapy is often indicated for patients with hypercalciuria, increased fluid intake is the cornerstone of management for patients with all types of kidney nephroliths. Calcium intake should be markedly reduced only in the presence of hypercalciuria and when calcium intake is > 2–3 g/day as is indicated. Patients should be advised to limit sodium intake to a maximum of 100–150 mEq/day (2–3 g). Consumption of animal protein should be < 1.5 g/kg/day, and foods high in oxalates (certain vegetables, tea, nuts, chocolate) should be avoided.

■ ACUTE AND CHRONIC TUBULOINTERSTITIAL DISEASE

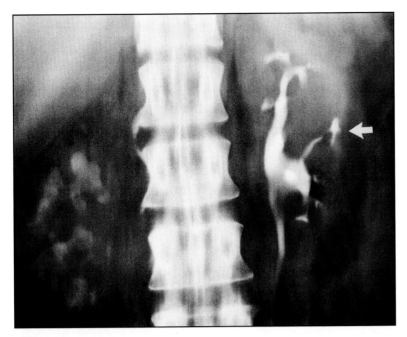

FIGURE 13-35.

Cortical scarring in tubulointerstitial nephritis. Acute and chronic tubulointerstitial disease may arise consequent to a wide variety of disorders, including bacterial infection, allergic or immunologic response, nephrotoxins, and metabolic and neoplastic diseases. In addition, the tubulo-interstitial area is frequently involved, secondarily, in glomerular and vascular diseases such as glomerulonephritis, ischemia, and vasculitis.

This intravenous pyelogram (tomographic image) shows several areas of cortical scarring and "clubbed" calyces (arrow) in the left kidney in a patient with chronic pyelonephritis. The right kidney is atrophic with dilated calyces. (*From* Boswell [10]; with permission.)

■ PRIMARY GLOMERULAR DISEASE

The Primary Glomerular Lesions

Minimal change disease (MCD)
Focal and segmental glomerulosclerosis with hyalinosis (FSGS)
Membranous glomerulonephritis (MGN)
Membranoproliferative glomerulonephritis (MPGN)
Mesangial proliferative glomerulonephritis (MesPGN)
Crescentic glomerulonephritis IgA nephropathy (CrGN)
IgA nephropathy
Fibrillary and immunotactoid glomerulonephritis

FIGURE 13-36.

The primary glomerular lesions. These lesions arise in the absence of multisystem involvement and may produce heavy proteinuria (nephrotic syndrome), rapidly progressive renal failure, or asymptomatic hematuria or proteinuria.

Glomerulonephritis

	Nephritis	Nephrotic Syndrome
Primary Glomerular Disease	Post-infectious glomerulonephritis	Minimal change disease
	IgA nephropathy	Focal glomerular sclerosis
	RPGN	Membranous nephropathy
	Anti-GBM	Membranoproliferative
	ANCA-positive	glomerulonephritis
		Type I
		Type II
Secondary Glomerular Disease	SLE	Diabetes
	Henoch-Schönlein purpura	Amyloid
	Microscopic polyangiitis	
	Wegener's granulomatosus	
	Essential mixed cryoglobulinemia	

FIGURE 13-37

Classification of glomerulonephritis. Glomerulonephritis and glomerular disease can occur without systemic symptoms; however, they can produce proteinuria severe enough to cause nephrotic syndrome. They also can cause rapidly progressive kidney failure, with the patient presenting with acute renal failure or, conversely, asymptomatic proteinuria and hematuria. ANCA—antineutrophil cytoplasmic antibody; GBM—glomerular basement membrane; RPGN—rapidly progressive glomerulonephritis; SLE—systemic lupus erythematosus.

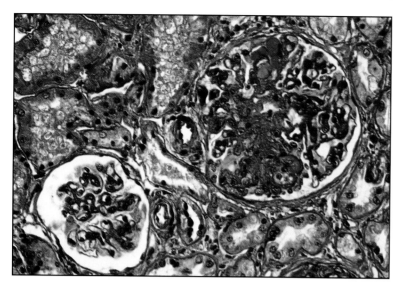

FIGURE 13-38.

FIGURE 13-38.

Focal and segmental glomerulosclerosis. Patients with this disorder present with heavy proteinuria (usually nonselective), hypertension and meaturia, and renal functional impairment. The nephrotic syndrome often does not respond to corticosteroid therapy, and there is progression to chronic renal failure over many years, although in some patients this may occur in only a few years. This glomerulopathy is defined primarily by its light microscopic appearance. Only a portion of the glomerular population, initially in the deep cortex, are affected. The abnormal glomeruli exhibit segmental obliteration of capillaries by increased extracellular matrix/basement membrane material, collapsed capillary walls, or large insudative lesions (hyalinosis), which are composed of IgM and complement (C3). The other glomeruli are usually enlarged, although they may be of normal size. In some patients, mesangial hypercellularity may be a feature. Focal tubular atrophy with interstitial fibrosis is invariably present. (*Courtesy of* Arthur Cohen.)

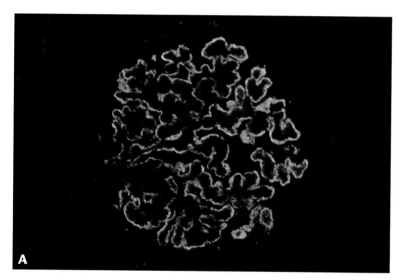

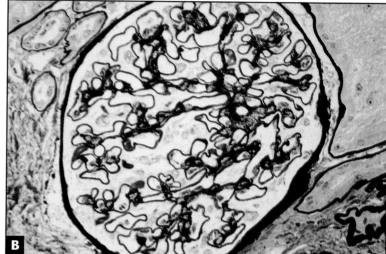

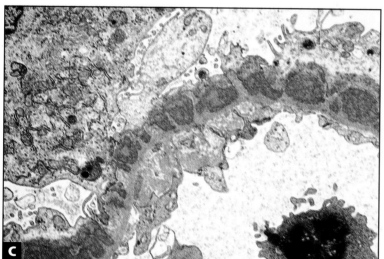

FIGURE 13-39.

Membranous glomerulonephritis. Membranous glomerulonephritis is an immune-complex–mediated glomerulonephritis, with the immune deposits localized to subepithelial aspects of virtually all glomerular capillary walls. It is the most common cause of

nephrotic syndrome in adults in developed countries. In most (75%) instances, the disease is idiopathic and the antigens of the immune complexes are unknown. In the remainder, membranous glomerulonephritis is associated with well-defined disease, often with an immunologic basis, *eg*, systemic lupus erythematosus, hepatitis B or C infection, some solid malignancies (especially carcinomas), or drug therapy such as gold, penicillamine, captopril, and some nonsteroidal anti-inflammatory reagents. Treatment is controversial.

The changes by light and electron microscopy mirror one another quite well and represent morphologic progression likely dependent on duration of disease. At all stages, the immunofluorescence discloses the presence of uniform granular capillary wall deposits of IgG and C3 (**A**). In the early stage, the deposits are small and without other capillary wall changes; hence, by light microscopy, glomeruli are often normal in appearance (**B**). By electron microscopy, there are small electron-dense deposits (*arrows*) in the subepithelial aspects of the capillary walls. In the intermediate stage, the deposits are partially encircled by basement membrane material (**C**), an abnormality that, when viewed with periodic acid-methenamine–stained sections, appears as "spikes" of basement membrane perpendicular to the basement membrane, with adjacent nonstaining deposits.

(Continued)

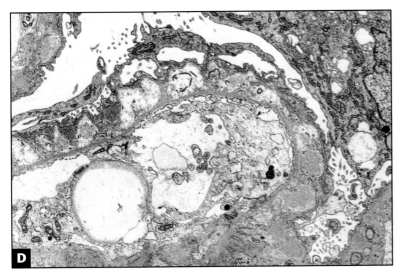

FIGURE 13-39. (CONTINUED)
Similar features are evident by electron microscopy, with dense deposits and intervening basement membrane. In late lesions, the deposits are completely surrounded by basement membranes and are undergoing resorption (**D**). (*Courtesy of* Arthur Cohen.)

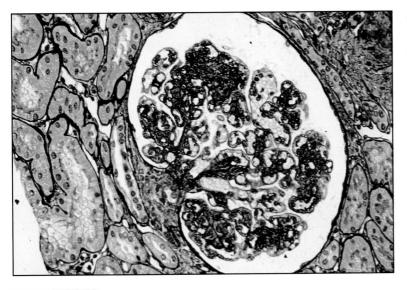

FIGURE 13-40.
Membranoproliferative glomerulonephritis, type I. Patients with this type of immune-complex–mediated glomerulonephritis often present with nephrotic syndrome accompanied by hematuria and depressed levels of serum complement (C3). The morphology is varied with at least three pathologic subtypes, only two of which

are at all common. The first, known as membranoproliferative (mesangiocapillary) glomerulonephritis, type I, is a primary glomerulopathy that is most common in children and adolescents. The same pattern of injury may be observed during the course of many diseases with chronic antigenemic states; these include systemic lupus erythematosus and hepatitis C viral and other infections. In membranoproliferative glomerulonephritis type I, glomeruli are enlarged with increased mesangial cellularity and variably increased matrix, resulting in lobular architecture. Capillary walls are thickened, often with double contours, an abnormality resulting from peripheral migration and interposition of mesangium. Immunofluorescence discloses granular to confluent granular deposits of C3, IgG, and IgM in peripheral capillary walls and in mesangial regions. The characteristic finding by electron microscopy is in the capillary walls. Between the basement membrane and endothelial cells are the following in order inward: epithelial cell, basement membrane, electron-dense deposits, mesangial cell cytoplasm, mesangial matrix, and endothelial cell. Electron-dense deposits are also in central mesangial regions. Subepithelial deposits may be present, albeit typically in small numbers. The electron-dense deposits may contain an organized (fibrillar) substructure, especially in association with hepatitis C infection and cryoglobulinemia. (*Courtesy of* Arthur Cohen.)

Classification of Membranoproliferative Glomerulonephritis: Type I

Primary (idiopathic)
Secondary
    Hepatitis C (with or without cryoglobulinemia)
    Hepatitis B
    SLE
    Light- or heavy-chain nephropathy
    Sickle-cell disease
    Sjögren's syndrome
    Sarcoidosis
    Shunt nephritis
    Anti-trypsin deficiency
    Quartan malaria
    Chronic thrombotic microangiopathy

FIGURE 13-41.
Classification of membranoproliferative glomerulonephritis, type I. Note the wide variety of underlying causes for the lesion of membranoproliferative glomerulonephritis. Hepatitis C, with or without cryoglobulinemia accounts for a majority of cases. SLE—systemic lupus erythematosus. (*Courtesy of* Arthur Cohen.)

Serum Complement Concentrations in Glomerular Lesions

Lesion	Serum Concentration			
	C3	C4	C'H50	Other
Minimal change disease	nl	nl	nl	—
Focal sclerosis	nl	nl	nl	—
Membranous glomerulonephritis (idiopathic)	nl	nl	nl	—
IgA nephropathy	nl	nl	nl	—
Membranoproliferative glomerulonephritis				
Type I	↓↓	↓	↓	—
Type II	↓↓↓	nl	↓	C3Nef+
Acute post-streptococcal GN	↓↓	nl	↓	ASLOT+
Lupus nephritis (WHO class IV)	↓↓-↓↓↓	↓↓-↓↓↓	↓	Anti-dsDNA+
(WHO class V)	nl or ↓	nl or ↓	nl or ↓	Anti-dsDNA+
Cryoglobulinemia (hepatitis C)	nl or ↓	↓↓↓	↓↓	Cryoglobulins, hepatitis C ab+
Amyloid	nl	nl	nl	—
Vasculitis	nl or ↑	nl or ↑	nl	ANCA+

FIGURE 13-42.

Serum complement concentrations in glomerular lesions. The table shows the serum complement component concentration (C3 and C4) and serum hemolytic complement activity (C'H50) in various primary and secondary glomerular lesions. Note the limited number of disorders associated with a low C3 or C4 level. nl—normal; occ—occasionally decreased; ↓—mildly decreased; ↓↓—moderately decreased; ↓↓↓—severely decreased; ↑—increased. (*Courtesy of* Arthur Cohen.)

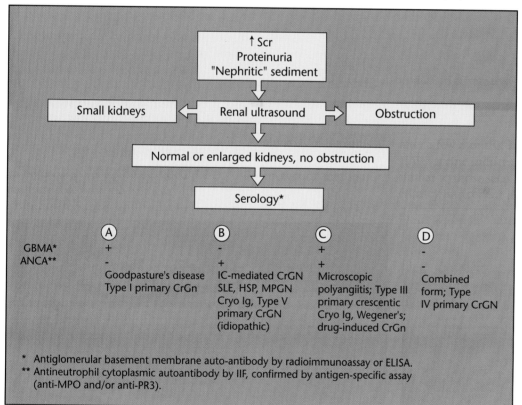

FIGURE 13-43.

Evaluation of rapidly progressive glomerulonephritis. This algorithm illustrates a diagnostic approach for the various causes of rapidly progressive glomerulonephritis, utilizing serologic studies, especially measurement of circulating, antiglomerular basement membrane autoantibody (AGBM), antineutrophil cytoplasmic autoantibody (ANCA). Anti-MPO—antimyeloperoxidase autoantibodies; anti-PR3—antiproteinase-3 autoantibodies; CrGN—crescentic glomerulonephritis; Cryo Ig—cryoimmunoglobulinemia; HSP—Henoch-Schönlein purpura; IC—immune complex; MPGN—membranoproliferative GN; SLE—systemic lupus erythematosus.

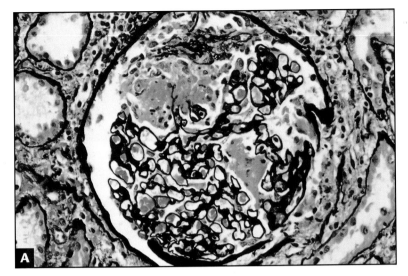

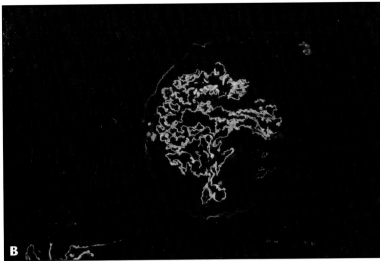

FIGURE 13-44.

Crescentic glomerulonephritis. A crescent is the accumulation of cells and extracellular material in the urinary space of a glomerulus. The cells are composed of parietal and visceral epithelium, as well as monocytes and other blood cells, and the extracellular material is composed of fibrin, collagen, and basement membrane material. In the early stages, the crescents consist of cells and fibrin, whereas in the latter stages the crescents undergo organization, with disappearance of fibrin and replacement by collagen. Crescents represent morphologic consequences of severe capillary-wall damage. In the vast majority of instances, there are small or large areas of destruction of capillary walls (cells and basement membranes) (*arrow*), thereby allowing fibrin and other large molecular weight substances as well as blood cells to pass readily from capillary lumina into the urinary space (**A**). Immunofluorescence frequently discloses fibrin in the urinary space. The proliferating cells in Bowman's space ultimately give rise to the typical "crescent." Whereas crescents may complicate many forms of glomerulonephritis, crescents are most commonly associated with either antiglomerular basement membrane (AGBM)

antibodies or antineutrophil cytoplasmic antibodies (ANCA). The clinical manifestations are typically of rapidly progressive glomerulonephritis with moderate proteinuria, hematuria, oliguria, and uremia. The immunomorphologic features depend upon the basic disease process. In both AGBM-antibody–induced disease and ANCA-associated crescentic glomerulonephritis, the glomeruli without crescents by light microscopy often have a normal appearance. It is the remaining glomeruli that are involved with crescents. AGBM disease is characterized by linear deposits of IgG (**B**) and often complement in all capillary basement membranes and, in approximately two-thirds of affected patients, in tubular basement membranes. The ANCA-associated lesion typically has little or no immune deposits by immunofluorescence; hence, the term "pauci-immune" crescentic glomerulonephritis. Neither of these disorders has diagnostic ultrastructural abnormalities; as with light microscopy, defects in capillary wall continuity are easily identified. Both AGBM- and ANCA-associated crescentic glomerulonephritis can be complicated by pulmonary hemorrhage. (*Courtesy of* Arthur Cohen.)

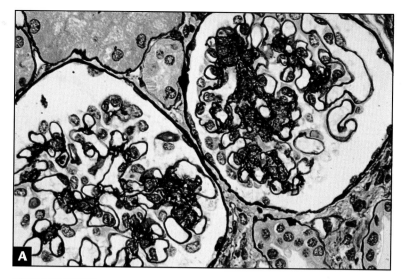
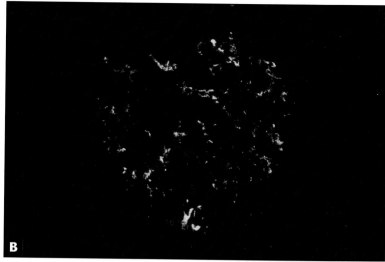

FIGURE 13-45.

IgA nephropathy. IgA nephropathy is a chronic glomerular disease in which IgA deposits are the dominant or sole component of deposits that localize in mesangial regions of all glomeruli and, in severe or acute instances, in the capillary walls. This disorder may have a variety of clinical presentations, although recurrent macroscopic hematuria often coincident with or immediately following upper respiratory infections, with persistent microscopic hematuria and low-grade proteinuria between episodes of gross hematuria, is the typical presenting manifestation. Approximately 20% to 25% of patients develop end-stage renal disease greater than 20 years following onset. By light microscopy, there is widening and often an increase in cellularity in mesangial regions, a process that sometimes affects some lobules of some glomeruli to a greater degree than others; this feature gives rise to the term *focal proliferative*

glomerulonephritis for this disorder (**A**). In advanced cases, segmental sclerosis is often present and is associated with heavy proteinuria. During the acute episodes, crescents may be present. Large round paramesangial fuchsinophilic deposits are often identified with Masson's trichrome or other similar stains.

Immunofluorescence defines the disease; there are granular mesangial deposits of IgA with associated C3 and IgG and/or IgM, the last two often in lesser degrees of intensity than IgA (**B**). The electron microscopic abnormalities are typically those of large rounded electron-dense deposits in paramesangial zones of most, if not all, lobules. Capillary wall deposits (subepithelial or subendothelial) may be present, especially in association with acute episodes. In addition, capillary basement membranes may show segmental thinning and rarefaction. (*Courtesy of* Arthur Cohen.)

SECONDARY GLOMERULAR DISEASE

World Health Organization Classification of Lupus Nephritis

		Microscopy	
Class	**Light Microscopy**	**Immunofluorescence**	**Electron Microscopy**
I	Normal	Mesangial Ig, C3	Mesangial ED deposits
II	Mesangial hypercellularity or widening	Mesangial Ig, C3	Mesangial ED deposits
III	Focal segmental proliferative, necrotizing, sclerotic lesions	Mesangial and focal capillary wall, Ig, C3	Mesangial and focal SEn
IV	Diffuse glomerulonephritis with mesangial, endocapillary or membranoproliferative lesions	Mesangial and diffuse capillary wall Ig, C3	ED deposits
V	Diffuse membranous glomerulonephritis with or without superimposed II, III, or IV lesions	Diffuse capillary wall Ig, C3	Mesangial and diffuse SEp ED deposits
VI	Advanced sclerosing glomerulonephritis	± Ig deposits	± ED deposits

FIGURE 13-46.

Lupus nephritis. Lupus nephritis consists of a variety of glomerular, tubulointerstitial, and vascular lesions arising as a consequence of this multisystem, immune complex–mediated autoimmune disorder. The immune deposits are believed to consist of autoantibody and endogenous (auto) antigens, principally double-stranded DNA

or oligonucleotides derived from DNA or nucleosomes. Shown here is the World Health Organization classification of lupus nephritis (with light, immunohistologic, and electron microscopic features). ED—electron-dense; Ig—immunoglobin; SEn—subendothelial; SEp—subepithelial.

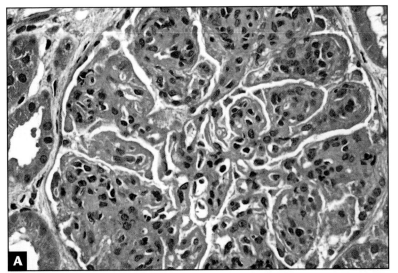

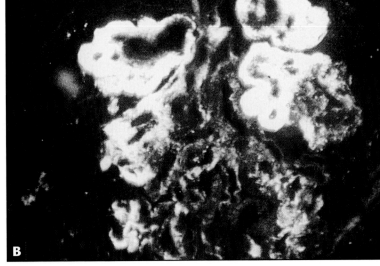

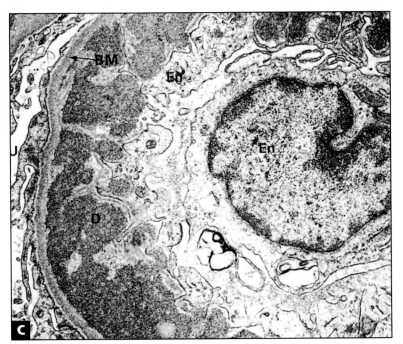

FIGURE 13-47.

World Health Organization class IV lupus nephritis. **A,** Light microscopy. **B,** Immunohistology. **C,** Electron microscopy. Note diffuse endocapillary proliferation, extensive capillary wall Ig deposits, and mesangial and peripheral capillary subendothelial electron dense deposits. BM—basement membrane. (*From* Churg *et al.* [11]; with permission.)

HIV Nephropathy

Epidemiology

90% Black

Predominantly male

25%–50% have history of IV drug abuse

Also reported in Haitians (heterosexual transmission), children (vertical transmission), and homosexuals

Clinical Manifestations

Usually in patients with AIDS, but may occur in patients with ARC or with asymptomatic HIV infection

Nephrotic syndrome, often with massive (> 10 g) proteinuria

Rapidly advancing renal failure (3–6 months)

Peripheral edema often absent despite nephrotic proteinuria

Lipids (cholesterol) may be normal

Hypertension infrequent

Kidneys normal or large by ultrasound

Pathology

Principal lesion: focal and segmental glomerulosclerosis

Other reported lesions

    Mesangial hyperplasia

    IgA nephropathy*

    Membranoproliferative GN*

    Lupus-like diffuse proliferative GN

    HUS-TTP

    Minimal change disease

    Polyarteritis-vasculitis syndromes

*Slower progression; more common in whites.

FIGURE 13-48.

Key features of the epidemiology and clinical manifestations of HIV nephropathy. Nephropathy of HIV can take several forms. It can be present with nephrotic syndrome with or without renal failure. The kidney can be involved with a secondary infection such as cytomegalovirus or hepatitis, or the kidney can be injured by some of the antiretroviral drugs used to manage HIV. HIV nephropathy is a growing problem and a common cause of secondary renal involvement. ARC—AIDS-related complex; GN—glomerulonephritis; HUS—hemolytic-uremic syndrome; TTP—thrombotic thrombocytopenic purpura.

Glomerulonephritis Associated with Chronic HCV Infection

Native kidneys

    Cryoglobulinemic membranoproliferative GN (MPGN)

    MPGN Type 1

    Other (membranous, fibrillary GN)

Transplant kidneys

    MPGN Type I

    Cryoglobulinemic MPGN

    Membranous

    Thrombotic microangiopathy (with anticardiolipin antibodies)

Treatment Options for Chronic HCV-associated MPGN

No treatment

α-IFN

    Standard (3 mU TIW x 12–18 mos)

    High dose? (10 mU qd x2 wk, then qod x 6 wks)

    Chronic (3 mU continuously, with slow taper)

Combination antiviral

    α-IFN + Ribavirin

Other antiviral

    Amantadine

Immunosuppressive treatment

    Prednisone

    Prednisone/cyclophosphamide

    Plasma exchange

FIGURE 13-49.

Glomerulonephritis (GN) associated with chronic hepatitis C virus (HCV) infection. Hepatitis B and C can be associated with renal lesions including membranous and membranoproliferative glomerulonephritis (MPGN).

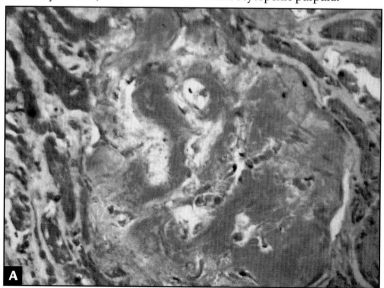

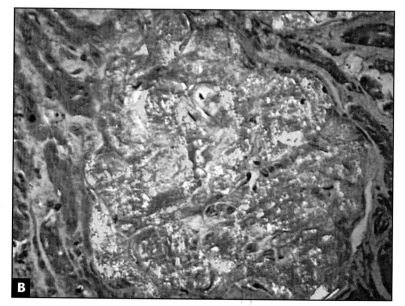

FIGURE 13-50.

Amyloidosis. Amyloidosis, either primary (AL type) or secondary (AA type), may involve the kidney (especially glomeruli). The amyloid fibrils stain Congo-red and demonstrate interwoven networks of 10- to 15-nM fibrils by electron microscopy. Primary amyloidosis appears to be due to excessive production of amy loidogenic light chains (related to multiple myeloma), whereas secondary amyloidosis is due to excessive production and decreased degradation of serum AA protein. A, Congo red stain. B, Congo red stain under polarized light. Note apple-green color of deposits.

(Continued)

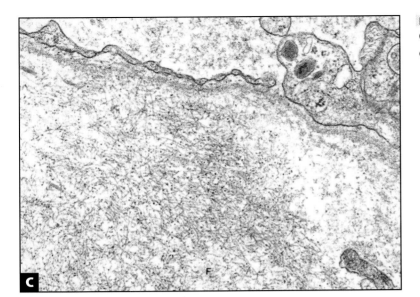

FIGURE 13-50. (CONTINUED)

C, Electron microscopy. Note interwoven fibrils, 10- to 15-nM in diameter. (*From* Churg *et al.* [11]; with permission.)

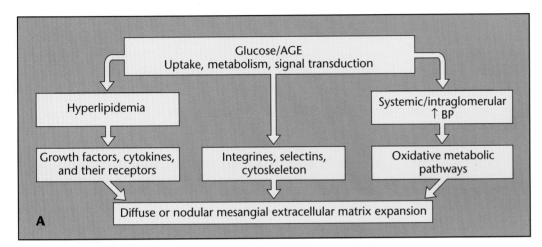

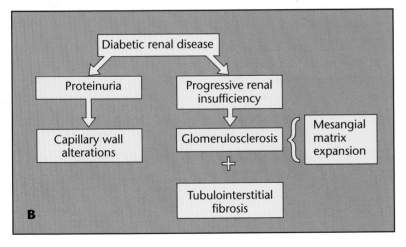

FIGURE 13-51.

Diabetic nephropathy. **A,** Pathogenesis of diabetic nephropathy. Nephropathy due to diabetes is the most common cause of end-stage renal disease in the United States. **B,** Progression of diabetic nephropathy. Patients with type 1 diabetes progress to renal failure over a defined period of time, usually 15–20 years; type 2 diabetes is a growing problem particularly in minority populations in the United States. The renal involvement in diabetes is the result of an accumulation of extracellular matrix material in the glomerulus with eventual occlusion of capillaries and loss of filtrating surface area. There is also injury to the mesangial, endothelial, and glomerular visceral epithelial cells due to intraglomerular hypertension, advanced glycosylation end products, increased secretion of growth factors and cytokines, and increased synthesis and decreased degradation of matrix protein.

Genetic factors also play a prominent role in diabetic nephropathy, particularly in type 2 diabetes. On light microscopy, the histopathology includes diffuse or nodular mesangial expansion with diffuse thickening of glomerular basement membranes. Immunofluorescence is occasionally positive, with a linear deposition of albumin or immunoglobulin along the glomerular basement membrane. This is not considered pathogenetically important. On electron microscopy, diffuse or nodular glomerulosclerosis and thickened basement membranes are seen. Clinically, diabetes presents in three phases. In phase 1, usually in the first seven years after the initial diagnosis of type 1 diabetes, there is no nephropathy. It is characterized by normal blood pressure and no albumin in the urine; however, the glomerular filtration rate is increased and kidney enlargement may be noted. In phase 2, or incipient nephropathy, microalbuminuria occurs. This is present in 25%–30% of diabetic patients with insulin-dependent diabetes approximately 7 to 15 years after the initial diagnosis.

Microalbuminuria (20–300 µg/min) is the earliest clinical manifestation of nephropathy and predicts development of overt nephropathy later. In both type 1 and type 2 diabetes, the occurrence of microalbuminuria is associated with an increased risk for cardiovascular morbidity and mortality. Phase 3 includes overt proteinuria. This occurs after 15–20 years of insulin-dependent diabetes mellitus. About 80% of patients with diabetes mellitus who develop microalbuminuria will develop nephrotic syndrome, azotemia, and end-stage renal disease approximately 7 years after the onset of overt proteinuria.

Progression to end-stage renal disease can be slowed by tight blood glucose and blood pressure control, restriction of dietary protein, and use of angiotensin-converting enzyme (ACE inhibitors) and AT_1-receptor blockers.

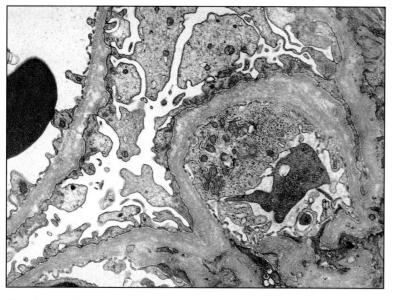

FIGURE 13-52.

Alport syndrome. Alport syndrome (hereditary nephritis) is a hereditary disorder in which glomerular and other basement membrane collagen is abnormal; it is characterized clinically by hematuria with progressive renal insufficiency and proteinuria. Neurosensory

hearing loss and abnormalities of eyes are present in many patients. The disease is inherited as an X-linked trait, although, in some families, autosomal recessive and perhaps autosomal dominant forms exist. It is clinically more severe in males than females. End-stage renal disease develops between the ages of 20 and 40 years. Some families also have ocular manifestations, thrombocytopenia with giant platelets, or esophageal leiomyomata. In the X-linked form, there are mutations in gene encoding the α 5 chain of type IV collagen (COL4A5). In the autosomal recessive form, mutations of either α 3 or α 4 chain genes have been described. By light microscopy, in the early stages of the disease, the glomeruli appear normal. However, with progression of the disease, increase in mesangial matrix and segmental sclerosis develop. Interstitial foam cells are common but are not diagnostic. Immunofluorescence is typically negative except in glomeruli with segmental sclerosis where segmental IgM and C3 are in sclerotic lesions. Ultrastructural findings are diagnostic and consist of profound abnormalities of glomerular basement membranes. They range from extremely thin and attenuated to considerably thickened, the latter with multiple layers of alternating medium and pale staining strata of basement membrane material often with incorporated dense granules, as can be seen in this figure. The subepithelial contour of the basement membrane is typically scalloped. (*Courtesy of* Arthur Cohen.)

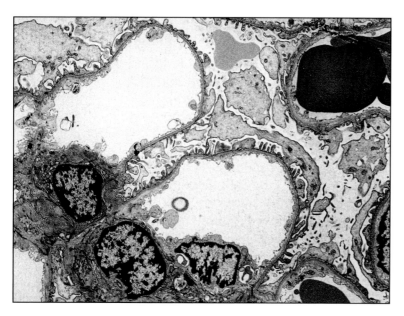

FIGURE 13-53.

Thin basement membrane nephropathy. Glomeruli with abnormally thin basement membranes may be a manifestations of benign familial hematuria or occur in individuals without a familial history of renal disease but with hematuria or low-grade proteinuria. Although the ultrastructural abnormalities have some similarities to some capillary basement membranes of Alport syndrome, these two glomerulopathies are not directly related to one another. Clinically, persistent microscopic hematuria or occasionally episodic gross hematuria are important features. Nonrenal abnormalities are absent. By light microscopy, glomeruli are normal and by immunofluorescence, there are no deposits. The electron microscopic abnormalities are diagnostic; all or virtually all glomerular basement membranes are markedly thin (less than 200 nm in adults without other features such as splitting, layering, or abnormal subepithelial contours). (*Courtesy of* Arthur Cohen.)

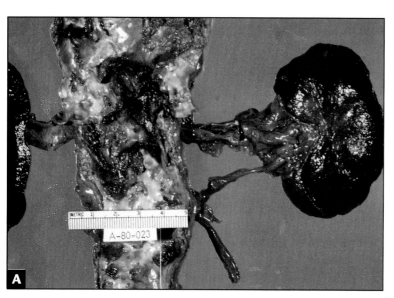

FIGURE 13-54.

Vascular occlusive disease and thrombosis. Atheroemboli (cholesterol emboli) are most commonly associated with intravascular instrumentation of patients with severe arteriosclerosis. Most commonly, aortic plaques are complicated with ulceration and often adherent fibrin (**A**). Portions of plaques are dislodged and travel distally in the aorta; because the kidneys receive a disproportionately large share of the cardiac output, they are a favored site of emboli. Typically, the emboli are in small arteries and arterioles, although glomerular involvement with a few cholesterol crystals in capillaries is not uncommon. Because of the size of the crystals, it is sometimes difficult, if not impossible, to identify them in glomerular capillaries in paraffin-embedded sections.   (*Continued*)

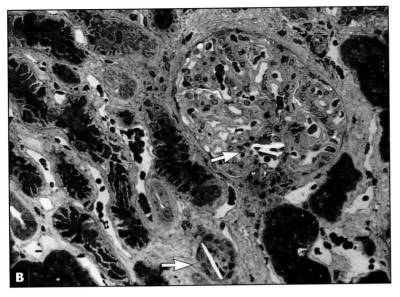

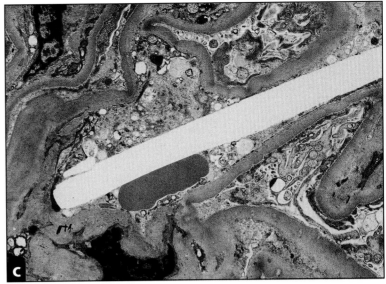

FIGURE 13-54. (*CONTINUED*)
However, in plastic-embedded sections prepared for electron microscopy, it is quite easy to detect them (**B**). By light microscopy, cholesterol is represented by empty crystalline spaces. In early stages, the crystals lie free in vascular lumina; with time, they are engulfed by multinucleated foreign body giant cells. In this light microscopic photograph, a few crystals are evident in glomerular capillary lumina and in an arteriole (*arrows* in *panel B*). In the electron micrograph, the elongated empty space represents dissolved cholesterol (**C**). Note that no cellular reaction is evident. (*Courtesy of* Arthur Cohen.)

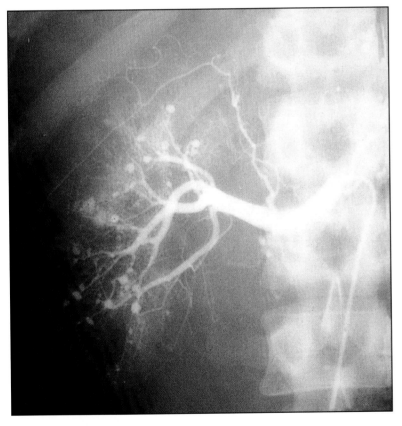

FIGURE 13-55.
Renal arterial aneurysms resulting from polyarteritis nodosa. A selective renal angiogram showing multiple small aneurysms of the interlobar and arcuate vessels in a patient with polyarteritis nodosa secondary to chronic hepatitis B infection. Such aneurysms seldom bleed spontaneously but they may produce segmental ischemia or infarction and are associated with high-renin hypertension.

■ ACUTE RENAL FAILURE

Causes of Acute Renal Failure

Pre-renal
  Volume depletion (hemorrhage, diarrhea, "third spacing")
  Congestive heart failure
  Arterial occlusion (emboli, thrombosis)
Intrinsic renal
  Glomerulonephritis
  Vasculitis
  Interstitial nephritis
  Microemboli (cholesterol)
  Acute tubular necrosis (nephrotoxic, ischemic)
  Intratubular obstruction (urate)
  Malignant nephrosclerosis (scleroderma, renal crisis)
  Hepatorenal syndrome
Post-renal
  Obstructive nephropathy (pelvis, ureter, bladder, urethra)

FIGURE 13-56.
Causes of acute renal failure.

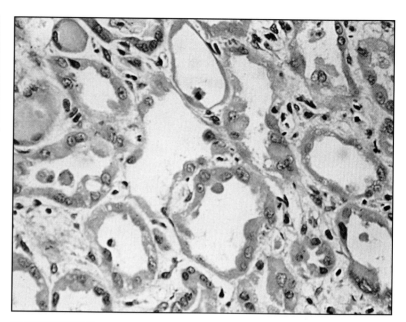

FIGURE 13-57.
Acute tubular necrosis. A light photomicrograph showing patchy tubular necrosis from a nephrotoxin. Note loss of brush border, desquamated cells in tubular lumina, and mild interstitial edema. These lesions can be seen after ischemia or nephrotoxicity. (*From* Brun and Olsen [12]; with permission.)

A. Urinary Sediment Findings in Acute Renal Failure

Pre-renal ARF	Normal, or with hyaline casts or rare granular casts
Post-renal ARF	Normal, or can have erythrocytes, leukocytes, and crystals
Renal	
Vascular	Erythrocytes, eosinophils—especially in atheroembolic disease
Glomerulonephritis	Erythrocytes, red cell casts, granular casts
Interstitial nephritis	Leukocytes, white cell casts, eosinophils
Tubular necrosis	Pigmented granular casts, renal tubular epithelial cells, granular casts

ARF—acute renal failure.

B. Spot Urine Chemistries in Acute Renal Failure

Na < 30 mEg/L, Fe_{Na} < 1%
  Pre-renal azotemia
  Hepatorenal syndrome
  NSAID use
  Early postradiocontrast
  Early sepsis
  Myoglobinuric ARF
  Glomerulonephritis
  Hemolytic uremic syndrome
  Thrombotic thrombocytopenic purpura
Na > 30 mEq/L, Fe_{Na} > 1%
  Acute tubular necrosis
  Glycosuria
  Bicarbonaturia
  Diuretic use

NSAID—nonsteroidal anti-inflammatory drug.

FIGURE 13-58.
Urinalysis (A) and urine chemistry (B) in acute renal failure (ARF). Prerenal failure is suggested when the urine sediment is normal or shows only scanty hyaline casts and the urine sodium concentration (U_{Na}^+) is < 30 mEq/L or the fractional excretion of sodium (Fe_{Na}^+) is less than 1% (FE_{Na} [%] = $U/P_{Na}^+ \div U/Pcr \times 100$). Parenchymal renal failure is associated with varied abnormal urinalyses (hematuria, proteinuria) and varied urine chemistry, depending on cause. Acute tubular necrosis (ATN) is suggested when brownish ("muddy") granular casts are seen in the urine sediment and the U_{Na}^+ is > 30 mEq/L or the Fe_{Na}^+ is > 1%. (*Courtesy of* Heather T. Sponsel and Robert J. Anderson.)

■ CYSTIC DISEASES OF THE KIDNEY

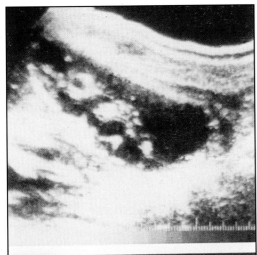

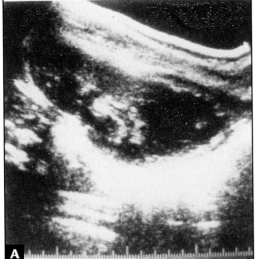

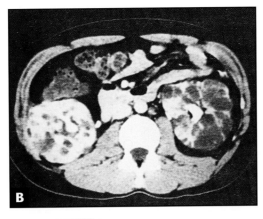

FIGURE 13-59.

Polycystic kidney disease (PKD). **A,** Ultrasonographic scans and **B,** computed tomographic image of kidneys of patients with PKD. The most common cystic disease of the kidney is autosomal dominant PKD (ADPKD), occurring in one in 1000 live births. Since the transmission is autosomal dominant, 50% of children from an affected parent carry the genetic abnormality. Penetration is virtually complete; carrying the gene is equivalent to having some phenotypic manifestations of the disease. The two main types of ADPKD share an identical phenotype. PKD1 is defined by an abnormality of the gene encoding the complex protein, polycystin-1, whereas PKD2 is an abnormality in the gene encoding polycystin-2. The precise relationship between the genetic abnormality and the clinical manifestations of this disease is at present unclear. PKD is diagnosed by finding cysts in the kidney on imaging studies. The most preferable diagnostic techniques for diagnosing PKD are renal ultrasound and CT scanning. A negative study in a patient younger than 30 years of age does not exclude the disease, so it is recommended that only adults at risk be tested.

Manifestations of ADPKD

Renal	Extrarenal
Hematuria	Cerebral aneurysm
Nephrolithiasis	Hepatic cysts
Flank, abdominal pain	Cardiac valve disease
Infection	Colonic diverticula
	Umbilical and inguinal hernia

FIGURE 13-60.

Clinical manifestations of autosomal dominant polycystic kidney disease (ADPKD). Clinically, patients with ADPKD present with hypertension, severe flank pain simulating renal colic, or gross hematuria. The clinical manifestations of polycystic kidney disease may be either renal or extrarenal. The most severe extrarenal complication of ADPKD is the presence of berry aneurysms, occurring in 5% to 10% of patients. These aneurysms seem to cluster within certain families. Noninvasive vascular studies using high-resolution computed tomography and magnetic resonance angiography can detect cysts > 5 mm. Aneurysms > 10 mm are at risk for rupture. Routine screening is not recommended because of an unacceptably high false-negative rate.

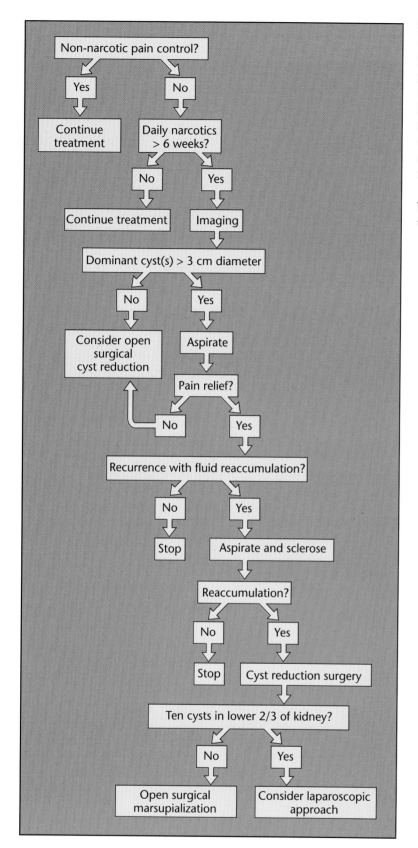

FIGURE 13-61.

Chronic abdominal or flank pain in patients with autosomal dominant polycystic kidney disease (ADPKD). Severe abdominal or flank pain is a frequent complaint of patients with polycystic kidney disease, presumably due to the progressive enlargement of both kidneys. However, the differential diagnosis of flank pain can be complicated because polycystic kidneys may bleed, with resulting clots passing through the ureter, or a cyst may rupture causing severe flank pain. These conditions are difficult to distinguish from nephrolithiasis.

Nephrolithiasis occurs in up to 20% of patients with ADPKD. These nephroliths usually are composed of either calcium oxalate or uric acid. They are managed similarly to other nephroliths.

■ DIALYSIS

Functions of the Kidney and Pathophysiology of Renal Failure

Function	Dysfunction
Salt, water, and acid-base balance	Salt, water, and acid-base balance
Water balance	Fluid retention and hyponatremia
Sodium balance	Edema, congestive heart failure, hypertension
Potassium balance	Hyperkalemia
Bicarbonate balance	Metabolic acidosis, osteodystrophy
Magnesium balance	Hypermagnesemia
Phosphate balance	Hyperphosphatemia, osteodystrophy
Excretion of nitrogenous end products	Excretion of nitrogenous end products
Urea	?Anorexia, nausea, pruritus, pericarditis, polyneuropathy, encephalopathy, thrombocytopathy
Creatinine	
Uric acid	
Amines	
Guanidine derivatives	
Endocrine-metabolic	Endocrine-metabolic
Conversion of vitamin D to active metabolite	Osteomalacia, osteodystrophy
Production of erythropoietin	Anemia
Renin	Hypertension

FIGURE 13-62.
Functions of the kidney and pathophysiology of renal failure.

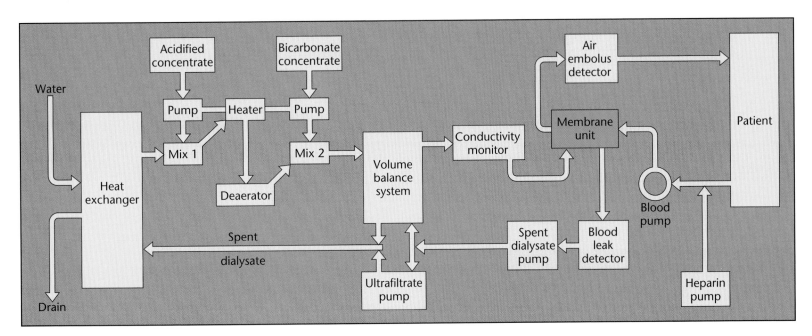

FIGURE 13-63.
Simplified schematic of typical hemodialysis system. In hemodialysis, blood from the patient is circulated through a synthetic extracorporeal membrane and returned to the patient. The opposite side of that membrane is washed with an electrolyte solution (dialysate) containing the normal constituents of plasma water. The apparatus contains a blood pump to circulate the blood through the system, proportioning pumps that mix a concentrated salt solution with water purified by reverse osmosis and/or deionization to produce the dialysate, a means of removing excess fluid from the blood (mismatching dialysate inflow and outflow to the dialysate compartment), and a series of pressure, conductivity, and air embolus monitors to protect the patient. Dialysate is warmed to body temperature by a heater.

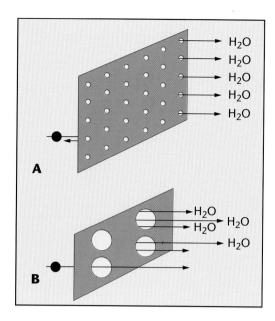

FIGURE 13-64.

Dialysis membranes with small and large pores. Although a general correlation exists between the (water) flux and the (middle molecular weight molecule) permeability of dialysis membranes, they are not synonymous. **A,** Membrane with numerous small pores that allow high water flux but no β_2-microglobulin transport. **B,** Membrane with a smaller surface area and fewer pores, with the pore size sufficiently large to allow β_2-microglobulin transport. The ultrafiltration coefficient and hence the water flux of the two membranes are equivalent.

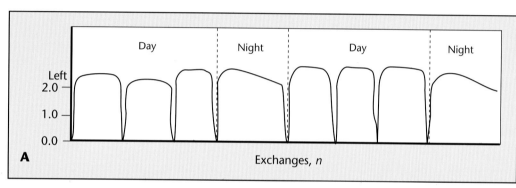

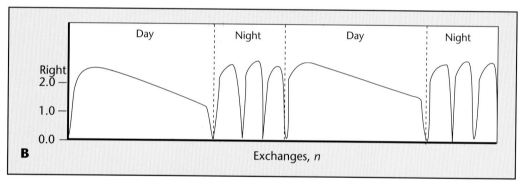

FIGURE 13-65.

Continuous peritoneal dialysis regimens. **A,** Continuous ambulatory peritoneal dialysis (CAPD); **B,** continuous cyclic peritoneal dialysis (CCPD) is shown. Multiple sequential exchanges are performed during the day and night so that dialysis occurs 24 hours a day, 7 days a week.

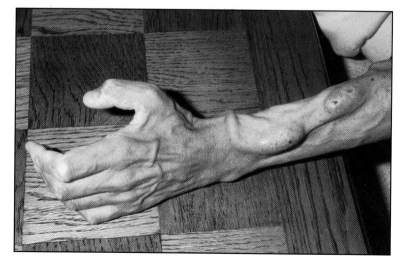

FIGURE 13-66.

The Brescia-Cimino (radial-cephalic) fistula. The radial-cephalic fistula offers many advantages. It is simple to create and preserves more proximal vessels for future access construction. The lower incidence of steal is likely the result of the lower flow rate associated with these accesses. Additionally, such accesses have low rates of thrombosis and infection. The photograph shows a mature Brescia-Cimino fistula in a patient with longstanding diabetes. The fistula outflow vein has numerous aneurysmal segments, and, although they are associated with some tendency toward flow stagnation, they are of no harm to the patient's dialysis life. They do, however, become obvious targets for the dialysis technical staff, who have a tendency to puncture them repeatedly rather than to utilize new needle insertion sites. The patient's arm also demonstrates marked muscle atrophy secondary to advanced diabetic neuropathy, which particularly involves the thenar eminence and the interosseus muscle groups. Complaints of weakness and loss of grip strength in the arm are common and may represent symptoms of steal. In this case, however, the symptoms are due to the intrinsic loss of muscle mass, rather than to steal.

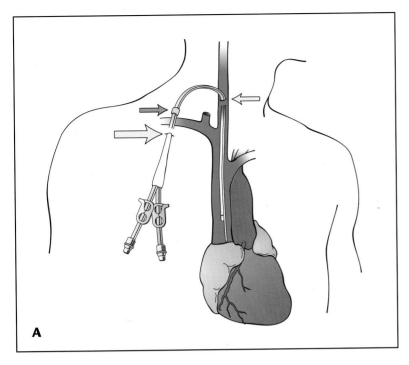

A

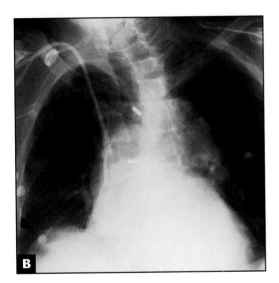

B

Right internal jugular vein catheters. The use of central vein catheters has grown significantly over the past several years. These catheters were at one time used only on a temporary basis and served as a "bridge" to permanent vascular access. Improvements in catheter design and function combined with ease of insertion have increased use of central vein catheters in dialysis units. To minimize the risk of central vein stenosis and subsequent thrombosis, central vein catheters should be inserted preferentially into the right internal jugular vein, regardless of whether they are being used for temporary or more permanent purposes. The typical position of a double-lumen catheter, **A**, is with its tip at the junction of the right atrium and the superior vena cava. The catheter has been "tunneled" underneath the skin so that the exit site (*large arrow*) is located just beneath the right clavicle and distant from the insertion site (*small arrow*). This catheter also has a cuff into which endothelial cells will grow and produce a biologic barrier to bacterial migration. **B**, Chest radiograph showing a dialysis central vein catheter that is composed of two separate single-lumen catheters that have been inserted into the right internal jugular vein. The distal tip of the venous catheter is positioned just above the right atrium. Care must be taken, however, to ensure proper placement of catheters with this type of design, because the two single lumens are radiographically indistinguishable.

Acceptable Methods to Measure Hemodialysis Adequacy*

Formal urea kinetic modeling (Kt/V) using computational software

$$Kt/V = -L_N (R-0.008 \times t)$$
$$+ (4-3.5 \times R)$$
$$\times Uf/w^t$$

Urea reduction ratio

*Recommended by the National Kidney Foundation Dialysis Outcomes Quality Initiative Clinical Practice Guidelines, which suggest a prescribed minimum Kt/V of 1.3 and a minimum urea reduction ratio of 70%.
tLn is the natural logarithm; R is postdialysis blood urea nitrogen (BUN)/predialysis BUN; t is time in hours, Uf is ultrafiltration volume in liters; w is postdialysis weight in kilograms.

Acceptable methods to measure hemodialysis adequacy as recommended in the Dialysis Outcomes Quality Initiative (DOQI) Clinical Practice Guidelines. These guidelines may change as new information on the benefit of increasing the dialysis prescription becomes available. For the present, however, they should be considered the minimum targets.

Complications of Hemodialysis

Complication	Differential diagnosis
Fever	Bacteremia, water-borne pyrogens, overheated dialysate
Hypotension	Excessive ultrafiltration, cardiac arrhythmia, air embolus, pericardial tamponade; hemorrhage (gastrointestinal, intracranial, retroperitoneal); anaphylactoid reaction
Hemolysis	Inadequate removal of chloramine from dialysate, failure of dialysis concentrate delivery system
Dementia	Incomplete removal of aluminum from dialysate water, prescription of aluminum antacids
Seizure	Excessive urea clearance (first treatment), failure of dialysis concentrate delivery system
Bleeding	Excessive heparin or other anticoagulant
Muscle cramps	Excessive ultrafiltration

FIGURE 13-69.

Complications associated with hemodialysis.

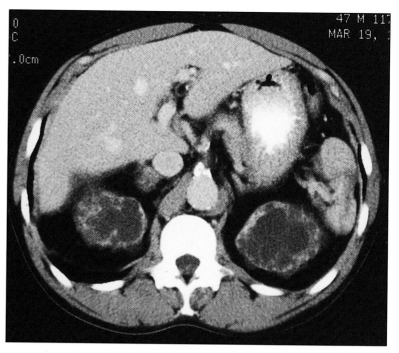

FIGURE 13-70.

Acquired cystic disease of the kidney. Abdominal computed tomography demonstrates cystic disease in this patient, who had focal segmental glomerulosclerosis complicated by protein C deficiency and renal vein thrombosis. Eleven years after the initial diagnosis, he developed renal failure requiring hemodialysis. Two years after starting dialysis, he developed hematuria, and these cysts were found. The appearance and clinical course are consistent with acquired cystic disease of the kidney. These cysts carry some risk of malignant transformation.

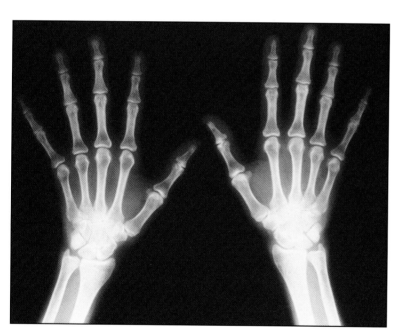

FIGURE 13-71.

Radiograph of the hands of a patient who has renal osteodystrophy. The hands demonstrate diffuse bilateral osteoporosis. The resorption of the distal phalanges is best seen in the first and second digits of the right hand. The radial side of the middle phalanges of the second and third digits bilaterally demonstrates subperiosteal bone resorption. Soft tissue calcification is present on the radial side of the proximal interphalangeal joint of the second digit of the left hand.

■ RENAL TRANSPLANTATION

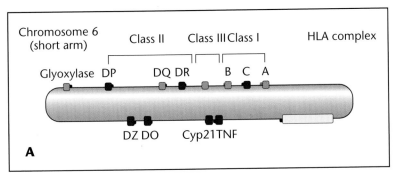

A

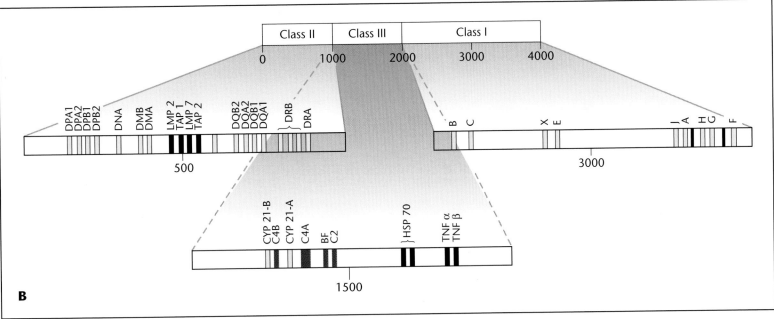

B

FIGURE 13-72.

The major histocompatibility complex (MHC) is a group of closely linked genes that was first appreciated because it was found to contain the structural genes for transplantation antigens. **A,** The MHC, located on the short arm of chromosome 6, is now recognized to include many other genes important in the regulation of immune responses. **B,** Regions of the MHC classes I, II, and III. The MHC can be divided into three regions, of which the class I and II regions contain the loci for the human histocompatibility antigen or human leukocyte antigen (HLA). Genes in the class I region encode the α or heavy chain of the class I antigens, HLA-A, B, and C. The class I region is composed of other genes, most of which are pseudogenes and are not expressed. The MHC class II region is more complex, with structural genes for both the α and β chains of the class II molecules. The class II region includes four DP genes, one DN gene, one DO gene, five DQ genes, and a varying number of DR genes (two to 10), depending on the halotype. Many other immune response genes are coded within the class III region. TNF—tumor necrosis factor.

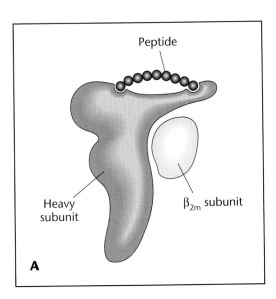

A

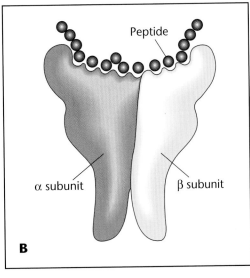

B

FIGURE 13-73.

The structure of class I and II molecules. Comparison of the crystalline structures of classes I and II molecules has revealed overall structural similarity, with a few significant differences. **A,** Class I molecules have a groove with deep anchor pockets at each end (a "pita pocket"). These pockets restrict the binding of peptides to those of eight to nine amino acid residues in length. **B,** The peptide-binding groove of class II molecules is more flexible and relatively open at one end, more like a "hotdog bun," permitting larger peptides from 13 to 25 amino acid residues in length to bind.

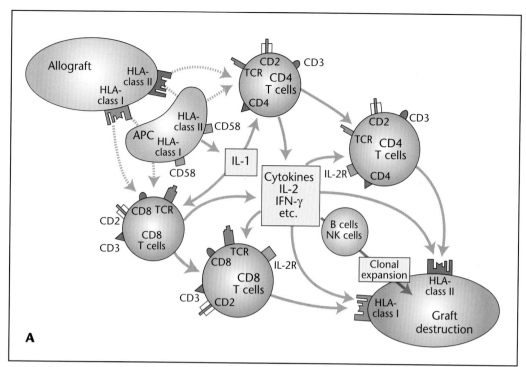

FIGURE 13-74.

Aspects of the rejection response. **A,** The immune response cascade. Rejection is a complex and redundant response to grafted tissue. The major targets of this response are the major histocompatibility complex (MHC) antigens, which are designated as human leukocyte antigens (HLAs) in humans. The HLA region on the short arm of chromosome 6 encompasses more than 3 million nucleotide base pairs. It encodes two structurally distinct classes of cell-surface molecules, termed class I (HLA-A, -B, and -C) and class II (-DR, -DQ, -DP).

B. Overview of Rejection Events

Antigen-presenting cells trigger CD4 and CD8 T cells

Both a local and systemic immune response develop

Cytokines recruit and activate nonspecific cells and accumulate in graft, which facilitates the following events:

Development of specific T cells, natural killer cells, or macrophage-mediated cytotoxicity

Allograft destruction

B, Overview of rejection events. T cells recognize foreign antigens only when the antigen or an immunogenic peptide is associated with a self-HLA molecule on the surface of an accessory cell called the antigen-presenting cell (APC). Helper T cells (CD4) are activated to proliferate, differentiate, and secrete a variety of cytokines. These cytokines increase expression of HLA class II antigens on engrafted tissues, stimulate B lymphocytes to produce antibodies against the allograft, and help cytotoxic T cells, macrophages, and natural killer cells develop cytotoxicity against the graft.

A. Varieties of Rejection

Types of Rejection	Time Taken	Cause
Hyperacute	Minutes to hours	Preformed antidonor antibodies and complement
Accelerated	Days	Reactivation of sensitized T cells
Acute	Days to weeks	Primary activation of T cells
Chronic	Months to years	Both immunologic and nonimmunologic factors

B. Immune Mechanisms of Renal Allograft Rejection

Type	Humoral	Cellular
Hyperacute	+++	-
Accelerated	++	+
Acute		
Cellular	+	+++
Vascular	+++	+
Chronic	++	+?

FIGURE 13-75.

Varieties of rejection, **A,** and immune mechanisms, **B.** On the basis of the pathologic process and the kinetics of the rejection response, rejection of renal allografts can be commonly divided into hyperacute, accelerated, acute, and chronic types.

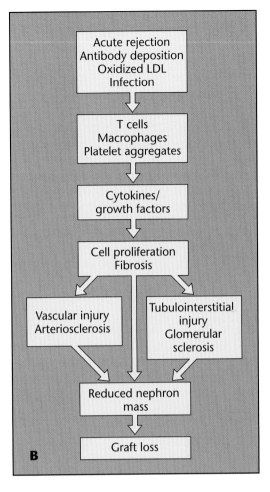

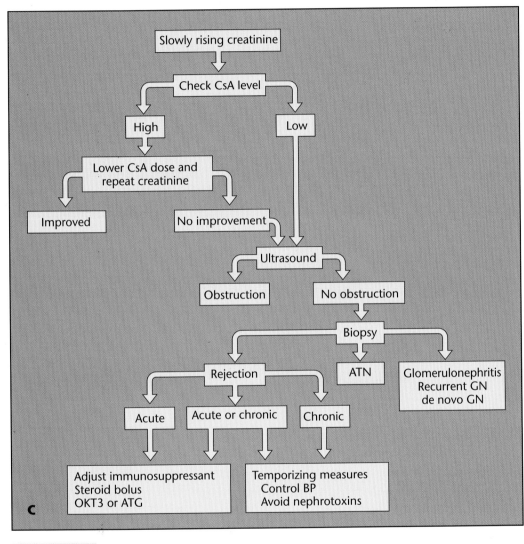

A. Chronic Allograft Rejection

Typical clinical presentation
- Gradual increase in creatinine (months)
- Non-nephrotic–range proteinuria
- No recent nephrotoxic events

Key pathologic features
- Interstitial fibrosis
- Arterial fibrosis and intimal thickening

FIGURE 13-76.

Features of chronic rejection. **A,** Typical presentation and pathologic features. Chronic rejection occurs during a span of months to years. It appears to be unresponsive to current treatment and has emerged as the major problem facing transplantation [14]. Because chronic rejection is thought to be the end result of uncontrolled repetitive acute rejection episodes or a slowly progressive inflammatory process, its onset may be as early as the first few weeks after transplantation or any time thereafter.

B, The likely sequence of events in chronic rejection and potential mediating factors for key steps. Progressive azotemia, proteinuria, and hypertension are the clinical hallmarks of chronic rejection. Immunologic and nonimmunologic mechanisms are thought to play a role in the pathogenesis of this entity. Immunologic

mechanisms include antibody-mediated tissue destruction that occurs possibly secondary to antibody-dependent cellular cytotoxicity leading to obliterative arteritis, growth factors derived from macrophages and platelets leading to fibrotic degeneration, and glomerular hypertension with hyperfiltration injury due to reduced nephron mass leading to progressive glomerular sclerosis. Nonimmunologic causes can also contribute to the decline in renal function. Atheromatous renovascular disease of the transplant kidney may also be responsible for a significant number of cases of progressive graft failure.

C, Diagnostic and therapeutic approach to chronic rejection. ATG— antithymocyte globulin; ATN—acute tubular necrosis; BP—blood pressure; CsA—cyclosporine; LDL—low-density lipoprotein.

A. Antirejection Therapy Regimens

Intravenous methylprednisolone, 0.5 or 1 g x 3 d
OKT3
Antithymocyte gamma globulin
Rabbit antithymocyte globulin
Humanized anti-CD25 (IL-2 receptor) intravenously every 2 wk
Anti–ICAM-1 and anti–LFA-1 antibodies

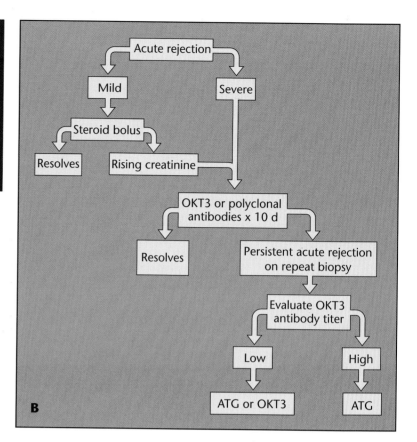

FIGURE 13-77.

Treatment of acute rejection. **A,** Typical antirejection therapy regimens. **B,** Treatment algorithm. A biopsy should be performed whenever possible. The first-line treatment for acute rejection in most centers is pulse methylprednisolone, 500 to 1000 mg, given intravenously daily for 3 to 5 days. The expected reversal rate for the first episode of acute cellular rejection is 60% to 70% with this regimen [15–17]. Steroid-resistant rejection is defined as a lack of improvement in urine output or the plasma creatinine concentration within 3 to 4 days. In this setting, OKT3 or polyclonal anti–T-cell antibodies should be considered [18]. The use of these potent therapies should be confined to acute rejections with acute components that are potentially reversible, *eg,* mononuclear interstitial cell infiltrate with tubulitis or endovasculitis with acute inflammatory endothelial infiltrate [19,20]. ATG—antithymocyte globulin; ICAM-1—intercellular adhesion molecule-1; LFA-1—leukocyte function-associated antigen-1.

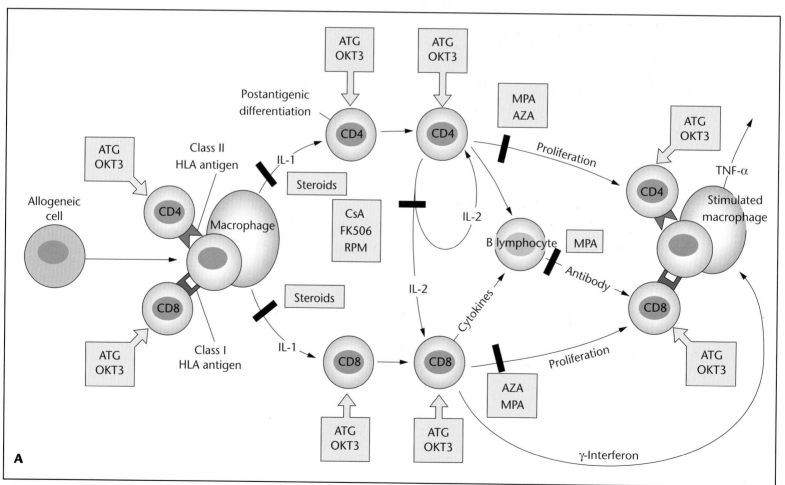

FIGURE 13-78.

Mechanism of action of immunosuppressive drugs. **A,** The sites of action of the commonly used immunosuppressive drugs. Immunosuppressive drugs interfere with allograft rejection at various sites in the rejection pathways. Glucocorticoids block the release of interleukin (IL)-1 by macrophages, cyclosporine (CsA) and FK506 interfere with IL-2 production from activated helper T cells, and azathioprine (AZA) and mycophenolate mofetil (MPA) prevent proliferation of cytotoxic and helper T cells.

(Continued)

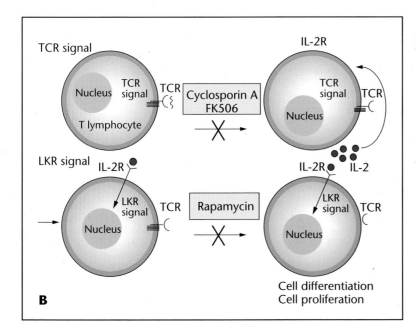

FIGURE 13-78. (*CONTINUED*)

B, Mechanism of action of CsA, FK506, and rapamycin (RPM). CsA and FK506 block the transduction of the signal from the T-cell receptor (TCR) after it has recognized antigen, which leads to the production of lymphokines such as IL-2, whereas RPM blocks the lymphokine receptor signal, *eg*, IL-2 plus IL-2 receptor (IL-2R), which leads to cell proliferation.

The addition of a prophylactic course of antithymocyte globulin (ATG) or OKT3 with delay of the administration of CsA or FK506 during the initial postoperative periods has been advocated by some groups. OKT3 prophylaxis was associated with a lower rate of early acute rejection and fewer rejection episodes per patient. Prophylactic use of these agents appears to be most effective in high-risk cadaver transplant recipients, including those who are sensitized or who have two HLA-DR mismatches or a prolonged cold ischemia time [21,22]. IFN-γ—interferon gamma; TNF–α—tumor necrosis factor-α.

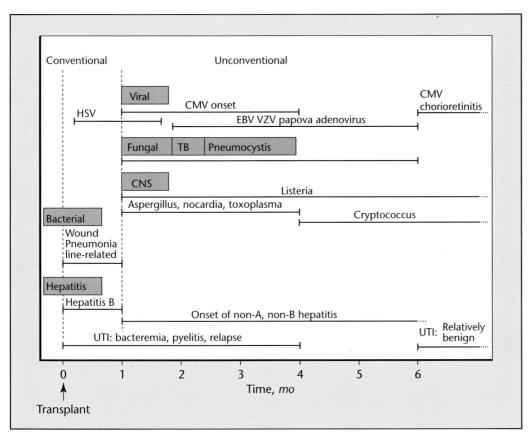

FIGURE 13-79.

Timetable for the occurrence of infection in the renal transplant patient. Exceptions to this chronology are frequent. CMV—cytomegalovirus; CNS—central nervous system; EBV—Epstein-Barr virus; HSV—herpes simplex virus; UTI—urinary tract infection; VZV—varicella-zoster virus. (*Adapted from* Rubin *et al.* [23].)

Classification of Infections Occurring in Transplant Patients

Infections related to technical complications*
   Transplantation of a contaminated allograft, anastomotic leak or stenosis, wound hematoma, intravenous line contamination, iatrogenic damage to the skin, mismanagement of endotracheal tube leading to aspiration, infection related to biliary, urinary, and drainage catheters
Infections related to excessive nosocomial hazard
   Aspergillus species, *Legionella* species, *Pseudomonas aeruginosa*, and other gram-negative bacilli, *Nocardia asteroides*
Infections related to particular exposures within the community
   Systemic mycotic infections in certain geographic areas
      Histoplasma capsulatum, Coccidioides immitis, Blastomyces dermatitidis, Strongyloides stercoralis
   Community-acquired opportunistic infection resulting from ubiquitous saphrophytes in the environment [†]
      Cryptococcus neoformans, Aspergillus species, *Nocardia asteroides, Pneumocystis carinii*
   Respiratory infections circulating in the community
      Mycobacterium tuberculosis, influenza, adenoviruses, parainfluenza, respiratory syncytial virus
   Infections acquired by the ingestion of contaminated food/water
      Salmonella species, *Listeria monocytogenes*
Viral infections of particular importance in transplant patients
      Herpes group viruses, hepatitis viruses, papillomavirus, HIV

*All lead to infection with gram-negative bacilli, *Staphylococcus* species, and/or *Candida* species.
[†]The incidence and severity of these infections and, to a lesser extent, the other infections listed, are related to the net state of immunosuppression present in a particular patient.

FIGURE 13-80.
Classifications of infections occurring in transplant patients. (*Adapted from* Rubin [24].)

Infections Transmitted to Transplant Recipients via the Donor Organ

Virus	Bacteria	Fungi	Parasitic
HIV, cytomegalovirus, herpes simplex virus, Epstein-Barr virus, hepatitis B virus, hepatitis C virus, hepatitis D virus (?), hepatitis G virus, adenovirus (?), parvovirus (?), papillomavirus, rabies, Creutzfeldt-Jakob	Aerobe (gram positive), aerobe (gram negative), anaerobes, *Mycobacterium tuberculosis*, atypical mycobacteria	*Candida albicans, Histoplasma capsulatum, Cryptococcus neoformans, Marosporium apiospermum*	Malaria toxoplasmosis, trypanosomiasis, strongyloidiasis

FIGURE 13-81.
Infections transmitted to transplant recipients via the donor organ.

Manifestations of CMV Disease in Renal Transplant Recipients

CMV disease

A. Syndrome: fever, leukopenia, malaise, lack of another cause

B. Organ specific: hepatitis, enteritis—duodenum, colon; pancreatitis; pneumonitis; interstitial nephritis, retinitis

C. Risk of CMV disease by donor

Recipient serostatus without antiviral prophylaxis

D/R	Infection*	Disease
D⁺R⁻	70%–100%	56%–80%
D⁺R⁺	50%–80%	27%–39%
D⁻R⁺		0%–27%
D⁻R⁻		5%

*Infection determined by new anti-CMV antibody development or a greater than fourfold rise in anti-CMV titers

FIGURE 13-82.

Manifestations of cytomegalovirus (CMV) disease in renal transplant recipients.

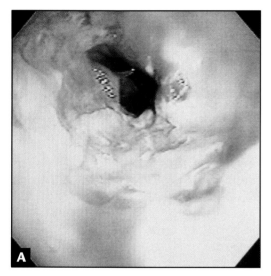
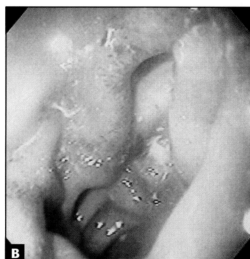

FIGURE 13-83.

Endoscopic aspects of cytomegalovirus (CMV) infection. **A**, CMV esophageal ulcers. **B**, CMV duodenal ulcers.

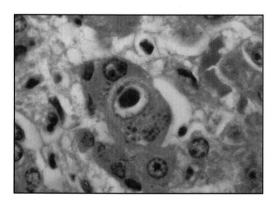

FIGURE 13-84.

Histologic lesion in cytomegalovirus infection.

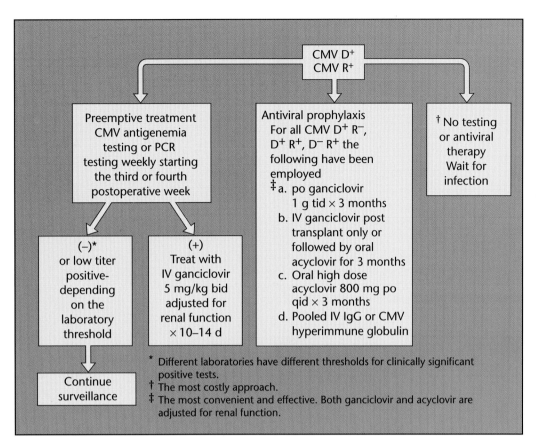

FIGURE 13-85.
The "prevention" of cytomegalovirus (CMV) disease. This figure shows the different strategies for the management of CMV-positive transplant recipients or recipients of CMV-positive organs.

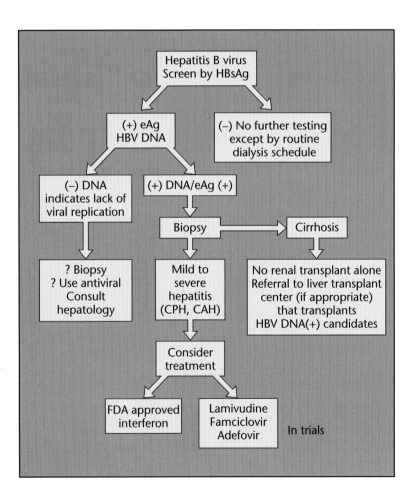

FIGURE 13-86.
Hepatitis B screening in renal transplant candidates. CAH—chronic active hepatitis; CPH—chronic persistent hepatitis; HBsAg—hepatitis B surface antigen; HBV—hepatitis B virus.

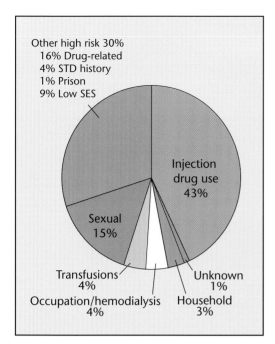

FIGURE 13-87.

Risk factors associated with reported cases of acute hepatitis C in the United States (1991 to 1995). Hepatitis C transplant infection prior to transplantation has not been definitively shown in most studies to markedly affect survival for at least 5 years following renal transplantation. Furthermore, hepatitis C–positive individuals who are otherwise good transplant candidates appear to have increased survival when transplanted, compared with staying on dialysis. Liver biopsies performed prior to transplantation have usually shown mild histological changes or chronic persistent hepatitis, but sequential biopsies have not been performed for a long enough period of time and compared with survival to outline the natural history. Transaminase levels do not help to predict histology or outcome. Death in hepatitis C–positive individuals is more often related to infection than in hepatitis C–negative transplant recipients. Post-transplant treatment with interferon alpha has led to an unacceptably high rate of both rejection and acute renal failure secondary to severe interstitial edema without tubulitis. Additionally, except for a few individuals, interferon has not resulted in long-term viral clearance. Most studies show the return of hepatitis C viremia within 1 month following cessation of interferon. At this point it appears that hepatitis G infections (also caused by an RNA virus) in renal transplant recipients, although occasionally associated with slight increases in chronic hepatitis, are not associated with decreased survival.

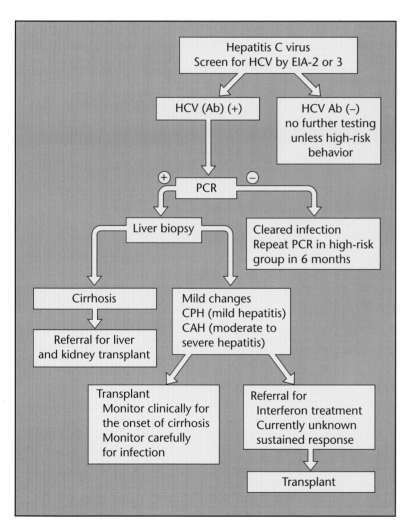

FIGURE 13-88.

Hepatitis C screening in renal transplant candidates. CAH—chronic active hepatitis; CPH—chronic persistent hepatitis; HCV(ab)—hepatitis C virus antibody; PCR—polymerase chain reaction.

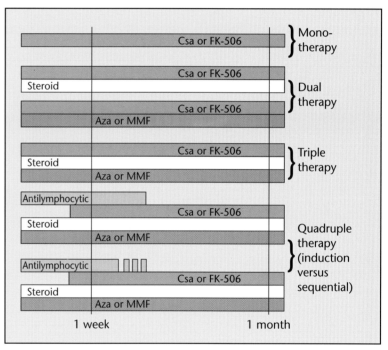

FIGURE 13-89.

Summary of strategies for combining immunosuppressive agents. Currently, monotherapy (usually cyclosporine [Csa]) is not used in the United States. Dual therapy (involving cyclosporine or tacrolimus) is used commonly in Europe. Most centers in the United States use triple or quadruple therapy (induction or sequential). Some centers continue the induction with the antilymphocytic biologic agent for a predetermined period (usually 10–14 days), overlapping with the initiation of cyclosporine (or tacrolimus). Alternatively, the biologic agent is discontinued and cyclosporine (or tacrolimus) begun as soon as the graft function reaches a determined threshold, resulting in no overlap of these two agents. In living donor transplants, azathioprine (Aza) is commonly begun a few days before surgery [25]. FK-506—tacrolimus; MMF—mycophenolate mofetil.

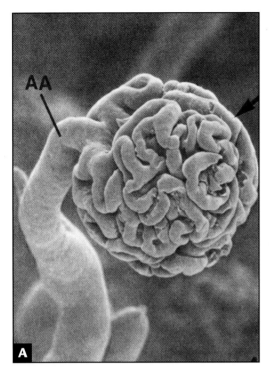

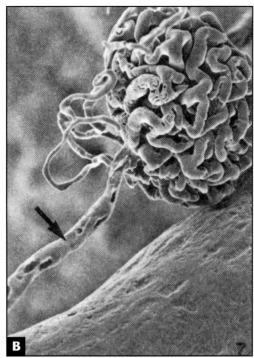

FIGURE 13-90.

Experimental model of the vasoconstrictive effect of cyclosporine. Some of the acute nephrotoxicity of cyclosporine is due to the significant yet reversible vasoconstrictive effect of the drug. **A,** Scanning electron micrograph of glomerulus of a rat not exposed to cyclosporine. Arrow indicates glomerular capillary loop. AA—afferent artery. **B,** After 14 days of cyclosporine treatment, the entire length of an afferent arteriole shows narrowing (magnification x 500). *Arrow* indicates afferent artery. (*From* English *et al.* [26].)

Clinically Relevant Drug Interactions with Immunosuppressive Drugs

Drug	Effect	Mechanism
Cyclosporin A and tacrolimus		
Diltiazem	Increased blood levels	Decreased metabolism (inhibition of cytochrome P-450-IIIA 4)
Nicardipine		
Verapamil		
Erythromycin	Increased blood levels	Decreased metabolism (inhibition of cytochrome P-450-IIIA 4)
Clarithromycin		
Ketoconazole	Increased blood levels	Decreased metabolism (inhibition of cytochrome P-450-IIIA 4)
Fluconazole		
Itraconazole		
Methylprednisolone (high dose only)	Increased blood levels	Unknown
Carbamazepine	Decreased blood levels	Increased metabolism (inhibition of cytochrome P-450-IIIA 4)
Phenobarbital		
Phenytoin		
Rifampin		
Aminoglycosides	Increased renal dysfunction	Additive nephrotoxicity
Amphotericin B		
Cimetidine	Increased serum creatinine	Competition for tubular secretion
Lovastatin	Decreased metabolism	Myositis, increased creatine phosphokinase, rhabdomyolysis
Azathioprine		
Allopurinol	Increased bone marrow toxicity	Inhibiting xanthine oxidase
Warfarin	Decreased anticoagulation effect	Increased prothrombin synthesis or activity
ACE inhibitors	Increased bone marrow toxicity	Not established
Mycophenolate mofetil		
Acyclovir-ganciclovir (high doses only)	Increased levels of acyclovir-ganciclovir and mycophenolate mofetil	Competition for tubular secretion
Antacids	Decreased absorption	Binding to mycophenolate mofetil
Cholestyramine	Decreased absorption	Interferes with enterohepatic circulation

ACE—angiotensin-converting enzyme.
Adapted from de Mattos *et al.* [27,28].

FIGURE 13-91.

Clinical relevant drug interactions with immunosuppressive agents. Close monitoring of drug levels is required periodically with concomitant use of drugs with potential interaction. Drug level monitoring is clinically available for cyclosporin A and tacrolimus. Monitoring of non-immunosuppressive drug level is also important when used with potential interacting immunosuppressive agents.

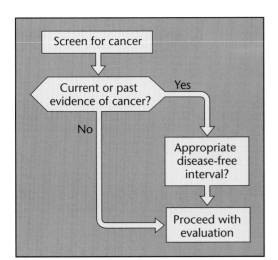

FIGURE 13-92.

Screening for cancer. An active malignancy is an absolute contraindication to transplantation. Effective screening measures for patients at risk include chest radiograph, mammogram, PAP test, stool Hemoccult, digital rectal examination, and flexible sigmoidoscopy examination. Patients who have had a life-threatening malignancy but are potentially cured may be candidates for transplantation when there has been an appropriate disease-free interval. This interval generally is at least 2 years, and longer in the case of some malignancies. (*Adapted from* Kasiske *et al.* [29].)

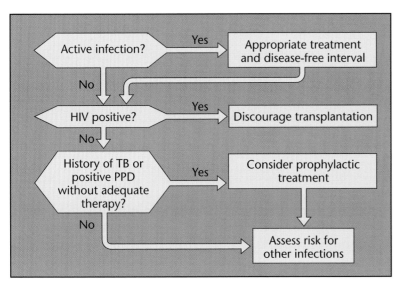

FIGURE 13-93.

Screening for infection. An active potentially life-threatening infection is a contraindication to transplantation. Patients with human immunodeficiency virus (HIV) are usually not candidates for transplantation. Patients with a history of tuberculosis (TB) or a positive purified protein derivative (PPD) skin test who have not been adequately treated should generally receive prophylactic therapy. (*Adapted from* Kasiske *et al.* [29].)

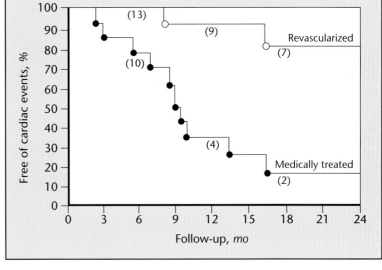

FIGURE 13-94.

Effects of surgical versus medical management of coronary disease before renal transplantation in candidates who have insulin-dependent diabetes. In this study, 26 patients with insulin-dependent diabetes who were found to have over 75% stenoses in one or more coronary arteries were randomly allocated to either medical management or a revascularization procedure before transplantation. Ten of the 13 patients who were managed medically and 2 of the 13 who had revascularization performed had a cardiovascular disease end point within a median of 8.4 months after transplantation ($P > 0.01$). These findings suggest that transplantation candidates who have diabetes should be screened for silent coronary artery disease because revascularization decreases morbidity and mortality after transplantation. The numbers in parentheses indicate the number of patients being followed at that time. (*Adapted from* Manske *et al.* [30].)

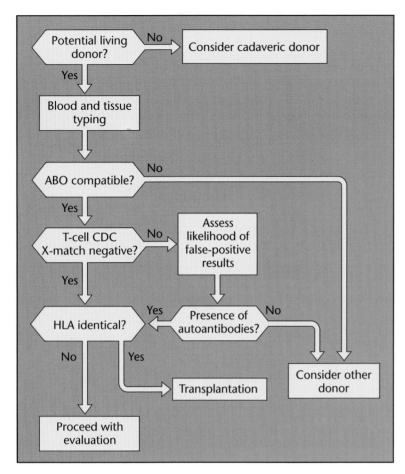

FIGURE 13-95.

Immunologic evaluation for living donor transplantation. Generally, transplantation donors and recipients must have compatible blood groups. Tissue typing is also carried out, and the degree of human leukocyte antigen (HLA) matching may be taken into account in selecting the best living donor when more than one donor is available. Just before transplantation, the recipient's serum is tested against donor cells to be certain no preformed antibodies are present in the recipient that may cause a hyperacute rejection. A positive cross-match (X-match) generally precludes transplantation from that donor. CDC—cell-dependent cytotoxicity. (*Adapted from* Kasiske *et al.* [29].)

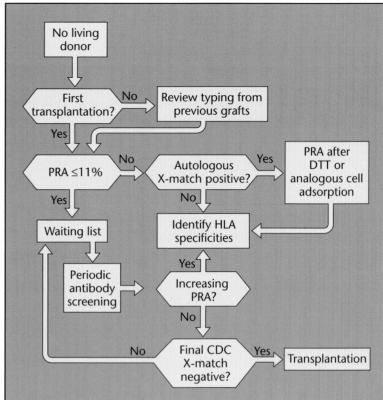

FIGURE 13-96.

Immunologic evaluation for cadaveric transplantation. Donors and recipients must have compatible blood groups. Tissue typing is carried out, and the degree of matching is used in the allocation of cadaveric organs. Some data suggest that the presence of human leukocyte antigen (HLA) mismatches that were also mismatched in a previous graft (especially at the DR locus) may lead to early graft loss. Thus, it may be wise to avoid these mismatches. When the percentage of panel reactive antibodies (PRA) is over 10%, tests may be carried out to determine whether some of the antibodies are autoreactive rather than alloreactive. Autoreactive antibodies may not increase the risk for graft loss as do alloreactive antibodies. The presence of high titers of alloreactive antibodies usually is due to previous pregnancies, transplantations, and blood transfusions. Determining antibody specificities may be useful in avoiding certain HLA antigens. In the highly sensitized patient (PRA > 50%) it may be difficult to find a complement-dependent cytotoxicity (CDC) cross-matched (X-match) negative donor. Avoiding blood transfusions may help the titer decrease over time. DTT—1,4-dithiothreitol (DTT). (*Adapted from* Kasiske *et al.* [29].)

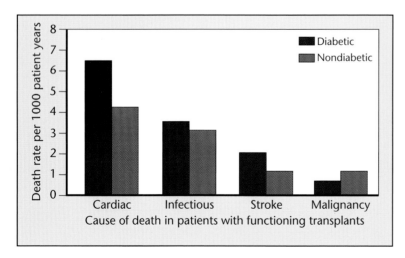

FIGURE 13-97.

Causes of death in renal allograft recipients. Cardiovascular diseases are the most common cause of death, largely reflecting the high prevalence of coronary artery disease in this population [31]. The risks are particularly high among recipients who have diabetes, as many as 50% of whom, even if asymptomatic, may have significant coronary disease at the time of transplantation evaluation [32]. Effective management of cardiac disease after transplantation mandates documentation of preexisting disease in patients at greatest risk [33].

Guidelines for Lipid-lowering Therapy

Diet Therapy

LDL Cholesterol, *mg/dL*	Initiation	Goal
No CHD and < 2 risk factors	≥ 160	< 160
No CHD and ≥ 2 risk factors	≥ 130	< 130
CHD	≥ 100	≤ 100

Diet plus Drug Therapy

LDL Cholesterol, *mg/dL*	Initiation	Goal
No CHD and < 2 risk factors	≥ 190	< 160
No CHD and ≥ 2 risk factors	≥ 160	< 130
CHD	≥ 130	≤ 100

FIGURE 13-98.

The indications for lipid-lowering therapy and its goals are based on the clinical history, risk factor profile, and low density lipoprotein (LDL) cholesterol level in individual patients. CHD—coronary heart disease.

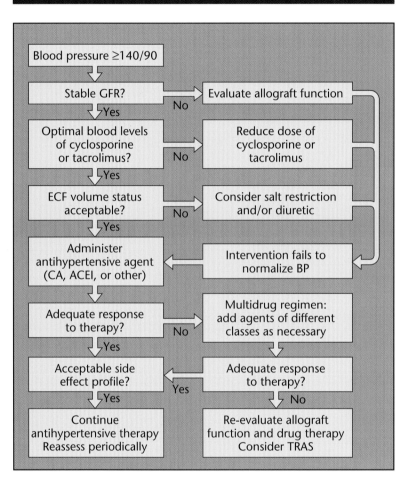

FIGURE 13-99.

Hypertension in the renal transplant recipient. In these patients it may be possible to approach diagnosis and therapy in a fairly standardized fashion. In transplant recipients with blood pressure readings consistently over 140/90 mm Hg, intervention is warranted. The initial approach includes assessment of allograft function, extracellular fluid volume (ECF) status, and immunosuppressive dosing. If these variables are stable, it is reasonable to proceed with antihypertensive therapy. Calcium antagonists (CA) are effective agents and may offer the added benefit of attenuating cyclosporine-induced changes in renal hemodynamics. Verapamil, diltiazem, nicardipine, and mibefradil increase blood levels of cyclosporine and tacrolimus and should be used with caution. Common problems with CAs that may limit their use include cost, refractory edema, and gingival hyperplasia. Angiotensin antagonists (ACEIs and receptor antagonists) are also effective; their use requires close monitoring of renal function, serum potassium levels, and hematocrit levels. Diuretics frequently are useful adjuncts to therapy in recipients owing to the salt retention that often accompanies cyclosporine use. Other antihypertensive medications offer no particular benefits or drawbacks and can be employed as needed. The rationale of multidrug therapy is to employ agents that block hypertensive responses via interruption of differing pathogenetic pathways. As antihypertensive drugs are added, this consideration should remain paramount [34,35]. GFR—glomerular filtration rate; TRAS—transplanted renal artery stenosis.

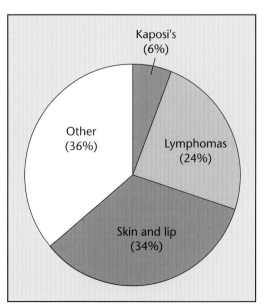

FIGURE 13-100.

Types and distribution of malignancies among renal transplant recipients in the current era of cyclosporine use. In these patients the risk of malignancy is increased approximately fourfold when compared with the general population [36]. Malignancies likely to be encountered in the transplantation recipient differ from those most common in the general population [37,38]. Lymphomas and Kaposi's sarcoma may evolve as a consequence of viral infections. Women are at an increased risk for cervical carcinoma, again related to infection (human papilloma virus). Surprisingly, the solid tumors most commonly seen in the general population (*eg*, of the breast, lung, colon, and prostate) do not occur with significantly greater frequency among transplant recipients. Nonetheless, long-term care of these patients should involve standard screening for these malignancies at appropriate intervals. (*Adapted from* Penn [37].)

■ REFERENCES

1. Johnson RJ, Feehally J, eds: *Comprehensive Clinical Nephrology*. St. Louis: Mosby; 1999.

2. JNC VI: The Sixth Report of the Joint National Committee on Detection, Evaluation, and Treatment of High Blood Pressure. *Arch Intern Med* 1993, 153:154–183.

3. Bauer JH, Reams GP: Mechanisms of action, pharmacology, and use of antihypertensive drugs. In *The Principles and Practice of Nephrology*. Edited by Jacobson HR, Striker GE, Klahr S. St. Louis: Mosby; 1995:399–415.

4. Bauer JH, Reams GP: Antihypertensive drugs. In *The Kidney* edn 5. Edited by Brenner BM. Philadelphia: W.B. Saunders Co.; 1995:2331–2381.

5. Hallet JW: Renal revascularization for the chronically occluded renal artery. In *Modern Management of Renovascular Hypertension and Renal Salvage*. Edited by Calligaro K, Dougherty R, Dean R. Baltimore: Williams and Wilkins; 1996:174.

6. Halperin M, Goldstein M: *Fluid, Electrolyte and Acid-Base Physiology: A Problem-Based Approach* edn 2. Philadelphia: WB Saunders; 1998:293.

7. Klahr S, Harris KPG: Obstructive Uropathy. In *The Kidney: Physiology and Pathophysiology* edn 2. Edited by Seldin OW, Giebisch G. New York: Raven Press; 1992:3327–3369.

8. Gonzalez J, Suki WN: Polyuria and nocturia. In *Textbook of Nephrology* edn 4. Edited by Massry S, Glassock R. Baltimore: Williams and Wilkins; 1995: 551:29.1.

9. Klahr S, Bander SJ: Obstructive uropathy. In *Textbook of Nephrology* edn 2. Edited by Massry SG, Glassock RJ. Orlando, FL: Williams and Wilkins; 1989:889–909.

10. Boswell WD: Radiology of the kidney. In *Textbook of Nephrology* edn 4. Edited by Massry S, Glassock R. Baltimore: Williams and Wilkins; 1995.

11. Churg J, Bernstein J, Glassock R: *Renal Disease: Classification and Atlas of Glomerular Diseases* edn 2. New York: Igaku-Shoin; 1995:159,161,163,173,189,191,315,321,381.

12. Brun C, Olsen S: *Atlas of Renal Biopsy*. Philadelphia: WB Saunders; 1981:135,171.

13. J Clin Immunol 1995, 15:184.

14. Shaikewitz ST, Chan L: Chronic renal transplant rejection. *Am J Kidney Dis* 1994, 23:884.

15. Gray D, Shepherd H, Daar A, *et al.*: Oral versus intravenous high dose steroid treatment of renal allograft rejection. *Lancet* 1978, 1:117.

16. Chan L, French ME, Beare J, *et al.*: Prospective trial of high dose versus low dose prednisone in renal transplantation. *Transpl Proc* 1980, 12:323.

17. Auphan N, DiDonato JA, Rosette C, *et al.*: Immunosuppression by glucocorticoids: inhibition of NF-κ activation through induction of IkBa. *Science* 1995, 270:286.

18. Ortho Multicenter Study Group: A randomized trial of OKT3 monoclonal antibody for acute rejection of cadaveric renal transplants. *N Engl J Med* 1985, 313:337.

19. Norman DJ, Shield CF, Henell KR, *et al.*: Effectiveness of a second course of OKT3 monoclonal anti-T cell antibody for treatment of renal allograft rejection. *Transplantation* 1988, 46:523.

20. Schroeder TJ, First MR: Monoclonal antibodies in organ transplantation. *Am J Kidney Dis* 1994, 23:138.

21. Chan L, Kam I: Outcome and complications of renal transplantation. In *Diseases of the Kidney* edn 6. Edited by Schrier RW, Gottschalk CW. Boston: Little, Brown; 1979.

22. Halloren PF, Lui SL, Miller L: Review of transplantation 1996. *Clin Transpl* 1996.

23. Rubin RH, Wolfson JS, Cosimi AB, *et al.*: Infection in the renal transplant recipient. *Am J Med* 1981, 70:405–411.

24. Rubin RH: Infectious disease complications of renal transplantation. *Kidney Int* 1993, 44:221–236.

25. Barry JM: Immunosuppressive drugs in renal transplantation: a review of the regimens. *Drug* 1992, 44:554–566.

26. English J, Evan A, Houghton DC, Bennett WM: Cyclosporine-induced acute renal dysfunction in the rat. *Transplantation* 1987, 44:135–141.

27. de Mattos AM, Olyaei AJ, Bennet WM: Pharmacology of immunosuppressive medications used in renal diseases and transplantation. *Am J Kid Dis* 1996, 28:631–637.

28. de Mattos AM, Olyaei AJ, Bennet WM: Mechanism and risks of immunosuppressive therapy. In *Immunologic Renal Disease*. Edited by Neilson EG, Couser WG. Philadelphia: Lippincott-Raven; 1996:861–885.

29. Kasiske BL, Ramos EL, Gaston RS, *et al.*: The evaluation of renal transplant candidates: clinical practice guidelines. *J Am Soc Nephrol* 1995, 6:1–34.

30. Manske CL, Wang Y, Rector T, *et al.*: Coronary revascularisation in insulin-dependent diabetic patients with chronic renal failure. *Lancet* 1992, 340:998–1002.

31. United States Renal Data System: 1996 Annual Data Report. Bethesda, MD: The National Institutes of Health; 1996.

32. Odorico JS, Knechtle SJ, Rayhill SC, *et al.*: The influence of native nephrectomy on the incidence of recurrent disease following renal transplantation for primary glomerulonephritis. *Transplantation* 1996, 61:228–234.

33. Watts RWE, Danpure CJ, De Pauw L, *et al.*: Combined liver-kidney and isolated liver transplantation in primary hyperoxaluria type 1. *Nephrol Dial Transplant* 1991, 6:502–511.

34. Kim EM, Striegel J, Kim Y, *et al.*: Recurrence of steroid resistant nephrotic syndrome in kidney transplants is associated with increased acute renal failure and acute rejection. *Kidney Int* 1994, 45:1440–1445.

35. Senggutuvan P, Cameron JS, Hartley RB, *et al.*: Recurrence of focal segmental glomerulosclerosis in transplanted kidneys: analysis of incidence and risk factors in 59 allografts. *Pediatr Nephrol* 1990, 4:21–8.

36. Gaya SBM, Rees AJ, Lechler RI, *et al.*: Malignant disease in patients with long-term renal transplantations. *Transplantation* 1995, 59:1705–1709.

37. Penn I: Cancers in cyclosporine-treated versus azathioprine-treated patients. *Transplantation Proc* 1996, 28:876–878.

38. Penn I: Occurrence of cancers in immunosuppressed organ transplantation recipients. In *Clinical Transplantations 1994*. Edited by Terasaki PI, Cecka JM, Los Angeles: UCLA Tissue Typing Laboratory; 1995:99–109.

chronic ischemic disease of, 16–21
conduction system of, 37, 38
contraction of, 22
failure of, 22–29
in aortic regurgitation, 65
in aortic stenosis, 64
myocarditis of, 35–36
sarcoidosis of, 33
transplantation of, 30
tumors of, 74–75
valvular disorders of, 57–67, 333
Heberden's nodes, 227
Heerfordt's syndrome, 110
Helicobacter pylori infection, 320
Hemangioma of liver, 534–535
Hematologic disorders, 449–467
in anemia, 249, 450–454, 463
in dysproteinemia, 462
in erythrocyte aplasia, 456
in hemochromatosis, 249, 457, 520–523
in hemophilia, 459
ichthyma gangrenosum in, 467
in infections, 456–457
in leukemia, 463–467
in mastocytosis, systemic, 467
in pancytopenia, 455
in polycythemia vera, 461
purpura in, 458
telangiectasia in, 459
in thrombocythemia, 461
in thrombocytopenia, 105, 459, 460
thrombotic microangiopathy in, 459
Hematuria, 544, 545
Hemochromatosis, 249, 457, 520–523
Hemodialysis, 578, 580–581
Hemolytic anemia, 453
Hemolytic-uremic syndrome, 460
Hemophilia, 459
Hemorrhage
cerebral, 334, 350, 365, 366
conjunctival, in endocarditis, 323
in fingernail, 330
gastrointestinal, 478, 530
subarachnoid, 350, 351
subconjunctival, 299
vitreous or preretinal, in diabetes mellitus, 146
Hemorrhoids, 484
Henoch-Schönlein purpura, 483
Heparin therapy
thrombocytopenia from, 105, 459
in venous thromboembolism, 103, 104–105
Hepatitis, 316–317, 501–516
alcoholic, 501, 524
autoimmune, 507–509
ischemic, 531
renal transplantation in, 588–589
Hepatitis A, 316, 501–502
Hepatitis B, 316, 503–505, 510–513
Hepatitis C, 505–506, 513–516
cirrhosis in, 316, 474, 513
hepatocellular carcinoma in, 316, 506, 538
histologic findings in, 508, 515
and kidney disorders, 571
renal transplantation in, 589
liver transplantation in, 540
natural history of, 316, 514
porphyria cutanea tarda in, 216, 515
Hepatitis D, 505
Hepatitis E, 503
Hepatocellular adenoma, 536, 537
Hepatocellular carcinoma, 537, 538–539
in hepatitis C, 316, 506, 538
Hepatotoxicity of drugs, 517
Hernia in ascites, 527
Herpes simplex virus infections, 189, 293
cervicitis in, 329
chronic mucocutaneous, 287
encephalitis in, 295, 352, 353
erythema multiforme in, 207, 208
genital, 309
gingivostomatitis in, 304
in HIV infection and AIDS, 189, 287
of lip, 185
whitlow in, 189
Herpes zoster virus infection, 189, 299

Histocompatibility complex, major, 581, 582
Histoplasma infections, 98, 312, 315, 326
HIV infection and AIDS, 280–288
cholangiopathy in, 492
fat redistribution in, 293
gastrointestinal disorders in, 286, 479
in cryptosporidiosis, 482
diarrhea in, 318, 320
esophageal, 473
Kaposi's sarcoma in, 283–284, 285, 479
nephropathy in, 571
neurologic disorders in, 287, 294, 295, 398
respiratory infections in, 98, 286, 310, 315
skin disorders in, 189, 281–283
HLA antigens
in renal transplantation, 592
in spondyloarthropathy, 241
Hughes' syndrome, 232
Huntington's disease, 386
Hydrocephalus, 348, 385
Hydronephrosis, 561
Hypercalcemia, 556
Hyperglycemic hyperosmolar syndrome, 135, 137
Hyperkalemia, 554
Hypermagnesemia, 560
Hypernatremia, 551
Hyperplasia
fibromuscular, hypertension in, 549, 550
of liver, 537
Hyperprolactinemia, 161–162
Hypertension, 48–56, 546–560
in atherosclerosis, 6, 52, 549
cerebral hemorrhage in, 365
in endocrine disorders, 548
in fibromuscular hyperplasia, 549, 550
kidneys in, 48–50, 52, 546–550
and renal transplantation, 593
mild, 56, 548
pathogenesis of, 48–51
portal, 526, 527–528, 530
esophageal varices in, 474, 530
pulmonary, 68–74
in mitral stenosis, 58
renovascular, 52, 550
secondary, 52–53, 549–550
treatment of, 55–56, 546–548
in emergencies and urgencies, 547
resistance to therapy in, 548
Hyperthyroidism, 123, 125, 127–129
Hypocalcemia, 555
Hypoglycemia, 149–150
Hypogonadism, hypogonadotropic, 163–164
Hypokalemia, 553
Hypomagnesemia, 560
Hyponatremia, 170–172, 551
Hypopituitarism, 158–160, 348
Hypothalamus, 156
and pituitary-adrenal axis, 165, 166
and pituitary-thyroid axis, 129, 133
Hypothyroidism, 123, 124–125, 130–133
Hypoxemia
in chronic obstructive pulmonary disease, 71, 82
in respiratory failure, 114–116

I

Ichthyma gangrenosum, 467
Ileum, Crohn's disease of, 481
Ileus, 484
Immune globulin, hepatitis A, 502
Immunobullous diseases, 213–214
Immunodeficiency syndrome, acquired. *See* HIV infection and AIDS
Immunoglobulin IgA nephropathy, 569
Immunosuppressive drugs in renal transplantation, 584–585, 589–590
Impetigo, 185, 187, 288, 324
Infarction
cerebral, 350, 358–359, 360
dementia in, 373
myocardial, 8–15, 23, 28
pulmonary, 101
Infections, 279–337
arthritis in, 246–248
cardiovascular, 330–337
cellulitis in, 188, 298, 300

of central nervous system, 294–296, 352–353, 395–400
cervicitis in, 329
diarrhea in, 318–320
of ear, 259–262, 302
external manifestations of, 322–326
of eye, 284–285, 299–300
gastrointestinal, 318–321
headache in, 410
HIV infection and AIDS in. *See* HIV infection and AIDS
leukocytes in, 456–457
of liver, 322
hepatitis in. *See* Hepatitis
of mouth, 303–305
in renal transplantation, 585–589
respiratory, 93–98, 310–315
in HIV infection and AIDS, 98, 286, 310, 315
sepsis in, 298
sexually transmitted, 305–310
sinusitis in, 296–297, 303
of skin, 187–191, 288–294
subperiosteal abscess in, 301
of urinary tract, 305–310, 327–328
vaginitis in, 307, 329, 349
Inoue balloon technique in mitral stenosis, 59
Insect bites and stings, 271–275
Lyme disease in, 247–248, 324–325, 399
neurotoxicity in, 404
Insulin
consequences of deficiency, 135–138
regulation of secretion, 133–134
resistance to, 140, 144
serum levels in obesity, 175
therapy in diabetes mellitus, 139, 141
Insulinoma, 497
Interferon therapy in hepatitis B, 513
Interstitial lung disease, 107–108
Io caterpillar stings, 272
Ipratropium in chronic obstructive pulmonary disease, 82
Iron, 175
accumulation in hemochromatosis, 457, 520–523
deficiency of, 450, 451
Irritable bowel syndrome, 490
Ischemia
cerebral, 350, 355–365, 373
coronary, 2–7
acute, 8–15
chronic, 16–21
Islet cells of pancreas
function of, 133–134
tumors of, 497
Isometheptene in migraine, 408
Isoniazid in tuberculosis, 97
Ixodes ticks, 247–248, 324–325

J

Janeway lesions, 323
Jaundice, 500–501
Jejunum, adenocarcinoma of, 483
Joint disorders, 248–250
arthritis. *See* Arthritis
differential diagnosis of, 218
in hemochromatosis, 249, 520
Jugular vein catheters in dialysis, 580
Juxtaglomerular apparatus in hypertension, 49, 50

K

Kaposi's sarcoma, 183
in HIV infection and AIDS, 283–284, 285, 479
Kawasaki disease, 330–332
Kayser-Fleischer rings, 345, 521
Keloids, 196
Kennedy's spinobulbar muscular atrophy, 346
Keratosis, 181, 195
Ketoacidosis, diabetic, 135–138
Kidneys, 543–593
in acid-base disorders, 557–559
acute failure of, 545, 575
in amyloidosis, 571–572
calculi in, 327, 562–563, 577
chronic failure of, 578–581
cysts of, 433, 576–577, 581
in diabetic nephropathy. *See* Nephropathy, diabetic
evaluation of disorders, 544–545